ROUTLEDGE HANDBOOK OF
GLOBAL MENTAL HEALTH NURSING

Psychiatric disorders have consistently been identified as serious and significant global burdens of disease, yet meeting the needs of people in mental distress has not often been a priority in health care. This important reference work sets out the knowledge base for understanding the state of mental health care globally and translating that into effective practice.

The *Routledge Handbook of Global Mental Health Nursing* provides a historical and contemporary context of mental health care, identifies and discusses evidence-based standards of care and strategies for mental health promotion and explores the need to deliver care from interdisciplinary and community-based models, placing these imperatives within a human rights and empowerment framework. It is made up of four core sections, which look at:

- key and emerging issues that affect global mental health practice and research, including the social context of health;
- evidence-based health promotion strategies for major areas of practice internationally;
- a range of country studies, reflecting different problems and approaches to mental health and mental health care internationally; and
- what constitutes empowering practice.

The only comprehensive work looking at global perspectives on mental health nursing, this is an invaluable reference for all students, academics and professionals involved in mental health research with an interest in global or cross-cultural issues.

Edilma L. Yearwood has served as a child, adolescent and family clinician, educator and researcher for over 40 years. She holds BS, MA and PhD degrees in Nursing and also completed a postdoctoral fellowship in Child and Family at New York University, USA. She is a Fellow, American Academy of Nursing (FAAN) and has received numerous awards from the International Society of Psychiatric Nurses (ISPN), most recently the Melva Jo Hendrix Lectureship award. She is Associate Editor of *Archives of Psychiatric Nursing* and is on the editorial board of the *Journal of Child and Adolescent Psychiatric Nursing* where she also wrote the Culture Bound Column. She is an editor and author of Yearwood, Pearson and Newland *Child and Adolescent Behavioral Health: A Resource for Advanced Practice Psychiatric and Primary Care Practitioners in Nursing* (2012). She is a faculty member and Chair, Department of Professional

Nursing Practice at Georgetown University, School of Nursing and Health Studies, USA. She teaches mental health nursing and undergraduate research to honors nursing students. Her research interests include mental health of immigrant youth, mood dysregulation, youth empowerment, community-based participatory action and social determinants of health. She serves as President of ISPN from 2016–2017.

Vicki P. Hines-Martin holds BS (Nursing), MA (Education), MSN (Psychiatric Nursing-Adult), and PhD (Nursing Research) degrees. She has received numerous awards and recognitions in Nursing including Fellow, American Nurses Association Ethnic/Racial Minority Clinical Fellowship Program, Lecturer, International Society of Psychiatric Mental Health Nurses Melva Jo Hendrix Lectureship and Fellow, American Academy of Nursing (ANA). Dr Hines-Martin has been a nurse for over 35 years and has served as a clinician, educator, author, university administrator and researcher throughout her career. She is currently a Professor and Director of the Office of Health Disparities and Community Engagement in Nursing and Director for Community Outreach for University Health Sciences at the University of Louisville School of Nursing in Louisville, Kentucky, USA. She teaches undergraduate and graduate students in the areas of mental health, nursing leadership, research, social determinants of health and community engagement. She also serves on professional and community boards that advocate for mental health and health equity among underserved and low-income populations.

"I welcome, at long last, a book on global mental health targeted to nurses, the front-line health worker for billions of people around the world. The roles that nurses can, and should, play in mental health care are diverse and this book addresses both well-trod, as well as, emerging concerns across the continuum of care from promotion to prevention to treatment. Importantly, at the heart of this diversity is the foundation of compassion and care, the hallmark of the nursing profession."

Vikram Patel, *FMedSci. Professor of International Mental Health and Wellcome Trust Principal Research Fellow in Clinical Science*

ROUTLEDGE HANDBOOK OF GLOBAL MENTAL HEALTH NURSING

Evidence, practice and empowerment

Edited by
Edilma L. Yearwood and
Vicki P. Hines-Martin

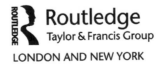

LONDON AND NEW YORK

First published 2017 by Routledge

2 Park Square, Milton Park, Abingdon, Oxfordshire OX14 4RN
52 Vanderbilt Avenue, New York, NY 10017

Routledge is an imprint of the Taylor & Francis Group, an informa business

First issued in paperback 2019

British Library Cataloguing-in-Publication Data
A catalogue record for this book is available from the British Library

Library of Congress Cataloging in Publication Data
Names: Yearwood, Edilma Lynch, editor. | Hines-Martin, Vicki, editor.
Title: Routledge handbook of global mental health nursing :
evidence, practice and empowerment / edited by Edilma Yearwood
and Vicki Hines-Martin.
Other titles: Handbook of global mental health nursing
Description: Abingdon, Oxon ; New York, NY : Routledge, 2016. |
Includes bibliographical references and index.
Identifiers: LCCN 2016010196| ISBN 9781138017610 (hardback) |
ISBN 9781315780344 (ebook)
Subjects: | MESH: Mental Disorders – nursing | Evidence-Based Nursing
| Mental Health Services
Classification: LCC RB170 | NLM WY 160 | DDC 616.89/0231 – dc23
LC record available at http://lccn.loc.gov/2016010196

ISBN: 978-1-138-01761-0 (hbk)
ISBN: 978-0-367-22408-0 (pbk)

Typeset in Bembo
by Florence Production Ltd, Stoodleigh, Devon, UK

CONTENTS

Contents

FIGURES

TABLES

ABOUT THE EDITORS

Edilma L. Yearwood, PhD, PMHCNS-BC, FAAN. Dr Yearwood has served as a child, adolescent and family clinician, educator and researcher for over 40 years. She holds BS, MA and PhD degrees in Nursing and also completed a postdoctoral fellowship in Child and Family at New York University. She is a Fellow, American Academy of Nursing (FAAN) and has received numerous awards from the International Society of Psychiatric Nurses (ISPN), most recently the Melva Jo Hendrix Lectureship award. She is an Associate Editor of *Archives of Psychiatric Nursing* and is on the editorial board of the *Journal of Child and Adolescent Psychiatric Nursing* where she also wrote the Culture Bound Column. She is an editor and author of Yearwood, Pearson and Newland *Child and Adolescent Behavioral Health: A Resource for Advanced Practice Psychiatric and Primary Care Practitioners in Nursing* (2012). She is a faculty member and Chair, Department of Professional Nursing Practice at Georgetown University, School of Nursing & Health Studies, USA. She teaches mental health nursing and undergraduate research to honours nursing students. Her research interests include mental health of immigrant youth, mood dysregulation, youth empowerment, community-based participatory action and social determinants of health. She serves as President of ISPN from 2016–2017.

Vicki P. Hines-Martin, PhD, CNS, RN, FAAN. Dr Hines-Martin holds BS (Nursing), MA (Education), MSN (Psychiatric Nursing-Adult), and PhD (Nursing Research) degrees. She has received numerous awards and recognitions in Nursing including Fellow, American Nurses Association Ethnic/Racial Minority Clinical Fellowship Program, Lecturer, International Society of Psychiatric Mental Health Nurses Melva Jo Hendrix Lectureship, and Fellow, American Academy of Nursing (ANA). Dr Hines-Martin has been a nurse for over 35 years and has served as a clinician, educator, author, university administrator and researcher throughout her career. She is currently a Professor and Director, Office of Health Disparities and Community Engagement in Nursing and Director for Community Outreach for University Health Sciences at the University of Louisville School of Nursing in Louisville, Kentucky, USA. She teaches undergraduate and graduate students in the areas of mental health, nursing leadership, research, social determinants of health and community engagement. She also serves on professional and community boards which advocate for mental health and health equity among underserved and low-income populations.

NOTES ON CONTRIBUTORS

Jason Anuik, CPMHN(C), RN, BN, BSc. Adolescent Inpatient Psychiatry, Foothills Medical Centre, Alberta Health Services, Canada. Mr Anuik has been a registered nurse specialising in adolescent inpatient psychiatry for the past 10 years. Jason received his Bachelor of Nursing from the University of Calgary in 2006 and the Canadian Certification in Psychiatric-Mental Health Nursing (CPMHN(C)) in 2011. Jason currently practises on a 14-bed inpatient adolescent psychiatry unit in Calgary, Alberta, Canada.

Wendy Austin, BScN, MEd (Counselling), PhD, RN. Professor Emeritus, Nursing and the Dossetor Health Ethics Centre, University of Alberta, Canada. Dr Austin, a Canada Research Chair (Relational Ethics in Health Care) from 2003–2013, is a founding co-director of the UA's PAHO/WHO Collaborating Centre (Nursing and Mental Health), a former President of the Canadian Federation of Mental Health Nurses, and served on the Board of the International Academy of Law & Mental Health.

Leilani Marie Ayala, MSN, RN, PMHCNS-BC, PMHNP-BC. UCLA-Resnick Neuropsychiatric Hospital. Ms Ayala is an ANCC Board Certified Clinical Nurse Specialist in Child and Adolescent Psychiatry and Family Psychiatric Nurse Practitioner. She completed her post-graduate studies at the University of Virginia School of Nursing. She currently works at UCLA-Resnick Neuropsychiatric Hospital as a Nursing Professional Development Specialist.

Catherine Batscha DNP, PMHNP-BC, PMHCNS-BC. University of Louisville. Dr Batscha is an Assistant Professor at the University of Louisville School of Nursing. She has worked as an advanced practice psychiatric nurse in inpatient, outpatient and residential settings for more than 30 years and has researched metabolic syndrome, transitions of care and interventions to improve mental health of caregivers.

Sarah Benbow, RN, MScN, PhD. School of Nursing, Fanshawe College, London, Ontario, Canada. Dr Benbow is a nursing professor who specialises in mental health nursing, with a clinical background in acute, chronic and forensic psychiatric settings. Her research focuses on issues of social justice, health promotion and policy with a particular focus on the health of marginalised groups.

Maureen Bentley, MSN, RN, PMHNP–BC. Indiana University School of Nursing. Ms Bentley is an experienced clinician, educator and researcher. Her work includes serving diverse communities and populations as a clinician with a community health centre. She is adjunct lecturer and researcher with Indiana University School of Nursing, where her research focus is on interprofessional collaboration of delivery of health care.

Kunsook S. Bernstein, RN, PhD, PMHNP–BC, FAAN. Hunter College, City University of New York, Hunter–Bellevue School of Nursing. Dr Bernstein is Professor and Psychiatric Nurse Practitioner Program Coordinator. She is a researcher, educator and advanced mental health practitioner who specialises in depression and mental health disparity. Her research has been focused on Asian Americans' mental health issues and also has served as NYS Behavioral Health Advisory Council member advocating and promoting mental health and substance abuse issues among minority population in New York State.

Spencer R. Case, Master of Science in Global Health, RAND Corporation. Mr Case works in health policy research at the RAND Corporation. In 2014 he completed his MS in Global Health at Georgetown University where he researched culture and treating mental health problems in West Africa. Before Georgetown he served on the DSM-5 development team at the American Psychiatric Association.

Andrew Cashin, RN, MHN, NP, Dip App Sci, BHSC, GCert PTT, GCert Hpol, MN, PhD, FACNP, FACMHN, FCN. School of Health and Human Sciences, Southern Cross University, Australia. Dr Cashin is Professor of Nursing at Southern Cross University. He is a credentialled mental health nurse and endorsed and practising mental health nurse practitioner who conducts a practice in the Southern Cross University Health Clinic for people with Autism Spectrum Disorders.

Teresa McEnroe Clare, BSN, MSN, APRN. Georgetown University, School of Nursing and Health Studies, Washington, DC. Ms Clare is a graduate of Georgetown University's Undergraduate Nursing Program and the Gerontological Nurse Practitioner Master's Program. She has taught in the Nursing Department since 2005. She is a member of the Gerontological Society of America and Sigma Theta Tau, Tau Chapter.

María Cristina Cometto, RN, MHSSM, MBE, PhD. Professor and Director Centre for Studies, Research and Development of Human Resources for Health (CEIDRHUS), School of Public Health, National University of Córdoba, Argentina. Dr Cometto is Professor in the Nursing School and Coordinator of the International Network of Nursing and Patient Safety 2006 to the present. She serves as Southern Cone Vice President ALADEFE, 2008–2012 and President Tribunbal of Ethics, Nursing Association of Cordoba, Argentina, 2011–2013.

Mary L. Corbett, RN APRN-C. University of Louisville, School of Nursing. Ms Corbett is Research Coordinator for the Caregivers Program of Research at the University of Louisville in Kentucky, USA.

Cheryl Forchuk, RN PhD. Western University & Lawson Health Research Institute, Ontario, Canada. Dr Cheryl Forchuk is a Distinguished University Professor at the Arthur Labatt Family School of Nursing and Department of Psychiatry, Western University. She is Assistant Director for Lawson Health Research Institute (Lawson), the research arm of the London Ontario hospitals, and Group Leader of Mental Health Research at Lawson.

Jessica Gill, RN, PhD. Lasker Clinical Research Scholar, National Institutes of Health, Rockville, MD, USA. Dr Gill is a tenure track investigator at the National Institutes of Health (NIH) and co-director of the biomarkers core for the Center for Neurosciences and Regenerative Medicine. Dr Gill examines the biological mechanisms of a variety of disorders and symptoms including: traumatic brain injury (TBI), and related comorbidities including post-traumatic stress disorder (PTSD), post-concussive disorder (PCD), depression and neurological deficits.

Patricia Fabiana Goméz, RN, MMH, SFST, PhD. Professor of the Department of Mental Health School of Nursing, National University of Cordoba, Argentina. Dr Gomez is Professor in the Nursing School, National University of Cordoba, where she has served as Coordinator International Network of Nursing in Mental Health since 2006. She was faculty representative, Council, School of Nursing, National University of Cordoba, 2011–2014; served as Vice President, Tribunal of Ethics Nursing Association of Cordoba, Argentina, 2011–2013 and is Director, University Institute of Human Systems Sciences, 1999 to present.

Molly Hall, University of Louisville School of Nursing. Ms Hall is an Administrative Specialist to the Associate Dean of the Undergraduate Programs at the University of Louisville School of Nursing. She has been a mental health services consumer since the age of 7 years old and a mental health advocate for 8 years.

Marc Haspeslagh, Registered Psychiatric Nurse, Master in Hospital Management, Master in Statistics, PhD in Biomedical Science, AZ-Sint-Jan Brugge-Oostende, Brugge, Belgium. Dr Haspeslagh graduated as a registered psychiatric nurse in 1979 and worked on the psychiatric unit of the general hospital Sint-Jan in Brugge. He became head nurse of the unit and promoted to nurse manager. He developed the business intelligence unit of the hospital and is now internal audit and accreditation advisor.

Michael Hazelton, PhD, RN. School of Nursing and Midwifery, The University of Newcastle, Australia. Dr Michael Hazelton is Professor of Mental Health Nursing at the University of Newcastle. He is the author of numerous publications on mental health; is a past editor of the *International Journal of Mental Health Nursing* and is a Life Member of the Australian College of Mental Health Nurses.

Hermi Hyacinth Hewitt, PhD, MPH, BScN, RN, RM, FAAN. Associate Dean and Professor of the Caribbean School of Nursing (CSON), University of Technology (UTech), Jamaica. Dr Hewitt's research includes Caribbean nursing history, Carica papaya use in chronic skin ulcer care, HIV risk reduction among adolescents, and quality of life for persons with asthma and mental health. Her book entitled, *Trailblazers in Nursing Education: A Caribbean Perspectives* is used by scholars globally. The Government of Jamaica awarded her the Order of Distinction (OD), in recognition of her excellent contribution to nursing education.

Sara Horton-Deutsch, PhD, RN, PMHCNS, FAAN, ANEF. University of Colorado College of Nursing. Dr Horton-Deutsch is a Professor, Watson Caring Science Endowed Chair, and an established leader in the psychiatric mental health nursing community. She has a sound international reputation and is known for her work in leadership development and advancing the art and science of reflective pedagogies and mindfulness in nursing education and practice.

Irene Eunhee Kim, DNP, MS, NPP, RN, PMHNP-BC, PMHCNS-BC. New York City Children's Center. Dr Irene Kim is a psychotherapist and a psychopharmacologist, who specialises in children and adolescents. She is also a clinical faculty and her academic interest is culturally specific preventive mental health programmes for children and their families. She is a mental health activist who works for underprivileged Asian American families.

Katelyn Klein, RN, BSN. Georgetown University School of Medicine, Washington, DC. Ms Klein is a global health and critical care nurse. After practising in various US settings, she moved to rural Malawi where she cared for adult and pediatric patients with an array of physical and mental illnesses. She is currently a Doctor of Medicine candidate at Georgetown University.

Angela Barron McBride, PhD, RN, FAAN. Indiana University School of Nursing, USA. Dr McBride is Distinguished Professor and University Dean Emerita at Indiana University School of Nursing. She is also a member of the Indiana University Health Board, and chairs the board's Committee on Quality and Patient Safety. She is known for her contributions to psychiatric-mental health nursing and leadership development.

Rose McMaster, Registered Nurse; Diploma of Applied Science (Nursing); Graduate Diploma in Education (Nursing); Master of Nursing (Honours); PhD candidate, Australian Catholic University, North Sydney campus. Ms McMaster is a registered general nurse, with psychiatric qualifications, who has worked in generalist and mental health settings. She has been involved in teaching undergraduate and post-graduate nursing students for over 20 years. Areas of research interest include social inclusion and vulnerable populations.

Silvina Malvárez, RN, MMIH, MMH, PhD. School of Public Health, National University of Córdoba, Argentina. Dr Malvarez served as Professor/Director Nursing School, National University of Córdoba, Argentina, 1973–2002. She was also Regional Advisor on Nursing Personnel Development, Pan American Health Organization PAHO/WHO, 2002–2013. She served as Latin American representative to the Global Panel for the Future of Nursing, STTI; member of the Global Advisory Group on Nursing Human Resources, ICN and was founder and developer of the Nursing Networks Initiative of the Americas.

Kerry Mawson, RN, MHSc, Grad Cert HigherEd. Australian Catholic University and Mental Health Drug and Alcohol Northern Sydney Local Health District Australia. Ms Mawson is a registered nurse with qualifications in drug and alcohol, mental health and counselling. Kerry has worked in a variety of areas including mental health and addiction. She has been involved in teaching mental health for 10 years and is also a nurse counsellor and research assistant at a major teaching hospital.

Magdala Habib Farid Maximos, RN, PhD. Professor of Psychiatric and Mental Health Nursing, Faculty of Nursing, Alexandria University, Egypt. Dr Maximos received her bachelor's, master of science, and doctoral degree in psychiatric nursing from Alexandria University. She has taught in undergraduate, graduate and doctoral programmes in nursing in Egypt, Jordan and United Arab Emirates. She has 35 years of experience in psychiatric nursing including teaching, conducting research and treating persons with psychiatric disorders.

Pamela A. Minarik, PhD, RN, CNS, FAAN. Samuel Merritt University, Oakland, California. Dr Minarik is a certified Clinical Nurse Specialist (CNS) in California and professor at Samuel Merritt University, California. She teaches in Accelerated Bachelor of Science in Nursing and Doctor of Nursing Practice (DNP) programmes. A Professor Emeritus, Aomori University of Health and Welfare, Japan, she annually teaches at multiple universities in Japan.

Madeline A. Naegle, PhD, CNS-PMH-BC, FAAN. College of Nursing, New York University. Dr Naegle is a Professor at NYU's College of Nursing. Her work has focused on education and policy in the specialties of psychiatric-mental health and addictions nursing and is a national spokesperson on the issue of impaired nursing practice for the American Nurses Association. She writes frequently on the specialty of addictions nursing and substance misuse and alcohol related disorders in older adults. Dr Naegle is Director, NYU College of Nursing WHO Collaborating Center on Geriatric Nursing Education.

Yoko Nakayama, RN, PHN, PhD. Professor, Graduate School of Nursing, University of Kochi, Japan. Dr Nakayama is a faculty member of the Disaster Nursing Global Leader Degree Program (www.dngl.jp/archives/en_members/) and Professor, Graduate School of Nursing, University of Kochi, Japan. Dr Nakayama is currently engaged in psychiatric research about the aftereffects of the 2011 Great East Japan earthquake, tsunami and radiation-hazard disaster in Fukushima Prefecture, Japan.

Deena A. Nardi, PhD, PMHCNS-BC, FAAN. University of St Francis, Joliet, IL. Dr Nardi is Director, DNP Program, University of St Francis; board member, *Journal of Psychosocial Nursing and Mental Health Services*; and therapist, Mindful Living Telecounseling and Consultation Services. Her social science research, policy papers and editorials advocate for universal single payer insurance, preventing gun violence and global nursing.

Ukamaka M. Oruche, PhD, RN, PMHCNS-BC. Indiana University School of Nursing. Dr Ukamaka Marian Oruche is an Assistant Professor at Indiana University School of Nursing in Indianapolis, USA. Her research advances the care of family members of adolescents with mental disorders. Her influence extends to Nigeria where she co-directs a health-service project focused on management of chronic conditions for underserved populations.

Geraldine S. Pearson, PHD, PMH-CNS, FAAN. University of Connecticut School of Medicine. Dr Pearson is an Associate Professor in the Department of Psychiatry. She was formerly the editor of *Perspectives in Psychiatric Care* and is now editor of the *Journal of the American Psychiatric Nurses Association*. Her professional interests involve mental health needs of underserved children and adolescents and particularly, those individuals involved in juvenile justice.

Steven Pryjmachuk, PhD PGDipEd RN (Mental Health) CPsychol SFHEA, School of Nursing, Midwifery & Social Work, The University of Manchester, Manchester. Dr Pryjmachuk is a UK-based nurse educator and researcher who has published widely, particularly around children and young people's mental health, occupational stress in nursing and student support and guidance. He is the editor of a core mental health-nursing textbook and is the Vice Chair (Chair-elect) of Mental Health Nurse Academics UK.

Andrea Pusey Murray, PhD Post Grad Dip in Education, MPH, BSc (Hons), Post Diplomas in Psychiatric Nursing, Nursing Administration, RN. Kingston, Jamaica. Dr Pusey-Murray is a Lecturer and Program Director for the undergraduate nursing programme at the Caribbean School of Nursing, University of Technology, Jamaica. She has published peer-reviewed articles in journals such as *Biomedical Science and Engineering* and *Mental Health in Family Medicine*. Her research interests are in mental health, sexually transmitted infections and education.

Karen M. Robinson, PhD, PMHCNS-BC, FAAN. Institute of Sustainable Health and Optimal Aging, University of Louisville School of Nursing, Louisville, Kentucky. Dr Robinson is

Director, Memory Wellness Initiative, Institute of Sustainable Health and Optimal Aging and Gerontology Professor Emerita. Dr Robinson is an expert in care of persons with dementia (PWD) and their caregivers. She is the Founder of the Caregiver's Program of Research and directs an initiative that provides evidence-based education and support to caregivers of PWD and their family members. She publishes extensively in the interdisciplinary literature.

Ann J. Sheridan, PhD, M.Ed, BNS, RPN, RGN, RNT. School of Nursing, Midwifery and Health Systems, University College Dublin, Ireland. Dr Sheridan is an experienced lecturer and researcher in psychiatric/mental health nursing, supervising graduate research students at master's, doctoral and PhD levels. Current research areas are palliative care needs of people with a diagnosed mental illness and an 18-year cohort study of first episode psychosis examining indicators of personal, clinical and functional recovery.

Peter Shine, Master of Public Health, Master of Health Science in Health Promotion, Clinical Associate Professor of Australian Catholic University (ACU) and Northern Sydney Local Health District (NSLHD) Aboriginal Health Service. Mr Shine is a Gomeroi Aboriginal man from north-western NSW. He is a strong advocate for Aboriginal health equity, Aboriginal and Torres Strait Islander peoples and dismantling institutional and individual racism from all societies. Peter is the Director of the Aboriginal Health Service in NSLHD and has assisted in creating one of the most successful Aboriginal Health Services in NSW.

Victoria Soltis-Jarrett, PhD, PMHCNS/NP-BC, FAANP. University of North Carolina at Chapel Hill School of Nursing. Dr Victoria Soltis-Jarrett is the Carol Morde Ross Distinguished Professor of PMHN and has practised psychiatric nursing for over 30 years, focusing her clinical practice, educational pedagogy and scholarship on rural mental health care, integrating behavioural health into primary, acute and long-term care settings, participatory research and community engagement.

Wafa'a Ta'an, RN, BScN, MScN, PhD. Research Coordinator at LAWSON Health Research Institute, London, Ontario, Canada. Dr Ta'an has international experience studying and working in the field of psychiatric mental health nursing in Jordan, UK and Canada. Distinguished academic achievements include receiving several funds and awards from highly reputable organisations since high school up to and including during PhD study.

Malene Terp, PhD student, MScN, RN. Aalborg University Hospital – Psychiatry Unit for Psychiatric Research, Denmark. Ms Terp is a mental health nurse by background. Her research interest is in ubiquitous person-centered care, including participatory methods and approaches to co-design services with, and not for, end-users.

Deborah V. Thomas, EdD, APRN, PMHCNS-BC, PMHNP-BC, CMP. Professor, Coordinator of Graduate Psychiatric Nursing Specialty, University of Louisville School of Nursing. Dr Thomas has been a psychiatric nurse since 1986, and an APRN since 1992. Currently, she is director of the graduate psychiatric nurse practitioner programme at the University of Louisville School of Nursing. She is owner of Here and Now Psychiatric Services, Center for Pharmacogenomic Studies and The Parenting Institute, a comprehensive psychiatric private practice since 1992.

Lily van Rhyn, PhD, RN. School of Nursing, University of the Free State, Bloemfontein, South Africa. Dr van Rhyn is senior lecturer and head of the research portfolio in the School of Nursing. She teaches a module in research methodology and supervises masters and doctoral students. She is involved in teaching child and adolescent psychiatric nursing and mentoring a junior staff member to assume responsibility for managing the programme, the only one of its kind in the country, at the end of 2017. Dr van Rhyn has a part-time practice in child and adolescent mental health and offers workshops on a variety of topics in this field.

Idalia Venter, PhD. Mental Health Nursing, School of Nursing University of the Free State, South Africa. Dr Venter teaches Primary Mental Health. She has been involved in the organised nursing profession in South Africa including its transformation when South Africa changed to a democracy.

Roberta Waite, EdD, PMHCNS-BC, FAAN, ANEF. Drexel University, College of Nursing and Health Professions, Doctoral Nursing Department, Philadelphia, Pennsylvania. Dr Waite, Professor and Assistant Dean of Academic Integration and Evaluation of Community Programs at Drexel University, also holds a secondary appointment in the Health Systems and Science Research Department. Her educational research focuses on leadership development of students in the health professions and her clinical scholarship explores social determinants of health using a life-course development perspective examining adult ADHD and psychological trauma and adversity.

Melanie Walters, RN, PMHNP-BC. University of Louisville School of Nursing. Ms Walters is a second-year PhD student and graduate research assistant. Research interests include effects of cognitive impairment on self-management and parent–child attachment in individuals with stable persistent mental illness.

REVIEWERS

Kelley Anderson, PhD, FNP, Associate Professor, Georgetown University School of Nursing & Health Studies.

Pamela Galehouse, PhD, RN, PMHCNS-BC, Associate Professor and CNL Program Director, Seton Hall University School of Nursing.

Catherine Kane, PhD, RN, FAAN, Professor of Nursing University of Virginia School of Nursing.

Beverly Malone, PhD, RN, FAAN, CEO, National League for Nursing, Washington, DC.

Jamesetta A. Newland, PhD, FNP-BC, FAANP, DPNAP, Clinical Associate Professor, New York University College of Nursing.

Evelyn Parrish, PhD, PMHNP-BC, Professor, Eastern Kentucky University School of Nursing.

Sally Raphel MS, APRN-PMH, FAAN, Johns Hopkins University School of Nursing.

Joan B. Riley, MS, MSN, FNP-BC, FAAN, Associate Professor, School of Nursing & Health Studies, Georgetown University.

Karen Gulseth Schepp, PhD, RN, PMHCNS-BC, FAAN, Chair and Professor, Psychosocial and Community Health, University of Washington School of Nursing, Seattle, WA.

Victoria Soltis-Jarrett, PhD, RN, PMH-NP, University of North Carolina at Chapel Hill.

Carol Taylor, PhD, RN, Professor, Georgetown University School of Nursing & Health Studies.

Arayna Yearwood, PhD in Education, International and Multicultural/Multilingual Educator, Paris, France.

PART I

Historical and contemporary mental health nursing

1

OVERVIEW OF MENTAL HEALTH IN LOW-, MIDDLE- AND HIGH-INCOME GLOBAL COMMUNITIES

Edilma L. Yearwood and Spencer R. Case

Arthur Kleinman asserted that a significant barrier to global mental health is moral in that individuals with mental illness exist within poor environmental conditions and that governments, as stewards of its citizenry, have failed to protect them (2009).

Introduction

Global mental health is an emerging science and the scientists and clinicians engaged in this work are aggressively working to bring this neglected issue to the forefront. Their actions are motivated by the knowledge that the extent of poor mental health is widespread with catastrophic public health impact, and that significant challenges to well-being exist for individuals, families and communities particularly those living in poorly resourced environments. More than 450 million people globally suffer from mental health challenges with 1 in 4 individuals affected by a mental illness (WHO, 2010a); however, two thirds of those in need of mental health treatment never receive it (WHO, 2001a). Mental illness constitutes roughly 13 percent of the global burden of disease, outpacing cardiovascular disease and cancer (WHO, 2001a) with depression expected to be the second highest cause of disease burden in middle-income countries by 2030 (WHO, 2010a). Suicide is ranked as the third leading cause of death in 15- to 44-year-olds and the second cause of death in 10- to 24-year-olds (WHO, 2014), a statistic that translates into 800,000 to one million deaths annually.

Globally, more than 40 percent of countries have no mental health policy (WHO, 2001a) and additionally, one-third of countries allocate less than 1 percent of their health budgets to mental health. There are fewer available mental health beds to address existing needs, with ranges of 5–50 beds per 100,000 population depending on low-, middle-, or high-income country status (WHO, 2014). Globally, nurses are the most prevalent health care professionals and constitute the largest group working in mental health (Morris, Lora, McBain, & Saxena, 2011). However, we argue that nurses are not being fully utilized as resources in mental health promotion and prevention efforts across all countries.

The assertion made in 2005 that, "there can be no health without mental health," (WHO, 2005, p. 11) endorsed and supported by the World Health Organization (WHO), appears to have been a timely catalyst for an increased focus on obtaining prevalence data on mental, neurological and substance use disorders globally, and for bringing about widespread discussion of mental health and prevention of *mental ill health*. However, variability exists across countries at multiple levels when looking at drivers known to promote or impede mental health or well-being. At the macro system level, areas that are the responsibility of governments include ensuring healthy economic conditions, developing and enforcing humanistic policies, valuing comprehensive well-being of its citizenry and promoting knowledge by making education accessible for all. These factors provide a basic underlying framework for health, including mental health. Building on these, safeguarding human rights as a fundamental underpinning of well-being, early case finding, ensuring availability of treatment resources (human, materials and services), stigma elimination, supportive cultural attitudes, consumer awareness, mental health literacy and mental health promotion strategies are critical ingredients to further support mental health. The process of global mental health awareness and promotion, research, and developing evidence-based treatment strategies to fit specific resource-able and culturally distinct contexts is developmentally in its infancy across different global communities. New models of treatment must be developed, including intentional integration of mental health care in primary care, task sharing through the use of traditional healers and non-specialist workers in low resourced environments, and expanded use of technology to begin to meet the vast mental health needs that exist and that cannot be managed with the existing number of trained mental health care providers who primarily reside in cities or more populated regions within countries. Without healthy human contributors to societal development, the specific community, state, region or country remains at a disadvantage, fails to flourish and lags behind comparable entities across multiple measures of overall health, including mental health.

Non-communicable disease burden, of which mental health is a component, increased from 36 percent to 49 percent in low- and middle-income countries from 1990–2010. During the same time frame, non-communicable disease burden in high-income countries saw only a 4 percent increase (Charlson *et al.*, 2015). Cause specific deaths (one underlying cause) resulted in 775,000 deaths attributable to Alzheimer's and other dementias, alcohol abuse and epilepsy. Excess deaths (due to multiple factors) accounted for over 8 million deaths and were associated with alcohol use disorder, schizophrenia, Alzheimer's and other dementias and opioid misuse. Other mental disorders such as bipolar, major depression, autism, and intellectual disability resulted in 4.5 million deaths (Charlson *et al.*, 2015).

This chapter will provide the framework for understanding the emergent field of global mental health as will be described throughout this text, define common terminology, discuss incidence and prevalence of major neuropsychiatric disorders, describe characteristics of low-, middle-, and high-income countries, illustrate consequences of unmet mental health needs and identify individuals and organizations leading the global mental health movement.

The purpose of this textbook is to provide a nursing perspective on the global mental health crisis, describe prevention, mental health promotion and evidence-based treatments, and present several in country exemplars with individuals and groups experiencing mental and behavioral health challenges. Nurses, as the largest health care profession globally can make significant contributions to improving mental health across all income communities and the profession can play a more significant role in the movement for global mental health and the evolution of global mental health science.

Low-, middle-, and high-income countries

On an annual basis the World Bank determines Gross National Income status of World Bank members and other countries with populations greater than 30,000. The three factors examined are country income level, region of the world in which the country is situated and country lending status.

Low-income countries are defined as countries with citizen incomes of $1035 or less annually. Examples of countries in this category include the Central African Republic, Democratic Republic of the Congo, Cambodia, Afghanistan, Ethiopia, Haiti, and Uganda.

Middle-income countries are countries in which citizens on average earn between $1036 and $12,615. Examples of countries in this category are Angola, Brazil, China, Columbia, Costa Rica, Cuba, Turkey, and the Dominican Republic.

High-income countries are countries in which citizens on average earn greater than $12,616 annually. Countries in this category include the United States, Canada, England, Australia, France, Germany, Belgium, and Argentina (World Bank, n.d.).

Mental health and mental illness

Mental health has been defined as, "a state of well-being in which an individual realizes his or her own abilities, can cope with the normal stresses of life, can work productively, and is able to make a contribution to his or her community" (WHO, 2001b, p. 1). While mental health is achievable in individuals across the lifespan, it is increasingly clear that overall psychological wellness or mental well-being is dependent on factors frequently outside the control of the individual. These external factors termed social determinants of health (SDH) include environmental conditions that exist where people are born, live, work, and play; socio-economic status such as poverty; access to education and subsequent health literacy; race and gender; early childhood experiences associated with social advantages or disadvantages; availability of and access to resources including health care services; lack of or ineffective policies, and individuals and communities who have been disempowered (Braverman *et al.*, 2011; Friel & Marmot, 2011). In addition, biological risk for mental illness exists, rendering some more vulnerable as most psychiatric disorders have a genetic basis and frequently originate in childhood or adolescence. Recently there has been a push to replace the term mental health simply with well-being due to the stigma associated with the terminologies of mental health and mental illness. Both terms, mental health and well-being will be used in this textbook.

Mental illness, at times referred to as mental ill health, is a brain disease manifested when the individual experiences alteration in thinking, mood or behavior often accompanied by distress and/or impairment in functioning, disability or mortality (WHO, 2013). Addressing and ameliorating individual vulnerabilities across multiple areas must become the focus of effective interventions to avoid or mitigate mental ill health. The burdens associated with mental disorders include poor health literacy, poor quality of life, inability to achieve one's potential, isolation, and potential for shorter life expectancy. There are an estimated 450 million people worldwide living with a mental illness and of that number, approximately 50–85 percent who are in need of mental health services do not receive them (Demyttnaere *et al.*, 2004). In low-income countries less than 1 percent of health spending is allocated to mental health. In middle-income countries approximately 2.5 percent is spent on mental health, and in high-income countries, 5 percent of health care dollars are earmarked for mental health services (WHO, 2011).

Along with the sparse allocation of financial resources dedicated to mental health promotion and treatment, many countries are either missing written policies or plans, or have outdated documentation outlining a vision for ensuring the mental health of its citizenry. In addition, accurate data collection on prevalence, monitoring of services and research on treatment effectiveness are missing, primarily in low- and middle-income countries. Variability across countries in the area of data collection methodology impacts the quality, accuracy and completeness of what truly exists and what is known. Without these data, it is difficult to make a compelling case for reallocation of funds even if they were available (WHO, 2013). Global mental health scientists are aggressively striving to rectify this situation.

Global Burden of Disease (GBD) represents epidemiological data reflecting risk factors, mortality, morbidity, health and injuries associated with disease burden. GBD incorporates prevalence and disability to arrive at an estimate of years lived with disability (YLDs). In addition it collects data on number of years that are lost to premature mortality (YLLs). The sum of both of these factors yields to disability-adjusted life years (DALYs). The 2010 GBD survey indicated that mental, neurological, and substance use disorders were the leading cause of YLDs, accounting for more than 10 percent of the global burden of disease (Whiteford *et al.*, 2013; Whiteford, Ferrari, Degenhardt, & Feigin, 2015). These chronic and non-communicable diseases more significantly impact low- and middle-income countries. Table 1.1 illustrates the WHO GBD for neuropsychiatric disorders and Table 1.2 provides a comparison between WHO and the Institute for Health Metrics and Evaluation (IHME) across neurologic, mental, behavioral, self-harm, and interpersonal violence dimensions.

Table 1.1 Global burden of disease: how the WHO Mental Health Atlas 2011 calculated the global burden of disease for mental ill health

WHO
Neuropsychiatric disorders (as reported in the WHO Mental Health Atlas 2011 Country Profiles)

The following disorders were used to calculate the global burden of disease (DALYs) for mental ill health in the WHO *Mental Health Atlas 2011* country profiles. (Note: the WHO does not use the term "neuropsychiatric disorders" in the most recent classifications for the GBD.)

Unipolar depressive disorders
Bipolar affective disorder
Schizophrenia
Epilepsy
Alcohol use disorders
Alzheimer and other dementias
Parkinson's disease
Multiple sclerosis
Drug use disorders
Post-traumatic stress disorder
Obsessive-compulsive disorder
Panic disorder
Insomnia (primary)
Migraine

www.who.int/healthinfo/global_burden_disease/2004_report_update/en/
www.who.int/mental_health/evidence/atlas/profiles/en/

Table 1.2 Comparison between WHO and the Institute for Health Metrics and Evaluation (IHME) across neurologic, mental, behavioral, self-harm, and interpersonal violence dimensions

Organization: IHME	*Organization: WHO*
Classification: "neurological disorders"	*Classification: "neurologic conditions"*
Alzheimer's disease and other dementias	Alzheimer's disease and other dementias
Parkinson's disease	Parkinson's disease
Epilepsy	Epilepsy
Multiple sclerosis	Multiple sclerosis
Migraine	Migraine
Tension-type headache	Non-migraine headache
Other neurological disorders	Other neurological conditions
http://viz.healthmetricsandevaluation.org/gbd-compare/#	www.who.int/healthinfo/global_burden_disease/estimates_regional/en/index1.html
IHME	*WHO*
"Mental and behavioral disorders"	*"Mental and behavioral disorders"*
Schizophrenia	Unipolar depressive disorders
Alcohol use disorders	Bipolar disorder
Drug use disorders	Schizophrenia
Opioid use disorders	Alcohol use disorders
Cocaine use disorders	Drug use disorders
Amphetamine use disorders	Anxiety disorders
Cannabis use disorders	Eating disorders
Other drug use disorders	Pervasive developmental disorders
Unipolar depressive disorders	Childhood behavioral disorders
Major depressive disorder	Idiopathic intellectual disability
Dysthymia	Other mental and behavioral disorders
Bipolar affective disorder	
Anxiety disorders	
Eating disorders	
Pervasive development disorders	
Autism	
Asperger's syndrome	
Childhood behavioral disorders	
Attention-deficit hyperactivity disorder	
Conduct disorder	
Idiopathic intellectual disability	
Other mental and behavioral disorders	
http://viz.healthmetricsandevaluation.org/gbd-compare/#	www.who.int/healthinfo/global_burden_disease/estimates_regional/en/index1.html
IHME	*WHO*
"Self-harm and interpersonal violence" Note: the IHME does not use the term "suicide"	*"Intentional injuries"* Note: the WHO does not use the term "suicide"
Self-harm	Self-harm
Interpersonal violence	Interpersonal violence
Assault by firearm	Collective violence and legal intervention
Assault by sharp object	
Assault	
http://viz.healthmetricsandevaluation.org/gbd-compare/#	www.who.int/healthinfo/global_burden_disease/estimates_regional/en/index1.html

General information on calculating the burden of disease for mental ill health (unrelated to the WHO *Mental Health Atlas 2011*)

There are two global health authorities that calculate the global burden of disease (GBD) for mental ill health, the Institute for Health Metrics and Evaluation (IHME) and the World Health Organization (WHO). The IHME and the WHO calculate the GBD for mental ill health by classifying conditions according to type, and both organizations classify conditions differently. The GBD can be reported according to Disability Adjusted-Life Years (DALYs) where one DALY equates to one lost year of "healthy" life.

> The sum of these DALYs across the population, or the burden of disease, can be thought of as a measurement of the gap between current health status and an ideal health situation where the entire population lives to an advanced age, free of disease and disability. DALYs for a disease or health condition are calculated as the sum of the Years of Life Lost (YLL) due to premature mortality in the population and the Years Lost due to Disability (YLD) for people living with the health condition or its consequences.
>
> *(World Health Organization, n.d.)*

Overview of mental health challenges

Mental, neurological/neurodevelopmental and substance use disorders all present challenges to individuals, families, and communities, impacting global burden of disease, economies, and overall health across multiple environments. Low- and middle-income countries are particularly challenged to adequately assess prevalence, develop and implement evidence-based treatments, have adequate human and treatment resources, and to provide long-term supports to maintain mental health. Each of these categories is briefly described below and will be explored in greater length throughout this book.

Mental health disorders

Mental health disorders are a set of symptoms associated with a DSM-5 or ICD-10 diagnosis in which there is significant disturbance in an individual's cognition, emotion regulation, or behavior that impacts functioning. Mental disorders are caused by genetic, social, and environmental factors. They are usually chronic and contribute to disease burden due to early onset, prevalence, impairment, persistence, and associated co-morbidities. Mental disorders contribute to distress in social, learning, occupational, relational, or other important activities. Examples of mental disorders include mood dysregulations such as major depression and bipolar disorder, schizophrenia, anxiety disorders such as post-traumatic stress, generalized anxiety, obsessive-compulsive, panic, and somatization disorders (APA, 2013; Collins, Patel, & Joestl, 2011; Hyman, Chisholm, Kessler, Patel, & Whiteford, 2006; Whiteford *et al.*, 2015).

Neurological/neurodevelopmental disorders

Neurological/neurodevelopmental disorders are disorders of the brain, spinal cord, or nerves that impact memory, learning, mood, movement, and one or more of our senses. The etiology of these disorders are varied and include genetics, poor nervous system development, degenerative diseases, injury, seizures, infections, tumors, or poor blood flow (NINDS, n.d.). Disorders in this category include Alzheimer's and other dementias, epilepsy or seizure disorders, autism, learning and intellectual disabilities, attention deficit disorder, Parkinson's disease, and acute ischemic strokes (Chandra *et al.*, 2006; NINDS, n.d.).

Substance use disorders

Alcohol, tobacco, and illicit drug use is a significant public health crisis across the lifespan and across all income countries globally. Substance use should be examined looking at volume and frequency of consumption, dependence and tolerance, impaired control, consequences to health, safety, quality of life, relationships, and productivity (Rehm, Chisholm, Room, & Lopez, 2006). Substances include alcohol, opiates such as heroin, opium and analgesics, stimulants such as cocaine and methamphetamines, inhalants and hallucinogens, among others.

WHO Mental Health Gap Action Programme (mhGAP) developed evidence-based management and scaling up guidelines for use when intervening with mental, neurological, substance use and child and adolescent disorders along with clinical practice recommendations applicable to low- and middle-income communities (Dua *et al.*, 2011; mhGAP, 2008). In addition, the Institute of Medicine supported development of core care competencies for non-specialist health workers in low- and middle-income countries. The competencies focused on the major mental, neurological and substance use disorders causing the greatest burden such as depression, psychosis, seizure, and alcohol use disorders (Collins, Musisi, Frehywot, & Patel, 2015). The competencies identified provider skills and characteristics to effectively manage the disorders, screening strategies, knowledge of what is assessed during screening, knowing when to refer to providers with additional training, and awareness of basic care needed (Collins *et al.*, 2015).

Table 1.3 provides an additional portrait of multiple factors impacting mental health in various countries and provides a visual comparison. The table includes among other factors, GBD, population literacy, presence or absence of mental health policies, resources (psychiatrists, mental health nurses, inpatient and community treatment facilities, and suicide rates).

An upper middle-class country exemplar

China, with a population of 1.3 billion people, reportedly has over 100 million people with mental health challenges (Tse, Ran, Huang, & Zhu, 2013), but accurate data is difficult to obtain. With this volume of individuals and families in need of treatment, the current 4 percent of health budget allocated for mental health along with the lack of inpatient resources created a crisis, which resulted in critical changes. The health budget targeting mental health has recently been doubled, resulting in mental health surveillance and work plans to target surveillance data, and additionally, the first National Mental Health Law has been passed. The law supports voluntary treatment, prevention and rehabilitation, expands the role of non-governmental organizations (NGOs) in providing services, promotes scientific research and international collaboration, puts in place social services to support individuals and families in need and provides resources to finance services (Phillips *et al.*, 2013; Zhou & Xiao, 2015).

Ultimately, unmet mental health needs have serious consequences. Table 1.4 provides a brief list of these effects on individuals. These consequences will be discussed throughout this textbook, reiterating the urgency for an intentional and comprehensive approach to eliminating challenges associated with achieving mental health and well-being.

Table 1.3 Mental health landscape: mental health aspects by country according to population and gross national income per capita

GNI per capita grouping (US$) **Country** (population in millions) / World Bank Region	1 % GBD MIH	2 TE on health as % of GDP	3 TE on MH as % of HB	4 % Literate	5 LE at birth	6 MH policy	7 Psych./ 100k	8 MH nurse/ 100k	9 Psych. hosp.	10 Comm. res.	11 MH OP Fac.	12 Suicides/ 100k
Low-income: GNI per capita of $1,035 or less.												
*Bangladesh (156.6) South Asia	11.2	3.41	0.44	M: 73 F: 76	M: 69 F: 71	Yes	0.07	0.20	1	11	60	UN
*Ethiopia (89.2) Sub-Saharan Africa	5.8	4.26	UN	M: 62 F: 39	M: 61 F: 64	No	0.04	0.59	1	1	57	UN
*Congo, Dem. Rep. (71.1) Sub-Saharan Africa	4.7	2.04	UN	M: 69 F: 62	M: 48 F: 51	Yes	0.066	0.236	6	0	1	UN
Lower-middle-income: GNI per capita of $1,036 to $4,085.												
India (1,276.5) South Asia	11.6	4.16	0.06	M: 88 F: 74	M: 65 F: 68	No	0.301	0.166	43	UN	4000	M: 12.2 F: 9.1
Indonesia (248.5) East Asia and Pacific	10.7	2.36	UN	M: 97 F: 96	M: 68 F: 72	Yes	0.01	UN	48	UN	UN	UN
Pakistan (190.7) South Asia	11.9	2.62	UN	M: 79 F: 59	M: 65 F: 67	Yes	0.185	7.384	5	0	3729	UN
Upper-middle-income: GNI per capita of $4,086 to $12,615.												
China (1,357.4) East Asia and Pacific	17.6	4.55	UN	M: 99 F: 99	M: 73 F: 77	Yes	1.53	2.65	780	UN	UN	M: 13.85 F: 12.29

Brazil (195.5) Latin America and the Caribbean	20.3	9.05	2.38	M: 97 F: 99	M: 71 F: 78	Yes	3.07	1.6	208	564	860	M: 7.3 F: 1.9
Mexico (117.6) Latin America and the Caribbean	19.4	6.47	0.65	M: 98 F: 98	M: 75 F: 79	Yes	1.57	2.62	46	UN	28	M: 6.8 F: 1.3
**Cuba (11.3) Latin America and the Caribbean	25.2	11.28	UN	M: 100 F: 100	M: 76 F: 80	Yes	10.85	29.6	24	UN	402	M: 19.6 F: 4.9
High-income (non–OECD): GNI per capita of $12,616 or more.												
Russian Federation (143.5) Europe and Central Asia	15.6	5.44	UN	M: 100 F: 100	M: 64 F: 76	Yes	11.61	46.26	360	11	4173	M: 53.9 F: 9.5
Saudi Arabia (30.1) Middle East and North Africa	14	4.97	3.89	M: 98 F: 96	M: 73 F: 75	Yes	2.91	13.41	20	2	94	UN
United Arab Emirates (9.3) Middle East and North Africa	19.9	2.81	UN	M: 94 F: 97	M: 76 F: 78	No	0.3	2.12	1	0	3	UN

Sources:
2012 World Bank GNI per capita Country Classifications: http://data.worldbank.org/news/2015-country-classifications
Organization for Economic and Co-operation and Development, About the OECD: www.oecd.org/about/
Population Reference Bureau: 2013 World Population Data Sheet: www.prb.org/pdf13/2013-population-data-sheet_eng.pdf
UN least developed country list: http://unctad.org/en/pages/aldc/Least%20Developed%20Countries/UN-list-of-Least-Developed-Countries.aspx
WHO Mental Health Atlas 2011: www.who.int/mental_health/publications/mental_health_atlas_2011/en/
WHO Mental Health Atlas 2011 Country Profiles: www.who.int/mental_health/evidence/atlas/profiles/en/#U

Notes:
UN = information unavailable
*Country meets 2013 UN criteria for least developed country
**Cuba is notable in terms of health resources

Table indicators by column:

GNI per capita grouping (US$): Countries represent the three largest countries (2013 populations) per 2012 World Bank income group. The high-income grouping only includes non-OECD countries.

1 **% GBD MIH:** % of the global burden of disease (GBD), measured in disability-adjusted life year (DALYs) due to mental ill health (neuropsychiatric disorders).
2 **TE on Health as % of GDP:** Total government expenditure on health as a percentage of GDP.
3 **TE on MH as % of HB:** Total government expenditure on mental health as a % of the health budget.
4 **% Literate:** Literacy rate (%) for males and females.
5 **LE at Birth:** Life expectancy at birth (years).
6 **MH policy:** Mental health policy in existence, yes or no.
7 **Psych. /100k:** Psychiatrists per 100,000 people.
8 **MH nurse /100k:** Mental health nurses per 100,000 people.
9 **Psych. hosp.:** Total number of psychiatric hospitals in the country.
10 **Comm. res.:** Total number of community residential facilities in the country.
11 **MH OP fac.:** Total number of mental health outpatient facilities.
12 **Suicides/100k:** Suicide rate per 100,000 people, males and females.

2012 World Bank analytical income groups (World Bank Atlas Method) (US$): Countries classified according to 2012 gross national income (GNI) per capita. Low-income countries are those with a GNI per capita of $1,035; lower middle-income countries are those with a GNI per capita of more than $1,036 but less than $4,085; upper middle-income countries are those with a GNI per capita of more than $4,086 but less than $12,615; high-income countries are those with a GNI per capita of $12,616 or more. **Note:** Income classifications are set each year on July 1. (http://data.worldbank.org/news/2015-country-classifications)

What is the OECD: The Organization for Economic and Co-operation and Development (OECD) is a group of 34 economically advanced, and democratically and market oriented countries that "promote policies to improve economic and social wellbeing around the world." High-income non-OECD countries are represented in the table because although average GNI per capita may be over $12,616, other development indicators such as health and education may be less substantial when compared to OECD member countries. (www.oecd.org/about/)

Table limitations:

- The table only represents data for countries with the largest populations according to GNI grouping.
- OECD countries are not included.
- Missing data ("UN") from the WHO Mental Health Atlas 2011 country profiles.
- The WHO Mental Health Atlas 2011 country profile reports data from multiple sources, some of which may not be the most recent.
- The WHO Mental Health Atlas 2011 survey terminologies may have been interpreted differently across countries.
- Column 1: The WHO Mental Health Atlas 2011 GBD calculations for "neuropsychiatric disorders" include: unipolar depressive disorders; bipolar affective disorder; schizophrenia; epilepsy; alcohol use disorders; Alzheimer's disease and other dementias; Parkinson's disease; multiple sclerosis; drug use disorders; post-traumatic stress disorder; obsessive-compulsive disorder; panic disorder; insomnia (primary); migraine. Therefore, multiple mental and behavioral disorders may not included in the WHO GBD calculation (WHO (2008), The Global Burden of Disease: 2004 Update). www.who.int/healthinfo/global_burden_disease/ 2004_report_update/en/ Geneva: WHO.)

Table 1.4 Consequences of unmet mental health needs

Chronicity of symptoms
Decreased productivity (GBD; DALYs)
Exacerbation of symptoms
Isolation
Loss (relationships, work, status, self-esteem)
Poor economic status
Poor quality of life
Poor self-concept
Suffering
Victim of stigma

Global mental health advocates

Numerous organizations have begun to include concepts associated with advancing mental health in their mission, have developed goals to achieve improvement in psychological well-being of individuals, and have identified strategies to improve conditions that contribute to overall community well-being. These organizations include the United Nations (UN), the World Health Organization (WHO), regional WHO offices (in the Americas, Africa, Eastern Mediterranean, Europe, South-East Asia, and Western Pacific), the National Institute of Mental Health (NIMH), Non-Governmental Organizations (NGOs), the World Bank, Human Rights organizations, religious institutions and the London School of Hygiene and Tropical Diseases. While these steps are crucial and laudable, the overwhelming needs and low resource status of some countries makes this work daunting.

The Millennium Development Goals (MDGs) developed by the UN in 2000 identified goals that were complementary to the social determinants of health but did not specifically identify or include mental health or psychological well-being as a goal. Work on achieving the MDGs spanned the period 2000 to 2015. The UN is now in the process of replacing MDGs with Sustainable Development Goals (SDGs). The goals of the original MDGs were to: 1) eradicate extreme poverty and hunger; 2) achieve universal primary education; 3) promote gender equality and empower women; 4) reduce child mortality; 5) improve maternal health; 6) combat HIV/AIDS, Malaria and other diseases; 7) ensure environment sustainability, and 8) develop global partnerships for development (UN-WHO Policy Analysis, 2010). More recently the Movement for Global Mental Health asked the UN to include three components in the new SDG's that relate to social determinants of health. These include:

1 Promote protection of human rights and prevent discrimination against people with mental illness and psychosocial disability.
2 Bridge the massive mental health treatment gap and improve access to health and social care.
3 Integrate attention to mental health into development initiatives.

(Eaton, Kakuma, Wright, & Minas, 2014)

The SDGs will be constructed with broad input from ministers of health, health care professionals, consumers and advocacy groups from around the world and are expected to be aligned with identified goals of participating low-, middle-, and high-income countries. The broad guiding principles driving goal development for this next round of global health goals include human rights, treatment gaps, equality, and sustainability.

As the mental health crisis continues and expands into all age groups and across borders, it is important to identify seminal works, movements, and organizations that are intentionally working to improve mental health for all. The focus has been on acquiring accurate prevalence data, developing community-involved interventions, training lay individuals from the community and culture to deliver interventions and support those with mental and behavioral challenges, working to decrease stigma, and providing research-informed education to promote mental health literacy in both professional and lay communities. The following is a partial resource list illustrative of this work.

Seminal documents, organizations and advocacy groups in the field of mental health promotion

1 *mhGAP*: The Mental Health Gap Action Programme of the World Health Organization works to promote government and stakeholder action to scale up services and interventions to provide care for those challenged by mental, neurological, and substance use disorders. mhGAP developed the *Mental Health GAP Evidence-Based Treatment Intervention Guidelines for Mental, Neurological and Substance Use Disorders in Non-Specialized Health Settings* (WHO, 2010b) and the *mhGAP Humanitarian Intervention Guide* (WHO, 2015).

2 *WHO*: The World Health Organization was established in 1948 by the United Nations and identified as the leading authority worldwide to direct and coordinate the health of all nations within the United Nations. The mission of WHO "in the area of mental health is to reduce the burden of mental disorders and to promote the mental health of the population worldwide" (WHO, 2011). To accomplish its mission, the WHO promotes leadership, research, health standards, importance of using evidence to inform actions and treatments, disease surveillance and response, technical support, education, and monitoring of health conditions. It provides a significant body of work on its website on a variety of health and mental health related topics. WHO has been at the forefront in responsiveness to both communicable and non-communicable diseases, health systems, health promotion and preparedness.

3 *Mental Health Atlas*: The *Mental Health Atlas* series is a publication of the WHO that was started in 2001. Subsequent versions of the document were in 2005, 2011 and most recently, 2014. The goal of the Atlas series is to "collect, compile and disseminate relevant information on mental health resources available within countries" (WHO, 2011). This evidence-based document chronicles global trends in the field to support advocacy and action to support an increase in resources, direct research activities, and ultimately catalyze a positive change in conditions.

4 *The Lancet Series*: The *Lancet Mental Health* Series of 2007 and 2011 was a groundbreaking set of scholarly papers that brought together researchers and scientists from around the world who engaged in methodical and comprehensive descriptions of initial and updated mental health conditions in low-, middle-, and high-income countries. The authors of many of the papers continue to conduct research and disseminate updated data on a variety of mental health issues. The series can be accessed at: www.thelancet.com/series/global-mental-health and www.thelancet.com/series/global-mental-health-2011.

5 *Human Rights Advocacy*: Human Rights Advocacy groups work to advocate for victims of human rights violations. Globally most countries have ratified international treaties endorsing human rights and humanitarian laws.

6 *Movement for Global Mental Health*: The Movement for Global Mental Health (MGMH) is a network of individuals and organizations, whose goal is to improve services for people with mental and psychosocial disabilities worldwide. MGMH prioritizes their work in low- and middle-income countries with a focus on scientific evidence and human rights protection. Additional information can be obtained at www.globalmentalhealth.org.

7 *Grand Challenges Canada*: The Grand Challenges Canada was established in 2010 to support Bold Ideas and Big Impact global research. The research must identify a barrier that if removed would help solve a significant problem in a developing country. Global mental health is one of the portfolios funded. Additional information can be obtained at www.grandchallenges.ca/grand-challenges/global-mental-health.

8 *National Institute of Mental Health (NIMH) (USA)*: NIMH strives to promote understanding and treatment of mental illnesses by engaging in and advancing basic and clinical research aimed at prevention, recovery and cure. NIMH is the largest organization in the world that endeavors to comprehend brain science and human experiences that contribute to behaviors. The 2016 NIMH operating budget is $31.3 billion dollars. Additional information can be obtained at www.nimh.nih.gov.

9 *Substance Abuse and Mental Health Services Administration (SAMHSA) (USA)*: SAMHSA was established in 1992 to advance behavioral health and decrease the impact of substance abuse and mental illness in communities within the United States.

   The 2016 budget of 3.7 billion dollars will target goals of building strong communities, strengthen crisis systems, increase the behavioral health workforce, develop strategies to combat prescription drug and opioid abuse and support behavioral health needs in tribal communities. Additional data can be obtained at www.samhsa.gov.

10 *Pan American Health Organization (PAHO)*: Founded in 1902, PAHO is an international public health agency and Regional Office for the Americas of the World Health Organization that provides technical support and fosters partnerships in countries in the Americas, Canada and the Caribbean. Their Non-Communicable Diseases and Mental Health branch focuses on prevention and control of non-communicable diseases, identifying and mitigating risk factors for mental, neurological, and substance abuse disorders that are culture specific. It raises public awareness, supports capacity building, and promotes policies, programs and services to enhance mental health. Additional information about PAHO can be obtained at www.paho.org.

11 *Center for Global Mental Health* (www.centreforglobalmentalhealth.org) *at the London School of Hygiene and Tropical Medicine* (www.lshtm.ac.uk): A renowned center that focuses on public and global health research, scholarship and education with a goal of translating knowledge to practice and policy.

12 *WHO MiND: Mental Health IN Development*: This is a WHO Quality Rights online tool of national and international resources used to end discrimination and violations against those with mental and behavioral disabilities. Additional information can be obtained at ww.who.int/mental_health/policy/contact/en/.

13. WHO AIMS: This is an assessment tool to determine the overall quality of mental health systems. The tool focuses on six domains containing 156 items. Additional information about AIMS can be found at www.who.int/mental_health/WHO-AIMS/en.

14. WHO comprehensive mental health action plan (2013–2020) as shown in Table 1.5.

Conclusion

For the past 15 years there has been an intentional and dynamic focus on bringing an accurate picture of global mental health needs to the forefront and to the attention of those in positions

Table 1.5 WHO comprehensive mental health action plan (2013–2020)

Obective 1: To strengthen effective leadership and governance for mental health	Target 1.1: 80% of countries will have developed or updated their policies or plans for mental health in line with international and regional human rights instruments (by the year 2020)	88 countries, equivalent to 56% of those countries who responded, or 45% of all WHO Member States. Value is based on a self-rating checklist (see Section 2.1 of report)
	Target 1.2: 50% of countries will have developed or updated their law for mental health in line with international and regional human rights instruments (by the year 2020)	65 countries, equivalent to 42% of those countries who responded, or 34% of all WHO Member States. Value is based on a self-rating checklist (see Section 2.2 of report)
Objective 2: To provide comprehensive, integrated and responsive mental health and social care services in community-based settings	Target 2: Service coverage for severe mental disorders will have increased by 20% (by the year 2020)	Not computable from Atlas 2014 data, but expected to be less than 25%, based on treatment gap and service uptake studies
Objective 3: To implement strategies for promotion and prevention in mental health	Target 3.1: 80% of countries will have at least two functioning national, multisectoral mental health promotion and prevention programmes (by the year 2020)	80 countries, equivalent to 48% of those countries who responded, or 41% of all WHO Member States. Value is based on a self-completed inventory of current programmes (see Section 4 of report)
	Target 3.2: The rate of suicide in countries will be reduced by 10% (by the year 2020)	11.4 per 100,000 population. Value is based on age-standardized global estimate (see WHO report on suicide, 2014)
Objective 4: To strengthen information systems, evidence and research for mental health	Target 4: 80% of countries will be routinely collecting and reporting at least a core set of mental health indicators every two years through their national health and social information systems (by the year 2020)	64 countries, equivalent to 42% of those countries who responded, or 33% of all WHO Member States. Value is based on a self-rated ability to regularly compile mental health specific data that covers at least the public sector (see Section 1 of report)

Source: Reprinted from *Mental Health Atlas 2014 with permission from the World Health Organization.*

to make necessary changes in the plight of those affected by mental ill health. These efforts are in response to a real crisis wherein only one out of four individuals globally is receiving treatment for their mental health needs. Stigma, poor knowledge of the etiology of mental, neurologic and substance use disorders, and an exclusive and long-standing focus on physical illnesses and communicable diseases have placed contributions to mental ill health at the bottom of the list of health-related priorities. However, it is increasingly clear that overall health or well-being is intertwined with both one's physical and mental health. Unfortunately, significant disparities exist across low-, middle-, and high-income countries in the areas of mental health literacy, treatment resources (human, facilities, and medications), accuracy of prevalence data, access, stigma, and engagement in research, to inform culturally congruent mental health treatment interventions.

At the forefront of the global mental health movement are the World Health Organization, researchers from the UK, Australia, the United States and Canada, non-governmental organizations and the World Bank, among others. Concerted efforts have been under way to disseminate information in multiple venues in order to call attention to the crisis surrounding a significant increase in global mental ill health and the companion threats to individual well-being.

Globally, as stated earlier, nurses are recognized as constituting the largest number of health care providers in all countries, and represent an untapped resource in the movement to impact positive changes in mental health. In addition to supporting and showcasing the aforementioned trailblazers in the global mental health movement, this textbook will acquaint the reader with data, primarily from mental health nurses, about successful strategies engaged in with this population; endorse evidence-based interventions for use in low-, middle-, and high-income environments, and offer new ways of thinking and intervening with individuals challenged by their emotional and mental health vulnerabilities. Many of the mental health nurse scientists who contributed to this textbook support a strong focus on prevention, mental health promotion, mental health literacy, integration of mental health into primary care, and working aggressively with communities to decrease stigma, while providing culturally sensitive mental health care with individuals and groups within diverse communities. This textbook is a unique contribution to the nursing literature in that it offers nurses and other health care providers real-life and relevant experiences from the field about mental health across different countries, shares the voices of nurses working in different environments as they strive to promote mental health, and presents innovative strategies to assist with navigation of policy, practice, research, and advocacy roles. This textbook can serve as a tool kit when working with consumers, other mental health professionals, and those outside of the health care field who are engaged in developing a greater understanding of mental health, mental ill health, and the process of mental health promotion.

References

American Psychiatric Association (APA). (2013). *Diagnostic and Statistical Manual of Mental Disorders* (5th ed.). Arlington, VA: Author.

Braveman, P., Egerter, S., & Williams, D. (2011). The social determinants of health: Coming of age. *Annual Review of Public Health*, *32*, 381–398.

Chandra, V., Pandav, R., Laxminarayan, R., Tanner, C., Manyam, B., Rajkumar, S., Silberberg, D., Brayne, C., Chow, J., Herman, S., Hourihan, F., Kasner, S., Morillo, L., Ogunniyi, A., Theodore, W., & Zhang, Z. (2006). Neurological disorders. In *WHO Disease Control Priorities Related to Mental, Neurological, Developmental and Substance Abuse Disorders* (pp. 21–37). Geneva: WHO.

Charlson, F.J., Baxter, A.J., Dua, T., Degenhardt, L., Whiteford, H., & Vos, T. (2015). Excess mortality from mental, neurological and substance use disorders in the global burden of disease study 2010. *Epidemiology and Psychiatric Sciences*, *24*(2), 121–140.

Collins, P., Patel, V., & Joestl, S. (2011). Grand challenges in global mental health. *Nature*, *475*, 27–30.

Collins, P. Musisi, S., Frehywot, S., & Patel, V. (2015). The core competencies for mental, neurological, and substance use disorder care in sub-Saharan Africa. *Global Health Action*, *8*: 26682.

Demyttenaere, K., Bruffaerts, R., Posada-Villa, J. Gasquet, I., Kovess, V., Lepine, J.P., Chatterji, S. (2004). Prevalence, severity, and unmet need for treatment of mental disorders in the World Health Organization World Mental Health Surveys. *JAMA*, *291*(21), 2581–2590.

Dua, T., Barbui, C., Clark, N., Fleischmann, A., Poznyak, V., van Ommeren, M., Saxena, S. (2011). Evidence-based guidelines for mental, neurological, and substance use disorders in low-and middle-income countries: Summary of WHO recommendations. *PLoS Medicine, 8*(11), e1001122.

Eaton, J., Kakuma, R., Wright, A., & Minas, H. (2014). A position statement on mental health in the post-2015 development agenda. *International Journal of Mental Health Systems,* 8, 28.

Friel, S. & Marmot, M. (2011). Action on the social determinants of health and health inequities goes global. *Annual Review of Public Health, 32,* 225–236.

Hyman, S., Chisholm, D., Kessler, R., Patel, V., & Whiteford, H. (2006). Mental disorders. In *WHO Disease Control Priorities Related to Mental, Neurological, Developmental and Substance Abuse Disorders* (pp. 1–20). Geneva: WHO.

Kleinman, A. (2009). Global mental health: A failure of humanity. *The Lancet, 374*(9690), 603–604.

Mental Health Gap Action Programme (mhGAP). (2008). *Scaling Up Care for Mental, Neurological, and Substance Use Disorders.* Geneva: WHO.

Morris, J., Lora, A., McBain, R., & Saxena, S. (2011). Global mental health resources and services: A WHO survey of 184 countries. *Public Health Reviews,* 34(2).

National Institute of Neurological Disorders and Stroke (NINDS). (n.d.). Available at www.ninds.nih.gov (accessed May 25, 2016).

Phillips, M., Chen, H., Diesfeld, K., Xie, B., Cheng, H., Mellsop, G., & Liu, X. (2013). China's new mental health law: Reframing involuntary treatment. *American Journal of Psychiatry, 170*(6), 588–591.

Population Reference Bureau. (2013). 2013 World population data sheet. Available at www.prb.org/pdf13/2013-population-data-sheet_eng.pdf (accessed May 25, 2016).

Rehm, J., Chisholm, D., Room, R., & Lopez, A. (2006). Substance abuse disorders. In *WHO Disease Control Priorities Related to Mental, Neurological, Developmental and Substance Abuse Disorders* (pp. 57–100). Geneva: WHO.

Tse, S., Ran, M., Huang, Y., & Zhu, S. (2013). The urgency of now: Building a recovery-oriented, community mental health service in China. *Psychiatric Services, 64*(7), 613–616.

UN-WHO Policy Analysis. (2010). Available at www.who.int/mental_health/policy/mhtargeting/mh_policyanalysis_who_undesa.pdf (accessed May 25, 2016).

Whiteford, H., Ferrari, A., Degenhardt, L., & Feigin, V. (2015). The global burden of mental, neurological and substance use disorders: An analysis from the global burden of disease study 2010. *PLoS ONE,* 10(2): e0116820.

Whiteford, H., Degenhardt, L., Rehm, J., Baxter, A., Ferrari, A., Erskine, H., Vos, T. (2013). Global burden of disease attributable to mental and substance use disorders: Findings from the Global Burden of Disease Study 2010. Available at http://dx.doi.org/10.1016/S0140-6736(13)61611-6 (accessed May 25, 2016).

World Bank. (n.d.). Country classifications. Available at data.worldbank.org/news/2015-country-classifications (accessed May 25, 2016).

World Health Organization (2015). Metrics: Disability-adjusted life year (DALY). Available at www.who.-int/healthinfo/global_burden_disease/metrics_daly/en/(accessed May 25, 2016).

World Health Organization Health Report. (2001a). Mental health: New understanding, new hope. Available at www.who.int/whr2001/media_centre/press_release/en/(accessed May 25, 2016).

World Health Organization. (2001b). *Strengthening Mental Health Promotion.* Geneva: WHO.

World Health Organization. (2005). Available at www.euro.who.int/__data/assets/pdf_file/0008/96452/E87301.pdf (accessed May 25, 2016).

World Health Organization. (2008). The global burden of disease-2004 update. Available at www.who.int/healthinfo/global_burden_disease/2004_report_update/en (accessed May 25, 2016).

World Health Organization. (2010a). *People with Mental Disabilities Cannot Be Forgotten.* Geneva: WHO.

World Health Organization. (2010b). *Mental Health GAP Intervention Guide for Mental, Neurological and Substance Use Disorders in Non-Specialized Health Settings: Mental Health Gap Action Programme (mhGAP).* Geneva: WHO.

World Health Organization. (2011). *Mental Health Atlas 2011.* Geneva: WHO.

World Health Organization. (2013*). Investing in Mental Health: Evidence for Action.* Geneva: WHO.

World Health Organization. (2014). *Mental Health Atlas 2014.* Geneva: WHO.

World Health Organization. (2015). *mhGAP Humanitarian Intervention Guide.* Geneva: WHO.

Zhou, W., & Xiao, S. (2015). Reporting on China's mental health surveillance. *American Journal of Psychiatry, 172*(4), 314–315.

2

HISTORICAL OVERVIEW OF PSYCHIATRIC/MENTAL HEALTH CARE

Ann J. Sheridan

Introduction

Historically, the treatment and care of the mentally ill has been influenced by societal, cultural, political, religious and scientific factors. Beliefs about the nature of lunacy, insanity and subsequently mental illness, while divergent across the globe, demonstrate a concordance that has served to determine how those with mental illness have been cared for by the societies in which they live. As societies began the interrelated processes of industrialisation and urbanisation, an increasing drive towards classification and segregation of various groups within society including prisoners, vagrants, the poor, the sick and ultimately the mentally ill, emerged.

The purpose of this chapter is to provide the historical context of the care and institutional treatment of the mentally ill from a global perspective. In doing so this chapter will examine a number of critical concepts including the emergence of segregation of the mentally ill as a group across cultures, the impact of colonisation on systems of care and definitions of mental illness and subsequently health; and how the origins of systems of mental health/psychiatric care have influenced our current thinking about those who experience mental illness and how they are cared for. According to Berrios (1996), this systematisation of mental health care was a result of the need to provide formal services to compensate for the weakening of self-sufficient, subsistent communities due to economic migration and the degree of structure required to provide funded professional services. This chapter will also briefly examine some of the central debates in mental health/psychiatric care to emerge over the past half a century and that have become dominant in influencing care in the twenty-first century.

Origins of care systems

Early origins

Internationally, the origins of psychiatric/mental health systems of care are attributed to the emergence of institutions built to provide care to the sick and to house the poor, abandoned and insane. Earliest accounts of such institutions originate in the Islamic Middle East and North Africa where hospitals for the provision of care to the sick were established. In dealing with the mentally ill, these institutions adopted Greek medical traditions focusing on physical rather than spiritual causes and treatment of mental illness (Cohen, Patel & Minas, 2014). Institutional care for the sick including the mentally ill continued to extend across the East, Middle East and into Europe as part of the Moorish invasion into Spain. While originating within the Islamic tradition, accounts of institutions to provide for the sick and the mentally ill established by Catholic religious organisations and provision grounded within other Christian traditions, are available for France, Belgium, Italy, Spain and Sweden (Cohen *et al.*, 2014). The earliest account of an institution established to treat the mentally ill in the Americas is in Mexico and this is likely to have been a feature of the colonisation of Mexico by the Spanish (Cohen *et al.*, 2014). In China, earliest accounts of provision for the mentally ill is in the Tang Dynasty (618–907 AD), when homeless widows, orphans and the mentally ill were cared for in the Bei Tian Fang, a type of charity facility administrated by monks (Liu *et al.*, 2011). Institutional care continued to extend across the Americas with the first hospital established to provide care of the mentally ill in North America opening in Virginia in 1773 (Grob, 1994). Colonisation across Europe, the Americas, Australia, India, Indochina and Africa continued to influence the spread and embedding of institutions as the primary means for providing care to the mentally ill and during the 1800s the asylum system was firmly established throughout Europe and North America, continuing to be consolidated during the early years of the twentieth century (Nolan & Sheridan, 2001; Patel, Minas, Cohen & Prince, 2014; Scull, 1993; Sheridan, 2006; Shorter, 1997; Shorter, 2005). As discussed in the case exemplar of Jamaica (Chapter 21), long-term institutionalization of the mentally ill was also a common practice in the Caribbean. It appears that no Western country was spared the rapid construction and apparently insatiable demand for accommodation of the mentally ill within these institutions, and these Western systems of care were transported globally through colonisation (Wright, 1997).

Colonialism

Colonialism, a process with a long history globally, has been instrumental in influencing the health systems and mental health services of many countries. Colonialism can be described as a process that erodes the indigenous political, cultural, social, economic and health-related customs of a country. It has been defined by Kelm (1998) as a process involving the establishment of external political control and economic dispossession; geographic incursion, social-cultural dislocation ultimately resulting in the creation of ideological formulations around race and skin colour that positions the coloniser at a higher evolutionary level than the colonised (Kelm 1998, p. xviii). For many countries the history of colonization is a disturbing one with decimation of the indigenous population through warfare, disease, dispossession of property and possessions as well as an active suppression of culture, religion, language and identity (Kirmayer *et al.*, 2000). Conceptualisations of health and health care have also been closely interrelated with the goals of colonialism. Colonisers frequently utilised as justification for colonisation, at least in part, the poor health status of the indigenous population and the need to provide adequate health care, thus portraying the colonisation process as 'doing good'. The belief that Western perspectives of health, illness and treatment were superior to local knowledge and practices served to legitimise the ideological position of the colonisers while dispossessing the indigenous population and specific action-focused groups, often faith-based, who saw this as a specific noble mission.

However, when examining the origins of mental health care from a global perspective, it is also necessary to appreciate that it is unlikely that the system of institutional care for the mentally ill emerged as a singular response to mental illness. Rather, it emerged within the wider social, political, economic and cultural context, including colonisation, during an era when societies, most likely due to the demands associated with increasing systematisation around formal employment, urbanisation and industrialisation, sought solutions to managing complex population health and social care needs. During these times various other institutions were being established to enable societies and communities to deal with different groups with particular needs including orphans, the poor, the sick and criminals. Thus while institutionalisation can be viewed as a societal response to population need, it is not one that was applied exclusively to providing for a great confinement of the mentally ill. Prior to the establishment of asylums for the insane, those mentally ill people requiring institutional care were regularly placed across the full spectrum of existing institutions. With the advent of the insane asylum, those considered mentally ill and who were most likely considered unsuitable and or unresponsive to the overriding aims of the institutions in which they were currently residing, were dispatched to these newly emerging special institutions. Thus, rather than viewing the emergence of the system of care for mental illness as one designed specifically to implement the segregation and confinement of the mentally ill, it may more correctly be viewed as an extension to, or specialisation of, an already existing system of institutional provision (Edington, 2013; Wright, 1997).

Mental illness and specialisation

Whereas the origins of mental health/psychiatric care can be broadly located in the emergence of the institutions built to contain the mentally ill, locating beliefs and conceptualisations of mental illness is more problematic. It is evident that throughout recorded history different beliefs about the origins and or causes of mental illness have been attributed to a range of factors influenced by social, cultural and religious beliefs and practices. These beliefs were also influenced by the thinking, considered scientific during those times, that 'madness' was viewed as mysterious and as a frightening disease located within the realms of the supernatural and associated with the power of a deity (Berrios & Freeman, 1991; Finnane, 1981; Nolan & Sheridan, 2001).

Notions of illness as divine retribution or favouritism, possession by malevolent spirits or shamanism, as witchcraft, resulting from astrological misalignment, or as a moral failing on the part of the individual or their family, were all seen as plausible explanations (Scull, 1993). The beliefs that human character, morality and temperament were governed by four fluids or bodily humours (blood, phlegm, yellow bile and black bile) was also utilised as an explanation of mental illness (Berrios, 1996; Berrios & Freeman, 1991; Malcolm, 1989). The disequilibrium of bodily humours, their associated release of vapours and accompanying symptoms served as one early method of classifying illness types and of determining treatment approaches (Berrios, 1996).

The advent of Westernised medical specialisations, a phenomenon of the nineteenth century, emerged from the belief that scientific knowledge was central to understanding illness and that eventually through scientific exploration and proof, all illness could be treated and cured. Prior to the nineteenth century a variety of methods to treat insanity already existed. These methods, such as those based upon the beliefs that mental illness was the result of physical factors including the disequilibrium of bodily humours, sought to address the causes through treatments such as purging, emetics and bleeding (Berrios, 1996; Berrios & Freeman, 1991; Finnane, 1981). Where belief systems employed supernatural or spiritual conceptualisations, alleviation of suffering was sought through the utilisation of religious and spiritual rituals or to calm the person through the use of water. Medicinal compounds such as herbal remedies and later drugs such as opium and laudanum and a variety of external physical restraints, were also utilised in an attempt to treat or alleviate suffering or to contain and manage the person (Finnane, 1981; Freeman, 1999;

Robins, 1986; Sadowsky, 2003). The emergence of specialised asylums for the treatment and care of the insane along with the adoption of a dominant bio-scientific ideology, fostered the belief that like physical illnesses, mental illness could be treated and cured. However, it soon became apparent that these physical interventions failed to live up to expectations of being a cure for mental illness.

Rather than relying on physical interventions, some of which were sufficiently barbaric to kill the patient, the nature of the ideologies underpinning asylum care began to change and the milieu created within the institution of the asylum began to be considered as the essential therapeutic element. Thus during the early part of the eighteenth century an era of reform emerged, which shifted ideas away from physical and or biological causation towards a more psychological and socially focused understanding of mental illness. It is important to recognise at this juncture that institutional provision for the mentally ill while evident across Europe and America, and to a lesser extent China, was non-existent in the vast majority of other countries. In many countries including those in Africa, in India and Japan, institutional provision for the mentally ill emerged as a direct result of colonisation. Thus for a significant proportion of the world's population, being identified as mentally ill and receiving treatment and care for mental illness, was the preserve of families, communities and local medical and spiritual healers (Ellis, 2015; Porter & Wright, 2003). Within Western cultures, the emergence of a psycho-social conception of causation for mental illness resulted in the adoption of a gentler and more refined approach to treatment and care. The subsequent advent of 'moral treatment' placed emphasis on the value of providing an environment in which the patient was exposed to humane and compassionate treatment. Patients were exposed to friendly association and encouraged to discuss their difficulties with specially trained attendants and physicians. Moral treatment also placed emphasis upon dietary factors and on balancing physical and mental activity in terms of productive and purposeful leisure and occupational pursuits (Berrios, 1996; Berrios & Freeman, 1991; Finnane, 1981; Nolan & Sheridan, 2001). While the drive towards moral management appears to have emanated within a Western context, there is evidence that within the earliest institutions developed to provide care and grounded with Islamic traditions, a relaxed atmosphere for the provision of care was adopted and attention to the care milieu was achieved through the use of gardens and fountains along with careful attention to diet (Patel *et al.*, 2014).

Eugenics

During the nineteenth and early twentieth centuries, the advancement of the positivist ethic that highly valued knowledge based on observable facts began to gain prominence. Within the newly emerging mental asylum system, it became evident that while moral management had had some success, it was far from efficacious in treating the majority of asylum inmates, a significant proportion of whom at that time were suffering from tertiary syphilis (Turner, 1999). As the nineteenth century progressed the numbers within insane asylums continued to rise and new explanations of causation for mental illness were required. The explanations that gained importance during the second half of the nineteenth century were framed as a variant of Darwinian evolution, which emphasised the potential for retrogression or degeneration as well as evolution. This idea, that both humans and society had the potential for 'retrogression' as well as evolution, became influential in explanations of causation of a range of social ills including poverty, criminality and mental illness. The concept of degeneration, popularised by Benedict Augustus Morel (1809–1873), suggested that psychological disorders along with the majority of deviations of human behaviour were the expression of an abnormal constitution and that this could be inherited (Shorter, 2005). Moreover, it was considered that this abnormal constitution was liable to progressive deterioration. In contrast with the other areas of medicine, the causes of mental illness were not evident in the dissected brains of deceased mentally ill patients. This inability to locate the cause of mental illness, or to attribute causation to pathological changes within the brain, provided the impetus for theories of degeneration to offer proof for the origin of mental disorders. The rise of degeneration as an explanation for mental illness shifted the locus of cause from something that could be identified, treated and ultimately cured, to an aspect of human nature. Thus degeneration firmly located cause within the nature of the individual, consequently the psychiatrist and psychiatric care system possessed a degree of powerlessness to treat or effect a cure (Robb, 1996; Zubin, Oppenheimer & Neugebauer, 1985).

What the system could do, however, was to prevent the spread of degeneration in society leading ultimately to the rise of the Eugenics movement. The Eugenics movement was the innovation of Darwin's cousin, Francis Galton and was seen by many as the answer to racial and social degeneration. In general, eugenics sought to increase those features of the population deemed most desirable including those from the middle class and intellectuals; and to reduce or preferably eliminate those features of the population deemed undesirable such as poverty, crime and mental illness (Robb, 1996). The movement sought to apply scientific principles of natural biology to human society and thereby strengthen the human race. The belief that prevention of mental illness and mental retardation could be achieved through prevention of procreation ultimately resulted in programmes of forcible sterilisation of the mentally ill and other 'undesirable' groups. The movement gained international popularity and became active in Holland, Sweden, Belgium, Germany, Switzerland, Britain and the United States, where programmes of forcible sterilisation were implemented in an attempt to eliminate degeneration and protect society (Birn & Molina, 2005; Schneider, 2011; Stern, 2005). The desire for the elimination of degeneration among certain groups and classes within society subsequently underpinned the idea of 'lives not worth living' and the promulgation of euthanasia for those deemed 'mentally dead'.

During the Nazi regime in Germany these ideas were linked to racial purity resulting in the atrocities perpetrated during World War II against the mentally ill, homosexuals, intellectually disabled and most notably the Jewish population (Benedict & Kuhla, 1999; Schneider, 2011).

Treatment and interventions

Physical interventions

In psychiatry, the nature of effective therapeutic intervention has long been the subject of debate. As in general medicine prior to the discovery of effective treatments such as antibiotics, different rigid ideologies existed as to what constituted effective therapy and this characteristic is evident when the bulk of clinical disorders can neither be effectively treated nor specifically explained. In the years preceding World War II, various physical treatments such as malarial and insulin therapy, electroconvulsive therapy, surgical intervention for focal sepsis and psychosurgery all seemed to offer hope of effective treatment for the mentally ill (Braslow, 1997; Scull, 2005; El-Hai, 2005). However, none of these treatments lived up to the expectations held of them. By far the most controversial treatments were surgical interventions and the use of electroconvulsive therapy. Developments in bacteriology also prompted a consideration that foci of infection may be causative in mental illness and this hypothesis gathered significant support. Developments occurring in other branches of medicine at the time coupled with the fact that a significant proportion of the residents of mental hospitals were experiencing the end stages of syphilitic infection – general paralysis of the insane – the hypothesis of infection as a causative factor in mental illness appeared to be a reasonable one. Various procedures aimed at removing 'foci of infection' were instituted in psychiatric institutions around the world. However, poor results and high mortality rates resulted in the diminishing of this intervention (El-Hai, 2005; Scull, 2005).

Trepanation – the drilling of holes in the skull – has existed in many cultures and was often performed to allow the release of demons thought to cause mental illness. In the early years of the twentieth century procedures aimed at reducing anxiety and neurotic symptoms were undertaken, initially on chimpanzees and subsequently on humans in an attempt to improve outcomes for patients. The procedure, originally named by Egas Moniz as Prefrontal Leucotomy and subsequently revised and re-named as Trans Orbital Leucotomy by Walter Freeman, became a popular approach to treating persistent mental illness (El-Hai, 2005). While such procedures were undertaken in various countries, ethical concerns about the uncertain outcomes for patients as well as the potential to utilise the procedure as a form of social and political control resulted in its abandonment.

The origins of electroconvulsive therapy, like many other experimental therapies of the time, was based upon the observation that patients who experienced seizures were often relieved of symptoms of mental illness, at least for a period of time. Originating as a chemical therapy using intramuscular injections of camphor in oil or metrazol, the use of electrical stimulation was subsequently introduced by Ugo Cerletti and Luigi Bini, who in 1938 identified that inducing epileptic type seizures relieved symptoms of depression in humans (Fink, 1999). Subsequently muscle relaxants and anaesthesia were used to alleviate unintended side effects associated with electroconvulsive therapy. In the majority of countries, while psychosurgical interventions are only undertaken in highly controlled and prescribed circumstances, electroconvulsive therapy continues to be utilised and although its use has significantly diminished over the past 50 years, it remains an effective, if controversial, treatment in a range of psychiatric conditions including depression, bipolar mania, schizophrenia and severe suicidal behaviours.

One of the most significant and far-reaching developments to impact psychiatric/mental health care was the discovery and development of a range of drug therapies. While herbal medicines had been used with varying degrees of effectiveness in a variety of countries and cultures, from the 1950s onwards, a wide range of psychotherapeutic agents have been developed to treat a range of mental illnesses. Originating with the development of Chlorpromazine (Thorazine) in the early 1950s, the demonstration that a drug could modify disturbed thoughts associated with psychotic processes was a breakthrough in the treatment of serious mental illnesses. Subsequent developments of neuroleptic medications that had less sedative effects added to the range of drug choices. As with the development of neuroleptics, the development of antidepressants and anxiolytics offered relief to a large cohort of people experiencing anxiety and depression. In addition to relieving symptoms of illness, a significant impact of pharmacological interventions in psychiatric/mental health care was the opportunity for patients to be discharged from hospital in much shorter time periods, thus reducing costs and the range of inconveniences associated with extended hospital stays. Treatment as an outpatient also became an option for patients and in this respect pharmacological interventions supported the development of outpatient and community-based care. Utilising medications, particularly for conditions such as anxiety, patients started to receive treatments from physicians other than psychiatrists.

Psycho–social interventions

The need to deal with large numbers of traumatised victims, displaced persons and refugees during and after World War II presented policy makers and health care professionals with the challenge of finding new approaches to addressing the emergent range of needs. The emergence of group therapy during the War, and its apparent effectiveness in assisting recovery and enabling soldiers to return to active duty, was seen to offer an alternative approach to physical interventions. As a result, the focus of interventions now began to shift towards a more psycho-dynamic approach. In the post-war period challenges continued to emerge including alarming rates of overcrowding within psychiatric hospitals, shortages of staff, particularly psychiatric nurses, and long lengths of stay, coupled with a serious lack of financial resources. Together, these issues converged within the international context to provide the momentum for a fundamental review of the existing systems of psychiatric care (Webster, 1991).

The recognition of the importance of the environment within which care was delivered was not however a new concept. The 'moral' management of patients promoted by Tuke at York and Pinel in Paris in the eighteenth century, and in the original institutions grounded with Islamic traditions, had recognised the value of providing an environment in which patients benefited by being exposed to friendly associations, discussion of their difficulties and productive and purposeful activity (Digby, 1984). The re-emergence of interest in the concept of the care environment began during the early years of the twentieth century, while later the works of Jones (1953), Barton (1959) and Goffman (1961) are identified as significant in focusing attention on the negative effects of institutions and their prevailing systems of rule, regulations and paternalistic attitudes, while promoting a recognition of the care environment as a potential therapeutic entity. The therapeutic value of community and the recognition of the nature of the relationship between patient and mental health professionals also gathered momentum as did the utilisation of techniques aimed at altering behaviour through addressing cognitive processes.

Increasing uniformity and globalisation in mental health care

In the years leading up to World War II, significant events occurred including an exodus of psychiatric practitioners, principally psychiatrists and psychoanalysts leaving Germany, Austria, Poland and other European countries and settling in the United States, Britain, Israel and other countries in South America and Canada (Berrios & Freeman, 1991). This exodus resulted in the transmission of ideas, principally psychoanalysis, which originated in and were central to conceptualisations of psychology, mental illness and treatments particularly within German, Austrian and French psychiatry, and these became a dominant paradigm, particularly in the United States. While psychoanalysis was also established in other countries, its sphere of influence particularly given the establishment of national health services in a range of countries during the post-war period, was relatively small. While Western ideas on psychiatric/mental health care were influential globally primarily through the effects of colonisation and the attendant acculturation processes, in the aftermath of World War II, advances in technology and tele-communications and increasing ease of international travel, along with the influence of media such as the film industry emanating principally from the United States of America and the United Kingdom, resulted in a greater degree of uniformity of psychiatric care across the globe. Likewise the influence of international organisations such as the World Health Organization and its sponsorship of the translation of technical terms and classification systems such as International Classification of Disease (ICD) have contributed to increasing uniformity in global mental health care, treatment and research (Lamensdorf Ofori-Atta & Linden, 1995; Crammer, 1999).

Western psychiatry with its changing systems and structures continues to be influential globally. Taking China as an example, prior to the founding of the People's Republic, Western-style hospitals had been in operation since the late nineteenth century with the original institution founded and funded by the American missionary John Kerr. In the aftermath of the founding of the People's Republic in 1949, a programme of extension of psychiatric hospitals was undertaken across all provinces and some community-based services were established. However, the advent of economic reforms in China resulted in the encouragement of existing hospitals to operate as profit-making entities, and this change in ethos along with the closure of not-for-profit institutions and services resulted in the decimation of the mental health services nationally (Liu *et al.*, 2011). In recent years, China has begun to rebuild its mental health care system. However, rather than seeking to establish a system based on its own diverse cultural and ethnic needs, it has engaged in a deliberate way with Western ideology of psychiatric care and services. In particular China is engaging with Australia, the USA and Britain to help it establish modern community-based mental health services and to support it in building human resource capacity within mental health systems (Liu *et al.*, 2011).

Moving away from institutional care provision towards a community-based model became a significant global issue in psychiatric/mental health care during the middle years of the twentieth century. However, the interpretation of what constitutes community care is diverse and remains variable across countries. In some countries community care is viewed as the provision of specialist mental health care within a community-based context and integrating the hospital provision as part of that approach. In other countries, community care is regarded as embedding mental health care within a public health care framework and providing generalist mental health promotion, support and care through networks of community-based organisations including a wide range of community-based health care professionals. In some countries both approaches in various combinations are utilised. The absence of an agreed-upon framework for community care or care in the community is understandable given the diversity of health systems and models of funding health care globally, as well as the diversity of societies and communities.

Psychiatric mental health nursing

The development of psychiatric/mental health nursing is closely aligned with the development of the asylum as a means of providing care for the insane. While the asylum system brought with it the demand for a workforce to ensure its optimal functioning, the care of the insane within these early asylums was provided primarily by untrained personnel. As psychiatry began to emerge in the second half of the nineteenth century along with the medicalization of insanity, it was accompanied by a desire to establish an associated group of workers similar to those existing in hospitals caring for the physically sick (Scull, 1979). During the early years of the profession of psychiatric/mental health nursing, the practice of nursing was focused primarily on the smooth running of the institution, supervision of patients, provision of physical care and assisting and supporting the work of doctors. Thus the clinical elements of the role of psychiatric nurses practising in the early years were generally limited to a specific range of treatments and tasks located firmly within a biophysical approach to care.

In 1956, the World Health Organisation (WHO) addressed specifically the issue of psychiatric nursing and provided a seminal international report on the topic. The impetus for addressing psychiatric nursing emanated from the Expert Group on Mental Health in 1953 (WHO, 1953). An explicit intention of the 1956 WHO report was the desire to drive change in the existing patterns of psychiatric nursing practice away from the predominant custodial-based approach towards a therapeutic and interpersonally based one. While recognising the existence of limitations in terms of national and local, social, cultural and economic determinants, and the impact of these on the eventual role of the psychiatric nurse, the report was to prove instrumental in directing changes in psychiatric/mental health nursing globally over the coming two decades.

In delimiting the future role of the psychiatric nurse, the expert committee drew heavily on the dual theoretical concepts of interpersonal relations and therapeutic community, with elements of the nurse's role outlined viewed as being an integral part of the therapeutic programme, concerned with the promotion of individualised care and competence in the use of group skills. The nursing structures required to achieve the desired changes were identified, as were the educational preparation and training of nurses at different levels within these structures. Other issues addressed, albeit briefly, were the need for personal, professional and practice development in psychiatric nursing along with the development of specialist nurses, viewed as a means of achieving changes within the profession and contributing overall to mental health care.

The report of the expert committee represents the beginning of a shift in the global practice, education and regulation of psychiatric nursing. Although still dependent upon changes in the nature and practice of psychiatry for identification of a distinctive role, there is evidence of a move towards highlighting the unique contribution of nurses to the care of the mentally ill and the definition of a distinctive body of knowledge based in interpersonal relations to underpin and guide psychiatric nursing practice.

The work of Peplau (1952) and her conceptualisation of the interactional or interpersonal nature of nursing was significant and groundbreaking at the time it was first published; and was in stark contrast to the prevailing belief that pathological processes were the primary basis of mental illness, and that the nurse's role was exclusively associated with assisting the doctor to fix that condition (O'Toole & Welt, 1994). In defining nursing Peplau attempted to identify the unique focus of nursing, and in her initial definition she considered nursing as:

> a significant therapeutic, interpersonal process (which) functions co-operatively with other human processes that make health possible for individuals and communities . . . Nursing is an educative instrument, a maturing force, that aims to promote forward movement of personality in the direction of creative, constructive, productive, personal and community living.
>
> *(Peplau, 1952, pp. 3–17)*

Elaborating and refining this definition in 1969, Peplau considered that, 'Nursing can take as its unique focus the reactions of the patient or client to the circumstances of his illness or health problem thus overlapping medicine only when dealing with disease processes more directly' (Peplau, 1969, pp. 42–55). The role of the psychiatric nurse, as described by Peplau (1952, 1965, 1969), was conceptualised as a complex set of sub-roles, which required the nurse to constantly negotiate between differing sets of norms, rules and expectations. From Peplau's perspective, a central organising set of concepts or processes could be distinguished, which in effect can be viewed as a 'supra' or 'meta-process' incorporating all others, and this was interpersonal relations. As an organising concept, interpersonal relations provided the meta-framework into which all other dimensions of the nurse's role could be incorporated or subsumed.

The transition of the role of the psychiatric/mental health nurse away from the existing custodial model towards a therapeutic one continued to be the subject of attention, and in 1963 WHO published *The Nurse in Mental Health Practice: Report on a Technical Conference* (John, Leite-Ribeiro & Buckle, 1963). The basis of this report was a pre-conference questionnaire distributed to a large number of psychiatric hospitals throughout Europe. The report, while acknowledging challenges in delimiting the role required of the nurse in mental health practice, considered attempting to 'spell out in more detail' the role of the psychiatric nurse if changes were to be effected and the most compelling 'argument of all' was that the needs of patients with psychiatric disorders were being inadequately met (John *et al.*, 1963).

In line with the report of the Expert Committee in 1956, and consistent with the work of Peplau (1952, 1964), it was recognised that the nurse's role encompassed a series of sub-roles, and was ultimately influenced by the practice location. Discrete skills or areas of competence were identified and these related to specific practice settings including the psychiatric institution, general hospital and extramural mental health services. This latter included health promotion, working with families and working in community settings. Again the primary emphasis was on the therapeutic function of the nurse based within a framework of interpersonal relations. Explicit recommendations were also made with regard to pre- and post-registration education and with regard to the need to prepare some nurses to function at higher levels of specialisation.

During the decades of the 1950s 1960s and early 1970s, the psychiatric nursing literature focused on the nature of psychiatric nursing and the multi-dimensional role of the psychiatric nurse (Altschul, 1972, 1984; Cormack, 1976, 1983; DeSalvo Rankin 1986; John *et al.*, 1961, 1963; Peplau, 1952, 1964, 1965; Robinson 1986; Travelbee, 1971). The key elements identifiable in this literature were defining of psychiatric nursing as an interpersonal process, and of the role of the psychiatric nurse as a therapeutic agent. With the re-orientation of services away from custodial and institutionally based systems, the nursing literature altered its focus to reflect the emerging types of clinical activities undertaken by psychiatric nurses such as behavioural psychotherapy and the nurses' roles within community-based services (Berkowitz & Heinl, 1984; Brooker, 1984; Brooker & Simmonds, 1985; Carr, Butterworth & Hodges, 1980; Marks, Connolly & Hallam, 1973; Marks, Hallam, Connolly & Philpott 1977; Paykel, Mangen, Griffith & Burns, 1982; Sladden 1979; Strang 1982; Wooff, Goldberg & Fryers, 1986).

Contemporary views

The recovery model

Over the past four decades the emergence of the consumer/survivor in the psychiatric/mental health care movement has gathered momentum across a number of countries. Influenced by de-institutionalisation, the anti-psychiatry movement and the rise of consumerism, such groups have emerged as a force challenging existing conceptions of mental illness and service provision. While initially threatening to mental health professionals, over recent years there is a greater sense of collaboration between survivor/consumer groups and psychiatric/mental health care professionals, along with a shifting of approach towards a more patient-centred focus on care.

Associated with the consumer/survivor movement and influenced by it, the concept of recovery as a philosophy in psychiatric/mental health care can be traced to the 1930s (Onken, Craig, Ridgway, Ralph & Cook, 2007), with its contemporary form emerging from the International Pilot Study of Schizophrenia which began to challenge the 'taken for granted' assumptions that serious mental illnesses, particularly schizophrenia, were progressive diseases without the possibility of recovery. Since the 1970s, and particularly over the past two decades, the notion of recovery has gained considerably in strength and prominence (Davidson, O'Connell, Tondora, Lawless & Evans, 2005). The movement towards accepting that recovery is possible was also inspired by political groups such as women's liberation and the black and gay rights movements (Roberts & Wolfson, 2004; Schiff, 2004).

In many respects, the recovery movement is, in essence, political in that it aims to promote the power of the 'patient' to challenge notions of dictatorial treatment and negative professional opinions. Moreover, it aims to promote the individual with mental health difficulties to the centre of his or her treatment, leading to a view that *recovery is a lived experience of moving through and beyond the limitations of one's disorder*. Reliance on conceptions of enduring mental health issues as synonymous with chronic illness, which placed individuals in the 'segregated company of like-damaged others' (Hopper, 2007, p. 870), is changing and recovery is now recognised as being more than symptom remission accompanied by an associated improvement in functioning.

In contrast, the shift to more 'personal' or 'survivor based' ideas of recovery draws upon the documented 'life journeys' of people who have experienced serious and persistent mental health problems, as well as their recovery journeys. Instead of focusing on the elimination of symptoms, this view emphasises the rebuilding of a worthwhile life; the reclaiming of valued social roles, and the (re)establishing of a positive self-identity (Tew *et al.*, 2011). Recovering from severe mental illness is a process of individual self-discovery that involves developing a positive sense of self and personal meaning in life, despite the presence of psychiatric symptoms and their consequences (Roe & Chopra, 2003). Hope, a sense of personal empowerment, and a desire to get well are central to recovery. From this perspective, recovery can be seen to be both a journey of personal change and a process of social (re)engagement. Regardless of its origin, 'recovery' is almost always understood as an individual process, one that can be helped along by professionals, family members, or a community of concern, but that ultimately has to be taken up by the person themself (Weisser, Morrow & Jamer, 2011). Internal aspects of recovery include concepts such as hope, personal growth and a positive sense of self; these elements can be helped along by supports such as family support, peer support and meaningful activity, whereas external factors, when mentioned, include having enough money to live and a house to live in (Pevalin & Goldberg, 2003; Spaniol, Wewiorski, Gagne & Anthony, 2002). Less attention has been given, however, to the structural changes needed within society to ensure that social environments are created that support recovery including adequate income, housing and social environments that are free of discrimination and provide access to crucial resources (Tew *et al.*, 2011; Weisser *et al.*, 2011). Despite this, there is evidence that new understandings of recovery are emerging, which are beginning to address these limitations.

Concluding thoughts: the road ahead

Despite the long history of various forms and philosophies of mental health service development across the world, services for people with mental health needs and challenges are still not adequately developed. Significant proportions of the global population who have mental health related needs do not have access to mental health care. A significant number of low-income countries have either an absence of mental health legislation and policy to direct mental health provision or where legislation and policy does exist, it frequently remains inadequate to address the mental health needs of the population with efforts instead being diverted to other public health agenda (Jack-Ide, Uys & Middleton, 2012). Globally, funding of psychiatric/mental health services is grossly under-resourced and it is estimated that between 32 per cent and 78 per cent of those with serious mental disorders do not receive any treatment (Wang *et al.*, 2007). Lack of political support, stigma, inadequate management, overburdened health services and, at times, resistance from policy-makers and health workers have hampered the development of coherent mental health care systems in many countries globally. In the industrialised countries pressures for other services, including higher profile acute physical health care to 'save lives' from conditions such as cancer, still gain far greater empathy and investment, with inadequate recognition of the burden on those with mental health needs, their families and their carers. Too often it needs a marketing frenzy around a scandal, such as revelations of poor quality of care, to trigger a remedy and then it can too often be a short-term containment. In the developing world, where governments and aid donors are struggling to find adequate investment across economic, agricultural, housing and health needs, mental health has been and continues to be low on the list of priorities.

Misunderstandings and prejudices about the nature of mental disorders and their treatment have further complicated progress. For example, many people think that mental disorders affect only a small subgroup of the population, but the reality is that up to 25 per cent of people will have a diagnosable mental disorder at some point during their lifetime (Kessler *et al.*, 2009). Others think that mental disorders cannot be treated, even though effective treatments do exist and can be successfully delivered in outpatient settings. Some may believe that some people with mental disorders are violent or unstable and therefore should be locked away, or are less deserving of investment than those with physical illness hence should be merely 'contained' as in the past, while in fact the vast majority of affected individuals are nonviolent and capable of living productively within their communities (WHO, 2009).

Maybe in our continuous quest for perceived wisdom from traditional academic and political sources, we should look wider to the example of Bhutan, where the King has stimulated the development of a Gross National Happiness Index, analysed down to a local level, with international aid agency support, as the basis for governance and investment (Ura, Alkire, Zangmo & Wangdi, 2012). Covering a wide range of aspects from literacy to environment, mental health status as part of psychological well-being is built into this using a well-known tool, Goldberg's General Health Questionnaire (GHQ-12). Only when mental health is seen in this sense as part of the national good, based on the understanding that 'Health is outcome of relational balance between mind and body, between persons and the environment' (Ura *et al.*, 2012, p. 16) and brought as such into government and investment values, using modern therapies in the context of societal understanding, will mental health services gain their just and adequate position.

Mental health, and services to support this, has been the concern of societies globally since early times. However, the quest for economic, scientific and policy conformity have led to fashions and phases of provision, and frequently to under-investment and to low esteem of the services and their recipients. Mental health problems will at some stage in their life affect one person in four, and therefore mental health services are a core societal issue. These services need to be designed and empowered to meet personal and societal needs, linking the science of health and the support of civil society.

References

Altschul, A. (1972). *Patient–nurse interaction: A study of interaction patterns in acute psychiatric wards*. Edinburgh, Scotland: Churchill Livingstone.

Altschul, A. (1984) Does good practice need good principles? *One Nursing Times*, 80(29), 36–38.

Barton, R. (1959). *Institutional neurosis*. Bristol, UK: J. Wright & Son.

Benedict, S. & Kuhla, J. (1999). Nurses' participation in the euthanasia programs of Nazi Germany. *Western Journal of Nursing Research*, 21(2), 246–263.

Berkowitz, R. & Heinl, P. (1984). The management of schizophrenic patients: The nurses' view. *Journal of Advanced Nursing*, 9(1), 23–33.

Berrios, G.E. (1996). *The history of mental symptoms: Descriptive psychopathology since the nineteenth century*. Cambridge, UK: Cambridge University Press.

Berrios, G. & Freeman, H. (eds). (1991). *150 years of British psychiatry, 1841–1991*. London: Royal College of Psychiatrists.

Birn, A.E. & Molina, N. (2005). In the name of public health. *American Journal of Public Health*, 95(7), 1095–1097.

Braslow, J. (1997). *Mental ills and bodily cures: Psychiatric treatment in the first half of the twentieth century*. Berkeley, CA: University of California Press.

Brooker, C.G. (1984). Some problems associated with the measurement of community psychiatric nurse intervention. *Journal of Advanced Nursing*, 9(2), 165–174.

Brooker, C.G. & Simmonds, S.M. (1985). A study to compare two models of community psychiatric nursing care delivery. *Journal of Advanced Nursing*, 10(3), 217–223.

Carr, P.J., Butterworth, A. & Hodges, B.E. (1980). *Community psychiatric nursing*. Edinburgh, Scotland: Churchill Livingstone.

Cohen, A., Patel, V. & Minas H. (2014). A brief history of global mental health. In V. Patel, H. Minas, A. Cohen & M. J. Prince (eds), *Global mental health principles and practice* (pp. 3–26). Oxford: Oxford University Press.

Cormack, D. (1976) *Psychiatric nursing observed*. London: Royal College of Nursing.

Cormack, D. (1983). *Psychiatric nursing described*. London: Churchill Livingstone.

Crammer, J. (1999). The impact of world events 1941–1950. In H. Freeman (ed.), *A century of psychiatry* (pp. 117–135). London: Mosby.

Davidson, L., O'Connell, M.J., Tondora, J., Lawless, M. & Evans, A. C. (2005). Recovery in serious mental illness: A new wine or just a new bottle? *Professional Psychology: Research and Practice*, 36(5), 480–487.

DeSalvo Rankin, E.A. (ed.). (1986). The nursing clinics of North America. *Psychiatric/Mental Health Nursing*, 21, 381–386.

Digby, A. (1984). The changing profile of a nineteenth-century asylum: The York Retreat. *Psychological Medicine*, 14(4), 739–748.

Edington, C. (2013) Going in and getting out of the colonial asylum: Families and psychiatric care in French Indochina. *Comparative Studies in Society and Health*, 55(3), 725–755.

El-Hai, J. (2005). *The lobotomist: A maverick medical genius and his tragic quest to rid the world of mental illness*. Hoboken, NJ: John Wiley & Sons.

Ellis, H.A. (2015). Obeah-illness versus psychiatric entities among Jamaican immigrants: Cultural and clinical perspectives for psychiatric mental health professionals. *Archives of Psychiatric Nursing*, 29(2), 83–89.

Fink, M. (1999). Convulsive therapy. In H. Freeman (ed.), *A century of psychiatry* (pp. 229–232). London: Mosby.

Finnane, M. (1981). *Insanity and the insane in post-famine Ireland*. London: Croom Helm.

Freeman, H. (ed.). (1999). *A century of psychiatry*. London: Mosby.

Goffman, E. (1961). *Asylums: Essays on the social situation of mental patients and other inmates*. Garden City, NY: Anchor Books.

Grob, G.N. (1994). *The mad among us: A history of the care of America's mentally ill*. New York: The Free Press.

Hopper, K. (2007). Rethinking social recovery in schizophrenia: What a capabilities approach might offer. *Social Science and Medicine*, 65(5), 868–879.

Jack-Ide, I. O., Uys, L.R. & Middelton, L.E. (2012). A comparative study of mental health services in two African countries: South Africa and Nigeria. *International Journal of Nursing and Midwifery*, 4(4), 50–57.

John, A.L., Leite-Ribeiro, M.O. & Buckle, D. (1963). The nurse in mental health practice: Report on a technical conference, Copenhagen, 15–24 November 1961. Geneva, Switzerland: World Health Organization. Retrieved 19 September 2014 from http://whqlibdoc.who.int/php/WHO_PHP_22_%28part1%29.pdf.

Jones, M. (1953). *The therapeutic community: A new treatment method in psychiatry*. New York: Basic Books.

Kelm, M.E. (1998). *Colonising bodies: Aboriginal health and healing in British Colombia, 1900–1950*. Vancouver, Canada: University of British Colombia Press.

Kessler, R.C., Aguilar-Gaxiola, S., Alonso, J., Chatterji, S., Lee, S., Ormel, J., Üstün, T.B. & Wang, P.S. (2009). The global burden of mental disorders: An update from the WHO World Mental Health (WMH) Surveys. *Epidemiologia e Psichiatria Sociale*, 18(1), 23–33.

Kirmayer, L.J., Brass, G.M. & Tait, CL. (2000). The mental health of Aboriginal peoples: transformations of identity and community. *Canadian Journal of Psychiatry*, 45(7), 607–616.

Lamensdorf Ofori-Atta, A.M. & Linden, W. (1995). The effect of social change on causal beliefs of mental disorders and treatment preference in Ghana. *Social Science and Medicine*, 40(9), 1231–1242.

Liu, J., Ma, H., He, Y.L., Xie, B., Xu, Y.F., Tang, H.Y., Tang, H.Y., Li, M., Hao, W., Wang, X.D., Zhang, M.Y., Ng, C.H., Goding, M., Fraser, J., Herrman, H., Chiu, H.F., Chan, S.S., Chiu, E., Yu, X. & Yu, X. (2011). Mental health system in China: history, recent service reform and future challenges. *World Psychiatry*, 10(3), 210–216.

Malcolm, E. (1989). *Swift's hospital: A history of St. Patrick's Hospital, Dublin, 1746–1989*. Dublin, Ireland: Gill & Macmillan.

Marks, I.M., Connolly, J. & Hallam, R.S. (1973). Psychiatric nurse as therapist. *British Medical Journal*, 3(5872), 156–160.

Marks, I.M., Hallam, R.S., Connolly, J. & Philpott, R. (1977). *Nursing in behavioural psychotherapy*. London: Royal College of Nursing.

Nolan, P. & Sheridan, A. (2001). In search of the history of Irish psychiatric nursing. *International History of Nursing Journal*, 6(2), 35–43.

Onken, S.J., Craig, C.M., Ridgway, P., Ralph, R.O. & Cook, J. A. (2007). An analysis of the definitions and elements of recovery: A review of the literature. *Psychiatric Rehabilitation Journal*, 31(1), 9–22.

O'Toole, A.W. & Welt S.R. (1994). *Hildegard E. Peplau, selected works interpersonal theory in nursing*. London: Macmillan.

Patel, V., Minas, H., Cohen, A. & Prince, M.J. (2014). *Global mental health principles and practice*. Oxford: Oxford University Press.

Paykel, E.S., Mangen, S.P., Griffith, J.H. & Burns, T.P. (1982). Community psychiatric nursing for neurotic patients: A controlled trial. *British Journal of Psychiatry*, 140, 573–581.

Peplau, H.E. (1952). *Interpersonal relations in nursing: A conceptual frame of reference for psychodynamic nursing*. New York: Putman.

Peplau, H.E. (1964). General application of theory and techniques of psychotherapy in nursing situations. In A.W. O'Toole & S.R. Welt (eds), *Hildegard E. Peplau, selected works interpersonal theory in nursing* (pp. 99–107 of Chapter 7). London: Macmillan.

Peplau, H.E. (1965). Interpersonal relationships: The purpose and characteristics of professional nursing. In A.W. O'Toole & S.R. Welt (eds), *Hildegard E. Peplau, selected works interpersonal theory in nursing* (pp. 42–55 of Chapter 3). London: Macmillan.

Peplau, H.E. (1969). Theory: The professional dimension. In A.W. O'Toole & S.R. Welt (eds), *Hildegard E. Peplau, selected works interpersonal theory in nursing* (pp. 21–41 of Chapter 2). London: Macmillan.

Pevalin, D.J. & Goldberg, D.P. (2003). Social precursors to onset and recovery from episodes of common mental illness. *Psychological Medicine*, 33(2), 299–306.

Porter, R. Wright, D. (eds). (2003). *The confinement of the insane: International perspectives, 1800–1965*. Cambridge, UK: Cambridge University Press.

Robb, G. (1996). The way of all flesh: Degeneration, eugenics and the gospel of free love. *Journal of the History of Sexuality*, 6(4), 589–603.

Roberts, G. & Wolfson, P. (2004) The rediscovery of recovery: Open to all. *Advances in Psychiatric Treatment*, 10, 37–49

Robins, J. (1986), *Fools and mad: A history of the insane in Ireland*. Dublin, Ireland: Institute of Public Administration.

Robinson, L. (1986). The future of psychiatric/mental health nursing. *Nursing Clinics of North America*, 21(3), 537–543.

Roe, D. & Chopra, M. (2003). Beyond coping with mental illness: Toward personal growth. *American Journal of Orthopsychiatry*, 73(3), 334–44.

Sadowsky, J. (2003). Confinements and colonialism in Nigeria. In R. Porter & D. Wright (eds), *The confinement of the insane: International perspectives, 1800–1965* (pp. 299–314 of Chapter 12). Cambridge, UK: Cambridge University Press.

Schiff, A C. (2004) Recovery and mental illness: Analysis and personal reflections. *Psychiatric Rehabilitation Journal*, 27(3), 212–219.

Schneider, F. (2011). *Psychiatrie im Nationalsozialismus: Erinnerung und Verantwortung (Psychiatry under National Socialism: Remembrance and responsibility)*. Berlin, Germany: Springer.

Scull, A. (1979). *Museums of Madness: The Social Organization of Insanity in Nineteenth Century England*. London: Allen Lane; New York: St Martin's Press.

Scull, A. (1993). *The most solitary of afflictions: Madness and society in Britain, 1700–1900*. New Haven, CT: Yale University Press.

Scull, A. (2005). *Madhouse: A tragic tale of megalomania and modern medicine*. New Haven, CT: Yale University Press.

Sheridan, A.J. (2006). The impact of political transition on psychiatric nursing – a case study of twentieth-century Ireland. *Nursing Inquiry*, 13(4), 289–299.

Shorter, E. (1997) *A History of psychiatry: From the Era of the Asylum to the Age of Prozac*. New York: John Wiley & Sons,

Shorter, E. (2005). *A historical dictionary of psychiatry*. Oxford: Oxford University Press.

Sladden, S. (1979). *Psychiatric nursing in the community*. Edinburgh, UK: Churchill Livingstone.

Spaniol, l., Wewiorski, N.J., Gagne, C. & Anthony, W. (2002). The process of recovery from schizophrenia. *International Review of Psychiatry*, 14(4), 327–336.

Stern, A. M. (2005). Sterilized in the name of public health: Race, immigration and reproductive control in modern California. *American Journal of Public Health*, 95(7), 1128–1138.

Strang, J. (1982) Psychotherapy by Nurses – some special characteristics. *Journal of Advanced Nursing*, 7, 167–171.

Tew, J., Ramon, S., Slade, M., Bird, V., Melton, J. & Le Boutillier, C. (2011). Social factors and recovery from mental health difficulties: A review of the evidence. *British Journal of Social Work*, 42(3), 443–460.

Travelbee, J. (1971). *Interpersonal aspects of nursing*. Philadelphia, PA: F.A. Davis Company.

Turner, T. (1999). Chapter 1: The century begins. The Early 1900 and Before. In H. Freeman (ed.), *A century of psychiatry* (pp. 1–30). London: Mosby.

Ura, K., Alkire, S. Zangmo, T. and Wangdi K. (eds). (2012). *A Short Guide to Gross National Happiness Index*. Centre for Bhutam Studies, Thimphu, Bhutan. Retrieved 3 June 2014 from www.-grossnationalhappiness.com/wp-content/uploads/2012/04/Short-GNH-Index-edited.pdf

Wang, P.S., Aguilar-Gaxiola, S., Alonso, J., Angermeyer, M.C., Borges, G., Bromet, E.J., Bruffaerts, R., de Girlolamo, G., deGraaf, R., Gureje, O., Haro, J.M., Karam, E.G., Kessler, R.C., Kovess, V., Lane, M.C., Lee, S., Levinson, D., Ono, Y., Petukhova, M., Posada-Villa, J., Seedat, S. & Wells, J.E. (2007). Worldwide use of mental health services for anxiety, mood and substance disorders: Results from 17 countries in the WHO World Mental Health (WMH) Surveys. *The Lancet*, 370(9590), 841–850.

Webster, C. (1991). Psychiatry and the early National Health Service: The role of the Mental Health Standing Advisory Committee. In G. Berrios & H. Freeman (eds), *150 Years of British Psychiatry 1841–1991* (pp. 1841–1991). London: Royal College of Psychiatrists.

Weisser, J., Morrow, M. & Jamer, B. (2011). *A critical exploration of social inequities in the mental health recovery literature*. Vancouver, Canada: Centre for the Study of Gender, Social Inequities and Mental Health (CGSM).

Wooff, K., Goldberg, D.P. & Fryers, T. (1986). Patients in receipt of community psychiatric nursing care in Salford 1976–1982. *Psychological Medicine*, 16, 407–414.

World Health Organization. (1953). *Technical report series No. 73: The community mental hospital: Third report of the Expert Committee on Mental Health*. Geneva, Switzerland: World Health Organization.

World Health Organization. (1956). *Technical report series No. 105: Expert committee on psychiatric nursing: First report*. Geneva, Switzerland: World Health Organization.

World Health Organization. (2009). *Improving health systems and services for mental health*. Geneva, Switzerland: World Health Organization.

Wright, D. (1997). Getting out of the asylum: Understanding the confinement of the insane in the nineteenth century. *Social History of Medicine*, 10(1), 137–155.

Zubin, J., Oppenheimer, G. & Neugebauer, R. (1985). Degeneration theory and the stigma of schizophrenia. *Biological Psychiatry*, 20(11), 1145–1148.

3

MENTAL HEALTH PROMOTION

Vicki P. Hines-Martin

Introduction

Mental health and illness have increasingly become a priority in global discussions because of their impact on individuals, families and communities. Mental illness or mental ill health has an impact on quality of life, lost days of productivity and economics status of citizens regardless of their setting (see Chapter 1). Current strategies to support the mental health of citizens have centered on recognition and treatment of those who are acutely ill and support for those who have persistent mental illness to attain and maintain their highest level of functioning. Conducting research and using evidence-based care strategies has been a goal to better address those who have mental health needs (WHO, 2015a).

Even as nurses and other providers strive to accomplish those goals, there is a clear recognition that resources to address the importance and enormity of this health care priority are inadequate to meet the need regardless of whether the setting is within a low-, middle-, or high-resource environment. In addition, as with other areas of health, there are many social determinants that impact health and place a variety of populations at higher risk for mental illness (see Chapter 4 on social determinants of health). Those two factors, *mental health resources* and *social determinants as a risk factor* have supported a start in the transformation of mental health care over the last 10–15 years. Also contributing to this change is the recognition that negative mental health can be mediated or prevented in many instances through proactive strategies such as targeted *mental health promotion, disease prevention* and *early intervention*. Mental health and how to support well-being among a variety of populations is now being viewed in the same way that other conditions such as cardiovascular disease and diabetes are being viewed. The care for populations at risk for these conditions clearly has a strong emphasis on minimizing the risks for and intervening early when beginning symptoms are identified. Central to this approach is engagement and education of individuals and populations in the process.

What is health promotion?

Health is a state of balance; an equilibrium that an individual has established within identified social and physical environments. Health allows the individual to adequately cope with demands of life while experiencing overall positive emotions and satisfaction. Within this definition is the concept of well-being (adapted from Sartorius, 2006 and Centers for Disease Control, 2013).

The identified definition is well suited to the aims of health promotion. Health promotion is the process of enabling people to increase control over, and to improve, their health. It moves beyond a focus on individual behaviour towards a wide range of social and environmental interventions (WHO, 2015b). Health promotion and disease prevention programs focus on keeping people healthy. Health promotion engages and empowers individuals and communities to participate in healthy behaviors, and make changes that reduce the risk of developing chronic diseases and other morbidities. Early intervention is defined as the recognition of symptoms indicative of negative health concerns, problems or conditions at early onset; upon identification, facilitating the use of appropriate resources to prevent problem progression and increasing severity (Substance Abuse and Mental Health Services Administration, 2014).

For the purposes of this chapter, the term health promotion will include functions of health promotion, disease prevention and early intervention as the focus for nursing actions. The goal for health promotion is empowerment. Empowerment describes a process through which individuals, groups, organizations, or communities gain self-reliance and abilities to enhance their quality of life.

Health promotion is multifocal in its approach and targets change at the micro (individual/ family) through macro (institutional and societal) levels of the environment to address modifiable risks that affect health. Usual strategies for health promotion programs include:

- *Communication* that focuses on raising awareness about healthy behaviors and engaging the public in partnership. Examples of communication strategies include lay advisory groups, public service campaigns (through a variety of media strategies), health fairs, etc.
- *Education* empowers populations toward health behavior change through increased knowledge. Examples of education strategies include peer counselors/navigators, trainings, and support groups.
- *Environmental* efforts include modifying structures or environments to make healthy decisions and resources more readily available to large populations. Examples would include conditions supporting access to clean water and non-smoking environments.
- *Policy* includes regulating or mandating activities by organizations or public agencies that encourage healthy decision-making such as immunizations.

Health promotion strategies are influenced by the approach that serves as its theoretical foundation. Effective practice depends on using theories and strategies that are appropriate to a situation. This *situation appropriateness* underlies any intervention that is culturally and socially congruent with the targeted population. There are many theories on which health promotion can be based. The following are some theories/models that focus on health promotion. The following theory/model descriptions are from the *Theory at a Glance: A Guide for Health Promotion Practice* publication (National Cancer Institute (NCI), 2005).

Individual or intrapersonal level of health promotion focuses on intrapersonal factors (those that are internal to the individual themselves). Intrapersonal factors include knowledge, attitudes, beliefs, values, self-concept, past experience, and skills.

- *The Health Belief Model (HBM)* addresses the individual's perceptions of the threat posed by a health problem (susceptibility, severity), the benefits of avoiding the threat, and factors influencing the decision to act (barriers, cues to action, and self-efficacy).
- *The Stages of Change (Transtheoretical) Model* describes individuals' motivation and readiness to change a behavior.

- *The Theory of Planned Behavior (TPB)* examines the relationship between an individual's beliefs, attitudes, intentions, behavior, and perceived control over that behavior.
- *The Precaution Adoption Process Model (PAPM)* names seven stages in an individual's journey from awareness to action. It begins with lack of awareness and advances through subsequent stages of becoming aware, deciding whether or not to act, acting, and maintaining the behavior.

(NCI, 2005, pp. 9–10)

Interpersonal level theory of health behavior recognizes that individuals exist within, and are influenced by, the context in which they live. The opinions, and influence of other valued people influences the individual's feelings and behavior, and the individual has a mutual effect on those people.

- *Social Cognitive Theory (SCT)* describes a dynamic, ongoing process in which personal factors, environmental factors, and human behavior exert influence upon each other. According to SCT, three main factors affect the likelihood that a person will change a health behavior: (1) self-efficacy; (2) goals; and (3) outcome expectancies.

(NCI, 2005, p. 19)

Community level models identify that social systems and their functioning affect people; and that those people can affect social systems. The focus of these models is to mobilize community members and organizations toward change that improves health. The strength of these models is community participation in identifying and implementing strategies that work in a variety of settings, such as health care institutions, schools, worksites, and in the community. Within this model, community can be a geographic area but also may be a population or group that holds a common interest, identity or shared characteristics or circumstances.

- *Community organization and other participatory models* emphasize community-driven approaches to assessing and solving health and social problems.
- *Diffusion of Innovations Theory* addresses how new ideas, products, and social practices spread within an organization, community, or society, or from one society to another.

(NCI, 2005, p. 30)

Nursing functioning is well suited to any of these models and most nurses are adept at health promotion especially as it relates to physical health conditions. However, health promotion in the area of mental health can be a challenge. The evidence for health promotion with individuals that have health concerns other than mental health is much more abundant. In addition, health promotion that may be much more readily accepted in other areas of health, may not be as acceptable when discussing mental health due to stigma. However, much can be learned from the evidence and expert opinions that are now being published in the area of mental health promotion.

What is mental health promotion?

Mental health is a "state of well-being in which the individual realizes his or her own abilities, can cope with the normal stresses of life, can work productively and fruitfully, and is able to make a contribution to his or her community" (WHO 2001, p. 1). Mental health promotion includes "*strategies* to promote the mental well-being of those who are not at risk, those who are at increased risk and those who are suffering or recovering from mental health problems" (WHO 2004). With an understanding of the social determinants of mental health, improving and supporting mental health also requires policies and programs in government and business sectors including education, employment, law, transportation, environment, housing, and social service provision, as well as specific activities in the health field relating to the prevention and treatment of a variety of illnesses (WHO, 2014).

The mental health promotion literature has most prominently been published in relation to the life span perspective with a focus on early childhood and school-age children with the greatest growth beginning in conjunction with publication of the document *Child and Adolescent Mental Health Policies and Plans* (WHO, 2005). Research has focused on supporting adaptive, and addressing maladaptive, interactions between parents and children (Chartier *et al.*, 2015; Gyungjoo *et al.*, 2013), promotion in school and community settings even with children who are at high risk due to environmental circumstances ((Barry, Clarke, Jenkins, & Patel, 2013; Puskar *et al.*, 2006). These exemplars and other research in this area have contributed to evidence about mental health promotion strategies aimed at creating a sense of attachment and connectedness and belonging; promoting resilience and developing competencies (efficacy and coping); supporting a positive and safe school environment; teaching and reinforcing positive behaviors and decision-making; encouraging pro-social behavior; educating adult care providers about influences on child development and early symptom/problem recognition; identifying and linking school-based mental health supports; and providing access to early intervention resources for children and their families when available (Campion, Bhui & Bhugra, 2012).

Mental health promotion literature focused on other points in the life span is much less developed. Adults in the workplace are an important area for focused direction about mental health promotion. The WHO (2006) identified the following,

> Work is an essential feature of most people's adult life, and has personal, economic and social value. Work substantially contributes to a person's identity; it provides income for an individual and his or her family, and can make a person feel that he or she is playing a useful role in society. It is also an important source of social support. Participation in work also contributes to the economic and social development of communities. . . . Work is important for mental health and indeed the right to work in just and favourable conditions and with protection from unemployment is enshrined in the United Nations Universal Declaration of Human Rights (Article 23). Work produces personal and health benefits, while the absence or loss of work can potentially damage a person's mental health.
>
> *(WHO, 2005b, p. 9)*

Although WHO and other national and international organizations identify the importance of work for individuals, families and society, there is mixed evidence regarding mental health promotion interventions to assist workers with work-related stressors or interventions for individuals who are unemployed and/or experience stress due to economic pressures. Evidence to identify successful organizational changes to reduce stress for those who are employed as health care workers and teachers has not been strong according to the Cochrane Database for Systematic Reviews (Naghieh *et al.*, 2015; Ruotsalainen *et al.*, 2015). Strategies such as changing work conditions, increasing communication skills, changing work schedules, changing organizational characteristics such as providing job promotion and performance bonuses and mentoring support were used in a variety of studies. Only one study that used relaxation techniques (such as meditation) showed strong evidence for use as a mental health promotion strategy for professional workers (Ruotsalainen *et al.*, 2015).

The workforce literature discusses the benefits of effective interventions that reduce the strain of unemployment including counseling to improve coping skills, and improving employment opportunities for low-income groups that provide social and job seeking skills training for at-risk youth entering the workforce (Tandon *et al.*, 2015). Recent health research literature now focuses on this population but provides limited support to the benefit of mental health promotion activities in relation to the stress of unemployment. Walhlbeck and McDaid (2012), in their discussion on alleviating the mental health impact of economic crisis, identify that the impact is significant worldwide. They also identify strategies such as family and parental support, suicide prevention and first aid, and income resource information as critical strategies. Within that discussion, limited evidence is provided, however, to identify the effectiveness of these strategies. Schuring *et al.* (2009) in a study of the effectiveness of a health promotion program for long-term unemployed individuals with physical health conditions, identified that interventions that were implemented in this study resulted in no changes in perceptions of physical or mental health status among participants. In addition, scores on measures of physical and mental health showed no statistical difference after the intervention.

In addition to the populations just discussed, people with mental health conditions also experience disadvantage entering the work place, which has implications for mental health. The Bazelon Center for Mental Health Law in its 2014 report entitled *Getting to Work: Promoting Employment of People with Mental Illness* provided a synthesis of data and estimated that only 22 percent of people with serious mental illness were employed, with about half of these individuals working full-time. This number is less than one-third of those employed who did not have a serious mental health condition (Bazelon, 2014).

These numbers reflect a particularly significant problem since mental health conditions affect so many people worldwide. Individuals with mental health conditions who are employed benefit in a variety of ways. Bazelon (2014) identifies that employment fosters social acceptance and integration into the community. Individuals gain a sense of purpose, self-esteem, and self-worth. Employment reduces poverty and dependence on others, empowering people to become self-sufficient, and live independently. It improves clinical outcomes, including reducing symptoms of a person's mental illness, and lessens the need for supportive resources. The Bazelon report (Bazelon, 2014) also identifies that about one half of people with serious mental illness who participated in a national survey reported the primary barriers to employment to be stigma and discrimination, and fear of losing benefits, and approximately one quarter of those surveyed cited inadequate treatment, and lack of vocational services, which served as insurmountable barriers (Bazelon, 2014).

Evidence for workplace mental health promotion initiatives is limited and what is available must be strengthened to serve as a foundation for change. Adult functioning in relation to the workplace, mental health and mental health promotion hold great potential for clinical and organizational research, and community partnership to identify and address important areas for mental health promotion that are effective and contextually appropriate.

Mental health promotion can be initiated through the screening of at-risk populations. Evidence for the importance of mental health screening is demonstrated in this section with two populations; aging adults and high-school girls.

With the growing numbers among the aging population, mental health promotion within this group has become increasingly important. The WHO identifies that the world population of older adults will double between 2000 and 2050 and will result in approximately 2 billion people over the age of 60 (WHO, 2013). The CDC (2008) in its report of findings about the

US aging population identifies that anxiety, severe cognitive impairment, and mood disorders are most common within this age group. "Risk factors for late-onset depression included widowhood, physical illness, low educational attainment (less than high school), impaired functional status, and heavy alcohol consumption" (CDC, 2008, p. 6). Men within this age group are more likely to commit suicide than any other population group (CDC, 2008). These conditions are under-recognized by health care professionals and have significant effects on mental and physical functioning in aging. The Hartford Institute for Geriatric Nursing identifies that

> persons drinking at (high) levels (are at risk for) negative outcomes for physical and mental health such as falls, stroke, depression, and gastrointestinal problems. Older drinkers taking prescription medications are at greater risk. Use of prescription drugs and alcohol in combination is not an uncommon occurrence.
>
> *(Naegle, 2012, p. 1)*

Recommendations by the CDC, the Hartford Institute, WHO, and other organizations focused on this population identify that mental health and substance abuse screenings are an essential part of care. Some of the recommendations about screening also provide direction on tools that can be used in any setting: for depression screening, the Patient Health Questionnaire (PHQ -9), which includes 9 questions and for alcohol abuse screening, the Short Michigan Alcoholism Screening Instrument Geriatric Version (SMAST-G), which includes 24 questions with yes/no responses. Both of these self-report instruments are easily incorporated into any health care environment and have been identified as valid in numerous studies. For more information about these screening instruments see van Steenbergen-Weijenburg *et al.* (2010); Sullivan and Fleming (1997); and Spitzer, Williams, and Kroenke (1995). Other screening measures are available for use and may be identified as more suitable based on cultural and social context.

Another at-risk population are females, especially those who live within contexts in which their roles are circumscribed and/or restricted based on their gender. These restrictions may be based on religion, culture or tradition (see Chapters 4 and 19 on social determinants of health and violence). El- Sayed Desouky, Abdellatif Ibrahem, and Salah Omar (2015) conducted a study of 1,024 Saudi adolescent girls and investigated the prevalence of psychiatric disorders (depression, anxiety, and obsessive compulsive disorder) within this population. The girls were aged 15–17 years and findings from this study identified that 54.9 percent had symptoms of anxiety, 42.9 percent had depressive symptoms, and 23.1 percent had symptoms of obsessive-compulsive disorder. There was a statistically significant co-morbidity between these conditions, meaning that many had symptoms of more than one of these disorders. Explanations for the incidence of these disorders in this sample were as follows. The author identified that some factors may be related to parental restriction of girls versus boys in regard to permissible behavior; lower expectations for girls related to competencies and achievement; and stress faced by Saudi females resulting from cultural and social factors. One important limitation of this reported study was the restriction on the researcher. As females they were not allowed to study males and therefore were unable to gather data for comparison between males and female prevalence of the identified disorders. The primary recommendation from the investigators resulting from this study is the need for mental health screenings for this population.

Increasingly the literature has identified the benefit of working with communities around mental health issues in the use of lay people in mental health promotion roles as navigators, educators and cultural experts. Patel *et al.* (2011) have been at the forefront in relation to identification and utilization of lay individuals in these capacities within communities with low resources. Although peer support has been used by many in relation to individuals with severe and persistent mental illness, data about mental illness resulted in increased recognition that mental health needs far exceeded the mental health resources. Patel *et al.* (2010) undertook innovative work to expand the scale of lay-worker delivered mental health resources which has served as a foundation for change in how peer support is used. Patel *et al.* (2011) identified that trained lay personnel can reduce incidence of the most prevalent mental conditions, suicide, and mental health disability days within a primary care setting. Other studies have supported the usefulness of lay workers on mental health promotion and care (Patel *et al.*, 2010; Shinde *et al.*, 2013).

As previously discussed, use of theory in health promotion strategies is well established and is beneficial in that an appropriate theory can help a health promotion strategy identify influential factors to consider and assist in making the chosen interventions situation (or culturally and socially) specific.

In their nursing intervention study of elderly Iranian women, Alaviani, Khosravan, Alami, and Moshki (2015) focused on the prevention of loneliness and social isolation and included 150 women. The study was constructed using the principles of the Pender Health Promotion model. The Health Promotion Model is a nursing model based on social cognitive theory. According to this theory, cognitive perception factors (such as perceived benefits and barriers) have influence on involvement in health promotion behaviors. In addition, the person already possesses interpersonal factors (like demographic factors, effective interpersonal factors, and behavioral factors). The theory proposes that an intervention that takes into account the interaction of all these factors can affect cognitive perception processes and result in healthier behaviors. Using this model, a quasi-experimental study employing a multi-modal intervention was used with the experimental group. Both the experimental and control groups were measured before and after the intervention period using questionnaires that measured perceived barriers, benefits, self-efficacy, and interpersonal influences on behaviors associated with loneliness and social isolation. Findings from this study indicate that there was significant decrease in perceived loneliness and improved ability to make social contact in the experimental group, which illustrated the benefit of this theory-driven mental health promotion study.

Mental health promotion, engagement and patient-centered care

The US Institute of Medicine (IOM, 2001) defines patient-centered care as: "Providing care that is respectful of and responsive to individual patient preferences, needs, and values, and ensuring that patient values guide all clinical decisions" (IOM, 2001, p. 2). Patients must be viewed as persons in context within their own social worlds, and therefore listened to, informed, respected, and involved in their care and, to whatever extent possible, have their wishes adhered to as part of the health care process. The IOM proposed 10 simple rules for improved patient-centered health care delivery; the following have particular application to mental health promotion.

- Care has a focus on supporting the highest level of health possible.
- Care is adapted according to patient needs and values.
- Knowledge and information on which care is based is shared with those involved.
- Decision making about therapeutic approaches is evidence-based.
- Cooperation among providers is a priority to accomplish positive health outcomes.

(IOM, 2001, p. 2)

The ICN in its statement on the definition of nursing identifies that the profession has an inherent focus on patient- or person-centered care and the following points of emphasis were particularly supportive of that message. ICN states that nursing encompasses autonomous and collaborative care of individuals of all ages, families, groups, and communities, sick or well, and in all settings. Nursing includes the promotion of health, and prevention of illness. Advocacy, promotion of a safe environment, research, participation in shaping health policy and in patient and health systems management, and education are also key nursing roles.

Both the IOM statement on patient-centered care and the ICN definition of nursing articulate the need to partner with individuals who are the focus of care (individually or collectively) to address health needs and accomplish identified health goals. The process must be one that involves mutual give and take, in context with the person's perception and circumstances, as well as active participation by all. When this process is successful, the care recipient becomes invested as a partner in the process, which is called engagement. Engagement and patient-centered care also require the collaboration of health care and non-health care personnel to fully accomplish the health care goals. Therefore, interprofessional collaboration is vital with nursing often functioning as the hub, facilitator, gatekeeper, or director of that collaboration. This function is particularly critical in the area of mental health promotion.

Literature on mental health promotion with a perspective on person-centered care, engagement and interprofessional practice illustrate the importance of these concepts on mental health outcomes.

With mental health promotion, the focus for partnerships is often communities or populations. Engagement of those populations to identify needs, strengths, and perspectives requires a consensus building process whereby mutually agreed upon priorities are identified. This process can focus on organizational coalition building (Maurer, Dardess, Carman, Frazier, & Smeeding, 2012; Ng, Fraser, Goding, Paroissien, & Ryan, 2013), or the development of appropriate mental health priorities for culturally diverse and/or at-risk populations (American Indian/Alasaka Native Indian Health Services Office of Clinical and Preventive Services, 2011; Hinton, Kavanagh, Barclay, Chenhall, & Nagel, 2015). Nurses have the right and the responsibility to serve as advocates, members or leaders in policy development groups and opportunities are at many levels regardless of the setting. However, large sectors of the nursing profession are constrained in how to implement engagement by contextual factors (geography, economics, social norms, etc.). All nurses can, and do, function with individuals and families. Most importantly, Interprofessional collaboration, person-centered care and engagement can be implemented successfully with nursing as the lead in those instances.

Markle-Reid *et al.* (2014) describe a nurse-led intervention for home-based elders, which was directed at depression prevention. The 1-year project with 142 participants incorporated patient, family/supports and collaboration of a personal support worker. The intervention included education, counseling and assessment. Study findings indicated that participants had improved recognition and management of depression, increased participant physical and pleasurable activities, social support, quality of life, and ability to manage other chronic health conditions. Nursing education improved the participants' and family knowledge of the symptoms of depression, available treatments, and available community resources.

Mental health promotion and implications for nursing

The data about influences on mental health and the universal support in the literature for mental health promotion clearly identify that this care strategy should be a priority in nursing regardless of the setting or the educational level of nurses. Nursing has an advantage in that health promotion has historically been one of the essential strategies within the profession. Nurses work with populations in support of their health.

The International Council of Nurses (ICN) has identified the priorities for nurses and mental health. ICN states that

> people worldwide suffer from mental disorders and all people are at risk of mental health problems, often due to stressful lifestyles, dysfunctional relationships, civil conflict, violence, physical illness, infection or trauma . . . Nurses are integral to holistic approaches to mental health promotion, prevention, care, treatment and rehabilitation of people living with mental health problems and support of their families and communities.
>
> *(ICN, 2008, p. 2)*

In the ICN/WHO joint statement on Developing Nursing Resources on Mental Health (2002), they identified that nurses are the largest group of health care providers in the world, and that they can serve an essential function in the provision of mental health care delivery. The statement also identifies that education is needed to help nurses better understand this rapidly developing field and their role in it. Specific recommendations were as follows:

- Increase education for nurses in the areas of
  - advocacy;
  - community mental health;
  - legal issues/human rights;
  - working with patients and their families in a variety of settings;
  - development of mental health policies;
  - public health models (for population health); and
  - promotion of mental health.
- Increase nursing involvement in the development of mental health policy by:
  - developing the vision for care delivery;
  - establishing models of care; and
  - improving consultation in policy and planning.

Nurses have been increasingly active in these areas since the 2002 statement. Nurses have added to the literature on mental health promotion by exploring mental health promotion and graduate education in multicultural settings (Khanlou, 2003), advocating for increased nursing involvement in mental health promotion (Calloway, 2007), conducting research on new approaches to mental health promotion (Alviani *et al.*, 2015; Chartier *et al.*, 2015; Melnyk *et al.*, 2015), and leading dialogue on expanded roles for the nurse and developing a vision for care delivery in this important area (Wand, 2011).

Nursing is at a pivotal point in time when there is a synergy within and across nations to view "there is no health without mental health" (WHO, 2016). Collaborative groups have developed and continue to develop focused in this area. Table 3.1 provides examples of several groups with a dedicated focus on mental health.

Mental health promotion is both old and new. Terminology and expectations evolve as health care groups better understand the importance of this area of health care provision and as health providers especially nurses better understand their role in mental health promotion. Nurses are the largest group of providers who have always seen the benefit of promoting health. It is now the time for us to communicate our strengths in this area and better focus our attention on using our expertise in supporting health through evidence-based mental health promotion.

Table 3.1 Examples of groups with a dedicated focus on mental health

Organization	Website (URL)
Centre for Global Mental Health (multi-site resource)	www.centreforglobalmentalhealth.org/global-mental-health-websites
European Network for Mental Health Promotion	www.mentalhealthpromotion.net/?i=portal.en.about
Portico. Canada's mental health and addiction network	www.porticonetwork.ca/
International Council of Nurses (see mental health page)	www.icn.ch/
Mental Health America US	www.mentalhealthamerica.net/
Mental Health Information Centre (South Africa)	www.mentalhealthsa.co.za/
Pan American Health Organization (see mental health page)	www.paho.org/hq/
The WHO Pacific Islands Mental Health Network (PIMHnet)	www.who.int/mental_health/policy/pimhnet/en/
National Asian American Pacific Islander Mental Health Association US	http://naapimha.org/

References

Alaviani M., Khosravan, S., Alami, A., & Moshki, M. (2015). The effect of a multi-strategy program on developing social behaviors based on Pender's health promotion model to prevent loneliness of old women referred to Gonabad urban health centers. *International Journal of Community Based Nursing and Midwifery, 3*(2), 132–140.

American Indian/Alaska Native Indian Health Services Office of Clinical and Preventive Services (2011). *Behavioral Health Briefing Book.* Washington, DC: US Department of Health and Human Services Division of Behavioral Health.

Barry, M.M., Clarke, A.M., Jenkins, R., & Patel, V. (2013). A systematic review of the effectiveness of mental health promotion interventions for young people in low- and middle-income countries. *BMC Public Health, 13*, 835.

Bazelon Center for Mental Health Law. (2014). *Getting to Work: Promoting Employment of People with Mental Illness.* Washington DC: Judge David l. Bazelon Center for Mental Health Law.

Calloway, S. (2007). Mental health promotion: Is nursing dropping the ball? *Journal of Professional Nursing, 23*(2), 105–109.

Campion, J., Bhui, K., & Bhigra, D. (2012). European Psychiatric Association (EPA) guidance on prevention of mental disorders. *European Psychiatry, 28*, 68–70.

Centers for Disease Control (2013). *Health Related Quality of Life: Well-Being Concepts.* Accessed at www.cdc.gov/hrqol/wellbeing.htm. Retrieved on September 10, 2015.

Centers for Disease Control and Prevention and National Association of Chronic Disease Directors. (2008). *The State of Mental Health and Aging in America Issue Brief 1: What Do the Data Tell Us?* Atlanta, GA: National Association of Chronic Disease Directors. Accessed at www.cdc.gov/aging/pdf/mental_health.pdf. Retrieved on September 10, 2015.

Chartier, M., Attawar, D., Volk, J., Cooper, M., Quddus, F., & McCarthy, J.A. (2015). Postpartum mental health promotion: Perspectives from mothers and home visitors. *Public Health Nursing, 32*(6), 671–679.

El-Sayed Desouky, D., Abdellatif Ibrahem, R., & Salah Omar, M. (2015). Prevalence and comorbidity of depression, anxiety and obsessive compulsive disorders among Saudi secondary school girls, Taif Area, KSA. *Archive of Iranian Medicine, 18*(4), 234–238.

Gyungjoo, L., McCreary, L. Breitmayer, B., Kim, M.J., & Yang, S. (2013). Promoting mother–infant interaction and infant mental health in low-income Korean families: Attachment-based cognitive behavioural approach. *Journal for Specialists in Pediatric Nursing, 18*(4), 265–276.

Hinton, R., Kavanagh, D., Barclay, L., Chenhall, R., & Nagel, T. (2015). Developing a best practice pathway to support improvements in Indigenous Australians' mental health and well-being: A qualitative study. *BMJ Open, 5*, e007938.

Institute of Medicine (IOM) Committee of the Quality of Health Care in America (2001). Crossing the quality chasm: New health care system for the twenty-first century—Brief report. Washington, DC: National Academies Press. Accessed at http://iom.nationalacademies.org/Reports/2001/Crossing-the-Quality-Chasm-A-New-Health-System-for-the-21st-Century.aspx. Retrieved on September 1, 2015.

International Council of Nurses (ICN) (2008). Position statement: Mental health. Accessed at www.icn.ch/images/stories/documents/publications/position_statements/A09_Mental_Health.pdf. Retrieved on September 14, 2015.

International Council of Nurses (ICN) and World Health Organization (WHO) (2002). *Developing Nursing Resources for Mental Health: Nursing Matters. Mental Health Policy, Planning and Service Development: Integrating Systems & Services, Integrating People*. Geneva: The WHO Mind Project, Mental Improvement for Nations Development of Mental health & Substance Abuse.

Khanlou, N. (2003). Mental health promotion education in multicultural settings. *Nurse Education Today 23*, 96–103.

Markle-Reid, M., McAiney, C., Forbes, D., Thabane, L., Gibson, M., Browne, G., Hoch, J.S., Peirce, T., & Busing, B. (2014). An interprofessional nurse-led mental health promotion intervention for older home care clients with depressive symptoms. *BMC Geriatrics, 14*, 62.

Maurer M., Dardess, P., Carman. K.L., Frazier. K., & Smeeding, L. (2012). *Guide to Patient and Family Engagement: Environmental Scan Report*. Rockville, MD: Agency for Healthcare Research and Quality; Prepared by the American Institutes for Research under contract HHSA 290–200–600019. Accessed at www.ahrq.gov/research/findings/final-reports/ptfamilyscan/index.html. Retrieved on August 29, 2015.

Melnyk, B.M., Amaya, M. Szalacha, l.A., Hoying, J., Taylor, T., & Bowersox, K. (2015). Feasibility, acceptability and preliminary effects of the COPE mental health outcomes and academic performance in freshman college students: A randomized control pilot study. *Journal of Child and Adolescent Psychiatric Nursing, 28*, 147–154.

Naegle, M. (2012). *Try This: Best Practices in Nursing Care to Older Adults. Alcohol Use, Screening and Assessment for Older Adults*. New York: Hartford Institute for Geriatric Nursing, School of Nursing, New York University.

Naghieh, A., Montgomery, P., Bonell, C., Thompson, M., & Aber, J.L. (2015). Organisational interventions for improving wellbeing and reducing work-related stress in teachers. *Cochane Database of Systematic Reviews, 4*. Accessed at http://onlinelibrary.wiley.com/doi/10.1002/14651858.CD010306.pub2/full. Retrieved on July 24, 2016.

National Cancer Institute (2005). *Theory at a Glance: A Guide for Health Promotion Practice*. Bethesda, MD: US Department of Health and Human Services, National Institutes of Health.

Ng, C., Fraser, J., Goding, M., Paroissien, D., & Ryan, B. (2013). Partnerships for community mental health in the Asia-Pacific: Principles and best-practice models across different sectors. *Australasian Psychiatry, 21*(1), 38–45.

Patel, V., Weiss, H.A., Chowdhary, N., Naik, S., Pednekar, S., Chatterjee, S., DeSilva, M.J., Bhat, B., Araya, R., King, M., Simon, G., Verdeli, H., & Kirkwood, B.R. (2010). Effectiveness of an intervention led by lay health counsellors for depression and anxiety. *The Lancet, 18*(374), 2086–2095.

Patel, V., Weiss, Naik, S., Pednekar, S., Chatterjee, S., Bhat, B., Araya, R., King, M., Simon, G., Verdeli, H., & Kirkwood, B.R. (2011). Lay health worker led intervention for depressive and anxiety disorders in India: Impact on clinical and disability outcomes over 12 months. *British Journal of Psychiatry, 199*(6), 3459–3466.

Puskar, K.R., Stark. K.H., Fertman, C., Bernardo, L.M., Engberg, R.A., & Barton, R.S. (2006). School-based mental health promotion: Nursing interventions for depressive symptoms in rural adolescents. *California Journal of Health Promotion, 4*(4), 13–20.

Ruotsalainen, J.H., Verbeek, J.H., Mariné, A., & Serra, C. (2015). Preventing occupational stress in healthcare workers. *Cochane Database of Systematic Reviews, 4*. Accessed at http://onlinelibrary.wiley.com/doi/10.1002/14651858.CD002892.pub5/full. Retrieved on July 24, 2016.

Sartorious, N. (2006). The meaning of health and its promotion. *Croatian Medical Journal 47*(4), 662–664.

Schuring, M., Burdorf, A., Voorham, A.J., der Weduwe, K., & Mackenbach, J.P. (2009). Effectiveness of a health promotion programme for long-term unemployed subjects with health problems: A randomised controlled trial. *Journal of Epidemiology and Community Health, 63*(11), 893–899.

Shinde, S., Andrew, G., Bangash, O., Cohen, A., Kirkwood, B., & Patel, V. (2013). The impact of a lay counselor led collaborative care intervention for common mental health disorders. *Social Science and Medicine, 88,* 48–55.

Spitzer, R., Williams, J., & Kroenke, K. (1995). *Patient Health Questionnaire Screeners.* New York: Pfizer. Accessed at www.phqscreeners.com/overview.aspx. Retrieved on September 6, 2015.

Substance Abuse and Mental Health Services Administration-SAMHSA (2014). Prevention of substance abuse and mental illness. Accessed at www.samhsa.gov/prevention. Retrieved on August 22, 2015.

Sullivan, E., & Fleming, M. (1997). *A Guide to Substance Abuse Services for Primary Care Clinicians. Treatment Improvement Protocol (TIP) Series No. 24.* Rockville, MD: US Department of Health and Human Services, Public Health Service Substance Abuse and Mental Health Services Administration Center for Substance Abuse Treatment. Accessed at www.ncbi.nlm.nih.gov/books/NBK64827/pdf/Bookshelf_NBK 64827.pdf. Retrieved on September 5, 2015.

Tandon, S.D., Clay, E., Mitchell, L., Tucker, M., & Sonnestein, F.L. (2015). Depression outcomes associated with an intervention implemented in employment training programs for low-income adolescents and young adults. *JAMA Psychiatry, 72*(1), 31–39.

van Steenbergen-Weijenburg, K.M., de Vroege, L., Ploeger R., Brais, J.W., Vloedbeld, M.G., Veneman, T.F., Hakkaart-van Roijen, L., Rutten, F.F.H., Beekman, A.T.F., & van der Feltz-Cornelis, C.M. (2010). Validation of the PHQ-9 as a screening instrument for depression in diabetes patients in specialized outpatient clinics. *BMC Health Services Research, 10,* 235.

Wahlbeck, K., & McDaid, D. (2012). Actions to alleviate the mental health impact of the economic crisis. *World Psychiatry, 11*(3), 139–145.

Wand, T. (2011). Real mental health promotion requires a reorientation of nursing education, practice and research. *Journal of Psychiatric and Mental Health Nursing, 18,* 131–138.

WHO (2001). *Strengthening Mental Health Promotion: Fact Sheet No. 220.* Geneva: World Health Organization.

WHO (2004). *Prevention of Mental Disorders. Effective Interventions and Policy Options: Summary Report.* Geneva: World Health Organization, Department of Mental Health and Substance Abuse and the Prevention Research Centre of the Universities of Jijmegen and Maastricht.

WHO (2005). *Child and Adolescent Mental Health Policies and Plans: Who Mental Health Policy and Service Guidance Package: Module 11.* Geneva: WHO.

WHO (2006). *Mental Health Policies and Programmes in the Workplace: Mental Health Policy and Service Package.* Geneva: WHO.

WHO (2013). *Mental Health and Older Adults: Fact Sheet No. 381.* Geneva: World Health Organization. Accessed at www.who.int/mediacentre/factsheets/fs381/en/. Retrieved on September 9, 2015.

WHO (2014). *Health in all Policies: Helsinki Statement. Framework for Country Action. The 8th Global Conference on Health Promotion.* Geneva: World Health Organization and Finland Ministry of Social Affairs and Health.

WHO (2015a). *Health Topics: Health Promotion.* Accessed at www.who.int/topics/health_promotion/en/. Retrieved on September 8, 2015.

WHO (2015b). *WHO Mental Health Gap Action Programme (mhGAP).* Accessed at www.who.int/mental_health/mhgap/en/. Retrieved on September 9, 2015.

WHO (2016). *Mental health: Strengthening Our Response Fact Sheet.* Geneva: WHO. Accessed at www.who.int/mediacentre/factsheets/fs220/en/. Retrieved on July 24, 2016.

4

SOCIAL DETERMINANTS OF MENTAL HEALTH

Edilma L. Yearwood and Vicki P. Hines-Martin

Introduction

Social determinants of health (SDH) are, circumstances in which people are born, grow, live, work, and age, and the absence or presence of systems available to deal with overall health and illness of its citizenry (WHO, 2008). Structural drivers are the circumstances that affect distribution of power; income; ability to obtain goods and services; ability to access health care and the ability to attend school to earn an education, with the knowledge that doing so has the potential to propel individuals out of low socio-economic status (WHO, 2008). Economics, politics and social policies are key drivers of environmental conditions that either support or impede healthy or unhealthy living conditions. Health and mental health are determined by multiple factors including individual characteristics, genetics, and the effects of SDH factors. SDH are increasingly recognized as modifiable and complex social factors that must be examined when looking at both protective factors and barriers to mental health and well-being. Cumulative exposure to negative SDH factors is known to take its toll on individuals and groups primarily in low- and middle-income communities.

As health and mental health are linked, the focus of this chapter will be on exploring how SDH affects mental health in low-resource communities, describing why awareness of exposure to SDH factors should be incorporated in routine assessment of individuals and families with mental, neurological and substance use vulnerabilities, describing how SDH is linked to SDMH and examining the evidence related to global mental health research incorporating elements of SDH.

Elements of SDMH

Social determinants of health are conditions and circumstances that are dynamic and complex. Prolonged and cumulative exposure to poor or negative SDH factors place individuals at risk for physical and mental ill health. The conceptual framework illustrating the SDMH developed by Lund, Stansfeld, and De Silva (2014) is found in Figure 4.1 and provides a clear illustration of this concept. The researchers identified six categories in both distal and proximal factors that comprise SDMH.

Distal or macro level categories include:

1   *built environments* (adequate and safe housing, recreational structures/facilities, transportation, access to affordable and healthy foods);
2   *community economic status* (such as deprivation/inequality, jobs);
3   *community social capital* (access to social relationships and memberships in groups, health care services, human and other resources, culture, language/interpreter services);
4   *community stability*, diversity and density;
5   *Biological characteristics*; and
6   *Environmental conditions* such as natural disasters, presence of toxic or hazardous conditions, climate change, migration (acculturation challenges), and exposure to prolonged war or conflicts.

Proximal or micro factors include:

1   household/family structure;
2   employment, under-employment or unemployment status;
3   access to education and early childhood enrichment opportunities;
4   access to social capital and social support;
5   being a victim of stigma;
6   gender, ethnicity, race and age including experience of bias and discrimination;
7   genetics and physical health status; and
8   trauma exposure/victimization.

(Marmot & Allen, 2014; Swartz, Kilian, Twesigye, Attah, & Chiliza, 2014; WHO, 2008)

It has long been recognized that mental health is supported by healthy relationships, social inclusion and the absence of stigma victimization. Mental health recovery models embrace social integration and opportunities for those with either vulnerabilities or disabilities to lead a normalized existence within their own communities. Grand Challenges in Global Mental Health identified the second most complex challenge in low-, middle-, and high-income countries as being the development of culturally informed methods to eliminate stigma, discrimination, and social exclusion across multiple settings (Collins *et al.*, 2011). Characteristics of social integration include personal capacity and social opportunity to: (a) engage in relationships and dialogue with familiar and unfamiliar community members; (b) participate in activities; and, (c) have a voice in civic and other community building actions (Baumgartner & Susser, 2013). For example, researchers in India strongly urge attention to economic and political forces within poorly resourced countries to better understand globalized mental health and well-being and further state that it is only through redistribution of resources that impactful changes in prevention and mental health promotion will occur (Das & Rao, 2012).

The Convention on the Rights of Persons with Disabilities was convened by the United Nations and in 2006 developed a position statement to "promote, protect and ensure" human rights and freedom of individuals with disabilities. Individuals with mental ill health are recognized as having a disability and therefore have fundamental rights to access social inclusion, social integration and civic engagement opportunities (Baumgartner & Susser, 2013).

Brazil is recognized as one of the countries with a more developed, sensitive, and progressive social policy history. In 2002 Brazil developed the National Policy of Health for People with Disabilities, which provides guidelines of care for individuals with disabilities. Fiorati and Elui (2015) conducted a small study looking at social inclusion of individuals with disabilities in Ribeirao Preto, SP, Brazil between 2011 and 2012. Disabilities included stroke, cerebral palsy,

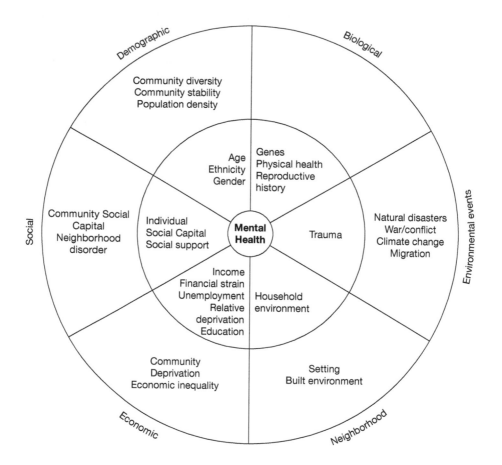

Figure 4.1 Social determinants of mental health: a conceptual framework

Source: From *Global Mental Health – Principles and Practice* edited by Patel, Minas, Cohen, and Martin (2014) Fig. 7.1 p. 119. By permission of Oxford University Press.

traumatic brain disease and cognitive deficits secondary to childhood meningitis. There was no indication from the sample that any of the participants had a mental or substance use disorder. Analysis of the 10 individuals included in the study determined that participants had challenges centered on accessing health care services, that there was a lack of specific health care services to meet their unique needs, and that there was poor coordination across services. The researchers concluded that inclusion is linked to SDH, specifically social equality, ability to access care, and opportunities for participation in social integration activities.

Actions targeting SDMH can promote awareness, advocacy, change, and ideally should result in responsive social policy development and enforcement. The ultimate goal of these actions is social justice and equity in order to intentionally support mental health and well-being (Embrett & Randall, 2014; Friel & Marmot, 2011). Health equity can be fostered when disparities in health between advantaged and less advantaged individuals are minimized or eliminated.

Knowledge of SDMH is critical for all health care workers (professional and non-specialist) because it provides a realistic context of additional factors (in addition to their psychological symptoms) that individuals who are struggling with mental, neurological, and substance use disorders are navigating. It may explain issues of recidivism, non-adherence, mistrust, lack of social scaffolds, and poor mental health literacy in this population. Awareness of these vulnerabilities can inform interventions that can be individually tailored to reflect consumer-specific realities.

Research needs

Given the complexity of factors associated with SDMH, research conducted in this area has not received adequate financial support and has not been conducted in the most applicable environments such as low- and middle-income countries. Most data obtained to date have been conducted in high-income countries and cannot be generalized to low resource environments and diverse cultures. Researchers have recommended that research on SDMH be longitudinal, descriptive, focus on the impact of social policies impacting mental health and assess effectiveness of non-specialist health workers in delivering interventions for mental, neurological and substance use disorders (Braveman, Egerter, & Williams, 2011; Patel, 2012). Given the significant influence of culture on community environments in low- and middle-income countries, community-based participatory research (CBPR) is a recommended research methodology and would be congruent with tenets of social justice, respect and inclusion when working with vulnerable individuals and populations. While it is acknowledged that the highest standard of research is randomized clinical trials that are deemed rigorous evidence of intervention effectiveness, poorly resourced environments require research methods that answer relevant clinical questions and incorporate realistic consumer experiences, which can be complex and multi-faceted.

Few robust tools exist to measure social integration in low- and middle-income countries, and this offers another potential area for conducting inquiry. A useful tool must provide data on communication, interactions with people known and not known within communities, participation in one's community and a perceived sense of belonging and connectedness. The DSM-5 does include the World Health Organization Disability Assessment Schedule WHODAS-2.0, which offers a potentially useful tool to obtain some elements of social integration (2013).

SDH and SDMH influence individuals across the life span. The negative impact can be cumulative and result in disparities in health, health decision-making and health outcomes. Central to understanding how SDH influence these outcomes is recognizing that all of the SDH are affected by the *social position* (associated with amount of resources/supports, level of education, degree of political influence/power, etc.) of individuals and communities. The WHO in their publication *Social Determinants of Mental Health* (2014) report using the growing body of international literature to clearly identify that the more compromised the social position experienced by individuals and populations, the higher the risk for health disparities and negative health outcomes especially poor mental health. Some population subgroups (e.g. refugees/immigrants/minority ethnic/racial and sexual orientation populations, etc.) experience a higher risk of mental health challenges because of greater exposure and vulnerability to detrimental social and ecological circumstances. This higher risk is further exacerbated for women regardless of the setting (WHO & Calouste Gulbenkian Foundation, 2014).

Mental health and many common mental disorders are influenced by socioeconomic and contextual factors that are encountered beginning before birth and progressing into early and older childhood, adolescence, during family building and working years, and into aging. The greater the inequality in those socioeconomic and contextual factors throughout the life span, the higher the inequality in risk for the development of mental and physical health conditions (Fisher & Baum, 2010; Paananen, Ristikar, Merikukka, & Gissler, 2013; Victorino & Gauthier, 2009; WHO, 2013).

Because SDH affect individuals and communities across the life span, the WHO and most nations that strive to improve the health of their citizens have identified *health equity* as their guiding principle. Health equity is "defined as the absence of unfair and avoidable or remediable differences in health among social groups . . . In essence, health inequities are health differences that are socially produced, systematic in their distribution across the population, and unfair" (Solar & Irwin, 2010, p. 14). The realization of the human right to health implies the empowerment of deprived communities to exercise the greatest possible control over the factors that determine their health (Solar & Irwin, 2010).

Because SDH affect can be chronic stressors across an entire lifetime, early childhood risk factors are critical to recognize and rectify if at all possible. For example, significant stressors or depression experienced by the mother in sensitive development periods prior to a child's birth affect the development of the child in terms of a greater risk of being underweight and underdeveloped, with low birth weight itself being identified as an increased risk factor for depression in later life (Forsyth *et al.*, 2013; Nugent, Tyrka, Carpenter, & Price, 2011).In utero, exposure to the mother's stress affects development of the child's biological stress regulatory systems through which stress responses are controlled. This prenatal effect places the child at higher risk for dysregulation of the stress response after birth (DiPietro, 2004; Uher, 2014).

Although children may have disadvantages based on prenatal exposure, the effects this exposure has on the child can be cushioned to some degree by social support from a caring individual and a stable environment, which is essential for healthy social and emotional growth. Secure attachment to a constant care provider in the early years is essential for the child as a mediator against mental health concerns and to support healthy coping with stressors (Russell, Ford, Tamsin, Rosenberg, & Kelly, 2014).

Persistent exposure to stressors over time as the child grows results in stress response changes that have physiological effects on multiple body systems including the brain, and affect physical functioning in ways that are damaging to health (Chetty, *et al.*, 2014). This accumulation of exposure to stress results in inequitable mental and physical health outcomes.

The impact of the mother on the emotional and mental development of the child cannot be overstated.

The WHO (2014) reports that

> [a] systematic review of studies in low- and middle-income countries estimated prevalence of common perinatal mental disorders among women to be 16 percent before birth and 20 percent postnatally. Risk factors for common perinatal disorders include socioeconomic disadvantage; unintended pregnancy; being younger; being unmarried; lacking intimate partner empathy and support; having hostile in-laws; experiencing intimate partner violence; having insufficient emotional and practical support; in some settings, giving birth to a female, and having a history of mental health problems. Protective factors include having more education, having a permanent job, being a member of the ethnic majority and having a kind, trustworthy intimate partner. A large body of research has emphasized the importance of maternal education and emotional wellbeing for a wide range of outcomes for children, with lower maternal education and depression relating to increased infant mortality, physical problems (such as low birth weight and malnutrition, overweight children, and infections) and cognitive and emotional problems (such as lower scores on vocabulary tests, conduct problems, behavioral problems, lower cognitive scores, and mental health problems).
>
> *(WHO and Calouste, 2014, p. 19)*

The critical nature of the mother–child interaction in early childhood was further emphasized by the UCL Institute of Health Equity, which reported that

> lack of secure attachment, neglect, lack of quality stimulation, and conflict, negatively impact on future social behaviour, educational outcomes, employment status and mental and physical health. Children's exposure to neglect, direct physical and psychological abuse, and growing up in families with domestic violence was particularly damaging.
>
> *(Bell, Donkin, & Marmot, 2013, p. 24)*

For the older child and adolescent, education is also crucial in fostering emotional resilience and affecting future outcomes as adults that are associated with greater risks for mental health conditions such as jobs, income, and social engagement. Schools are also important as institutions for engagement of youth and for mental health promotion during critical periods of development. The literature on older children and adolescents also identifies that those who are from poorer backgrounds are more likely to have greater exposure to and experience within poor environments and stressful family contexts (Bell *et al.*, 2013). Poverty has a direct impact on learning as it can lead to poor/inadequate housing with no place to do homework or study. Without needed resources to learn, adequate nutrition and non-stressful family dynamics in which a child can focus on the learning process, their risk of failure is high, and likelihood of success is low. Parents who are employed not only diminish the likelihood of poverty, but also improve family dynamics, and provide a role model for children to emulate. Schools may also engage parents and collaborate to develop needed support and guidance on parenting strategies through the child and adolescent years (Huang, Cheng & Theise, 2013).

As individuals become adolescents, and begin the journey toward independence, they may engage in behaviors that are physically and emotionally risky (Victorino & Gauthier, 2009). During this stage of development the critical task for parents is to ensure that adolescents have important information to make informed decisions, and that they have protective factors including social and emotional support, and positive interactions with peers, family, and the community at large. Depressive symptoms among adolescents are associated with their history of adverse childhood experiences as well as their current experiences such as individual, community, and armed conflict; bullying, physical and sexual trauma; social isolation/upheaval; adolescent marriage and childbearing; and chemical misuse/abuse among others (Bell *et al.*, 2013). The potential layering of negative life experiences significantly erodes the foundation for adaptive coping during adult years. Further discussion of factors related to child and adolescent mental health can be found in Chapter 18.

During adulthood, mental health and well-being is significantly associated with the ability to acquire resources (adequate food, safe housing, reliable transportation, etc.) for self and family along with a sense of security and control over one's work life. Employment with low compensation, low levels of control over the work environment by workers, and job insecurity and unemployment have a significant harmful impact on mental health, resulting in stress, anxiety, and depression (Cayuela, Malmusi, Lopez-Jacob, Gotsens & Rondo, 2015, Sousa *et al.*, 2010). In contrast, employment, job security and a perception of control at work are protective of mental well-being increasing self-esteem, job satisfaction and productivity. Most importantly, employment should be adequate for, and conducive to, the development of a healthy family unit to combat the risks inherent in impoverished and unstable living, which has been demonstrated to be strongly associated with poor mental health for all members of a family unit (Bell *et al.*, 2013; WHO & Calouste Gulbenkian Foundation, 2014). Family structure and parenting style influence children's mental health and future outcomes across the life span. Adult mental health can be greatly influenced by the stressors encountered during adulthood especially when inequality is experienced in relation to barriers that affect the roles and tasks that are expectations as part of adulthood and family development (Liang *et al.*, 2012).

As adults age, they continue to bring with them all prior life experiences, both positive and negative. This cumulative life experience can function as a barrier to, or buffer for, satisfactory aging. The body of literature regarding mental health and aging has grown over the last 10 years, especially as it relates to factors that impact the mental health of this population worldwide (WHO, 2013). The available evidence that exists identifies inequalities in mental health related to gender, educational attainment, ethnicity/race, socioeconomic level, and physical health status. Women experience more negative mental health outcomes when experiencing social isolation and lack of interpersonal supports, and men are more vulnerable to negative outcomes based upon physical health. Extant research reports poorer outcomes for women than men across a range of mental health conditions (Kwan & mHealth Alliance, 2013; WHO & Calouste Gulbenkian Foundation, 2014). Life events that can trigger depression and are likely to be experienced in older age include loss and grief, poor physical health, loss of connection with family and friends, perceived loss of social position and identity, living alone, and lack of ability to be active in their physical environment (due to safety issues or health).

As stated throughout this book, mental health and physical health are interactive processes. For example, adults with physical health conditions such as heart disease and diabetes have higher rates of depression than those who are medically well. Also, untreated depression in a person with a chronic physical condition can have a negative effect on their physical condition and outcome (Alaba & Chola, 2013). These experiences are magnified in aging and can result in isolation, loss of independence, loneliness, poor self-concept, and psychological distress. Changes occurring during this period of life are further exacerbated by forces, which include personal, financial, access to resources, and presence or absence of applicable national policies (WHO & Calouste Gulbenkian Foundation, 2014). Some changes are occurring globally in this population, which are addressing the SDH and are known to impede improved mental health outcomes. These are more thoroughly discussed in Chapter 17.

Conclusion

The field of mental health is becoming increasingly aware that well-being and mental health are supported by multiple factors, and are not just driven by the individual's biology, genetic pool, or home environment. Individuals live in families, each family has its own unique characteristics and is situated in a community. In turn, communities have multiple characteristics, each of which can be eroded or supported by government actions, resources, collective actions of community members and the relationship between individual communities and their government and governing bodies. These systems are open and dynamic, and interrelate in both overt and covert ways. What is now known is that all of these proximal and distal factors can have an effect on the life experience of individuals and this in turn impacts their well-being. SDH and mental health are intertwined. In order to arrive at effective interventions across low, middle-, and high-income environments, mental health providers have to first assess and gain knowledge of the multiple factors that contribute to mental ill health. Our most useful action as health care providers in resource-poor environments may be directed at policy, advocacy, anti-stigma campaigns, and mental health literacy; all actions that target distal system factors that serve as barriers to positive mental health. All mental health providers must broaden their understanding of the drivers of poor mental health beyond the individual consumer and his or her family/immediate community.

References

Alaba, O., & Chola, V. (2013). The social determinants of multimorbidity in South Africa. *International Journal for Equity in Health, 12*, 63.

Baumgartner, J.N., & Susser, E. (2013). Social integration in global mental health: What is it and how can it be measured? *Epidemiology and Psychiatric Services, 22*(1), 29–37.

Bell, R., Donkin, A., & Marmot, M. (2013). *Tackling structural and social issues to reduce inequities in children's outcomes in low- to middle-income countries, Office of Research Discussion Paper No.2013–02,* Florence: UNICEF Office of Research.

Braveman, P., Egerter, S., & Williams, D. (2011). The social determinants of health: Coming of age. *Annual Review of Public Health, 32*, 381–398.

Cayuela, A., Malmusi, D., López-Jacob, M.J., Gotsens, M., & Ronda, E. (2015). The impact of education and socioeconomic and occupational conditions on self-perceived and mental health inequalities among immigrants and native workers in Spain. *Journal of Immigrant and Minority Health, 17*(6), 1906–1910.

Chetty S., Friedman, A.R., Taravosh-Lahn, K., Kirby, E.D., Mirescu, C, Guo, F., Krupik, D., Nicholas, A., Geraghty, A.C., Krishnamurthy, A., Tsai, M.-K., Covarrubias, D., Wong, A.T., Francis, D.D., Sapolsky, R.M., Palmer, T.D., Pleasure, D., & Kaufer, D. (2014). Stress and glucocorticoids promote oligodendrogenesis in the adult hippocampus. *Molecular Psychiatry, 19*(12), 1275–1283.

Collins, P., Patel, V., Joestl, S., March, D., Insel, T.R., Daar, A.S., Scientific Advisory Board and the Grand Challenges on Global Mental Health, & Stein, D.J. (2011). Grand challenges in global mental health. *Nature, 475*, 27–30.

Das, A., & Rao, M. (2012). Universal mental health: Re-evaluating the call for global mental health. *Critical Public Health, 22*(4), 383–389.

Di Pietro, J. (2004). The role of prenatal maternal stress in child development. *Current Directions in Psychological Science Johns Hopkins University, 13*(2), 71–74.

Embrett, M., & Randall, G. (2014). Social determinants of health and health equity policy research: Exploring the use, misuse, and nonuse of policy analysistheory. *Social Science & Medicine, 108*, 147–155.

Fiorati, R., & Elui, V. (2015). Social determinants of health, inequality and social inclusion among people with disabilities. *Rev. Latino-Am Enfermagen, 23*(2), 329–336.

Fisher, M., & Baum, F. (2010). The social determinants of mental health: Implications for research and health promotion. *Australian & New Zealand Journal of Psychiatry, 44*, 1057–1063.

Forsyth, J.K., Ellman, L.M., Tanskanen, A., Mustonen, U., Huttunen, M.O., Suvisaari, J., & Cannon, T.D. (2013). Genetic risk for schizophrenia, obstetric complications, and adolescent school outcome: evidence for gene-environment interaction. *Schizophr Bull, 39*(5): 1067–1076.

Friel, S., & Marmot, M. (2011). Action on the social determinants of health and health inequities goes global. *Annual Review of Public Health, 32*, 225–236.

Huang, K.Y., Cheng, S., & Theise, R. (2013). School contexts as social determinants of child health: Current practices and implications for future public health practice. *Public Health Reports Supplement 3, 128*, 21–28.

Kwan, A., & mHealth Alliance. (2013). *mHealth solutions for improving mental health and illnesses in the aging process.* Washington, DC: mHealth Alliance UN Foundation.

Liang, Y., Gong, Y.-H., Wen, X.-P., Guan, C.-P., Li, M.-C., Yin, P., & Wang, Z.Q. (2012) Social determinants of health and depression: A preliminary investigation from rural China. *PLoS ONE, 7*(1): e30553.

Lund, C., Stansfeld, S., & De Silva, M. (2014). Social determinants of mental health. In V. Patel, H. Minas, A. Cohen, & M. Prince (Eds.). *Global Mental Health, Principles and Practice*, pp. 116–136. New York: Oxford University Press.

Marmot, M., & Allen, J. (2014). Social determinants of health equity. *American Journal of Public Health, Supplement 4, 104*(S4), S517–519.

Nugent, N.R., Tyrka, A.R., Carpenter, L.L., & Price, L.H. (2011). Gene-environment interactions: Early life stress and risk for depressive and anxiety disorders. *Psychopharmacology, 214*(1), 175–196.

Paananen, R., Ristikari, T., Merikukka, M., & Gissler, M. (2013). Social determinants of mental health: A Finnish nationwide follow-up study on mental disorders. *Journal of Epidemiology and Community Health, 12*, 1025–1031.

Patel, V. (2012). Global mental health: From science to action. *Harvard Review of Psychiatry, 20*, 6–12.

Russell, G., Tamsin, A., Rosenberg, R., & Kelly, S. (2014). The association of attention deficit hyperactivity disorder with socioeconomic disadvantage: Alternative explanations and evidence. *Journal of Child Psychology & Psychiatry, 55*, 436–445.

Solar, O., & Irwin, A. (2010). *A conceptual framework for action on social determinants of health: Social determinants of health discussion paper 2 (policy and practice)*. Geneva: World Health Organization.

Sousa, E., Agudelo-Suarez, A., Benvides, F.G., Schenker, M., Garcia, A.M., Benach, J., Delclos, C. López-Jacob, M.J., Ruiz-Frutos, C., Ronda-Pérez, E., Porthé, V, & ITSAL Project (2010). Immigration, work and health in Spain: the influence of legal status and employment contract on reported health indicators. *International Journal of Public Health, 55*, 443–451.

Swartz, L., Kilian, S., Twesigye, J., Attah, D., & Chiliza, B. (2014). Language, culture, and task shifting-an emerging challenge for global mental health. *Global Health Action, 7*, 23433. Available at http://dx.doi.org/10.3402/gha.v7.23433 (accessed April 29, 2015).

Uher R. (2014). Gene-environment interactions in common mental disorders: An update and strategy for a genome-wide search. *Social Psychiatry Psychiatric Epidemiology, 49*(1), 3–14.

Victorino, C.C., & Gauthier, A.H. (2009). The social determinants of child health: Variations across health outcomes—population based cross sectional analysis. *BMC Pediatrics, 9*, 53.

World Health Organization. (2008). *Closing the gap in a generation: Health equity through action on the social determinants of health*. Geneva: World Health Organization.

World Health Organization. (2013). *Mental health and older adults: Fact sheet 381*. Geneva: World Health Organization.

World Health Organization & Calouste Gulbenkian Foundation. (2014). *Social determinants of mental health*. Geneva: World Health Organization.

5

THE EFFECTS OF CULTURE AND STIGMA ON MENTAL HEALTH

Deena A. Nardi, Roberta Waite and Edilma L. Yearwood

Introduction

This chapter uses an ecological model of the social determinants of health to present the implications of culture and stigma on the mental health of populations and associated recommended treatments. This model illustrates the interrelationships of diverse determinants of health and well-being and their impact on individuals, populations, and societies (Guy, 2007). Stigma and its role in preventing timely, effective treatment of mental health disorders are examined. In addition, resources are identified that can inform and support the cultural competencies of nurse providers of psychiatric mental health care in regional, national, and global arenas.

Optimizing global mental health outcomes requires a concerted commitment by many individuals worldwide to modify the core contributing factors of mental health challenges and disparities, including internal and external influences such as personal and societal stigma as well as cultural considerations. These cultural considerations influence decision-making at all levels of health care, from individual patient and consumer care to policy-making. Globally, addressing mental health concerns in a timely and effective manner requires greater emphasis due to the wide range of implications of untreated health concerns for individuals, families, communities, and ultimately, the world. Beyond individual facilitators and barriers to seeking mental health services, there is an associated unfair, unequitable, and unethical distribution of resource dissemination such as information and treatment provisions (Ngui, Khasakhala, Ndetei, & Roberts, 2010). Also lacking are mental health and primary care policies that are comprehensive and protective, from a legal and human rights perspective for individuals affected by mental disorders, including their families (Ngui *et al.*, 2010).

Stigma

Stigma, defined as myths and fallacies in thought and actions regarding mental illness, contributes to a significant level of discrimination and human rights abuses endured by individuals with mental conditions (Ngui *et al.*, 2011). In developing countries the encumbrance of mental disorders is magnified by extraordinary rates of stigma and discrimination as evidenced by the poor treatment those with mental ill health receive. Notably, these factors are major impediments in the delivery and utilization of mental health services regardless of a person's age (Kleintjes, Lund & Flisher, 2010). Stigma therefore affects: (1) an individual's willingness to disclose and seek help; (2) the quality of health care received; and (3) access to mental health services to support recovery (Kleintjes *et al.*, 2010). Moreover, there can be secondary stigma extended to the family as a result of association with individuals affected by mental illness. This can contribute to the family members mistreating, alienating, and/or rejecting the individual(s) affected by mental illness (Kleintjes *et al.*, 2010).

Stigma involves discrediting an individual or group, which results in labeling as "out" or apart from others. The stigma label affixed is negative and serves to separate or highlight a difference between the stigmatized individual or group and others, and this label results in discrimination, loss of status, low self-esteem, and limited or no access to social opportunities (Corrigan, 2004; Link & Phelan, 2006). An underlying and influential element of stigma is a power imbalance, with power exerted over the stigmatized individual (Bos, Pryor, Reeder, & Stutterheim, 2013). Stigma alleviation is particularly challenged by its existence at multiple levels, public, individual and structural, requiring a multi-layered approach to support a positive outcome (Corrigan, Druss, & Perlick, 2014).

Stigma and discrimination, against individuals with mental health challenges, leads to human rights violations in civil, cultural, economic, political, or social spheres (Drew *et al.*, 2011). Human rights are rights that no one should be able to exclude. Fundamentally, each individual should have the freedom to partake in community life while being able to live independently. Human rights therefore endorses that persons with mental illness have complete respect, dignity, and recognition as being human (Drew *et al.*, 2011). However, when stigmatizing views infiltrate the minds of policy makers and funders, development and investment in mental health can be stymied and this ultimately contributes to the low priority of global mental health in the world's public agenda (Kleintjes *et al.*, 2010). However, there are examples of positive policy decisions to improve mental health. Nepal has been improving awareness of mental health and related problems through its national mental health policy. Nepal has specifically addressed the following: providing care in the community, educating the public, connecting with communities, and monitoring community mental health through the introduction of mental health first aid (Jha, Kitchener, Pradhan, Shyangwa, & Nakarm, 2012).

Culture

Cultural values, beliefs and processes can significantly impact mental health. Myers (2010, p. 505) reports that culture is often perceived as "symbolic apparatuses of meaning making, representation, and transmission." This outlook is closely linked with political and economic practices within society and are recognized and lived in local domains and beyond. Culture is conveyed to individuals through "experience," or a "felt flow of interpersonal communications and engagements" that "take place in a local world" and are "thoroughly intersubjective" (Myers, 2010, p. 505). Therefore, everything individuals have learned and appreciated about their history reflecting customary behaviors and actions as well as personal beliefs is indicative of an individual's culture (Bryan & Morrow, 2011).

Arnault (2009) describes culture as being a set of interrelating, system-level, social practices that encompass four interconnected dimensions—cultural ideology, political/economic dimension, practice, and the body. *Cultural ideology* are beliefs and values held by individuals relating to what is good, right and normal; it denotes symbols, meanings, and values regarding what is significant and what behaviors are appropriate and accurate. *Political/economic* characteristics of culture comprise the social structures of the society including how families and organizations allocate resources, assign labor, and obtain and distribute capital/wealth. This dimension accounts for how individuals in a position of power and influence define proper social behavior and how public conduct will be controlled. Cultural ideology informs the political/economic dimension of culture since cultural beliefs and values define what is considered "good" and "right," and rationalizes to explain why certain individuals are able to hold positions of power and over whom. The culture of *practice*, embodiment of tradition, encompasses traditional behaviors, spatial organization, and relational behaviors. Two central features under the practice domain include power and ideals in gestures, language patterns, custom of dress, social space allotted, food selections, and health behaviors. Arnault (2009) relates that cultural practices are representations of both cultural ideology and political/economy at the personal or group level. Lastly, the *body* is perceived as cultural in three significant ways— individuals experience the body as the "individual body-self" based on cultural prescriptions and templates; each person experiences themselves as having as a social body, which is a natural symbol for culturally based thinking about relationships among nature, society and culture; and finally, the body is political, in that it is an artifact of, and is subject to, culturally based social and political control (Arnault, 2009, p. 261).

The overlapping cultural dimensions of *ideology, political/economic, and practice* exert their effects on the body, specifically how these dimensions are lived through the body (Arnault, 2009). Importantly, these cultural forces occur in, and are shaped by, the geographic setting in which individuals live.

Given that culture encompasses the totality of principles, beliefs, abilities, customs, and institutions into which each member of society is born, being able to appreciate and understand the cultural context of individuals who receive mental health services is an essential professional competency. Culturally relevant proficiency and skills are necessary for ethical practice. An understanding of the impact of social context and worldviews on behavior is vital to the course of mental health service provision (Bryan & Morrow, 2011).

Description and discussion of the issues

Promoting global mental health enables the enhancement of healthy development across the life span including supporting individuals to realize educational, social, and economic goals. Moreover, optimizing mental health contributes to prevention of both communicable and noncommunicable health difficulties and early mortality (Jenkins, Baingana, Ahmad, McDaid, & Atun, 2011). Currently, however, the status of global mental health demonstrates a failure of humanity (Kleinman, 2009). The reality is that most individuals around the world, particularly those affected by mental illness living in developing countries, endure dreadful conditions beyond negative words that are stigmatizing. Kleinman (2009), a global mental health expert, has witnessed individuals with mental disorders in abysmal situations including being chained to beds; imprisoned in small cells constructed behind houses; isolated in concrete rooms with a hole in the floor for urine and feces in for-profit asylums; maltreated by traditional healers to the point of being starved and infected with tuberculosis; disfigured through burns as a consequence of inappropriate safeguarding from cooking fires; compelled to endure electroconvulsive therapy when psychotic; apprehended by the police; concealed by families; stoned by local youth; and treated in a manner devoid of dignity, respect, or protection by health care personnel. These behaviors and manners of treatment are readily apparent in small towns and villages as experienced by Kleinman (2009) and constitute some of the most inhumane treatment by man of his fellow human being.

Fundamentally, global mental health is a moral and human rights issue. Pertinent factors associated with principles underlying global mental health include: *mental capital, social capital,* and *political capital. Mental capital* is the cognitive and emotional effects that influence how well a person is able to contribute to society and is linked with positive mental health. Jenkins and colleagues (2011) state that positive mental health encompasses critical factors such as an improved sense of well-being; a belief in one's own worth and dignity including valuing others; personal assets such as self-esteem, hopefulness and sense of mastery and rationality; the capacity to initiate, cultivate, and endure mutually satisfying relations; and the ability to manage adversity. Collectively, these factors contribute to an individual's capability to enhance family dynamics, other social networks including the local community, and society in general (Jenkins *et al.*, 2011). Hence, mental health extends beyond the absence of symptoms or distress. Mental capital is also influenced by both mental health and physical health; they are interrelated, each influencing outcomes as indispensable aspects of an individual's general health. Importantly, they are an inseparable measure of public health. This endorses the modern-day phrase "there is no health without mental health" (Patel, 2012, p. 7). Thus, mental capital covers our conceptual understanding of "the bank account of the mind," encompassing "intellectual and emotional resources which can be built up or depleted or damaged through life" (Jenkins *et al.*, 2011, p. 70). Collective mental capital is undoubtedly significant for nations in quest of prosperous development.

Social capital is the helpfulness created by social networks including social relations and relates to the efficacy of participation in social reciprocity such as fundamental cultural practices of living a conventional lifestyle. This includes participation in marriage, work-related activities, academic functions, celebrations, commemorations, mourning rituals, and in commonplace experience in marketplaces, stores, and in other related ordinary activities (Jenkins *et al.*, 2011). Modern-day issues that affect social capital in many countries, and ultimately impacts mental health, include the impending rise of population growth and aging; marital and household breakdown; a growing number of orphans contributing to the growth in child-headed family units; and immigration both from rural to urban regions within a country as well as across international boundaries (Jenkins *et al.*, 2011). Additional issues that warrant attention and that influence social capital include fluctuating patterns of work availability, climate change, the threat of debt and amplified disparity in earnings, and increased alcohol and substance abuse. Issues that contribute to poor mental health will have an undesirable effect on physical health, and on expansive social and economic areas (Jenkins *et al.*, 2011).

Political capital includes access to political events and decision-making and is needed in order to tackle pervasive global mental health issues. Even with the high disease burden, global mental illness has not attained proportionate visibility, policy attention, or financial support (Tomlinson & Lund, 2012). Overarching steps that can support deserved attention in addressing our global mental health calamity include two central areas. First, political and international leaders must publicly and privately champion for improvement in global mental health in an unrelenting manner (Tomlinson & Lund, 2012). To date, there has been a low political will of countries to act on the evidence of global mental health disorders. Countries such as Brazil and India have exhibited some aptitude to establish their own health agendas independent of foreign contributors. These countries are also now allocating larger resources to mental health; however, these provisions continue to be inadequate based on the scale of unmet needs. In countries whose health policies are influenced by international donors, the potential to prioritize mental health can be obstructed by views that mental health is not urgent for individuals who are poor and reside in less-resourced countries (Patel, 2012). For example, 44 percent of African countries do not have a mental health policy and 33 percent do not have a mental health plan (Tomlinson

& Lund, 2012). Low- and middle-income countries struggle significantly with getting resources appropriate to the disease burden. As a global median 2.8 percent of health budgets are apportioned to mental health; however, broad variations exist with the mental health portion ranging from 0.53 percent for low-income countries to 5.10 percent for high-income countries. Second, and most importantly, not addressing global mental health is a social justice issue. Social justice advocates for "a societal state in which all members of a society have the same basic rights, security, opportunities, obligations, and social benefits" (Pope & Turner, 2009, p. 194).

Mental health treatment of populations

The increasing globalization of the world presents critical challenges as well as opportunities for psychiatric and mental health providers to effect positive change in perspectives and treatment. Globalization has brought disparate communities closer than ever before. The technologically enhanced instant interactions of different cultures provide access to new knowledge and more resources, yet it also creates new vulnerabilities to acts of terror, all forms of abuse, and the loss of cultural or political identity. Communities around the globe are confronting major issues that directly affect psychiatric/mental health and health care, including nurse and health provider migration; childhood poverty; malnourishment and ill health; rapid scientific and technological advances; political and financial destabilization; access to arms, explosives and guns; aging populations; and family, community, and political violence. These issues are experienced through the lenses of cultural-based attitudes, values and beliefs that influence the responses of individuals and communities to these stressors. Understanding the cultural influences on our patients' behaviors as well as our own improves nurses' ability to best respond to the needs of our patients, and to help them reach their personal health goals. This is a lifelong task, since the cultures in which we grow, work and live, are constantly interacting with other cultures, and changing in subtle, and not so subtle, ways. This purports that nurses must support and enhance their cultural competency through lifelong learning, continued self-awareness, and keeping a primary focus on the individual and individual's concerns when providing all level of care.

The relationship of culture to global mental health nursing

Nurses who are attentive to the cultural determinants of mental health will incorporate patient-centered information to actively shape and support their interpersonal communications, assessments, diagnosing, treatment planning, and follow-up. Nursing actions used to support treatment should be current, culturally adaptable to the populations served, relevant to the nurse's role in the system of care, and evidence based. Using an ecological perspective, these resources are used when negotiating the interrelated micro, exo and macro systems (Bronfenbrenner, 1979, 1994, 2005).

Microsystem resources that affect roles and experiences are used when working with the patients' symptoms, beliefs, perceptions, age, and health. Some microsystem resources are the nurse's own education and experience with each population, and the published assessment and intervention guidelines the nurse uses when working individually with the patient. Nurses must understand the laws and policies of the exosystem that the patient lives and works in in order to best support patients' return to their optimum level of health, return to work, and return to a degree of wellness in that society. Exosystem resources, connections and relationships, are used when communicating with social services, the work environment, or political bureaucracies. Nurses use the macrosystem resources (beliefs and customs) to clarify the attitudes, economics and ideologies of the patient's culture, and improve their general cultural understanding and competency. Their informed understandings of the influences of these interconnected systems serve to guide nurses' psychiatric evaluations and cultural assessments.

Culturally competent assessment

In order to optimize care, the nurse or health care provider should start with a basic assessment that includes a personal review of cultural factors that may influence care. If psychiatric services providers believe that understanding the patient's cultural context is essential for comprehensive and effective assessment, diagnosis, and treatment, then it follows that the initial psychiatric interview must include a cultural assessment from the individual's personal and lived experiences. This cultural assessment, also called "cultural formulation interview" or CFI, by the Multicultural Resource Centre (2014), as well as the American Psychiatric Association (2013b, p. 750), has become a key component of any psychiatric diagnostic evaluation. Table 5.1 illustrates questions that can be included while conducting a cultural assessment.

The CFI consists of categories of questions that enable the interviewer to examine the patient's culturally influenced definitions of the problem, its causes, the patient's social, economic and metaphysical supports including spirituality, coping behaviors, and help-seeking behaviors. Each section includes sample questions, with rationale and purpose, and a guide to approaching the patient that interviewers can use to elicit answers. The APA also offers supplementary modules to the CFI that providers may use in research, and for detailed cultural assessment with follow-up questions (American Psychiatric Association, 2013b). These modules, as well as the CFI, can be used initially for assessment, and throughout the care of the patient, as individual social networks, finances, and the supportive environment often change with time and circumstance. And since these changes affect health outcomes, they should be identified and incorporated into the plan of care in an iterative manner.

The CFI should be conducted during an initial assessment. Demographic data from the electronic health record, gathered prior to this interview, can then be used to tailor the interview questions to the patient's current situation. There are many versions of the CFI to guide the cultural assessment, and it is published in some form in many languages. The original CFI guide is published in the *Diagnostic and Statistical Manual of Mental Disorders*, fifth edition (DSM-5), and can be located in its Section III: Emerging Measures and Models (see American Psychiatric Association, 2013a, pp. 749–759). The DSM-5 is also cross-referenced to the International Classification of Diseases (ICD-9 and 10), and planned to be congruent with ICD-11 for global use by countries that are signatory to WHO and the UN (American Psychiatric Association, 2013a, pp. 10–11).

Resources for practice

Globally, there are approximately 150 national nurses associations (NNA) that are members of the International Council of Nurses (ICN), (International Council of Nurses, 2013). Each NNA provides information, guidelines and data to support and enhance the cultural competency of their country's nurses. Additionally, the country's national standards of psychiatric mental health practice, if they exist, also guide practice. It is well understood that countries with limited resources, must also develop practice standards. However, in the absence of standards, practice can be informed by using exemplars from around the world. For instance, the Canadian Nurses Association provides a link on their website to a nursing education framework for nurses caring for individuals of First Nations, Inuit and Métis populations. The purpose of the framework is to prepare nurses to work with indigenous peoples in Canada, through the fostering of

Table 5.1 The DSM-5 cultural formulation outline

Cultural classifications	Examples of question format	Intent to determine:
Culturally based values, beliefs, and practices (cultural identity)	1 Could you tell us about how this problem has affected you and your family? 2 Do you have an idea about what caused this problem? 3 Which part of this problem is most troubling?	1 Patient understanding of the problem 2 How the patient frames the problem 3 Prioritization and ranking of aspects of the problem
Cultural conceptualization of distress and supports	4 Why do you think you have this problem? 5 What does your family say contributes to this problem? 6 What or who helps you to cope with this problem? 7 Is there anything in the environment that contributes to this problem? 8 What is most important to you about your culture? 9 What aspects of your cultural background help you cope? 10 What aspects of our culture make the problem worse?	4 Meaning given to the problem 5 Perspectives of others close to patient 6 Social supports and supportive networks 7 Environmenmtal stressors 8 Aspects of cultural identity 9 Role of cultural identity in causing or alleviating distress 10 A probe to explore cultural identity
Psychosocial stressors, vulnerability and resilience	11 How do you cope with the problem? Can you give me an example? 12 People look for help from all sorts of sources. What resources or providers have you used to help with this problem? 13 What prevents you from getting help for this problem?	11 Relevant self-coping behaviors 12 Exploring actual and potential sources of support 13 Social barriers to help seeking behaviors
Cultural features of relationships	14 What kinds of help would be useful to you now to deal with this problem? 15 What kinds of help have been suggested to you? 16 Do you have any concerns about receiving help from this program that we can talk about now?	14 Perspective on what type of help/support is needed 15 Perspective on helpfulness of social network support 16 Perspectives on receiving meaningful help
Overall cultural assessment	Summarizes results of the CFI and how it can best be used to appropriately diagnose, treat, and manage the disorder with the patient	

Source: Adapted from the cultural formulation interview (American Psychiatric Association, 2013a). See the interview, pages 749–759, for specific questions and interview format.

"awareness, sensitivity, competence, and moreover the need for *cultural safety* in the care of clients, including First Nation, Inuit, and Métis peoples" (Hart-Waskeesikaw, 2009, p. 1).

The World Health Organization (WHO) proposed a comprehensive mental health action plan in 2012, and it was formally approved at the sixty-sixth World Health Assembly (World Health Organization, 2013). The action plan used two objectives whose outcomes would be directly related to the cultural competencies of mental health providers and all who practice in this field: " . . . (2) to provide comprehensive, integrated and responsive mental health and social care services in community-based settings; (3) to implement strategies for promotion and prevention in mental health" (World Health Organization, 2013, p. 6). Providing health and social services that promote and prevent mental health disorders requires responsiveness founded on commitment to, education about, and respect for, all populations served. These attributes are the hallmarks of culturally competent nursing care. The action plan began in 2013; its goals are scheduled to be accomplished by 2020. The plan can be accessed at http://apps.who.int/gb/ebwha/pdf_files/WHA66/A66_R8-en.pdf and includes actions and strategies that nursing leadership can use to promote mental health patient empowerment, as well as to improve provider responsiveness to vulnerable or marginalized populations who are at increased risk for poorer mental health outcomes.

Another example of the role of NNAs in supporting the cultural competencies of their country's nurses is the Trained Nurses Association of India, which provides links to its new initiatives to promote health care to rural populations. Its position statements on human rights and culturally appropriate health care, advocates for equitable access and treatment for women (Trained Nurses Association, 2013). In the US, a toolkit for teaching and enhancing cultural competency in master's and doctoral education that the American Association of Colleges of Nursing hosts on its webpage, and which can be accessed at www.aacn.nche.edu/education-resources/Cultural_Competency_Toolkit_Grad.pdf (AACN, 2011), provides references for health literacy and cross-cultural communication, and resources for faculty, students and practicing nurses.

There are many international organizations that provide strategies for culturally competent care to the global mental health provider community. These resources can be adapted to multicultural as well as distinct populations, and are useful to the lifelong learning of a diverse workforce, especially considering the immigration, migration, and rapid cultural changes produced by technology, which are experienced by all populations. Table 5.2 lists examples of the resources of the global community that are specific to psychiatric mental health care, the organization that sponsors each of the resources, and suggested uses.

Global standards for culturally competent mental health nursing practice

As the world shifts to an increasingly global perceptive on health care, there is a critical need for mental health nurses who can comfortably and competently work with diverse populations. The interactive influence of a number of factors such as the creation of the European Union, the global economy, the global migration of nurses and other health care providers, and the universal use of technology, especially web-based learning and entertainment, accelerates the interconnectedness of cultures. Another example of global interconnectedness is the increase in cross-border care. This term "cross-border care" refers to "medical services involving the movement of information, patients, and health care providers across national borders. These three elements—information, patients, and health care providers—are intertwined" (Nakajima, 2012, p. 6.) This practice is vibrant and growing. For instance, in the European Union, patients already have identified rights to cross-border health care (*Directive on Cross-Border Healthcare,*

Table 5.2 Global resources to support culturally competent mental health nursing practice

Organization	Host country and mission	Examples of resources
International Council of Nursing (ICN)	**Geneva, Switzerland** Ensures universal access to quality nursing care for all, sound global health policies, advancement of nursing knowledge	Nurses and Human Rights Position Paper (ICN, 2011). Global networking
International Society of Psychiatric–Mental Health Nurses (ISPN)	**Wisconsin, USA** To unify and strengthen the voice of psychiatric/mental health nurses	Advocacy Culturally competent curriculum guidelines Global networking
The Mental Health Consultation and Liaison Nurses Association of New South Wales and Australia Capital Territory	**Blacktown, NSW, Australia** Group of mental health nurses who provide liaison and consultation to medical and health care providers and settings. Membership services include networking and support	e-learning modules for Global Culturally and Linguistically Appropriate Services (CLAS) Standards in health and health care
Movement for Global Mental Health	**Melbourne, Australia** An evidence-based repository of articles, narratives, databases and other documents re human rights	Articles focused on the human rights of and advocacy for the mentally ill Databases
Multicultural Mental Health Resource Centre	**Calgary, Alberta, Canada** To improve access to quality mental health services for diverse populations	Cultural competence training, workshops and guidelines Mental health listserv CFI
Pacific Islands Mental Health Network (PIMHnet)	**Wellington, New Zealand** For the Western Pacific region of WHO nations. A network of Pacific Island countries to advocate, collaborate, and combine resources for effective mental health promotion and treatment	Publications Advocacy mhGAP Intervention Guide (mhGAP-IG)
Royal College of Nursing	**London, England, UK** Professional union; voice for nurses in the UK and abroad	Publications and e-learning to support transcultural nursing
Transcultural Nursing Society (TCS)	**Michigan, USA** Improve culturally congruent and competent health outcomes to improve health outcomes for people worldwide	Cultural competence resources Standards of practice for culturally competent nursing care
US Department of Health and Human Services Department of Minority Health	**US/Washington D.C.** To develop health policies and programs that assist in eliminating health disparities for racial and ethnic minorities.	Resources for CLAS standards in health and health care
World Health Organization (WHO)	**Geneva, Switzerland** The public health arm of the United Nations	Programmes for managing and intervening for mental health disorders
World Psychiatric Association (WPA)	**Chene-Bourg, Geneva, Switzerland** "To promote the advancement of psychiatry and mental health for all peoples of the world" (About the World Psychiatric Association, 2013)	Transcultural conferences and educational programmes Train the trainer workshops Journals

2011). In Canada, government approvals for Canadian nationals to receive health care in the USA have increased 450 percent (Cross-Border Care, 2012). In the USA, Blue Shield and Health Net California provide cross-border insurance policies to both US citizens and Mexican nationals (Schulz & Medlin, 2007), and the interest by other states in cross-border care in the US is growing. This increase in interconnectiveness of cross-border care, and global migration calls for standardization of at least a basic level of cultural competency that nurses can then use with the populations and cultures they serve.

There is a movement toward this basic standardization of culturally competent nursing care. The Horatio-European Psychiatric Nurses was formed in 2005, and in a few years its membership has grown to organizations from over 25 countries. Its purpose is to strengthen the voice and role of psychiatric mental health nursing in all aspects of patient care. Its expert panel of members developed the *Turku Declaration: A Consensus Document on Psychiatric-Mental Health Nursing Roles, Education and Practice* for all European PMHNs (Ward, 2011). This document outlines basic principles for PMH education, practice, and professional development. Although cultural skills are not mentioned specifically in the document, it emphasizes the central role of the PMH nurses in creating and using the therapeutic relationship with the patient, to provide patient-centered care, and to work within the patient's environment. To do this, PMH nurses must also use a cultural framework of understanding, and work within the culture of the patient.

Universally applicable guidelines for culturally competent nursing care practice were developed by a coalition from members of two professional nursing organizations (The Transcultural Nursing Society and the American Academy of Nurses' (AAN) Expert Panel on Global Nursing and Health) over a 6-year period, 2007–2013. Over 50 documents, including the United Nation's *Declaration of Human Rights* (United Nations, 2008), and the International Council of Nurses' (2006) *Code of Ethics*, were used in his effort. Their purpose was to enhance cultural competence in all nurses, as a priority of any nursing or health care. This document was first published in 2008, and comments from the international community of nurses were used to further refine the document. Its final version was published in the *Journal of Transcultural Nursing* in 2011 (Douglas, *et al.*, 2014). The International Council of Nursing (ICN) endorsed these guidelines in November 2013. They are mentioned in this chapter to provide examples for culturally competent nursing approaches to patient care.

Standards specific to global psychiatric mental health nursing have also been suggested, and published in the *Journal of Psychosocial Nursing and Mental Health Service* (Nardi, Waite, & Killian, 2012). The authors emphasized the need to adapt person-centered mental health care to cultural contexts; these contexts include the ecological, environmental, economic, educational, social, political, spiritual, and familial processes that interact to influence one's values, beliefs, and behaviors. Figure 5.1 depicts the complex systems the nurse must understand and negotiate in order to provide mental health care that is culturally safe and recognizes the human rights that the majority of United Nations member nations have recognized.

The triangle represents culturally congruent health care delivery, from its base of delivery, which derives first from the health care provider's individual and family systems background, based upon their values, beliefs, and behaviors, and their recognition of, and respect for these health care values, beliefs, and behaviors in their patient populations. This transformative process continues through to the point of delivery of culturally congruent health care. The layers of the triangle are not hierarchical, but filter through a transactional and dialectical process to the actual point of care represented at the point of the triangle. This point of care might be at the systems level, such as at a program, school, or hospital, or at a direct patient/provider/therapist level of interaction in a home or treatment program, at any number of politically or economically determined points of care delivery in countries and regions across the globe.

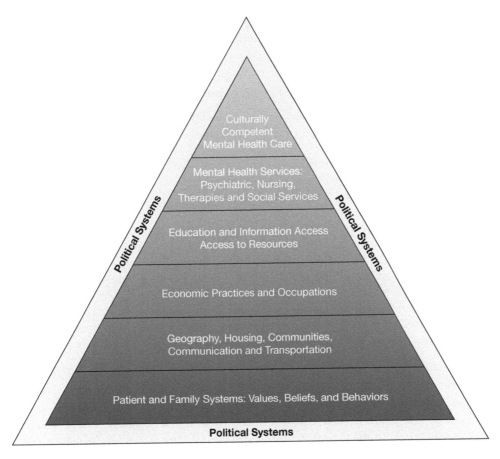

Figure 5.1 Culturally competent mental health care

Culturally competent approaches to mental health care

Providers of mental health care are practicing in a rapidly changing world, and an increasingly diverse society. Accordingly, mental health nurses can apply the guidelines for culturally competent nursing care when creating a therapeutic relationship with their patients, in order to facilitate assessment. This will also strengthen the therapeutic alliance between the patient, patient populations, and the therapist. However, the biggest impediment toward applying these global guidelines and resources to provide culturally competent nursing care is the very inequity in basic levels of nursing education and inconsistency in clinical training.

There is a severe shortage and unfair distribution of global mental health resources and clear obstacles to scaling up services for mental disorders which is informed by two principles—scientific support cost-effective treatments and a regard for the human rights of individuals affected by mental disorders. Transformational changes must occur to attempt to address the treatment gap. Present-day in many communities, mental health care is being delegated to non-specialist health workers who are educated to deliver interventions for particular mental disorders. Task shifting, the strategy of reasonable restructuring tasks among health workforce teams, has developed into an accepted practice for attending to shortages of specialist health resources (Patel, 2012). When applicable, highly qualified and educated health personnel share specific tasks with health workers having less preparation and fewer qualifications in order to make more effective use of the available human capital (Patel, 2012).

The role of mental health professionals and paraprofessionals

It is incumbent that to effectively address global mental health, the mental health community must have a strong engagement with the agenda at hand in diverse communities and pursue task-sharing strategies to meet the existing needs. Nursing, psychiatry, psychology, couple and family therapists, counselors, and other mental health professions and paraprofessionals, have a vital role to play. With shortages of professional health care providers, available human resources within communities must be "trained up" to provide basic mental health care that includes assessment, support, brief treatment and referral of complex cases to trained providers. Choosing members from the community who are knowledgeable about the fabric and socio-cultural processes in existence are invaluable as trusted cultural brokers, bring credibility to the topic of mental health, and can decrease the associated stigma. A multisite study, the PRogramme for Improving Mental health carE (PRIME) using non-specialist community workers in Uganda, South Africa, Ethiopia, India, Nepal found that the program was both accessible and feasible in providing mental health care within communities by trained lay workers. The success of the program was credited to availability and access to medications, inclusion of structured supervision, adequate initial training, and appropriate financial compensation for the work done (Mendenhall et al., 2014).

Experts need to deliver the supervision required for the successful enactment of task sharing; therefore, traditional work styles like functioning in silos is ill-advised and no longer compatible to meet modern-day needs of our world. Given that front-line mental health care will be shared with nonspecialist health workers, unique demands will be placed on mental health practitioners requiring them to learn and to become proficient in more diverse skill-sets including supervising nonspecialist health workers; be involved in monitoring and assessment for quality assurance of mental health care programs; obtain the management abilities fundamental for directing teams of health workers; and function as advocates for the human rights of individuals with mental disorders (Patel, 2012).

Mental health services

Even with evidence-based knowledge accrued worldwide about mental illness, the everyday experience for most individuals affected by mental disorders has been an indifferent health system that does little to answer to their needs, leading to estimates that up to three out of four affected persons in low- and middle-income countries do not receive the treatments known to help their conditions (Patel, 2012). For example, in sub-Saharan Africa the treatment disparity can surpass 90 percent, for schizophrenia and other psychoses, the most serious and incapacitating of mental disorders. This gap is scarcely unexpected, given that low- and middle-income countries control less than 20 percent of global mental health resources (Patel, 2012). In addition to improving access to evidence-based treatments in low-resource settings, the cultural suitability and appro-priateness of treatment is also relevant. This is particularly relevant for psychological treatments since these treatments have been established in high-income countries in distinctly dissimilar cultural contexts. A key example of a treatment viewed as unacceptable in contexts where local communities were unfamiliar with the approach was the use of talk therapy to address mental health problems. Service use by varied cultural groups is also influenced by stigma, competing work pressures, and low adherence often associated with costs due to time taken to attend sessions and the direct costs of transport to health facilities (Patel, Chowdhary, Rahman, & Verdeli, 2011). Ultimately, to both improve services rendered as well as health outcomes we need to:

- improve our understanding of the root causes of mental disorders;
- develop more effective prevention and early intervention strategies for global mental health that are grounded in evidence, are scalable, and can be shown to have an impact at the structural level;
- conduct research that incorporates a life-course approach recognizing the developmental origins of mental disorders;
- invest in research regarding the nature and treatment of mental disorders that is conducted in both high-income countries and in low- and middle-income countries;
- direct population-based studies that will help us to describe the phenotypes of mental disorders, as well as differences in the distribution of disorders between and within varied populations;
- intentionally engage in anti-stigma campaigns consistently and at multiple levels;
- acknowledge that mental health and environmental exposures, such as extreme poverty and war, are closely related to mental illness; and
- use a research framework that operationalizes principles of social justice and human rights.

(Tomlinson & Lund, 2012)

In summation, we must engage a diverse array of participants including mental health professionals and paraprofessionals, political advocates, global health activists, lay community workers, and individuals and families affected by mental disorders. This form of collective advocacy is needed when fighting for a common goal in order to guarantee that it stays in the foreground of global health efforts (Patel, 2012). Moreover, increasing community solidity and international governance structures need development to add to a more amalgamated voice concerning global mental health, reflecting the social determinants of health. A framework focused on integrated innovation is desirable so that global mental health communicates in a common language that is relevant to national and international policy-makers (Patel, 2012).

Recommendations

Mental health care that is culturally sensitive and respectful of the values, beliefs, and lifeways of patients requires providers who can serve as cultural brokers and change agents to reduce stigma related to psychiatric mental health disorders. Cultural brokers work within the culture of their patient populations to: (1) identify existing stigma related to psychiatric mental health disorders; (2) reduce stigma and its accompanying discrimination and discriminatory practices as much as possible; and most importantly (3) prevent continued stigma through developing, updating, and disseminating mental health education programs that are culturally relevant as well as empowering for the patient, their family, and their community. Change agents should partner with culturally diverse patients and patient populations to assist them in the development of a comprehensive assessment and plan that will preserve and respect their culture and decrease public, self, and structural stigma:

1 Consider culture and cultural influences on the values, lifeways, and behaviors of patients.
2 Promote patient empowerment and advocacy, as understood within diverse cultures and socioeconomic systems.

3   Engage with the immediate needs and agendas at hand in diverse communities.
4   Engage in anti-stigma activities that target consumers, communities, care providers, and policy makers.
5   Include health care education, as part of the overall treatment plan, including mental health care specific education, which is individualized to the patient's health care literacy needs, goals and cultural context.
6   Provide a plan for access to necessary information and culturally congruent resources for promoting, maintaining, sustaining mental health.
7   More effectively use the human capital available for providing mental health services through task shifting, management, and supervision of non-specialist mental health workers.
8   Use the economic, logistic, political and religious practices of the patient's culture and of the region to deliver culturally congruent treatment services.
9   Understand the political systems that regulate the transportation, economic, medical, and information services for the patient to provide relevant and congruent point of care treatment.
10 Support the patient's positive mental health, obtaining timely, effective treatment when needed, to preserve functional ability and overall productivity.
11 Protect the rights, responsibilities and decision-making of the patient.

Summary

An ecological model was used to guide the examination of the implications of culture and stigma on the mental health of populations, as well as the cultural-based attitudes, values, and beliefs that affect the responses of individuals and communities to these influences. Understanding cultural influences on patient behaviors as well as the provider's responses, improves the nurses' ability to best respond to patient needs, and to assist them in reaching their personal health goals. Therefore, being able to appreciate and understand the cultural context of individuals who receive mental health services is an essential professional competency.

Mental health is a social justice issue. Nursing practice must incorporate principles related to global mental health, including mental capital, social capital, access, equity, and political responsibility, in order to practice in a culturally relevant manner. Also, since stigma is a universally experienced occurrence that decreases access to mental health services and negatively affects mental health outcomes, each patient should be assessed for the effects of stigma. Nurses should advocate for the development and use of evidence-based mental health policies when practicing in countries that do not have a mental health policy or mental health plan. These proficiencies and skills are necessary for ethical practice.

Lastly, developing and maintaining sensitivity to, and respect for, the patient's culture-based attitudes, values, beliefs, and behaviors are lifelong tasks. Cultural competency is a process, not an end result, which requires motivation, self-awareness, and self-examination, a search for and use of knowledge, and a genuine desire to understand the patient from his/her perspective and experience. The culturally competent nurse provider of psychiatric and mental health care to facilitate assessment, interaction, education, and follow-up treatment should use local, national, and global resources. These resources include continuing education, support, and engagement from select mental health and nursing professional organizations, development and use of clinical guidelines for assessment and treatment, and ongoing feedback from the targeted population themselves. Use of these resources, coupled with nurses' understanding of and respect for the patient's cultural context is essential for delivery of comprehensive, appropriate mental health services, which include assessment, diagnosis, episodic and ongoing treatment, and long-term follow up with support and relevant linkages.

References

AACN Toolkit for master's and doctorate cultural competency in nursing education. (2011). American Association of College of Nursing. www.aacn.nche.edu/education-resources/Cultural_Competency_Toolkit_Grad.pdf.

About the World Psychiatric Association (WPA). (2013). http://wpanet.org/detail.php?section_id=5&content_id=4.

American Psychiatric Association. (2013a). *Diagnostic and Statistical Manual of Mental Disorders*. DSM-5. (5th ed.). Washington, DC: American Psychiatric Association.

American Psychiatric Association. (2013b). *Supplementary Modules to the Core Cultural Formulation Interview*. Washington, DC: American Psychiatric Association. www.psych.org/practice/dsm/dsm5/online-assessment-measures.

Arnault, D. (2009). Cultural determinants of help seeking: A model for research and practice. *Research Theory and Nursing Practice, 23*(4), 259–278.

Bos, A.E.R., Pryor, J.B., Reeder, G.D., & Stutterheim, S.E. (2013). Stigma: Advances in theory and research. *Basic and Applied Social Psychology, 35*(1). Doi: 10:1080/01973533.2012.746147.

Bronfenbrenner, U. (1979). *The Ecology of Human Development*. Cambridge, MA: Harvard University Press.

Bronfenbrenner, U. (1994). Ecological models of human development. *International Encyclopedia of Education, 3*(2), 1643–1647.

Bronfenbrenner, U. (Ed.). (2005). *Making Human Beings Human*. Thousand Oaks, CA: Sage.

Bryan C. & Morrow, C. (2011). Circumventing mental health stigma by embracing the warrior culture: Lessons learned from the Defender's Edge program. *Professional Psychology: Research and Practice, 42*(1), 16–23.

Corrigan, P. (2004). How stigma interferes with mental health care. *American Psychologist, 59*, 614–625.

Corrigan, P., Druss, B., & Perlick, D. (2014). The impact of mental illness stigma on seeking and participating in mental health care. *Psychological Science in the Public Interest, 15*(2), 37–70.

Cross-Border Care, Part 1. (2012). *Toronto Insider*. www.insidetoronto.com/community-story/46062-part-i-cross-border-care/.

Directive on Cross-Border Health Care Adopted. (2011). Council on the European Union. www.consilium.europa.eu/uedocs/cms_data/docs/pressdata/en/lsa/119514.pdf.

Douglas, M., Rosenkoetter, M., Hattar-Pollara, M., Lauderdale, J., Milstead, J., Nardi, D., & Purnell, L. (2014) Guidelines for implementing culturally competent nursing care. *Journal of Transcultural Nursing, 25*(109), 109–121.

Drew, N., Funk, M., Tang, S., Lamichhane, J., Chávez, E., Katontoka, S., Pathare, S., Lewis, O., Gostin, L., & Saraceno, B. (2011). Human rights violations of people with mental and psychosocial disabilities: An unresolved global crisis. *The Lancet, 378*, 1664–1675.

Guy, L. (2007). The ecological model: An overview for advocates. *Partners for social change, 9*(3), 1–6.

Hart-Waskeesikaw, F. (2009). *Cultural Competencies and Cultural Safety Nursing Education: A Framework for First Nation, Inuit and Métis Health Human Resources*. Ottawa, Ontario: Aboriginal Nurses Association of Canada. www.nurseone.ca/docs/NurseOne/FNIH%20Documents/B_CulturalCompetenceAndCulturalSafetyNsgEducation.pdf.

International Council of Nurses (ICN). (2006). *The ICN Code of Ethics for Nurses*. Geneva: Author. www.icn.ch/icncode.pdf.

International Council of Nurses (ICN). (2011). *Nurses and Human Rights*. www.icn.ch/images/stories/documents/publications/position_statements/E10_Nurses_Human_Rights.pdf.

International Council of Nurses (ICN). (2013). *About ICN*. www.icn.ch/about-icn/about-icn/.

Jenkins, R., Baingana, F., Ahmad, R., McDaid, D., & Atun, R. (2011). Mental health and the global agenda: Core conceptual issues. *Mental Health in Family Medicine, 8*(2), 69–82.

Jha, A., Kitchener, B., Pradhan, P., Shyangwa, P., & Nakarm, B. (2012). Mental Health First Aid Programme in Nepal. *Journal of Nepal Health Research Council, 10*(3), 258–260.

Kleinman, A. (2009). Global mental health: A failure of humanity. *The Lancet, 374*(9690), 603–604.

Kleintjes, S., Lund, C., & Flisher, A. (2010). A situational analysis of child and adolescent mental health services in Ghana, Uganda, South Africa, and Zambia. *African Journal of Psychiatry, 13*(2), 132–139.

Link, B.G., & Phelan, J.C. (2006). Stigma and its public health implications. *The Lancet, 367*, 528–529.

Mendenhall, E., De Silva, M., Hanton, C., Petersen, I., Shidhaye, R., Jordans, M., Luitel, N., Ssebunnya, J., Fekadu, A., Patel, V., Tomlinson, M., & Lund, C. (2014). Acceptability and feasibility of using non-specialist health workers to deliver mental health care: Stakeholder perceptions from the PRIME district sites in Ethiopia, India, Nepal, South Africa, and Uganda. *Social Science and Medicine, 118,* 33–42.

Multicultural Resource Centre. (2014). www.multiculturalmentalhealth.ca/clinical-tools/cultural-formulation/.

Myers, N. L. (2010). Culture, stress and recovery from schizophrenia: Lessons from the field for global mental health. *Culture, Medicine and Psychiatry, 34*(3), 500–28.

Nakajima, I. (2012) Cross border medical care and Telemedicine. *International Journal of E-Health and Telecommunications, 3*(1), para. 6. Doi: 10.4018/jehmc.2012010104.

Nardi, D., Waite, R. & Killian, P. (2012). Establishing standards for culturally competent mental health care. *Journal of Psychosocial Nursing and Mental Health Service, 50*(7), 3–5.

Ngui, E., Khasakhala, L. Ndetei, D., & Roberts, L. (2010). Mental disorders, health inequalities and ethics: A global perspective. *International Review of Psychiatry, 22*(3), 235–244.

Patel, V. (2012). Global mental health: From science to action. *Harvard Review of Psychiatry, 20*(1), 6–12.

Patel, N., Chowdhary, N., Rahman, A., & Verdeli, H. (2011). Improving access to psychological treatments: Lessons from developing countries. *Behavioral Research and Therapy, 49*(9), 523–528.

Pope, M., & Turner, S. (2009). North America's Native peoples: A social justice and trauma counseling approach. *Journal of Multicultural Counseling and Development, 37*(4), 194.

Schulz, A. & Medlin, C. (2007). Cross border health care plans. *Health Policy Monitor.* http://hpm.org/us/d7/4.pdf.

Trained Nurses Association of India. (2013). *Policy and position statement.* http://tnaionline.org/index.htm

Tomlinson, M., & Lund, C. (2012). Why does mental health not get the attention it deserves/an application of the Shiffman and Smith framework. *PLOS Medicine, 9*(2), e1001178.

United Nations. (2008). Office of the High Commissioner for Human Rights. *Universal Declaration of Human Rights: Dignity and Justice for All of Us.* www.un.org/en/universal-declaration-human-rights/.

Ward, M. (2011). *Turku Declaration: A Consensus Document on Psychiatric-Mental Health Nursing Roles, Education and Practice. Horatio-European Psychiatric Nurses.* www.horatio-web.eu/downloads/Horatio_Turku_Declaration_2011.pdf.

World Health Organization (WHO). (2013). Sixty-Sixth World Health Assembly. (May, 2013). *Comprehensive mental health action plan 2013–2020.* Document WHA66.8. http://apps.who.int/gb/ebwha/pdf_files/WHA66/A66_R8-en.pdf.

6

GLOBAL HEALTH ETHICS AND MENTAL HEALTH

Wendy Austin

Introduction

If ethics is "aiming at the 'good life' with and for others in just institutions," as suggested by philosopher Paul Ricoeur (1992, p. 192), how might we envision ethical action in a global community? What constitutes ethical health care when the moral horizon embraces the entire world? How do health professionals striving to be ethical re-orientate themselves to this broader understanding of their duties and responsibilities? The paramount risks to human health and well-being are now global ones with worldwide effects (Austin, 2001a). The undeniable interconnectedness of the global community, "There is no us and them anymore" (Ward, 2012, p. 6), requires a new way of thinking. The twenty-first century demands a global health ethic.

Within this new ethic, mental health may come "out of the shadows at last" (Kirby & Keon, 2006) and be recognized for its importance to human health and the global society. There is opportunity in this time of change to challenge the devastating discrimination associated with mental disorders that exists worldwide, injures the lives of many, and reaches to the level of governmental policy and funding. Health professionals can play a significant role in such a challenge. They will require an understanding of the language of global health ethics, of the current status of global mental health care, and of pressing ethical issues in the field of mental health. The goal for this chapter is to assist health professionals by identifying core concepts and key trends in global health ethics, relating them to mental health care, and providing some recommendations for action. It opens with an answer to what is global health ethics?

Global health ethics

"Global health ethics" is used with the emphasis on "global" to characterize health ethics issues related to global health phenomena and/or those that require action at a global level (Hunter & Dawson, 2011; Stapleton, Schröder-Bäck, Laaser, Meershoek, & Popa, 2014). Pandemics are a good example of such an issue. Global health ethics is also used with the emphasis on "ethics" to refer to a field of study within bioethics (Hunter & Dawson, 2011). This field's interests are wide-ranging, from health inequities to human cloning. Neither of these conceptualizations of global health ethics, however, fully embraces the reality that the world has become one community, a global village (McLuhan & Powers, 1989). The view from space has dramatically shown us that we reside together with other living things on one small planet.

Globalization is essentially a social process in which the social and cultural aspects of life are no longer powerfully shaped by geographical boundaries and constraints (Waters, 1995). Economic globalization has become a force impacting every nation (Friedman, 1999); the diversity created by the migration of people across the globe is transforming societies (Robertson, 2003). Threats to well-being in one part of the world (e.g., poverty, armed conflicts/terrorism, environmental degradation, political crises, corruption, as well as epidemics) can have significant consequences for others geographically distant. The key question of law—"What rules do we need to promote a peaceful and fair society?"—now requires a global answer (Andorno, 2009, p. 224). The World Economic Forum's *Global Risks* (2013) identifies water and food crises, increased incidence of extreme weather events, severe income disparity, and high un/under-employment as among the top 10 risks facing the global community. These are all threats to human health and health is high on the world's political agenda (Harman, 2012).

A global health ethics is needed that can provide moral guidance to world health systems and governance (Velji & Bryant, 2014). Is it possible, however, to achieve such an ethic given the diversity of human languages and cultures and the disparities in wealth and health? How may the current deficiencies in global governance be overcome? Finding answers will require significant worldwide dialogue and exploration. There are core concepts that are key to the vocabulary of global health ethics and to its evolution. They are introduced in the next section.

Core concepts in global health ethics

Although telecommunication allows us to connect quickly across great distances (at least for those with access), genuinely connecting across the diverse cultural, political, religious, and language differences of the global village remains highly challenging. There are, however, some elements that have significance across diversity and that are serving as components of a framework for a global health ethic. These include human dignity, human rights, social responsibility, social justice, and global health governance.

The universality of human dignity

The fundamental unity of human beings—made scientifically evident by the decoding of the human genome—and the inherent dignity of each member of the human family have been primary assumptions in international rights and ethics documents. Law and ethics scholar, Roberto Andorno (2009) finds that, when paired with human rights (which are grounded upon human dignity), the overarching principle of respect for human dignity provides a practical way to address bioethics issues at a global level. It is the best grounding for international biomedical legal standards. Nevertheless, the notion of "human dignity" is not universally accepted. It is considered by some health ethicists as a "useless concept" because it is "hopelessly vague" (Macklin, 2003, p. 1420). To date, there is no broadly accepted definition of human dignity in the global health ethics literature. Mark Lagon and Anthony Arend (2014), however, have developed a working definition by drawing from the many traditions that acknowledge human dignity: it is "the fundamental agency of human beings to apply their gift to thrive" (p. 16). It rests, they note, on the notions of "agency" (i.e., the capability of achieving one's potential) and "respect" (i.e., recognition that each person has inherent worth and a claim to equal opportunity). For human dignity to be meaningful, they argue, it must be "institutionalized in practice and governance" (Lagon & Arend, 2014, p. 16). Human dignity is fundamental to the concept of human rights.

Human rights

Human rights have become a language that makes engagement across the human community on fundamental issues possible (Ignatieff, 2001). "Human rights" reflect values that are based on the assumption that every human being has natural rights; that is, human individuals can make certain claims based entirely on their humanness (Austin, 2001b). In 1948 the United Nations' (UN) Universal Declaration of Human Rights (UDHR) formalized the recognition of every person's inherent freedom and equality in dignity and rights (UN General Assembly, 1948). The UDHR makes the respecting, protecting, and fulfilling of human rights the responsibility of nation states.

Within the UDHR, health is conceptualized as a right, moving it beyond a narrower medical perspective and emphasizing its social determinants. In Article 25 of the UDHR, the *right to health* is described as:

> The right to a standard of living adequate for the health and well-being of him [or her] and his [or her] family, including food, clothing, housing, and medical care and necessary social services, and the right to security in the event of unemployment, sickness, disability, widowhood, old age, or other lack of livelihood in circumstances beyond his [or her] control.
>
> *(UN General Assembly, 1948)*

Once a nation ratifies (i.e., formally approves) the UDHR, it is required to report to the UN on the ways in which it promotes the health of its people. In many respects, the UDHR remains aspirational. Although it is considered binding and nations are to monitor their progress in upholding the rights of their people, it is difficult to hold nations accountable. The UDHR lacks "enforcement machinery" (Benatar, 1998, p. 297). It does have rhetorical force, given that violations of the rights proclaimed within it are imbued with shame (Austin, 2001b).

Additional human rights instruments continue to be created. For instance, the International Covenant on Economic, Social and Cultural Rights (ICESCR) (UN, 1966) addresses not only the "right of everyone to the highest attainable standard of physical and mental health" (Article 12), but the right to many of the social determinants of health, such as an adequate standard of living, education, and social security. Freedoms related to health (e.g., right to be free from non-consensual or degrading treatment) and entitlements (e.g., access to essential medicines; right to have diseases prevented, treated, and controlled; equal and timely access to basic health services) are identified (OHCHR & WHO, 2008). A basic issue with such instruments is that they are not necessarily ratified (i.e. formally approved) by all nations. The United States, for example, signed the ICESCR in 1977, but has never ratified it.

Direct references to the right to health appear in the 1989 Convention on the Rights of the Child (e.g., the right to treatment and rehabilitation facilities; the requirement that states take measures to abolish traditional practices prejudicial to children's health). The 2006 Convention on the Rights of Persons with Disabilities, grounded upon a social model of disability, identifies what societies need to do to address social exclusion and defines the entitlements of persons living with disabilities, including psychosocial disability (UN, 2006). The Universal Declaration of the Human Genome and Human Rights, endorsed by the UN in 1998, addresses such issues as the potential for genetic discrimination and the implications of interventions (e.g., research, treatment, diagnosis) on a person's genome. The fact is that most, perhaps all, human rights instruments are relevant to the right to health: health is dependent on rights fulfillment.

The Declaration of Bioethics and Human Rights

In 2005, the Declaration of Bioethics and Human Rights (DBHR) was developed by the UN's Educational, Scientific and Cultural Organization (UNESCO) (UNESCO, 2005). Created by using principles of bioethics within a human rights framework, it is a legal (but nonbinding) instrument that addresses "ethical issues related to medicine, life sciences and associated technologies as applied to human beings, taking into account their social, legal and environmental dimensions" (UNESCO, 2005, p. 76). Upheld are the equality of all human beings in dignity and rights, their right to be treated justly without discrimination, the solidarity of the human community, and respect for diversity and pluralism. Humanity's interconnection with other living things is addressed along with its role in protecting the environment. There is emphasis on the sharing of scientific and technological benefits and specific goals related to access to quality health care and essential medicines. Reaction to this Declaration has ranged from appreciation of its achievement to profound doubt of its (Andorno, 2009) or any universal declaration's (Benatar, 2005) value. Specific articles are challenged, such as Article 3b, which states that the interest of individuals are of greater importance than the interests of science and society, a claim that is not universally accepted (Landman & Schüklenk, 2005) and that can be perceived as counter to some public health initiatives, like quarantine.

Social responsibility

Responsibility can be defined as "a moral obligation to behave correctly towards or in respect of a person or thing" ("Responsibility," 2014). The concept of social responsibility resides in the belief that individuals, organizations, communities, and governments have an ethical obligation to act in ways that support, not harm the well-being of their society. In a global society, how is social responsibility understood? The *cosmopolitan* perspective considers every individual as a world citizen who has a moral duty to assist others in need without proximity or nationality being a factor. The opposing or *anti-cosmopolitan* perspective regards morality as local and specific, delimited within a culture or community (e.g., a nation), although peaceful co-existence has moral worth (Stapleton *et al.*, 2014).

These perspectives are reflected in approaches to social responsibility known as the *humanitarian approach* and the *statist approach* (Toumi, 2014). The latter is congruent with the anti-cosmopolitan perspective: governments' responsibilities are for the well-being of their own citizens. It is acknowledged that interactions between states can create moral obligations, such as when one state's actions negatively impact the citizens of another (e.g., an oil spill caused by one state's shipping affects the environment of another). There is a "negative duty" not to harm the other, but there can be no expectation (i.e., "positive duty") that one state should help another, such as during a natural disaster. To do so is supererogatory (i.e. charity): no moral duty exists (Toumi, 2014). What is not acknowledged in this approach is the interdependence of contemporary states (Toumi, 2014). In the humanitarian perspective, location is not a factor (Lowry & Schüklenk, 2009). Those who are prosperous and able to do so have a moral obligation (a positive duty) to help those in need, as the dignity and worth (i.e., moral status) of each person is the same. Not acknowledged is the reality of competing interests, exploitive actions, and mutual hostilities that currently occur between nations (Toumi, 2014).

The drowning child in a shallow pond

Moral philosopher, Peter Singer (1997) created a scenario for his students to imagine. One morning on their way to class as they pass a shallow pond, they see a child is drowning.

Do they have any obligation to rescue the child? His students invariably believe that they do: there is no excuse not to do so. Muddy shoes and being late for class are trivial in comparison. Singer points out that everyone is in this position: we can save the lives of distant children at risk of dying of hunger or illness at little cost and no danger to ourselves by contributing to humanitarian aid. Why is this rescue not as morally necessary? Singer's scenario has become a classic metaphor regarding global moral obligation.

Singer's humanitarian position—that those who have "surplus" resources should use them to help those living in poverty—is supported by others like Peter Unger, author of *Living High and Letting Die: Our Illusion of Innocence* (1996), but some reject it entirely (Wisor, 2011). Neera Badhwar (2006), for example, finds the expectations of Singer and Unger to be "incompatible with that which makes life worth living: the pursuit of happiness" (p. 74) and against common sense. But what if we have metaphorically pushed the child into the pond? Thomas Pogge (2002) argues that this is the real case and thus responding with aid is a negative duty. He finds that systemic economic and political strategies have created poverty and that, not only should we harm less but we should help more, given that about one-third of the 18 million human deaths each year are due to preventable, poverty-related causes such as poor nutrition, unsafe water, and lack of vaccines, antibiotics, and other medicines. Globally, severe poverty could be eradicated with little economic cost: the rich half of the world's population would have to make do with 1 percent less of the global household income (96 percent rather than 97 percent). That this does not happen is to Pogge "morally indefensible" (2002, p. 241).

Solidarity

Solidarity has been named as the most important of all values for global health ethics (Benatar, Daar, & Singer, 2003). Without an attitude of unity, caring, and mutual support, it is possible that distant indignities, rights violations, injustices, and disparities will be ignored. A sense of solidarity evolves as we expand our capacity for empathy, that is, our ability to recognize the pain, degradation, and suffering of others and know that it matters to us (Rorty, 1999; Benatar, Daar, & Singer, 2003). The "sentiments of mutual belonging and of shared responsibility for the common future" and the "willingness to find amicable and enduring solutions" to conflicts are essential aspects of human solidarity (Bauman, 2008, p. 250). The sociologist, Zygmunt Bauman (2008) notes that acknowledgement of "the logic of global responsibility" is necessary to the addressing of planet-wide problems, but it takes us to where humankind has never been (2008, p. 252). As well, this necessary but formidable shift in thinking needs to take place in the early twenty-first century at a time when market capitalism is dominating most societies. The corporatization of society—termed "The McDonaldization of society" by sociologist George Ritzer (1993)—supports, at most, non-cosmopolitan approaches to responsibility. The worth of solidarity is negated. It seems that, for the vision of global solidarity among strangers to be realized as called for in the DBHR, the notion of the world as a collection of individual consumers must first be overcome.

Social justice

Social justice is fundamentally "the fair distribution of society's benefits and responsibilities and their consequences" (CNA, 2006, p. 7). Although not made an explicit goal of the UN until 1990, social justice has always been a prime concern, as evidenced in the articles of the UDHR. It needs to be: "Social injustice is killing people on a grand scale" (CSDH, 2008, p. 26). It creates risk for all, leading as it may to serious conflict within and between nations and/or the impediment of meaningful societal progress. Examination of social justice involves determination of the extent of population disparities, their causes, and potential strategies to eliminate them (CNA, 2006). Poverty is a crucial measure. It is estimated, based on multidimensional measures of poverty that 1.5 billion people in 91 countries live in poverty, along with the associated deprivations in living standards, health, and education (UN Development Programme, 2014). There exists great and rapidly growing economic disparity in the world: "The wealth of the world is divided in two; almost half going to the richest 1 percent; the other half to the remaining 99 percent" (Oxfam, 2014, p. 1). This widening of disparities is a major global trend that threatens social stability within nations, as well as global security (World Economic Forum, 2013). This widening gap between rich and poor is in urgent need of solutions. It underscores the call for international consensus on achieving universal social protection that is the focus of the 2014 UN Development Report.

Health equity

Equity is about fairness and "the just treatment of individuals in their own social context" (CNA, 2006, p. 8). Equity in health is about the fair opportunity to obtain one's full health potential. Although differences in health potential will always exist due to biological causes (e.g., genetics, age, gender), other differentials in health are preventable or remediable. Equity in health care is about "equal access to available care for equal need"; "equal utilization of care for equal need," and "equal quality of care for all" (Whitehead, 1992, p. 221). Inequity in health care is highly visible as when individuals who are members of a high-income population receive prolonged biomedical treatments supported by advanced technology to sustain their lives even when such treatments are of little benefit or futile, while others with less income struggle to meet basic needs or sustain their health (Benatar, 2013).

Addressing inequities in health and health care can be difficult. The Global Strategy of Health for All by the Year 2000, initiated by the World Health Assembly in 1981, failed to achieve its goals. Although the greatest threats to health are poverty, population growth, depletion of natural resources, global warming, and new and emerging infectious diseases, too often an international health approach (i.e., focused predominately on biomedical health care assistance) is taken in addressing health inequities, rather than a global health approach with its focus on health for all (Benatar, 2013). In 2008, the WHO's Commission on the Social Determinants of Health recommended three strategies be implemented for "Closing the Gap" in health equity: "improve daily living conditions"; "tackle inequitable distribution of power, money, and resources"; "measure and understand the problem and assess impact of action" (CSDH, 2008, p. 2).

Research is vital for closing the gap in health equity, but the reality is that significant imbalances and gaps exist in the field of health research itself (Pang, 2011). In 1990 the Commission on Health Research for Development reported results of a worldwide survey of health research, coining the term "10/90 gap" for the disparities found: only 10 per cent of the world's health resources are used for research into 90 per cent of the world's health problems (Ramsay, 2001). A decade later, The Global Forum for Health Research, the worldwide research network created as a response to the report, found that despite total funding increases, the disparities gap remained much the same (Ramsay, 2001). Although the "10/90 gap" is not currently accurate in a quantitative sense, the resources for health research on the needs of low- and middle-income countries remain extremely inadequate (Global Health Forum, 2011). Disparities exist, not only in funding for health, but disparities in access to the benefits of research, opportunities for using research outcomes effectively, and in research capacity development (Pang, 2011). Tikki Pang

(2011), Director of Research and Cooperation at the WHO argues for a new global health research agenda, one guided by key criteria that include: inclusiveness in setting priorities, balance between generation/utilization of knowledge and between new interventions/improvement of health systems, and equitable access to "the fruits of research" (p. 288). To make this agenda a reality will be a matter of good governance (Pang, 2011).

Global governance for health

Global governance for health has evolved over the last three centuries. It has moved from international standards developed to oversee sanitation and trade-related health issues and the work of non-governmental agencies in times of emergencies and conflicts (e.g., International Committee of the Red Cross) to institutions formed at the end of WWII (e.g., the World Health Organization (WHO), other UN agencies like UNICEF, and the World Bank) (Harman, 2012). The WHO has been the primary UN institution overseeing global health, with all nations as members. For global health issues, the WHO has "unrivalled normative authority, global influence, and legal powers" (Sridhar & Gostin, 2014, p. 117).

Governance for global health and global health research, however, increasingly involves complex public–private partnerships, such as The Global Fund, based in Geneva, which includes governments, civil society, and the private sector in a fight to end AIDS, TB and malaria (Harman, 2012). While these new partnerships mobilize awareness, monies, and expertise, they tend to focus predominately on one disease and are responsible only to their funders. Like celebrities, also new actors in global governance for health, they are not the best source for global health agenda setting (Harman, 2012), which requires addressing human resources, global health infrastructure, and the social, economic and environmental determinants of disease (Cooper, Kirton, & Stevenson, 2009). The WHO is having to adapt to a shifting global environment and the reality that health is critically influenced by policies made in other areas, such as environment, trade, and migration (Frenk & Moon, 2013). It may be losing its ability to set the global health agenda (Lidén, 2014).

Julio Frenk and Suerie Moon (2013), experts in global governance for health, identify four essential functions of the global health system: "production of global public goods" (e.g., research and development; standards); "management of externalities across countries" (e.g., surveillance and information sharing); "mobilization of global solidarity" (e.g., financing, technical cooperation); and "stewardship" (priority setting, mutual accountability) (p. 940). Their indicators for good governance in this area are "effectiveness, equity, efficiency in achieving outcomes" along with "credibility and legitimacy" in how decisions are made (Frenk & Moon, 2013, p. 939). A critical issue for current global governance is that there is no global government. The tools for collective action at national levels (e.g., taxation, democratic procedures, law enforcement), for the most part, do not—as yet—exist for the global village (Frenk & Moon, 2013).

Global health diplomacy

With the recognition that political and economic stability requires healthy populations, health has increasingly become a priority in states' foreign policy, security, and trade concerns. This has fostered the WHO's concept of *global health diplomacy*. This form of diplomacy encompasses negotiations about key systemic changes that impact global public health and is based on understanding health as a human right and as global public good. It offers a new lens through which to perceive the landscape of global health and foreign relations (Kickbusch, Novotny, Drager, Silberschmidt, & Alcazar, 2007).

Ethics and global mental health

Consideration of the core concepts of global health ethics in their application to mental health and mental health care allows for a portrait of the current global ethical issues in this area to be created. Thus, human dignity, human rights, social responsibility, social justice, and global governance for health will frame the following discussion of the status of the ethics of global mental health (GMH). Prior to this discussion, however, it is important to note that consensus has not been achieved on the worth of a global approach to mental health. Against the scientific arguments (from human biology, epidemiology, evidence-based medicine) and the ethical arguments (universality of human dignity and rights, health equity) for a global frame of reference in mental health are opposing perspectives that claim GHM primarily supports the expansion of Western psychiatry, medical empiricism, and the pharmaceutical industry (Summerfield, 2012) and/or that mental health is so contingent upon the "local" (i.e., ethno-cultural, social, community aspects) that a global approach is highly inappropriate (Bemme & D'souza, 2014). In their cogent presentation of such arguments regarding GMH, Doerte Bemme and Nicole D'souza (2014) move beyond them to suggest that GMH, conceived as situated within global health (not psychiatry) with a pluralistic vision of knowledge, an understanding of "community" as varying in scale (i.e., local to global), and emphasizing multidisciplinarity, may be explored for meaningful responses to a suffering humanity. The Movement for Global Mental Health (a coalition of institutions and individuals in over 100 countries) stipulates that appropriate mental health services are essential to every prosperous and humane society and that ensuring the rights of persons with mental disorders must become a top priority (Patel, Boyce, Collins, Saxena, & Horton, 2011). Ensuring the right of persons with mental disorders to lives of dignity is fundamental to global health ethics.

Human dignity

Persons with mental health challenges and disorders face—even in high-income countries—social exclusion, violations of their human rights, barriers to accessing effective care, and challenges in sustaining or improving their standard of living. This situation has been called "a global emergency on a par with the greatest human rights scandals" (Patel, 2011, p. 1441) and "a failure of humanity" (Kleinman, 2009, p. 603). Recognition that this failure is fundamentally a matter of ethics will be important to success in addressing it. In fact, Arthur Kleinman, a global mental health expert, argues that it will require a "moral transformation" as it is due to "prejudice, discrimination and lack of political will to commit adequate resources" (Kleinman, 2009, p. 603).

Research on mental health stigma in the global context (across 16 countries) reveals that, even in countries with low overall stigma, prejudice was associated with issues dealing with intimate settings (e.g. the family), vulnerable groups (e.g., children), and self-harm; there was unwillingness to have persons with mental disorders in positions of authority, uneasiness about interactions with them and about potential for violence. The researchers concluded that anti-stigma initiatives need to address tolerance and inclusion at a cultural level (Pescosolido, Medina, Martin, & Long, 2013). This appears to be true within the culture of health care services itself (see Chapter 5 for additional information about stigma).

Many persons with mental disorders, in numbers sufficient to form national and international organizations, call themselves "survivors." They are not referring to surviving their illness, as a person with cancer or cardiac disease may, they are saying that they have survived their treatment and care (Austin, Bergum, & Nuttgens, 2004). Responsive mental health services must evolve so that the changing needs of persons with mental disorders, from in-patient services for acute symptoms to community support for dealing with life constraints are addressed (Frese, Stanley, Kress, & Vogel-Scibilia, 2001). A review and synthesis of consumer literature (Horsfall, 2003), however, indicates that there is insufficient inclusion of health services requested by persons living with mental disorders and that persons using existing health services feel that professionals define them primarily by their diagnosis (Horsfall, 2003). Quality relationships with helpers is a key concern, as are related concerns of choice, individuality, and information (Edwards, 2000). Users of mental health services want to be heard (Hamilton & Roper, 2006; Happell, Manias, & Roper, 2004) and to be taken seriously (Edwards, 2000). The WHO asserts that primary care for mental health can reduce stigma and discrimination as persons with mental disorders are treated like those with other conditions and see the same health workers. Such commonality affects the perception of mental health problems and disorders by the persons experiencing them, their families and community, and by health workers who have become better educated and experienced in their care and treatment (WHO & Wonca, 2008).

The incarceration of persons with mental disorders in prisons and jails is a serious problem across the globe, with the mentally ill prisoner being doubly stigmatized (Chaimowitz, 2012). Treatment within correctional institutions can be poor or nonexistent. Correctional officers are usually not trained to provide mental health care; and some prisoners with mental disorders may be unable to adjust to a highly structured, rule-driven environment. Too often the strategies available for keeping the mentally ill prisoner safe involve segregation, seclusion, or restraints (Peternelj-Taylor, 2008). Persons with psychosocial disability are made incredibly vulnerable within prisons and jails; they need to be treated by the least restrictive means and their dignity preserved (Okasha, 2004). If societies are judged on their treatment of their most vulnerable members, then the mentally ill person under forensic purview will be a touchstone for evaluating the state of the global society as it evolves.

Embracing human dignity as a true value in global mental health care, rather than as a platitude, has the potential to support mental health professionals to work in genuine partnership with persons with mental disorders, their families and communities. Through mutual respect, the moral transformation called for by Kleinman (2009) can begin to be realized at the grassroots level. To secure the necessary political will to overcome the threats to human dignity from prejudice and discrimination, such stigma may need to be conceived and confronted as a human rights issue (Mehta & Thornicroft, 2014).

Human rights

Health law scholar, Lawrence Gostin (2001) points out that human rights is an important approach to global mental health because it encompasses two fundamental ideas: "human rights is the only source of law that legitimizes international scrutiny of mental health policies and practices within a sovereign country" and "human rights do not rely on government beneficence" (p. 264). As rights are possessed on the basis of one's humanity, a government cannot grant nor deny them but can be made accountable for violations of rights under international law. Gostin proposes that using human rights doctrine is a stronger response to advancing the dignity and welfare of persons with mental (psychosocial) disability than a health approach, as it is enforceable. He underscores three connections between mental health and human rights: human rights can be violated by mental health policies, programs, and practices; mental health is adversely affected by rights violations; and rights and mental health are complementary approaches to a flourishing human life (Gostin, 2001). As well as an instrument for advancing the civil and political rights and freedoms of persons with mental disability (e.g., areas related to liberty, privacy, and autonomy), human rights can support "the right to health" (Gostin, 2001). As noted previously in this chapter, duties related to upholding economic, social, and cultural rights, including the right to health, are imposed on nations by the ICESCR. For the right to health to be globally generalized, governments who have yet to ratify this covenant will need to do so.

Assistance for governments in developing and adopting strategies to protect the rights of people with mental disorders, particularly through mental health legislation, is provided by WHO through the Mental Health and Human Rights Project. Guidance materials include an international network of experts, a "checklist" for reviewing existing laws, technical support to countries, and a WHO (2005) *Resource Book on Mental Health, Human Rights and Legislation*. The latter is primarily a resource for those working with legislation, but is an excellent resource for health professionals as it includes details of human rights instruments and standards relevant to mental health. Mental health law can enable health policy to be developed, conceptually framed, and enforced, thus helping to ensure

> the establishment of high quality mental health facilities and services; access to quality mental health care; protection of human rights; patients' right to treatment; the development of robust procedural protections; the integration of persons with mental disorders into the community; and promotion of mental health throughout society.
>
> *(WHO, 2005, p. 4)*

Advocacy for the rights of persons living with disability is a global priority, recognized by the UN with the *Convention of the Rights of Persons with Disability* (UN General Assembly, 2007), an explicit acknowledgement of rights to respect, dignity, and an optimal quality of life. From the WHO's perspective, mental disorders are not synonymous with disability but persons with mental disorders may be considered to have a disability if they are experiencing the disorder as a long-term impairment that negatively affects their societal participation because of physiological and/or social constraints (WHO, 2005).

What do human rights mean to persons who have a psychosocial disability? Users of mental health services in low- and middle-income countries, self-identified as having a mental or psychosocial disability, describe human rights as ensuring "basic needs" are met, "human dignity" respected, and "freedom" to have a "decent life" as participants in society are upheld (Drew *et al.*, 2011, p. 1665–6). Their major concerns were identified as lack of access to basic mental health care and "ill treatment and abuse by health workers" (Drew *et al.*, 2011, p. 1664). Alleged human rights violations in mental health care reported to the Office of the United Nation's High Commissioner for Human Rights (OHCHR) include: poor conditions in psychiatric facilities, inadequate nutrition and sanitation, abusive treatment of patients, and persecution of health professionals due to their professional activities (OHCHR & WHO, 2008, p. 39). Further, the Pan American Health Organization (PAHO) finds that problems in psychiatric institutions in many countries involve "completely unregulated involuntary admission of patients"; "little control over the use of physical restraints or isolation of patients"; and "problems with court-ordered confinement of people with supposed mental disorders who have committed unlawful or criminal acts" (PAHO, 2009, p. 7). These are very serious threats to or violations of human rights. Yet, across low-, middle-, and high-income countries, the physical, mental, and emotional abuse of persons with mental disorders in hospitals and social care facilities goes underreported, making it "a hidden human rights emergency" (WHO, 2012,¶1). Such a state of affairs requires an urgent response by governments.

To support effective response, the WHO has initiated "WHO QualityRights: act, unite and empower for mental health" and a "QualityRights Toolkit" to assess and improve care and human rights in health and social care facilities (O'Hara, 2012). The focus is on five human rights: the right to an adequate standard of living and social protection; enjoyment of the highest attainable standard of physical and mental health; to exercise legal capacity and to personal liberty and the security of person; as well as freedom from torture or cruel, inhumane or degrading treatment or punishment and from exploitation, violence and abuse; and the right to live independently and be included in the community (WHO, 2012, Table 3, ¶2).

In 2013 on Human Rights Day, December 10 another WHO resource for mental health was launched: MINDbank (WHO, n.d.). Part of the Quality Rights initiative, it is an online platform with national and international resources related to mental health, addiction, disability, and human rights. Its purpose is to facilitate dialogue, advocacy, and research that support nations' reform of policies, laws, and service standards so that they are in line with international best practices and human rights.

The global acknowledgement of the grave situation in mental health care with regards to human rights violation and the new resources being developed to enable governments to address them are creating a more hopeful future for persons with mental disorders and their families and for the health professionals who strive to work in partnership with them to provide appropriate quality care.

Social responsibility

Social responsibility in a global society encompasses, at the very least, all of humanity. The Global Health Movement holds the assumption that humanity transcends geographical, statist, cultural boundaries, and that it is a moral imperative to act in response to the prejudice, discrimination, and inequities that threaten the dignity and rights of persons with mental disorders (Bemme & D'souza, 2014). Yet such responsibility may be staggering in its scope. Moral responsibility can be, as Bauman says, "cumbersome, incapacitating, joy-killing," and "insomnogenic" (1993, p. 242). When one recognizes the depth and span of social injustice, it can be "deeply unsettling," and "disorientating" (Harbin, 2014, p. 162). The philosopher, Ami Harbin (2014) points out that when responsibilities are very complex, require moral action at many levels, and when there is no assurance that a sufficient response exists, the ordinary agent may be overwhelmed and lose motivation to act. But disorientation does not need to overwhelm, she argues, when one can identify projects suiting one's capabilities, learn how to negotiate calls to act, and discover how to sustain one's motivation for doing so.

It may be that accepting the essential messiness of the ethical demand is a necessary wisdom, particularly for the global citizen. That wisdom and the knowledge that social responsibility is about interdependence and collectivity may sustain health professionals as they attempt to respond locally to global social injustice. They possess the asset of being experienced agents of social change. For example, nursing, like other health professions with a fiduciary (faithful) relationship with the public, has always held social responsibility as an obligation (Tyer-Viola *et al.*, 2009).

A tool for health professionals who are resisting disorientation at the extent of mental health injustices is Iris Young's (2006) social connection model of responsibility. Responsibility in this model is delineated by virtue of social roles (e.g., nurse, teacher, physician, citizen) and understood as shared with others. Young advises individuals to reflect upon structural injustices (i.e., morally unacceptable conditions) and decide what they can do. She offers a guide to such reflection: consideration of *interest, power, privilege,* and *collective ability.* One needs to choose where one's interest for action most strongly lies. What injustice seems most urgent to remedy? It might be the lack of mental health literacy in one's community or the need for housing for persons with a severe and persistent mental disorder. Both are global issues that can be impacted by local actions. What is one's potential to influence or effect positive change in this chosen interest? While a celebrity like Bono (singer and rock music group lead) is able to meet with world leaders and Angelina Jolie (movie star) can access the media to speak to millions, an individual health professional's options—writing a letter to the editor of a local or national newspaper, addressing the members of one's professional organization, contacting a government representative, or joining others to act collectively—may be more limited but can still be effective in making a difference. In what way is one privileged, that is, able to act without deprivation or negative consequences? For example, has one's education provided the knowledge and skills to support persons with psychosocial disability and their families to act themselves to effect change? Is a particular issue of injustice more readily addressed than another due to one's existing roles, connections, influence, or organizational membership? A group of nurse educators in a high-income country, for example, may be able to partner with nurse educators in a low- or middle-income county to assist them in developing particular mental health skills, resources, or research and, in turn, learn from them about their situation and challenges. This social connection approach can be a platform for health professionals to act on their social responsibility for mental health in a realistic, sustainable, and hopeful way.

Social justice

Mental, neurological, and substance (MNS) disorders are estimated, using the 2010 Global Burden of Disease (GBD) data, to be the leading cause of Years-Lived-with-Disability (Whiteford *et al.*, 2013). The GBD is an economic parameter calculated using the DALY (disability-adjusted-life-year), a measure of years of life lost to premature death and to time lived without full health (Murray & Lopez, 1996). Because mental health problems and disorders are nearly invisible when mortality rate is the statistic used, the GBD has been of major import in measuring the true toll of mental disorders in national and global contexts (Desjarlais, Eisenberg, Good, & Kleinman, 1995). It is now known that MNS disorders contribute nearly 14 percent of the GBD (Kleinman, 2013). The startling fact remains, however, that MNS disorders still receive less than 1 percent of health care services funding in most low- and middle-income countries, The *mental health treatment gap* (i.e., the difference between the prevalence of a disorder and the proportion of persons with it who receive treatment) remains large, even in high-income countries, where it is estimated that only one-third of persons with mood disorders get treated; in low-income countries the estimate is 1 in 10 (Eaton, De Silva, Rojas, & Patel, 2014).

The degree and effect of insufficient resources can be seen by examining a core component of mental health care—human resources. When the human resources for mental health were analyzed in 58 low- and middle-income countries, all but three had insufficient numbers of nurses in mental health settings and 93 percent of low-income countries and 59 percent of middle-income countries had a shortage of psychiatrists (Scheffler, 2011). Often those working in mental health services lack training in psychiatric clinical skills and ethics, making quality of care a serious problem (Kleinman, 2013). Investment in the global mental health workforce is urgently needed and represents a significant gap that must be addressed.

Unfortunately, mental health remains at the bottom of public health priorities everywhere, its importance unrecognized by policy makers, funders, and the public, mainly due to the stigma associated with mental illness (Caldas de Almeida, Minas, & Cayetano, 2014). Along with this substantial barrier and lack of trained workforce, other barriers to progress on just access to humane, effective mental health care include: the "complexity of and resistance to decentralization of mental health services," challenges to mental health integration into primary care settings, and insufficient public health perspectives in mental health leadership (Saraceno *et al.*, 2007, p. 1164).

According to the WHO, health systems must strive to meet legitimate expectations on the non-health aspects of health care across the domains of dignity, prompt attention, autonomy, choice of health care provider, clear communication, confidentiality, quality of basic amenities, and access to social support networks. Although *responsiveness* is highly relevant to mental health care services because of the "specific dependency and vulnerability" of its users, (Bramesfeld, Klippel, Seidel, Schwartz, & Dierks, 2007, p. 880), it may be a greater challenge to achieve there than anywhere else, given the prevailing barriers to care.

The increased vulnerability of users of mental health services is related not only to the devastating effect of mental health problems and mental disorders, and the associated stigma, but often also due to poverty. Poverty appears to be both a determinant and a consequence of poor mental health. Vijaya Murali & Femi Oyebode (2004) note that psychiatric conditions occur at higher rates in the world's poorest, with unemployment significantly increasing the risk for psychiatric disorders. There is epidemiological evidence that an inverse relationship exists globally between social class and mental illness. The reasons for this may be the downward social drift caused by the consequences of having a mental disorder; that the socio-economic adversity of lower-class living precipitates mental illness; or that persons from the lower social class have less mental health literacy and/or less access to effective treatment and services compared to those in higher social classes (Murali & Oyebode, 2004). There is evidence that "low education, food insecurity, inadequate housing, low social class, low socio-economic status and financial stress" are positively correlated with some mental disorders (e.g., depression, anxiety disorders) (Lund, 2014, p. 136).

The neglect of mental health in the global health arena is so extreme as to be unconscionable. It is noteworthy that Sophie Harman in her work, *Global Health Governance* (2012), when arguing that issues like HIV/AIDS and pandemic flu dominate global health to the neglect of other health priorities, fails to even mention mental health in her chapter, "Neglected Health." Despite the WHO slogan, "there is no health without mental health," authentic acceptance of this fact continues to be elusive. Indeed, it was in 1948 that the WHO's first director, Dr Brock Chisholm, a psychiatrist, stipulated that without mental health there is no true physical health (Kolappa, Henderson, & Kishore, 2013). Although it can be challenging to remain optimistic regarding positive change in this arena, strong and effective global governance for health offers a pathway to hope.

Global governance for health

Barriers to actualizing ethical, quality mental health care across the globe can seem insurmountable. However, much will be accomplished if the WHO Mental Health Action Plan 2013–2020 is fully enacted and its objectives met. These objectives involve strengthening leadership and governance; providing comprehensive, integrated, and responsive mental health and social care in community-based settings; implementing promotion and prevention in mental health; and strengthening information systems, evidence, and research (WHO, 2013). In the last two decades, resources have been created that can support the Action Plan, including *The World Health Report 2001: Mental Health: New Understanding, New Hope* (WHO, 2001); mhGAP intervention guidelines (WHO, 2010); informed calls for action by world experts in mental health (see *The Lancet* series on global mental health in 2007, 2011); the Grand Challenges in Mental Health research initiative (Collins *et al.*, 2011, 2013); and the Movement for Global Mental Health (Patel *et al.*, 2011). A major factor will be whether or not mental health is included in the post-2015 Sustainable Development Goals and whether governments commit to increased mental health budgets, particularly human resources (Lund, 2014). Ultimately, it will be political will and public advocacy that will determine the global governance for health's response to the emergency of failing mental health care.

Recommendations to health professionals

Develop a global state of mind

Crucial to global health ethics is "a global state of mind about the world and our place in it" (Benatar *et al.*, 2003, p. 129). This will require imagination. The philosopher, Charles Taylor (2004) explains that the social imaginary (i.e., the way one's life with others is perceived) is shaped by myths, tales, and images: what is (and is not) encountered in books, the press, and other media shapes how individuals understand their place in the world. These influences on social life will affect how (or if) a global society is envisioned. It may be pictured as individual consumers residing in a global shopping center or as global citizens living in an interconnected world. Metaphors are central to imaginative thinking. They allow perceptions to shift and the self and world to be seen in new ways (Lakoff & Johnson, 2003). The "global village" of Marshall McLuhan, for instance, suggests a re-vision of the world as local space (McLuhan & Powers, 1989). Imagined as a moral community that is evolving to become harmonious and just, the global village has possibilities as a healthy and safe home. People can come together, in the words of Richard Rorty in *Philosophy and Social Hope* (2003), through "an image of themselves as part of a great human adventure, one carried out on a global scale" (pp. 238–239), he was writing, however, about democracy.

Re-orientate one's vision of health and health ethics to encompass the global community

A global attitude to health and health ethics is necessary if they are to be understood in their full context. Questions need to be raised about what changes for ethical practice when "global" becomes a significant frame of reference (Austin, 2001a). What will it mean for resource allocation? For service delivery? For health systems development? This global attitude brings an expansion of moral responsibility. Fortunately, such responsibility is shared and trans-disciplinary in nature. It can be acted upon locally. And the basis of a global attitude is foundational to the health disciplines: ethical care is without discrimination related to race, religion, politics, gender, age, or other such attributes. It is moral space that is changing for health professionals, not values.

Raise consciousness of all regarding dignity and human rights in health care

Attentiveness to the dignity of all persons does much to support equality and to prevent or overcome discrimination in health care. This is particularly important in mental health due to the extensive prejudice and discrimination that can be the most devastating aspect of a psychiatric diagnosis. The promotion of right to health can be accomplished by helping patients/families and colleagues understand their rights, by helping the public to query and monitor health systems and services, and by influencing policy development through proactive contributions and critique and the mobilizing of professional associations (Austin, 2001b). Rights can be protected by health professionals through identification, documentation, and testimony about rights violations. Such action, however, can be dangerous. Health workers have been attacked for treatment and care of politically unpopular groups or for witnessing human rights violations. In 2013, for example, the UN Human Rights Council was called upon by the Safeguarding Health in Conflict Coalition, and other human rights groups to strengthen documentation and accountability for attacks on health workers, an increasing phenomenon (Physicians for Human Rights, 2013). One can keep informed and contribute support for human rights through groups such as Physicians for Human Rights, Global Lawyers and Physicians, and Human Rights Watch.

Acquire and/or contribute to capacity building for global health ethics

Knowledge regarding human rights, particularly as related to health, is necessary if one is to competently play a part in advocating for those with rights at risk. The need for education for global citizenship in the health disciplines is increasingly recognized, with considerable agreement existing in relation to the necessary competences. Actualization of such education, however, is not as common. A Brazilian study of nurse educators found that, while there was agreement about competencies to be included in global citizen curricula—"GBD," "health implications of migration, travel, and displacement," "social and environmental determinants of health," "health care in low-resource settings," "health as a human right and development resource," and "globalization of health and health care"—inclusion was not necessarily occurring (Ventura *et al.*, 2014, p. 182). Yet, if local and global health realities are to be transformed, the nascent clinician must be prepared for practice in a globalized world (Ventura *et al.*, 2014).

One popular strategy in the education of health professionals, particularly in high-income countries is the practicum abroad. Although this strategy can prove highly educational, it can be "morally problematic" (Dwyer, 2011, p. 325). Students may be ill prepared, stay for too brief a time, and disrupt the host health care system rather than benefit it (Dwyer, 2011). James Dwyer offers some points for reflection by students considering an out-of-country experience, including: knowledge of the language used in host region; knowledge of its history, culture, and social structures; appropriateness of length-of-stay and of their stage of training; the worth of the proposed project (a respectful partnership?; benefits and burdens fairly shared?); and motivation for going (2011, pp. 325–326). He raises an important question: Are there ways at home to promote global health? (2011, p. 326). Also helpful is Andrew Pinto's and Ross Upshur's (2009) global health ethics framework for educators of students going abroad for experience in a developing nation: the principles of humility (e.g., recognize own limitations); introspection (e.g., examination of motives, privileges); solidarity (e.g., consider the "global commons" and "global health goods); and social justice (e.g., equity, human rights, and the forces of globalization) (pp. 7–9).

Reflect upon your social responsibility as a health professional in a global community

What social injustices and health inequities inspire you to act? Consider this interest realistically and determine your best options for acting upon it. What group, association, or community offers a potential collective for activating your chosen action or project? If your talents, privileges, and connections are in the mental health arena, not only are there a myriad of injustices requiring remedy, but the time is ripe for change. There is opportunity to be part of a moral movement that will advocate for policies, funds, and sustainable programs in mental health, and for the research to support them (Kleinman, 2013).

Conclusion

The questions posed at the onset of the chapter—How might we envision ethical action in a global community? What constitutes ethical health care when the moral horizon embraces the entire world? How do health professionals striving to be ethical re-orientate themselves to this broader understanding of their duties and responsibilities?—remain open. They are questions humankind has not raised before and we will need to live through to the answers.

Some of the key concepts of a global health ethic, such as human dignity and human rights can appear to be too vague to be very useful. Yet most people intuit their meaning and understand their worth to human lives. These concepts form a basis for global dialogue. The DBHR, as imperfect as it is, offers a beginning and a basis for conversation about health ethics within a global society. The vision of a just world in this landmark document calls for respect and concern regarding "the interconnection between human beings and other forms of life," and our role in "the protection of the environment, the biosphere, and biodiversity" (UNESCO, 2005, Article 17).

Is there any reasonable basis for optimism that a just, harmonious, and healthy society is in the future of our planet? James Orbinski (2009), in his work *An Imperfect Offering: Humanitarian Action in the Twenty-First Century*, notes that he is frequently asked: "Are you still optimistic about the future?"; "How can you still have hope?"; and "What can we do?" His answer, learned from the writings of Vaclav Havel, former president of Czechoslovakia is: "While I am sometimes optimistic, I always try to be hopeful" (2009, p. 397). Orbinski concludes that, "Concretely, the most important thing we can do is actively and pragmatically assume our responsibility as citizens for the world in which we live" (2009, p. 400). This is what is demanded of the contemporary, ethical, mental health professional.

References

Andorno, R. (2009). Human dignity and human rights as a common ground for a global bioethics. *Journal of Medicine and Philosophy, 34*(3), 223–240.

Austin, W. (2001a). Nursing ethics in an era of globalization. *Advances in Nursing Science, 24*(2), 1–18.

Austin, W. (2001b). Using the human rights paradigm in health ethics: The problems and the possibilities. *Nursing Ethics, 8*(3), 183–195.

Austin, W., Bergum, V., & Nuttgens, S. (2004). Addressing oppression in psychiatric care: A relational ethics perspective. *Ethical Human Psychology and Psychiatry, 6*(1), 147–157.

Badhwar, N. (2006). International aid: When giving becomes a vice. *Social Philosophy and Policy, 23*(1), 69–101.

Bauman, Z. (1993). *Postmodern ethics.* Oxford: Blackwell.

Bauman, Z. (2008). *Does ethics have a chance in a world of consumers?* Cambridge, MA: Harvard University Press.

Bemme, D. & D'souza, N. (2014). Global mental health and its discontents: An inquiry into the making of *global* and *local* scale. *Transcultural Psychiatry, 51*(6), 850–874.

Benatar S. (1998). Global disparities in health and human rights: A critical commentary. *American Journal of Public Health, 88*(2), 295–300.

Benatar, S. (2005). The trouble with universal declarations. *Developing World Bioethics, 5*(3), 220–224.

Benatar, S. (2013). Global health and justice: Re-examining our values. *Bioethics, 27*(6), 297–304.

Benatar, S., Daar, A., & Singer, P. (2003). Global health ethics: The rationale for mutual caring. *International Affairs, 79*(1), 107–138.

Bramesfeld, A., Klippel, U., Seidel, G., Schwartz, F.W., & Dierks, M.L. (2007). How do patients expect the mental health service system to act? Testing the WHO responsiveness concept for its appropriateness in mental health care. *Social Science & Medicine, 65*, 880–889.

Caldas de Almeida, J., Minas, H., & Cayetano, C. (2014). Generating political commitment for mental health system development. In V. Patel, H. Minas, A. Cohen, & M. Prince (Eds.). *Global Mental Health: Principles and Practice* (pp. 450–468). Oxford: Oxford University Press.

Canadian Nurses Association (CNA) (February, 2006). *Social justice: A means to an end, an end in itself.* Ottawa, Canada: Authors.

Chaimowitz, G. (2012). Position paper: The criminalization of people with mental illness. *Canadian Journal of Psychiatry*, *57*(2), 1–6.

Collins, P.Y., Patel, V., Joestl, S.S., March, D., Insel, T.R., & Daar, A.S. (2011). Grand challenges in global mental health. *Nature*, *475*, 27–30.

Collins, P.Y., Insel, T.R., Chockalingam, A., Daar, A., Maddox, Y.T., Chockalingam, R., Daar, A., & Maddox, Y. T. (2013). Grand challenges in global mental health: Integration in research, policy, and practice. *PLoS Medicine 10*(4): e1001434.

Commission on Social Determinants of Health (CSDH) (2008). *Closing the gap in a generation: Health equity through action on the social determinants of health: WHO final report of the Commission on Social Determinants of Health*. Geneva, Switzerland: WHO.

Cooper, A.F., Kirton, J.J., & Stevenson, M.A. (2009). Critical cases in global health innovation. In A.F. Cooper & J.J. Kirton (Eds.). *Innovation in Global Health Governance: Critical Cases* pp. 3–22. Farnham, UK: Ashgate.

Desjarlais, R., Eisenberg, L., Good, B., & Kleinman, A. (1995). *World mental health: Problems and priorities in low-income countries*. Oxford: Oxford University Press.

Drew, N., Funk, M., Tang, S., Lamichhane, J., Chávez, E., Katontoka, S., Pathare, S., Lewis, O., Gostin, L., & Saraceno, B. (2011). Human rights violations of people with mental and psychosocial disabilities: An unresolved global crisis. *The Lancet*, *378*, 1664–1675.

Dwyer, J. (2011). Teaching global health ethics. In S. Benatar & G. Brock (Eds.). *Global Health and Global Health Ethics* (pp. 319–327). Cambridge, UK: Cambridge University Press.

Eaton, J., De Silva, M., Rojas, G., & Patel, V. (2014). Scaling up services for mental health. In V. Patel, H. Minas, A. Cohen, & M. Prince (Eds.). *Global Mental Health: Principles and Practice* (pp. 297–334). Oxford: Oxford University Press.

Edwards, K. (2000). Service users and mental health nursing. *Journal of Psychiatric and Mental Health Nursing*, *7*(6), 555–565.

Frenk, J. & Moon, S. (2013). Governance challenges in global health. *The New England Journal of Medicine*, *368*(10), 936–942

Frese, F.J., Stanley, J., Kraus, K., & Vogel-Scibilia, S. (2001). Integrating evidence-based practices and the recovery model. *Psychiatric Services*, *52*(11), 1462–1468.

Friedman, T. (1999). *The Lexus and the olive tree: understanding globalization*. New York: Farrar, Straus, & Giroux.

Global Health Forum. (2011). *What the Global Forum does*. www.globalforumhealth.org (accessed May 11, 2016).

Gostin, L. O. (2001). Beyond moral claims: A human rights approach in mental health. *Cambridge Quarterly of Healthcare Ethics*, *10*, 264–274.

Hamilton, E. & Roper, L. (2006). Troubling insight: Power and possibilities in mental health care. *Journal of Psychiatric and Mental Health Nursing*, *13*(4), 4416–422.

Happell, B., Manias, E., & Roper, C. (2004). Wanting to be heard: Mental health consumers' experiences of information about medication. *International Journal of Mental Health Nursing*, *13*(4), 242–248.

Harbin, A. (2014). The disorientations of acting against injustice. *Journal of Social Philosophy*, *45*(2), 162–181.

Harman, S. (2012). *Global health governance*. London: Routledge.

Horsfall, J. (2003). Consumer/service users: Is nursing listening? *Issues in Mental Health Nursing*, *24*(4), 381–396.

Hunter, D. & Dawson, A.J. (2011). Is there a need for a global health ethics? For and against. In S. Benatar & G. Brock (Eds.). *Global Health and Global Health Ethics* (pp. 77–88). Cambridge, UK: Cambridge University Press.

Ignatieff, M. (2001). *Human rights as polity and idolatry*. Princeton, NJ: Princeton University Press.

Kickbusch, I., Novotny, T.E., Drage, N., Siberschmidt, G., & Alcazar, S. (2007). Global health diplomacy: Training across disciplines. *Bulletin of the World Health Organization*, *85*(12), 971–973.

Kirby, M.J.L. & Keon, W. J. (2006). *Out of the shadows at last: Transforming mental health, mental illness, and addiction services in Canada*. www.parl.gc.ca/content/sen/committee/391/soci/rep/rep02may06-e.htm (accessed May 11, 2016).

Kleinman, A. (2009). Global mental health: A failure of humanity. *The Lancet*, *374*, 603–604.

Kleinman, A. (2013). Implementing global mental health. *Depression and Anxiety*, *30*, 503–505.

Kolappa, K., Henderson, D., & Kishore, S.P. (2013). No physical health without mental health: Lessons unlearned? *Bulletin of the World Health Organization, 91*(1), 3–3A.

Lagon, M.P., & Arend, A.C. (2014). Introduction: Human dignity in a neomedieval world. In Arend, A.C., Lagon, M.P., & De Gioia, J.J. *Human Dignity and the Future of Global Institutions* (pp. 1–22). Washington, DC: Georgetown University Press.

Lakoff, G., & Johnson, M. (2003). *Metaphors we live by.* Chicago, IL: University of Chicago Press.

Landman, W., & Schüklenk, U. (2005). From the editors. *Developing World Bioethics, 5*(3), iii–vi.

Lidén, J. (2014). The World Health Organization and global health governance: Post-1990. *Public Health, 128*, 141–147.

Lowry, C., & Schüklenk, U. (2009). Two models in global health ethics. *Public Health Ethics, 2*(3), 276–284.

Lund, C. (2014). Poverty and mental health: Towards a research agenda for low- and middle-income countries. Commentary on Tampubolon and Hanandita. *Social Science & Medicine, 111*, 134–136.

Macklin, R. (2003). Dignity is a useless concept. *British Medical Journal, 327*(7429), 1419–1420.

McLuhan, M., & Powers, B. (1989). *The global village: Transformation in world life and media in the 21ˢᵗ century.* Oxford: Oxford University Press.

Mehta, N., & Thornicroft, G. (2014). Stigma, discrimination, and promoting human rights. In V. Patel, H. Minas, A. Cohen, & M.J. Prince. (Eds.). *Global Mental Health: Principles and Practice* pp. 401–424. Oxford: Oxford University Press.

Murali, V. & Oyebode, F. (2004). Poverty, social inequality and mental health. *Advances in Psychiatric Treatment, 10*, 216–224.

Murray, C. J., & Lopez, A.D. (1996). *The global burden of disease.* Cambridge, MA: Harvard University Press.

O'Hara, M. (2012). Fighting for their rights. *Mental Health Today*, September–October, 8–9.

OHCHR & WHO (2008). *The right to health: Fact sheet 31.* Geneva, Switzerland: OHCHR.

Okasha, A. (2004). Mental patients in prisons: Punishment versus treatment? (Editorial). *World Psychiatry, 3*(1), 1–2.

Orbinski, J. (2009). *An imperfect offering: Humanitarian action in the twenty-first century.* Toronto, Canada: Anchor Books.

Oxfam International (2014) *Working for the few: Political capture and economic inequality.* Oxford: OxfamGB.

PanAmerican Health Organization (PAHO) (2009). *Strategy and plan of action on mental health.* Washington, DC: Author.

Pang, T. (2011). Global health research: Changing the agenda. In S. Benatar & G. Brock. (Eds.). *Global Health and Global Health Ethics* (pp. 285–292). Cambridge, UK: Cambridge University Press.

Patel, V. (2011). A renewed agenda for global mental health. *The Lancet, 378*, 1441–1442,

Patel, V., Boyce, N., Collins, P., Saxena, S., & Horton, R. (2011). A renewed agenda for global mental health, *The Lancet*, 378, 1441–1442.

Pescosolido, B.A., Medina, T.A., Martin, J.K., & Long, J.S. (2013). The backbone of stigma: Identifying the global core of public prejudice associated with mental illness. *American Journal of Public Health*, e1–e8. Doi: 10.2105/AJPH.2012.301147.

Peternelj-Taylor, C. (2008). Criminalization of the mentally ill. *Journal of Forensic Nursing, 4*(4), 185–187.

Physicians for Human Rights (2013, Sept. 20). *Press release: Human rights groups call to end impunity for attacks on health workers.* Geneva, Switzerland: Author.

Pinto, A.D. & Upshur, R.E.G. (2009). Global health ethics for students. *Developing World Bioethics, 9*(1), 1–10.

Pogge, T. (2002). *World poverty and human rights: Cosmopolitan responsibilities and reforms.* Cambridge: Polity Press.

Ramsay, S. (2001). No closure in sight for the 10/90 health-research gap. *The Lancet, 358*, 1348.

"Responsibility, 2014". *Oxford English Dictionary* (OED) Online. September 2014. Oxford University Press. www.oed.com/view/Entry/163862?redirectedFrom=responsibiliy (accessed November 7, 2014).

Ricoeur, P. (1992) [1990]. *Oneself as another.* K. Blamey (Trans.). Chicago, IL: University of Chicago Press.

Ritzer, G. (1993). *The McDonaldization of society.* Thousand Oaks, CA: Sage.

Robertson, R. (2003). *The three waves of globalization: A history of a developing global consciousness.* Nova Scotia, Canada: Fernwood.

Rorty, R. (1999). *Philosophy and social hope.* London: Penguin Books.

Saraceno, B., van Ommeren, M., Batniji, R., Cohen, A., Gureje, O., Mahoney, J., Sridhar, D., & Underhill, C. (2007). Global mental health 5: Barriers to improvement of mental health services in low-income and middle-income countries, *The Lancet, 370*, 1164–1174.

Scheffler, R.M. (2011). Human resources for mental health: Workforce shortages in low- and middle-income countries. *Human Resources for Health Observer, 8*, 1–56.

Singer, P. (1997). The drowning child and the expanding circle: As the world shrinks, so our capacity for effective moral action grows. *New Internationalist, 289*, 28.

Sridhar, D., & Gostin, L. (2014). World Health Organization: Past, present and future (Guest editorial). *Public Health, 128*, 117–118.

Stapleton, G., Schröder-Bäck, P., Laaser, U., Meershoek, A., & Popa, D. (2014). Global health ethics: An introduction to prominent theories and relevant topics. *Global Health Action*, 7: 23569. http://11dx.doi.org/10.3402/gha.v7.23569 (accessed May 11, 2016).

Summerfield, D. (2012). Afterword: Against "global mental health." *Transcultural Psychiatry, 49*(3–4), 519–530.

Taylor, C. (2004). *Modern social imaginaries*. London: Duke University Press.

Toumi, R. (2014). Globalization and health care: Global justice and the role of physicians. *Medicine, Health Care and Philosophy, 17*(1), 71–80.

Tyer-Viola, L., Nicholas, P.K., Corless, I.B., Barry, D.M., Hoyt, P., Fitzpatrick, J.J., & Davis, S.M. (2009). Social responsibility of nursing: A global perspective. *Policy, Politics, and Nursing Practice 10*(2), 110–119.

Unger, P. (1996). *Living high and letting die: Our illusion of innocence*. Oxford: Oxford University Press.

United Nations (2006). *Convention on the Rights of Persons with Disabilities*. www.un.org/disabilities/default.asp?navid=15&pid=150 (accessed November 1, 2014).

United Nations Development Programme (2014). *Human development report 2014: Sustaining human progress: reducing vulnerabilities and building resilience*. New York: Author.

United Nations Educational, Scientific and Cultural Organization (UNESCO) (2005). Universal Declaration of Bioethics and Human Rights. *Resolutions: Records of the General Conference 33rd Session*, Vol. 1, pp. 74–80. Paris: Author.

United Nations General Assembly (1948). *Universal declaration of human rights. General assembly resolution 217A (III), UN Doc A/810*. New York: United Nations General Assembly Official Records.

United Nations General Assembly (1966). *International Covenant on Economic, Social and Cultural Rights General Assembly Resolution 2200A (XXI)*. New York: United Nations General Assembly Official Records.

United Nations General Assembly (2007). *Convention on the rights of persons with disabilities: General resolution A/RES/61/106*. New York: United Nations General Assembly Official Records.

Velji, A., & Bryant, J. H. (2014). Global health ethics. In Markle, W.H., Fisher, M.A., & Smego, R.A. (Eds.). *Understanding Global Health 2nd ed.* (pp. 463–487). New York: McGraw-Hill Education.

Ventura, C., Mendes, I., Wilson, L., de Godoy, S., Tami-Maury, I., Zárate-Grajales, & Salas-Segura, S. (2014). Global health competencies according to nursing faculty from Brazilian higher education institutions. *Latin American Journal of Nursing, 22*(2), 179–186.

Ward, B. (2012). Challenges and opportunities in global health care research. *Health Innovation Report: Raising the bar on health systems performance, 6*, 6–9.

Waters, M. (1995). *Globalization*. London and New York: Routledge.

Whiteford, H., Degenhardt, L., Rehm, J., Baxter, A.J., Ferrari, A.J., Erskine, H. E., Charlson, F.J., Norman, R.E., Flaxman, A.D., Johns, N., Burstein, R., Murray, C.J.L., & Vos, T. (2013). Global burden of disease attributable to mental and substance use disorders: Findings form the Global Burden of Disease Study 2010, *The Lancet, 382*, 1575–1586.

Whitehead, M. (1992). The concepts and principles of equity and health. *International Journal of Health Services, 22*(3), 429–445.

Wisor, S. (2011). Against shallow ponds: An argument against Singer's approach to global poverty. *Journal of Global Ethics, 7*(1), 19–32.

World Economic Forum (2013). *Outlook on the global agenda 2014*. Geneva, Switzerland: Author

World Health Organization (n.d.). MINDbank: A database of mental health resources. www.WHO.int/mental_health/mindbank/en. (accessed May 11, 2016).

World Health Organization (2001). *The world health report 2001: Mental health: new understanding, new hope*. Geneva, Switzerland: Author.

World Health Organization (2005). *WHO resource book on mental health, human rights, and legislation*. Geneva, Switzerland: Author.

World Health Organization (2010). *mhGAP Intervention Guide for mental, neurological and substance use disorders in non-specialized health settings: Mental Health Gap Action Programme (mhGAP)*. Geneva, Switzerland: Author.

World Health Organization (2012). *WHO QualityRights Project: Addressing a human rights emergency.* (Project flyer). Geneva, Switzerland: Author. www.who.int/mental_health/policy/quality_rights/ QRs_flyer_2012.pdf?ua=1 (accessed May 11, 2016).

World Health Organization (2013). *Mental health action plan (2013–2020).* Geneva, Switzerland: Author. www.who.int/mental_health/action_plan_2013/en/ (accessed May 11, 2016).

World Health Organization & World Organization of Family Doctors (Wonca). (2008). *Integrating mental health into primary care: A global perspective.* Geneva and Singapore: Authors.

Young, I. (2006). Responsibility and global justice: A social connection model. *Social Philosophy and Politics, 23,* 102–130.

7

STANDARD OF MENTAL HEALTH CARE

Meeting consumer needs

Vicki P. Hines-Martin, Geraldine S. Pearson,
Melanie Walters and Molly Hall

Introduction

Integrating mental health care and consumer needs is a challenging, shifting process with decided historical trends resulting in a current consumer-driven movement that determines care. The variants with this are enormous and include the power differential between providers and patients, the policy-making political climate of health care, and the growing unwillingness of people to assume the role of patient just because they are suffering from a psychiatric disorder. Currently, in the United States, there is a growing move towards a requirement that consumer perspectives are the driving factor as services are organized and funded (Tomes, 2006).

Enlightened health care is hallmarked by the principle of "empowerment" or the right to make choices around health care (Tomes, 2006, p. 720). Certainly, the Patient Protection and Affordable Health Care Act (PPAHC) of 2010 enacted in the United States demanded that consumers have a more active role in planning their treatment and recovery (Johnson, Sanders, & Strange, 2014). The PPAHC essentially sees health care as a right and not a privilege. Implementation of this involves politically complex, fiscally driven systems officially tasked with meeting consumer needs. It is also influenced by an increasingly vocal and powerful consumer force around planning and funding care. Also termed the consumer/survivor movement in mental health, this historical move towards patient empowerment has had a significant influence on the decision-making inherent in care provision (Tomes, 2006). In the United States these changes in health care provision have the potential to make fundamental differences in the care received by consumers with psychiatric disorders.

The "principle of 'empowerment,' defined as having the right to make one's own health care choices, is now frequently invoked as one of the fundamental measures of enlightened health care" (Tomes, 2006, p. 720). In spite of this, the empowerment of individuals who need and use the health care system remains linked to a paternalistic system of physicians and policy makers with fiscal authority. The fiscal restructuring of health care, at least in the United States, has required that this paternalistic system undergo revision. This continues to be a work in progress.

While each country in the world establishes mental health standards that have wide variation and differences, the World Health Organization (WHO) has made mental health an integral part of its definition of health. "Good mental health enables people to realize their potential, cope with the normal stresses of life, work productively, and contribute to their communities" (Chan, 2013, p. 5). To this end the WHO has published a comprehensive document that takes a life-course approach to mental health, advocates universal health coverage, and has an emphasis on prevention. The four major objectives include:

- more effective leadership and governance for mental health;
- the provision of comprehensive, integrated mental health and social care services in community-based settings;
- implementation of strategies for promotion and prevention; and
- strengthened information systems, evidence and research.

(WHO, 2013, p. 5)

In May 2012 at the sixty-fifth World Health Assembly the resolution to address the global burden of mental disorders with a comprehensive, coordinated response from health and social sectors at the country level was established. This document offers an international blueprint for establishing mental health services at all levels of need and for low resource parts of the world. This document emphasizes that

determinants of mental health and mental disorders include not only individual attributes such as the ability to manage one's thoughts, emotions, behaviours and interactions with others, but also social, cultural, economic, political and environmental factors such as national policies, social protection, living standards, working conditions, and community social supports.

(WHO, 2013, p. 7)

The action plan is also reliant on the following six principles and approaches:

- universal health coverage;
- human rights;
- evidence-based practice;
- life-course approach;
- multisectoral approach; and
- empowerment of persons with mental disorders and psychosocial disabilities.

It is the last principle that has applicability to this chapter and focuses on collaborating with stakeholders and empowerment of individuals with mental health disorders. The WHO document emphasizes that in order to implement this empowerment there needs to be engagement with all relevant sectors and stakeholders when policies involving mental health issues are being planned and established. Sharing knowledge and developing mechanisms that improve coordinated care are essential. The emphasis is on building local capacity and raising awareness of mental health, law and human rights (WHO, 2013).

The document emphasizes the need for logistic, technical and financial support to build the capacity of organizations, while encouraging the development of independent local and national organizations composed of individuals with mental disorders and psychosocial disabilities. They must be involved in the development, implementation, and monitoring of mental health services.

Finally, they must be involved in the training of health workers who will deliver care to this population (WHO, 2013).

The reasons for developing standards of mental health care are inextricably linked to consumers, but they are not always defined specifically by consumers. The question could be raised: whose needs are being met by standards established by entities outside the ranks of consumers of mental health care? How are consumers determining standards of mental health care globally? This chapter will explore these issues while tracing the history of consumer-driven initiatives.

Historical perspective

The evolution of consumerism throughout the world has gradually shifted mental health treatment from a paternalistic care model in which providers determine patient care somewhat exclusively, towards a model in which consumers are influencing their care and their recovery (Ostrow & Adams, 2012). This is leading to changes in the ways standards of care are developed and implemented. Jaeger and Hoff (2012) note that concepts of recovery have been integrated into the mental health policy and service of many Anglophone countries. These include the United States, England, Scotland, Ireland, Australia, New Zealand, and Canada. Similar efforts around recovery from mental illness are reported from Hong Kong (Tse, Cheung, Kan, Ng, & Yau, 2012), Israel (Roe, Bril-Bamiv & Kravetz, 2012), and China (Wong, Zhuang, Pan, & He, 2014).

In the United States, there is a movement to transform the mental health treatment system to a consumer driven and recovery oriented model of care (Ostrow & Adams, 2012). Like most countries this is linked to the political, fiscal, and policy-driven practices that influence funding and perception of mental health care.

Influence of stigma

Consumerism in mental health is present internationally but references continue to identify the pervasive presence and influence of stigma and discrimination. Underneath all efforts at improving mental health treatment is the internationally pervasive fact that stigma is associated with mental disorders. This is a global public health problem (Griffiths, Carron-Arthur, Parsons, & Reid, 2014). Stigma is a particularly powerful force that keeps many consumers and their families silent. Social exclusions of individuals with mental health problems are prominent at home, work, personally, socially, in health care, and in the media (Thornicroft, Brohan, Kassam, & Lewis-Holmes, 2008; Link, Struening, Neese-Todd, Asmussen, & Phelan, 2001). Griffiths and colleagues (2014) in their meta-analysis of program effectiveness in reducing stigma, found that current stigma interventions were effective in reducing personal stigma. Previous research was based on efforts regarding specific diagnoses, predominantly depression and psychosis/schizophrenia (Corrigan, Edwards, Green, Diwan, & Penn, 2001). This meta-analysis confirmed that stigma can be reduced with a targeted intervention. The study used research from across the world although all studies were published in English, which eliminated several studies. It did not address the cultural influences operative in the research.

It is a logical premise that consumer needs would drive the development of mental health care at all levels including need assessment, delivery of service, and establishing the standard of care that informs the process. In all countries and cultures the concept of consumer need for mental health services and care is complex and rooted in issues involving stigma, advocacy, and level of care need.

Raines and Ellis (2014) note that the general public is remarkably disengaged in the process of mental health care. They acknowledge that advocacy organizations have played a significant role in legislation and regulations aimed at building mental health services and protecting rights and interests of the public. They also emphasize that reform has been dominated by the health care businesses rather than the consumers of the care.

Discussion of the issue: what is consumer-driven care?

An important driver to the current concept of consumer-driven care has been a historical movement called the antipsychiatry movement (Rismiller & Rismiller, 2006). This has involved a radical antipsychiatry movement largely focused on undermining organized psychiatry. This movement was based in the divisional differences between biological psychiatry and psychoanalytic psychiatry. Essentially psychoanalysis, which dominated psychiatric for decades, treated people subjectively, dynamically, and with protracted psychotherapy. In contrast, biological psychiatry has sought to identify the brain-based changes resulting in psychiatric illness (Rissmiller & Rissmiller, 2006). Most modern psychiatric providers would agree that the biological model has more credence in current psychiatry.

The remnants of the antipsychiatry movement, which did eventually fade in power, seemed to result in an active and increasingly powerful consumer voice, composed of former patients who believed they had been treated coercively, providers who did not believe in traditional psychiatry, and an evolving view that people with psychiatric disabilities were treated poorly and unfairly (Satel & Redding, 2005).

Rissmiller and Rissmiller (2006) note that the psychiatric profession has little constructive dialogue with radical consumerists. They note that these radical individuals and groups are seen as "extremist, having little scientific foundation and no defined leadership" (p. 866). However, these radical groups were effective in getting the United Nations General Assembly to adopt its 1991 principles for the Protection of Persons with Mental Illness and the Improvement of Mental Health Care (United Nations General Assembly, 1991).

International examples of consumer-driven care

The United States has tended to isolate itself in terms of policy and practice regarding recovery (Cox & O'Neil, 2008). Noting that the health care system in the United States differs from other care delivery systems in other developed and developing countries, Ostrow and Adams (2012) suggest that the United States could learn from the consumer-driven efforts in countries such as New Zealand and Finland. Scotland has incorporated the examples from other countries and consumer perspectives since 2000 to promote and support recovery beginning with the following priorities: learn from the uniqueness of each individual's experience, share stories to inspire hope, establish a Scottish evidence base, and use the evidence to contribute to the policy and practice development evidence base of influential factors that help and hinder recovery and well-being (Bradstreet & McBrierty, 2012). As this example illustrates, an international movement aggregating the findings of consumer-driven recovery-related outcomes is warranted.

Evidence and future directions for collaboration with populations who experience persistent mental illness

Several authors have examined perceptions of all consumers (Jeffs, Dhalla, Cardoso, & Bell, 2014; McKenzie, 2006; Tambuyzer & Van Audenhove, 2013). Despite divergent perspectives between the groups, providers acknowledge the importance of including clients in service evaluation and planning in order to inform their practice. Major themes that have arisen in these studies include: (a) autonomy; (b) skills of the provider; and (c) respect. Additionally, clients have indicated that a sense of belonging and social inclusion is integral to recovery and maintenance of optimal wellness (Brolin, Rask, Syren, Baigi, & Brunt, 2015; Chadwick, Street, McAndrew, & Deacon, 2012). This section provides a summary of some of the findings and recommendations.

Authors have identified several factors that affect client-perceived autonomy. For example, Barbato *et al.* (2014) surveyed clients of a large public mental health agency on the quality of service delivery. They found that clients assigned high priority to the idea of having a choice. Clients most frequently gave negative ratings regarding choice, reporting they had little comment or influence over who their provider was. Clients had positive evaluations, however, about the level of support they received through the nurse–patient relationship, and of the nurses' and staff skill level. The perception of independence seems to be associated with the client's sense of control and choice. For example, residents of ordinary housing with supplementary support have reported higher levels of autonomy and control than their supported housing counterparts (Brolin *et al.*, 2015). Perhaps the most frustrating factor that commonly occurs for this population is the endless waiting, in the office, on the phone, and in terms of accessing a first appointment with a provider (Barbato *et al.*, 2014; Zeber, Copeland, McCarthy, Bauer, & Kilbourne, 2009).

Sound knowledge of mental illness combined with high provider skill level culminates in a satisfying experience for the client, and develops clients' and families' trust in their provider. Integral to this competency is the provider's ability to identify at-risk clients, conduct thorough and accurate assessment, and identify appropriate treatment (Barbato *et al.*, 2014; Jeffs *et al.*, 2014). Barriers to access are commonly cited by clients and families as a highly problematic aspect of mental health care but this truth is complicated by system-level and personal factors such as staffing shortages and scarcity of client resources (McKenzie 2006; Zeber *et al.*, 2009). For children and clients new to mental health services, these barriers hinder early intervention and, in those instances, family caregivers express a sense of helplessness, feeling unable to advocate for their loved ones. Chadwick *et al.* (2012) performed a literature review consisting of six qualitative and three quantitative studies to examine the views of clients with mental disorders in terms of barriers to accessing physical health care. Three studies had reported improper diagnosis as a barrier. Similarly, using a case design and content analysis, Jeffs *et al.* (2014) explored recidivism of 16 medically complex clients. The clients reported improper diagnosis and treatment as the primary reasons for preventable readmissions. The authors emphasized the need for open and honest communication between client, family and provider. These findings indicate that providers must release preconceptions and biases, listening with unwavering attention to the information their clients disclose in order to initiate appropriate treatment.

The influence of effective communication transcends the procedural aspects of diagnosis and treatment, however. Effective communication encompasses the values and assumptions held by clients and providers, and is necessary for building and maintaining a solid working relationship with clients. The demonstration of respect toward clients by their providers is a salient aspect. Examining experiences of 20 clients with mental disorders, Shattell, McAllister, Hogan, and Thomas (2006) conducted an existential phenomenological study of being understood. The study revealed many clients generally felt misunderstood, and some of the underlying mechanisms were their personal feelings of inadequacy as well as discrimination. Feelings of being understood were equated with feelings of importance and of having an emotional or physical connection (e.g., hug) with their providers. In contrast to other studies that highlighted skillfulness in communication in diagnosis, clients valued the level of effort the provider puts forth in trying to understand them. Clients are cognizant of subtleties within the client–provider relationship and may internalize both positive and negative representations of that relationship. There is some evidence that providers may not be aware of the significance clients ascribe to the provider's nonverbal behavior.

Clients may use nonverbal behaviors to measure the level of respect and concern the provider has towards the client. Indeed, clients have described exemplars of how providers and support workers emanate respect (Schroeder, 2013; Shattell *et al.*, 2006), such as through active listening and presence, a nonjudgmental attitude, and spending the necessary time getting to know clients. Carless and Douglas (2012) provided detailed narrative accounts of three clients with mental disorders who were participating in physical activity groups. Clients reported that feeling accepted by other clients was important to facilitate an environment of trust and safety. Equally important to one client was the fact that the coach did not have any expectations for the group and treated the group as though they were incapable of learning the exercises. In this case, the dismissive attitude of the coach served to illuminate client weaknesses, compounding client feelings of inadequacy. When assisting clients to achieve goals, then, providers and other support workers must be aware of how their nonverbal behavior affects the overall atmosphere and subsequent client outcomes. Likewise, providers have been reported to exhibit overt controlling and coercive behaviors towards clients (Schroeder, 2013).

Forward thinking providers and organizations may reflect on these findings to refine the structures and approaches currently used in care delivery. In theory this sounds rational but implementation is multifaceted and complex. One method to achieve this outcome is through staff education. This education should include knowledge of mental illness for professionals who have less frequent exposure to the mentally ill population. Skill acquisition and maintenance in effective client–provider communication is paramount. Another important consideration is that underlying factors associated with the age and race of the client may influence perception of usefulness, and being respected and supported in mental health delivery systems (Schroeder, 2013; Woodward, Mowbray, Holter, & Bybee, 2007). On a broader level, Clossey and Rheinheimer (2014) suggest there is a strong relationship between organizational culture and client perceptions. Clients who receive mental health care from agencies where there is a high level of proficiency, engagement, functionality, and low levels of stress perceive a higher level of support for their recovery. Strategies to assist clients in developing a sense of autonomy include educating clients about their illness and treatment, keeping clients and caregivers abreast of necessary information, and including clients and family in decision-making (Barbato *et al.*, 2014; Tambuyzer & Van Audenhove, 2013).

In conclusion, Barbato *et al.* (2014) used the term "responsiveness" to describe a sort of conforming of organizations to wholeheartedly meet the identified needs of the clients they serve. This process of change may not occur quickly, but these strategies combined may yield the best formula for creating a culture of responsiveness in organizations, thereby leading to positive client outcomes in the long term.

The voice of consumers

As the reported literature has demonstrated, the voice of mental health care consumers at the individual, family, and community levels has increasingly been identified as critical to health care outcomes and standards of care. Investigators and clinicians have reported the impact of attention to how clients view mental illness, how they form therapeutic relationships, respond to treatment, and overcome barriers as key to improving access to and delivery of mental health services and positive outcomes. What is most powerful is the voice of consumers themselves.

Co-author, Molly Hall, is an administrative assistant in a school of nursing and has consented to provide a perspective on the journey she traveled toward, and during, mental health care treatment; what she perceived as the components she found most supportive of successful mental health care outcomes and what are important standards of "client driven care."

It started when I was about 8 years old. My mom said that she was told I had ADHD, which was the new thing at the time. I would come home from school . . . it was like night and day. When I came home from school—all hell broke loose. Before (I started on Ritalin) I came home it was a sunny day and then I walk in the door and there and it's a stormy day . . . and they put me on Ritalin. I don't know what Ritalin does, but my mom said it was like a mood stabilizer. I was on Ritalin through grade school, then they backed off that and put me back on again in High School my junior year. I always looked up my meds and wanted to know more about what I had. Then they thought after [I] could learn to control it after high school without meds. I started to work but I had no filter on my mouth and constructive criticism is ok but if you try to belittle me and I would go off . . . At one job I got so angry that I pushed over [a display of merchandise in the store that I was employed]. I feel there are degrees of illness and you may be able to hold things in most of the time. It's not fun on the inside and there are no doctors for that. Sometimes I hurt myself not to hurt others. During the 80s and 90s, I did not say anything to anyone about my problems, so most people I knew thought I had a "bad temper." About 10 years ago, I was told to go [to get treatment]. I was diagnosed with Bipolar disorder.

During that time she had negative emotional experiences with others as she tried to handle the mental health issues (mental health providers, work supervisors, and significant others).

[After working in the school of nursing for about 7 years], I became despondent [after a serious personal and financial crisis], trying to do everything . . . and I had to move to a one bedroom apartment and had to rehome my babies [pets]. I had pain pills [from a prior surgery], I had vodka—[I can] take everything but the kitchen sink. My son has a gun [and I had a plan to kill myself]. My babies are the only reasons I didn't do it. Things were so bad and I was talking with [a co-worker] and it scared her. She told [some of the mental health nursing faculty]. They came to me and made me promise to go [would not agree to be hospitalized]. I went to treatment first [with a psychiatric mental health nurse practitioner] and because of insurance hassles and I could not afford [out of pocket] I started to see [a psych MD].

Molly wanted to share these insights with mental health professionals.

Because you have a mental health diagnosis doesn't mean they cannot be a functional member of society. What they need is understanding—show that. (Mental health providers need to know) that 15 minutes in an office doesn't do it. Do not only ask me how I'm doing . . . Ask my safety net [family, friends, others] how I'm doing. I've been through all that and I'm still here. I can't stop it [my illness] but I can see it's coming. I've seen my depression slide, I can see it and I get in [to the doctor] and do not have to be hospitalized.

Because the guy [with a reported mental illness] shot up the movie theater I know they [people] are thinking I will shoot up people and just because I belong to this group [some of whom have been violent]—I will do the same thing. I understand discrimination. Everyone [doctor, nurses, and other people] need to be treated as a person—treat me as a person. I use humor to defuse a lot of situations and cover a lot of things—you cover that hurt cause people don't understand or don't want to understand. I know what ADHD looks like, I'm there and I want to help victims. We need more people who are—can identify to go into this field. If you've ever been discriminated against, you will never discriminate against others.

Individuals with mental health conditions bring with them families of origin, marital families and self-identified families and friends. Even as the client is designated as a consumer, so are those who function as supports, barriers and/or safety nets. Understanding their voice is equally important. An interview with a mother of an adult child with Bipolar and Anxiety Disorder brought out these perspectives and concerns about her experiences and standards of care.

I knew my child had special needs when she began school. She had difficulty reading, writing and organizing. I was OK having a child with a learning disability. We could work hard and handle that—which we did. I also began to see that she had difficulty making friends, understanding others' emotions and handling change. I was fortunate enough to have the education and financial means to get her into a school for the learning disabled and therapy along with medications. We made it through high school and into college where she studied hard, made good grades and graduated. However, [throughout that time] she still struggled with people and change. It became worse when she became an adult and was on her own. She became less likely to follow up with her therapy and medications. She made moves out of our state and the final move resulted in her hospitalization for Bipolar disorder and Generalized Anxiety disorder. She is back home and working her way back to health. I'm proud of her. It is stress-ful being a parent in the best of circumstance, it is disheartening to know your child struggles so and yet is so intelligent. Your heart breaks when you see her hope for a life she thinks her friends have and the one she saw as her future and her disappointment about where she is today. You worry about how to help her and support her inde-pendence and the "what ifs" as you grow older. You need to navigate being a part of her support system while communicating with her mental health provider within the bounds of confidentiality. So how does this fit with standards of care? From my perspective care means educating families who have children about what are signs that should warrant further assessment; helping teachers to better recognize conditions that are most prevalent in the age group they teach; educating adolescents and young adults about conditions, stressors and warning signs that help them with early self-identification and use of resources and educating all health care professionals that they play a part in mental health care for consumers and their families regardless of their setting. I know how tough it is to be a family member of someone with a mental health concern and I am a mental health nurse. I can't imagine the challenge of someone who didn't have the advantages I had.

Communities at risk are also targeted as consumers of mental health promotion and early intervention services and a priority that has been identified by the WHO and discussed in previous chapters. The Background paper, *Risks to mental health: An overview of vulnerabilities and risk factors* (2012), by WHO Secretariat for the Development of a Comprehensive Mental Health

Action Plan identifies the following factors as most influential in determining the risk for negative mental health.

> Mental health and well-being are influenced not only by individual attributes, but also by the social circumstances in which persons find themselves and the environment in which they live; these determinants interact with each other dynamically, and may threaten or protect an individual's mental health state. Risks to mental health manifest themselves at all stages in life. Taking a life-course perspective shows how risk exposures in the formative stages of life—including substance use in pregnancy, insecure attachment in infancy or family violence in childhood—can affect mental well-being or predispose towards mental disorder many years or even decades later. Depending on the local context, certain groups in society may be particularly susceptible to experiencing mental health problem, including households living in poverty, people with chronic health conditions, minority groups, and persons exposed to and/or displaced by war or conflict.
>
> *(WHO, 2012 p. 2)*

In addition, increasing numbers of nursing organizations (ICN, AAN and ISPN among others) have identified at-risk populations as consumers in need of mental health services, most of these being at the level of prevention and early intervention. Nursing plays a pivotal role in meeting their needs and recommendations are provided regarding what should be the standard of care to support the mental health of individuals, families and communities, and ameliorate risk factors (Pearson *et al.*, 2014 & 2015; WHO & ICN, 2007)

More effective leadership and governance for mental health

Just as consumer needs drive the development of mental health care, they need to drive the global leadership and governance process. The International Council of Nurses (2005) notes that all nurses worldwide are working under the constraints of economic limitations and political change. Decisions about health care are made within the confines of what countries can afford, resulting in changes in care delivery that pose both challenges and opportunities for nurses (ICN, 2005).

Sorensen, Iedema, and Severinsson (2008) note that nurses have to become "skilled multi-disciplinary team members with a capacity for professional advocacy and capable of contributing nursing's unique knowledge about patient care and patient care systems through which modern, complex and diverse health care is organized and managed" (p. 543). Leadership at all levels of policy and practice development flows from this skill set. Nurses must be part of health care redesign and provide leadership at all levels of practice and policy, beyond the bedside of the individual patient or family (Iedema, Ainsworth, & Grant, 2007).

Guidelines around governance and leadership are culturally dependent. All governments have differing objectives and requirements for the provision of mental health care. These are influenced by the cultural values about mental health and the pervasive stigma that exists worldwide. Additionally, the increasing fiscal restraints are pushing government and private systems to think creatively and make better use of health resources. It is within this context of change and increased cost effectiveness that nurses have unlimited opportunities to creatively and effectively contribute to the development of health policy.

The ICN gives explicit guidelines for nurses who want to increase their effectiveness and leadership in policy arenas. They suggest the following:

1   Keep abreast of developments, in the local community and country.
2   Write and publish.
3   Join special interest organizations that match your interests and share your positions.
4   Know who the key players are, such as politicians and officials in local, regional and national government.
5   Know the key nursing positions and networks that you might work with to have input into policy.
6   Identify nurses in influential positions outside nursing.
7   Communicate your position through: ongoing representation on policy-making committees or boards, lobbying, making submissions, and meeting with people in positions of influence.

(ICN, 2005, p. 12)

The ICN also suggests that nurses should insert themselves in government and policy-making bodies when it is clear that there is a contribution to be made. Nurses must understand the relevant health and public issues while strategizing policy development and change. Importantly, the ICN recommends partnering with other nursing organizations with similar policy views and values. Mentoring younger nurses and insuring that individuals representing the interests of the organization are well-informed are also essential components (ICN, 2005).

Nurses need to be educated about potential roles in policy development. This begins in basic nursing education and involves skill development for public speaking, negotiating, data analysis, strategic thinking and planning, and policy process. Development of leadership capacity is essential and begins early in the nursing education process (ICN, 2005).

Nurses have a prominent role in understanding that consumers have a right to greater involvement in their health care decisions. Wong (2015) notes that positive nursing leadership is pivotal to optimizing nursing practice that results in high quality patient care. Leaders at all levels must have the "vision, problem solving abilities and the relationship-building skills to navigate the dynamic contexts of organizations to obtain needed resources and support" (Wong, 2015, p. 277). This extends to inclusion of consumers in the decision-making processes around health care. Nursing knowledge results in the transformational leadership that changes and improves health care systems (Thyer, 2003). Essential to this is the growing and vocal consumer voice,which nursing leaders understand and consider.

The concept of global leadership commonalities was explored by Buckner and others (2014) as they described The Global Leadership Discussion sponsored by Sigma Theta Tau. Through a series of sponsored, international discussions, six framework elements were identified as significant to nursing leadership. These included creativity, change, collaboration, community, context, and courage. The commonality of the global policy process was identified and supported the ICN statement that modern "nurses must develop the skills and confidence that will earn the status required to influence health policy" (ICN, 2005, p. 4).

In summary, consumers of mental health services at all levels have become increasingly vocal and influential in determining new directions in service provision, needed skills of nurses and other health care providers who address mental health concerns. With this influence, consumers also play an essential role in the evolution of mental health standards of practice and resulting mental health outcomes. This evolution requires changes in education, collaboration, clinical practice, research and policy. As providers, nurses know and understand the needs of diverse groups of consumers; nurses have the perspective and practice, education, research and policy contexts essential to implementing change models. It is essential that nursing leaders be part of the global transformation of mental health services and evolving standards of consumer-driven care. For this to occur there needs to be targeted education at all levels of nursing preparation focusing on leadership, involvement with multi-disciplinary teams, and groups involved in policy development. Nursing leaders need to be nurtured and supported as they become involved in policy developing groups. This can only result in improved care for consumers.

References

Barbato, A., Bajoni, A., Rapisarda, F., D'Anza, V., De Luca, L.F., Inglese, C., & D'Avanzo, B. (2014). Quality assessment of mental health care by people with severe mental disorders: a participatory research project. *Community Mental Health Journal, 50*(4), 402–408.

Bradstreet, S., & Mcbrierty, R. (2012). Recovery in Scotland: Beyond service development. *International Review of Psychiatry*, 24(1), 64–69.

Brolin, R., Rask, M., Syren, S., Baigi, A., & Brunt, D. A. (2015). Satisfaction with housing and housing support for people with psychiatric disabilities. *Issues in Mental Health Nursing*, 36(1), 21–28.

Buckner, E.B., Anderson, D.J., Garzon, N., Hafsteinsdottir, T.B., Lai, C.K.Y., & Roshan, R. (2014). Perspectives on global nursing leadership: international experiences from the field. *International Nursing Review, 61*, 463–471.

Carless, D., & Douglas, K. (2012). The ethos of physical activity delivery in mental health: a narrative study of service user experiences. *Issues in Mental Health Nursing*, 33(3), 165–171.

Chadwick, A., Street, C., McAndrew, S., & Deacon, M. (2012). Minding our own bodies: reviewing the literature regarding the perceptions of service users diagnosed with serious mental illness on barriers to accessing physical health care. *International Journal of Mental Health Nursing*, 21(3), 211–219.

Chan, M. (2013). *Mental health action plan 2013–2020*. Geneva, Switzerland: World Health Organization.

Clossey, L. & Rheinheimer, D. (2014). Exploring the effect of organizational culture on consumer perceptions of agency support for mental health recovery. *Community Mental Health Journal, 50*(4), 427–434.

Corrigan, P.W., Edwards, A B., Green, A., Diwan, S.L., & Penn, D.L. (2001). Prejudice, social distance, and familiarity with mental illness. *Schizophrenia Bulletin*, 27, 219–225.

Cox, D., & O'Neil, A. (2008). The unhappy marriage between international relations theory and international law. *Global Change Peace and Security*, 20, 201–215.

Griffiths, K. M., Carron-Arthur, B., Parsons, A., & Reid, R. (2014). Effectiveness of programs for reducing the stigma associated with mental disorders: a meta-analysis of randomized controlled trials. *World Psychiatry*, 13, 161–175.

Iedema, R., Ainsworth, S., & Grant, D. (2007). The contemporary clinician-manager: performing professional values or entrepreneuralizing middle-management? In C. Caldas-Coulthard, & R. Iedema, (Eds.), *Identity Trouble: Critical Discourse and Contested Identities*, pp. 273–291. London: Palgrave-Macmillan.

International Council of Nurses (2005). Guidelines on shaping effective health policy. Available at: www.icn.ch/publications/guidelines (accessed April 28, 2015).

Jaeger, M., & Hoff, P. (2012). Recovery: conceptual and ethical aspects. *Current Opinion in Psychiatry*, 25(6), 497–502.

Jeffs, L., Dhalla, I., Cardoso, R., & Bell, C.M. (2014). The perspectives of patients, family members and health care professionals on readmissions: Preventable or inevitable? *Journal of Interprofessional Care*, 28(6), 507–512.

Johnson, T.J., Sanders, D.H., & Stange, J.L. (2014). The affordable care act for behavioral health consumers and families. *Journal of Social Work in Disability & Rehabilitation*, 13, 110–121.

Link, B.G., Struening, E.L., Neese-Todd, S., Asmussen, S., & Phelan, J.C. (2001). Stigma as a barrier to recovery: the consequences of stigma for the self-esteem of people with mental illnesses. *Psychiatric Services, 52*(12), 1621–1626.

McKenzie, L. H. (2006). Service users and carers' experiences of a psychosis service. *Journal of Psychiatric & Mental Health Nursing*, 13(6), 636–640.

Ostrow, L., & Adams, N. (2012). Recovery in the USA: from politics to peer support. *International Review of Psychiatry*, 24(1), 70–78.

Pearson, G.S., Evans, L.K., Hines-Martin, V.P., Yearwood, E.L., York, J.A., & Kane, C.F. (2014). Promoting the mental health of families. *Nursing Outlook, 62*, 225–227.

Pearson, G.S., Hines-Martin, V.P., Evans, L.K., York, J.A., Kane, C.F., & Yearwood, E.L. (2015). Addressing gaps in mental health needs of diverse, at-risk, underserved, and disenfranchised populations: a call for nursing action. *Archives of Psychiatric Nursing, 29*, 14–18.

Raines, L. & Ellis, A. (2014). Lessons learned from a Maryland citizen advocacy group's experience in impacting health reform: the seven Cs of effective citizen advocacy. *Journal of Social Work in Disability and Rehabilitation, 13*(1–2), 21–30.

Rissmiller, D.J. & Rissmiller, J.H. (2006). Evolution of the antipsychiatry movement into mental health consumerism. *Psychiatric Services, 57,* 863–866.

Roe, D., Bril-Bamiv, S., & Kravetz, S. (2012). Recovery in Israel: a legislative recovery response to the needs-rights paradox. *International Review of Psychiatry, 24*(1), 48–55.

Satel, S.L. & Redding, R.E. (2005). Sociopolitical trends in mental health care: the consumer/survivor movement and multiculturalism in B.J. Sadock and V.A. Sadock (Eds.). *Kaplan and Sadock's Comprehensive Textbook of Psychiatry, 8th edition.* Philadelphia PA: Lippincott, Williams &Wilkins.

Schroeder, R. (2013). The seriously mentally ill older adult: perceptions of the patient-provider relationship. *Perspectives in Psychiatric Care, 49*(1), 30–40.

Shattell, M.M., McAllister, S., Hogan, B., & Thomas, S.P. (2006). "She took the time to make sure she understood": mental health patients' experiences of being understood. *Archives of Psychiatric Nursing, 20*(5), 234–241.

Sorensen, R., Iedema, R., & Severinsson, E. (2008). Beyond profession: nursing leadership in contemporary health care. *Journal of Nursing Management, 16,* 535–544.

Tambuyzer, E. & Van Audenhove, C. (2013). Service user and family carer involvement in mental health care: divergent views. *Community Mental Health Journal, 49*(6), 675–685.

Thornicroft, G., Brohan, E., Kassam, A., & Lewis-Holmes, E. (2008). Reducing stigma and discrimination: candidate interventions. *International Journal of Mental Health Systems, 2,* 3.

Thyer, G. (2003). Dare to be different: transformational leadership may hold the key to reducing the nursing shortage. *Journal of Nursing Management, 11,* 73–79.

Tomes, N. (2006). The patient as a policy factor: a historical case study of the consumer/survivor movement in mental health. *Health Affairs, 25*(3), 720–729.

Tse, S., Cheung, E., Kan, A., Ng, R., & Yau, S. (2012). Recovery in Hong Kong: service user participation in mental health services. *International Review of Psychiatry, 24*(1), 40-7.

United Nations General Assembly (1991). The protection of persons with mental illness and the improvement of mental health care: A/RES/46/119. Available at www.un.org/documents/ga/res/46/a46r119.htm (accessed July 16, 2015).

Woodward, A.T., Mowbray, C.T., Holter, M.C., & Bybee, D. (2007). Racial differences in perceptions of social support in consumer-centered services. *Social Work Research, 31*(4), 221–228.

Wong, C.A. (2015). Editorial: connecting nursing leadership and patient outcomes: state of the science. *Journal of Nursing Management, 23,* 275–278.

Wong, D.F.K, Zhuang, X.Y., Pan, J.Y., & He, X.S. (2014). A critical review of mental health and mental health-related policies in China: more actions required. *International Journal of Social Welfare, 23*(2), 195–204.

World Health Organization (2013). *Mental Health Action Plan 2013–2010.* Geneva: World Health Organization.

World Health Organization & International Council of Nurses. (2007). Atlas: nurses in mental health 2007. Available at www.who.int/mental_health/evidence/nursing_atlas_2007.pdf (accessed July 5, 2015).

World Health Organization Secretariat for the Development of a Comprehensive Mental Health Action Plan (2012). Risks to mental health: an overview of vulnerabilities and risk factors. Available at www.-who.int/mental_health/mhgap/risks_to_mental_health_EN_27_08_12.pdf (accessed July 1, 2015).

Zeber, J.E., Copeland, L.A., McCarthy, J.F., Bauer, M.S., & Kilbourne, A.M. (2009). Perceived access to general medical and psychiatric care among veterans with bipolar disorder. *American Journal of Public Health, 99*(4), 720–727.

8

MENTAL HEALTH CARE NURSING STANDARDS

International perspectives

Sarah Benbow, Wafa'a Ta'an, Malene Terp,
Marc Haspeslagh and Cheryl Forchuk

Introduction

The purpose of this chapter is to describe similarities and differences in psychiatric mental health (PMH) nursing care and standards across diverse global contexts. This chapter is based on the experience of four authors residing in four different countries around the globe. Their experiences are bound to the mental health system of their countries and their own careers and practice environments. These examples reflect the authors' lens about psychiatric nursing care practice standards and the functioning of nurses within these countries. Specifically, sets of psychiatric nursing standards will be examined from differing cultural contexts: a North American country (Canada), a Middle Eastern country (Jordan), and two European countries (Belgium and Denmark). Definitions of the standards of mental health care will be provided and a description of PMH nursing within a contextual overview of mental health cares in each country (see Table 8.1). Current mental health issues and tensions that impact nursing and PMH nursing standards of practice will be explored. Recommendations for improving mental health care by increasing the role and visibility of psychiatric nurses will be addressed. The chapter will conclude by discussing the similarities and differences related to PMH nursing practice across these diverse contexts.

The purpose of PMH nursing standards is to describe and direct nursing care and to provide a framework for the practicing nurse. Essentially, standards are a framework, which outlines professional and ethical expectations. Standards can be legislative, or they can be professional and ethical guidelines, which may not be legally mandated. Implementation of standards is dependent on a variety of factors, but they are used to provide moral, ethical, legal, and professional guidance and are reflective of the current issues and trends, as well as nursing regulations in a particular area.

Canada

Canadian PMH care context: background and history

Under the Canadian Health Act (established in 1984), Canada's publicly funded health care system provides universal access and coverage to medically necessary hospital and physician services (Health Canada, 2010). Governed at the provincial level, Canada's health care system is based on *need* rather than the ability to pay, thus, necessary mental health services and hospitalizations are publicly funded. While Canada's system is based on the principles of universality, there is much question about the availability of mental health services to marginalized populations, such as those living in rural and remote Canada. Furthermore, other privatized mental health care options are available only to those who may have employment insurance coverage or the financial resources to pay.

Mental health care in Canada has changed dramatically throughout the years, as has the context in which psychiatric care is provided. Historically, and common to many countries, until the late nineteenth century people with mental illness were usually cared for by their families and religious groups or faced incarceration. Following this period, within Canada, "asylum care" became the responsibility of the government, specifically at the provincial level. This change began the institutionalization process in the 1900s. Many individuals once admitted into these facilities spent the rest of their lives there (Greenland, Griffin, & Hoffman, 2001).

In the early 1960s the deinstitutionalization period began. PMH care shifted with the availability of new psychotropic medications and the expansion of mental health treatment and promotion services from solely large provincial psychiatric facilities to general hospitals, outpatient clinics, and community-based services (Tipliski, 2002). Processes to de-stigmatize individuals with mental illness were also implemented, such as the establishment of a Mental Health Awareness Week, and the role that the Canadian Mental Health Association played in increasing awareness, access, and their engagement in advocacy. The psychiatric consumer-survivor movement emphasized peer support and political action in shaping mental health care and services. In the 1970s and 1980s, recovery and psychosocial rehabilitation models were beginning to influence mental health care. This movement recognized the *person* as opposed to the *illness*, while embracing holistic approaches with emphasis on the development of social skills with the ultimate aim of community (re)integration to optimize the potential for a meaningful life (Farkas, 2013).

PMH nursing in Canada

PMH nursing education in Canada is a component of general nursing baccalaureate and diploma programs (Canadian Federation of Mental Health Nurses, 2006). Four of the 10 Canadian provinces, British Columbia, Alberta, Saskatchewan, and Manitoba, offer specialized training and regulation for psychiatric mental health nurses who are titled *Registered Psychiatric Nurses*. Within the other six provinces of Ontario, Quebec, Nova Scotia, Prince Edward Island, Newfoundland, and New Brunswick, as well as the Territories of Yukon, Northwest Territories, and Nunavut, Registered Nurses and Registered Practical Nurses who work within PMH settings are trained within regular generic nursing education programs and are self-regulated within their respective regulatory provincial colleges and/or associations. All PMH nurses in Canada can receive specialization certification from the Canadian Nurses Association in the area of PMH nursing. Currently, across Canada, PMH nurses work in a variety of settings including: inpatient tertiary psychiatric facilities, mental health units within general hospitals, outpatient clinics, acute care emergency rooms, crisis management clinics/services, mental health organizations, within the criminal justice system, and within public health agencies.

Issues and tensions

PMH nurses across Canada share a number of foci as well as relevant issues. One of the most universal issues within PMH nursing is the continued societal stigma impacting individuals with mental illness (and subsequently the care that they receive). "The care of people with mental and behavioral disorders has always reflected prevailing social values related to the social perception of mental illness" (WHO, 2001a, p. 49). Individuals with mental illness remain one of the most excluded groups in society (Morgan, Burns, Fitzpatrick, Pinfold, & Priebe, 2007; Stuart, 2008). As summarized by Benbow, Rudnick, Forchuk, and Edwards (2014), this exclusion is evidenced by discrimination in employment, housing, and social sectors based on mental illness and/or disability status, which often intersect with poverty status. That is, individuals with mental illness who are dependent on governmental support programs often face economic insecurity. Societal stigma is recognized as an incredible barrier faced by individuals with mental illness (Benbow, 2009). The results of existing inequities, such as overrepresentation of individuals with mental illness in the homeless population (Kim *et al.*, 2007), criminal justice system (Canadian Psychiatric Association, 2011), and in employment discrimination (Benbow, Forchuk, & Ray, 2011) negatively impact their mental health and well-being.

Further, while deinstitutionalization and efforts toward community integration are positive aspects of a progressing mental health care system, mental health care consumers continue to face many barriers. Illness relapse rates, increased hospital admissions, limited availability of community supports, lack of access to basic human needs, such as food and shelter, and continued societal stigma negatively impact community integration and remain prime issues faced by this population and by the nurses who care for them (Benbow *et al.*, 2011; Forchuk, Nelson, & Hall, 2006).

Additional considerations for PMH nurses in Canada include the increasing diversity of populations being served. Providing culturally safe and sensitive care that ensures access and inclusivity for all is an increasingly important focus of PMH nursing. Access and treatment are impacted by language, ethnicity, age, newcomer status, and cultural values, among other factors (Health Commission of Canada, 2009). Another issue in PMH nursing is the rise in co-occurring (or co-morbid) disorders particularly the increase in substance use and dependence. The complexities in presentation and needs when co-occurring disorders are present require special consideration and unique treatment planning (Canadian Centre for Substance Abuse, 2009).

With many of these issues in mind, the Canadian Federation of Mental Health Nurses (CFMHN) developed *the Canadian Standards for Psychiatric-Mental Health Nursing: Standards of Practice*. The initial standards were released in 1995, and the current version is the fourth edition. The latest version further refined the previous documents and included data from focus groups with mental health consumers and their families held by the Standards Committee across the country, thus ensuring that the voices of mental health consumers were incorporated in the standards of practice (CFMHN, 2014).

PMH nursing standards of practice

With the purpose to guide and evaluate PMH nursing practice, there are seven standards of practice (CFMHN, 2014). Table 8.1 provides a summary of the standards, as originally outlined by CFMHN (2014).

Table 8.1 CFMHN PMH standards of nursing practice

Standard	Description
Standard 1: Provides competent professional care through the development of a therapeutic relationship	• The therapeutic relationship remains the crux of mental health nursing • Within this standard there is an emphasis on recognizing the influence that a variety of social and personal determinants of health have on the relationship and therapeutic process. It is important for the nurse to acknowledge the uniqueness and intersections that influence care • The nurse supports the resiliency, self-esteem, self-determination, and hope of the client
Standard 2: Performs/refines client assessments through the diagnostic and monitoring function	• Collaborating with the client, the nurse conducts holistic assessments and determines the most appropriate treatment plan to meet the client's needs
Standard 3: Administers and monitors therapeutic interventions	• Recognizing that many clients are at risk for harm to self and/or others, the nurse will use and monitor evidence-based interventions to provide safe and effective nursing care, including administration of medications • The nurse maintains every effort possible to include the client in treatment decisions • The nurse utilizes group process, client responses to therapeutic intervention, client's cultural values, and family input to shape treatment decisions
Standard 4: Effectively manages rapidly changing situations	• The nurse maintains the therapeutic relationship during rapidly changing situations while maintaining safety • The nurse utilizes a least restrain approach to care • The nurse evaluates responses to rapidly changing situations
Standard 5: Intervenes through the teaching-coaching function	• The nurse recognizes all interactions as potential teaching/learning situations • The nurse provides health promotion information to individuals, families, communities and populations
Standard 6: Monitors and ensures the quality of health care practices	• The nurse advocates for the clients' right to receive the least restrictive form of care, and supports the client's right to self-determination, while ensuring safety • The nurse advocates for continuous improvement to the organization/system • The nurse understands how social determinants impact the health of the client, community, and nursing practice
Standard 7: Practices within organizational and work-role structures	• The nurse participates in developing, implementing and critiquing mental health policy • The nurse advocates and supports a nursing leadership role • The nurse supports constructive and collaborative approaches to resolve differences within the health care teams • The nurse works in collaboration with consumer and advocacy groups for social action

Source: Canadian Federation of Mental Health Nurses, 2014, pp. 7–12.

The standards encompass consumer perspectives and emphasize collaboration with the client, as well as the nurses' role of advocacy. These aspects of the standards reiterate the client-centered shift in mental health care, as well as the continued need for advocacy due to the complex issues facing individuals with mental illness, families, and communities.

Moving into the future, it is clear that mental health (and illness) care requires a continued and strong recognition of the social determinants of health with emphasis on the unique barriers individuals with mental illness face. Demonstrating this, nurses can acknowledge and respond to the social and personal factors impacting one's mental well-being through advocacy at the micro, meso, and macro levels. For example, at the micro level nurses can ensure early assessment and identification of any social needs, such as homelessness, and can intervene to prevent discharge to homeless shelters and the streets (Forchuk, Russell, Kingston-MacClure, Turner, & Dill, 2006). At the intermediate level, nurses can engage in professional practice committees and committees at their place of employment to ensure current practices take social determinants of health into consideration in the care provided. At the macro level, nurses can engage in advocacy through nursing education and increasing awareness of social-political factors influencing the health of individuals with mental illness. This approach moves beyond the traditional and biomedical understandings and approaches to mental illness care, and embraces a person-centered and holistic understanding that one's illness experience is embedded within broader social contexts. PMH nursing standards in Canada will continue to evolve based on consumer involvement, changing issues, and necessary foci in continuing to refine and develop mental health nursing.

Jordan

Jordanian PMH care context: background and history

The political dynamicity of the area has influenced the history of Jordan at all levels, social, cultural, financial, and political, and the various functional systems in the country. The central location of Jordan in the Middle East has led to the immigration of an increasing number of refugees. People from neighboring war-torn countries, such as Iraq and Palestine, and Arab Spring-affected countries such as Syria, and Libya are moving to Jordan seeking a peaceful place to live. The net result is greater diversity of the Jordanian population in terms of backgrounds and country of origin. Within the health care sector, immigration has increased the demand for health care services.

Nursing as a profession started in Jordan approximately 60 years ago. The number of nurses in Jordan is estimated to be 29.5 per 10,000 people. This number is considered to be relatively high in the region, but low compared to Western countries, which also suffer from a nursing shortage (Jrasat, Samawi, & Wilson, 2005).

The history of mental health care can be traced back to the establishment of the first psychiatric mental health care facility in Jordan in 1968 (Hawamdeh, 2002), which makes this facility quite young compared to mental health care facilities in other countries. Before that, Jordanians relied on neighboring countries for mental health care, in addition to the commonly used traditional healing modalities such as visiting a religious person or a traditional healer. Given that mental health care is relatively new in Jordan compared to other Jordanian health care sectors, there is limited research available in the field of mental health care. Research programs that investigate nursing practices within Jordanian mental health care settings are greatly needed to advance the delivery of quality nursing care.

The current Jordanian mental health system is composed of services provided by public (Ministry of Health), university and private sectors, and the military services (Royal Medical Services). Mental health services in Jordan include hospitals, addiction centers, and outpatient mental health facilities. The major limitation of the Jordanian mental health care system is the absence of community-based psychiatric inpatient units or community residential facilities in the country. According to the WHO (2011) report, there are 8.27 beds per 100,000 people in Jordan's mental hospitals, which serve 45 patients per 100,000 people with an occupancy rate of 97 percent. Exact numbers of human resources for Jordanian mental health are unknown for both the public and private sectors. However, estimates based on existing data reveal relatively low numbers of mental health professionals per capita; there are an estimated 1.09 psychiatrists, 0.54 other medical doctors (not specialized in psychiatry), 3.95 nurses (both associated and registered nurses, not specialized in mental health), 0.27 psychologists, 0.3 social workers, and 0.09 occupational therapists per 100,000 inhabitants (WHO, 2011). Furthermore, human resources are disproportionately distributed, as a large percentage of mental health professionals work in mental hospitals near Amman, the capital city, where only 36 percent of the population live.

PMH nursing in Jordan

The profession of nursing is primarily regulated by two institutions, Jordan Nurses and Midwives Council (established in 1959), and the Jordanian Nursing Council (JNC) established in 2002, and led by Princess Muna Al-Hussein-President of the JNC.

According to the Jordanian Nursing Council (2006a), nurses in Jordan are classified as support worker, enrolled nurse, registered nurse, specialist nurse, and advanced practice nurse.

Support workers are also referred to as nursing assistant, auxiliary, and personal care worker. This term is applied to workers who assist directly in nursing care under the direct or indirect supervision of nurses. They are paid providers who are neither registered nor licensed by a regulatory body.

Enrolled nurse or licensed practical nurse (LPN) is a nurse authorized to provide limited nursing care under the supervision of a registered nurse. Registered nurse, qualified, or licensed nurse is a self-regulated care professional who has successfully completed an education program approved by the nursing council.

Specialist nurse is a nurse with advanced expertise in a branch of the nursing field including clinical, teaching, administration, research, and consultant roles. Advanced practice nurse or clinical nurse specialist is a registered nurse who has developed expert knowledge and clinical competencies for expanded practice. Different expectations and scopes of practice are identified for each group of nurses in regard to quality improvement, continuing education, enhancement of the profession, leadership and management, and therapeutic communication and interpersonal relationships.

Issues and tensions

Within the Ministry of Health, the main authorities are the Head of Mental Health Specialty and the Director of the National Centre for Mental Health: the largest governmental psychiatric hospital, which includes the National Center for Addiction and outpatient clinics. Although mental health services are available throughout the country, the structure is very centralized.

In general, there is a lack of PMH training for primary health care workers, and interactions between the primary care and mental health systems are rare. In 2010, Jordan was selected as one of the six countries for the pilot implementation of the Mental Health Gap Action Program (mhGAP), a WHO global program that aims to reduce the mental health treatment gap between what is needed and what is available, and integrate the mental health component into primary health care (PHC). While there are a large number of international NGOs and UN agencies providing psychosocial services, there are only a few local organizations providing these services, and training for mental health staff and psychosocial interventions is rarely provided (WHO, 2011). However, more attention is given to training PMH staff for the period between 2011 and 2013. The World Health Organization (WHO) is collaborating with the Jordanian Nursing Council and the Ministry of Health to provide continuous education for PMH working staff.

Other gaps in the system include the absence of mental health family associations in Jordan. In addition, public education and awareness campaigns are very rare. There are no coordinating bodies supervising mental health awareness campaigns and there is a lack of collaboration between mental health and other relevant sectors (WHO, 2011).

PMH nursing standards of practice

Until recently, there was no Jordanian *mental* health policy. However, there are four articles (art. 13, 14, 15, 16) about mental health and substance abuse included in the *General* Health Act. While specific mental health legislation does not presently exist in Jordan, there are a number of laws that may apply to individuals living with mental illness in the following areas: access to mental health care including access to the least restrictive care (as part of the health law); voluntary and involuntary treatment; law enforcement; and other judicial system issues for people with mental illness (WHO, 2011).

A blueprint for mental health service development was drafted in 1988 and included the following three areas: 1) establishing psychiatric outpatient clinics throughout the country; 2) providing mental health and psychiatry training for doctors, nurses, and mental health workers; and 3) extending mental health care to prisons. From 1988 until 2011, 64 outpatient psychiatric mental health clinics have been established throughout the country; however, the provided care in these facilities is mainly biomedical and needs further advancement. Training is being provided to mental health care professionals but yet is insufficient. Psychiatrists and other doctors receive education that is primarily focused on the rational use of drugs, whereas for nurses and psychologists the focus is on psychosocial interventions. Training on child mental health issues was minimally introduced and only given to psychiatrists. Further, an estimation of 1–20 percent of police officers received education on mental health within the years (2006–2011). Each prisoner with a psychiatric issue has at least one contact with a mental health care provider per month (WHO, 2011).

There are no Jordanian standards for PMH nursing. However, the standards of mental health services may be assessed through several means, including human rights monitoring. In Jordan, the National Centre for Human Rights and a few other non-governmental organizations (NGOs) carry out programs related to the monitoring of human rights in a number of contexts. Nonetheless, human rights standards have only been evaluated in some mental health facilities and only a small fraction of mental health workers receive human rights training. No mental health facility in Jordan receives regular annual human rights inspections, and no PMH staff working in inpatient facilities has received any training on the human rights protection of patients (WHO, 2011).

Another way to regulate PMH nursing practice is through the generic Nursing Professional Standards. Table 8.2 describes the nine standards endorsed by the Jordanian Nursing Council (2006b).

Table 8.2 Jordanian Nursing Council standards

Standard	Description
Standard 1: Professional responsibility and accountability	• The registered nurse is responsible for performing nursing practice in line with the nursing professional ethics approved by the Jordanian Nursing Council, bylaws of licensing agencies and of the employing institution
Standard 2: Practice based on nursing knowledge	• The registered nurse bases his/her nursing practice on knowledge derived from nursing science and other basic and human sciences
Standard 3: Nursing Performance Efficiency	• The registered nurse utilizes knowledge, skills, trends, and judgments in nursing practice
Standard 4: Communication and cooperation	• The registered nurse communicates and cooperates with the clients and the health team for providing nursing care
Standard 5: Compliance with professional ethics	• The registered nurse provides nursing care in line with the Nursing Professional Ethics Guide approved by the Council
Standard 6: Safe environment	• The registered nurse creates a safe environment for both clients and employees within the framework of public safety comprising infection control, protection against hazards, and medical waste management
Standard 7: Total quality management	• The registered nurse adopts a total quality management and continuous quality improvement philosophy as a general framework for upgrading nursing care
Standard 8: Scientific research	• The registered nurse/registered midwife relies on scientific research and evidence-based data for improving nursing care

Source: Jordanian Nursing Council, 2006b, pp. 5–21.

The registered nurse is responsible for practicing nursing in line with the nursing professional ethics approved by the Jordanian Nursing Council, bylaws of licensing agency, and of the employing agency (Jordanian Nursing Council, 2006b). Although standards and regulations are the building blocks for developing nursing practices, standards of care are very general and further detailed guidelines are needed. In addition, there are weaknesses in the commitment of applying these regulations among health care institutions (Jordanian Nursing Council, 2011).

Belgium

Belgian PMH care context: background and history

The political structure of Belgium (see Table 8.3) regulates health care at different levels. Health care in general, including mental health care; is primarily regulated through federal legislations. However, responsibilities are delegated to authorities of regions and communities such as Dutch, French, and German-speaking communities. Both regional and federal authorities are responsible for financing health care (Portal Belgium, 2012). The health care system is publicly funded by the contribution of every citizen in the compulsory social security system.

As in other countries, Belgium has a history of institutional PMH care provided in both general and psychiatric hospitals. Legislation on preventive ambulatory mental health care came in 1975. With the initiation of psychiatric care homes for elderly psychiatric patients came the development of housing initiatives for people with mental health issues who could not live independently (Belgian Bulletin, 1990). This legislation complemented and diversified the residential care facilities for psychiatric care in Belgium.

In 2002, all ministers with responsibility for health care agreed on the future policy for mental health. Major goals were that mental health care was to be deinstitutionalized; directed toward specific needs of target groups of patients; and that care would be organized along care circuits and care networks. A care network is an agreement between different care providers to deliver coordinated care for a specific patient population, e.g. those experiencing alcohol abuse or depression. A taskforce for mental health care was established to guide the implementation of this new policy. An experimental period then started, which included a variety of pilot projects pertaining to forensic, child and adolescent psychiatry, and transverse consultation between different care facilities, therapeutic projects, and reallocation of resources. Studies took place to best utilize the available resources and to evaluate the effectiveness of article 107 of the hospital law. Article 107 enabled the establishment and financing of care circuits and care networks (Belgian Bulletin, 2002).

Based on the results of the experiments, a new model for PMH care was established in 2008 that consisted of five functions:

1   a focus on prevention, promotion of mental health care, early detection, screening, and diagnosis;
2   use of ambulatory care teams for acute and chronic psychiatric disorders;
3   development of teams for rehabilitation and restoration of social integration;
4   establishment of intensive residential care units for acute and chronic psychiatric patients in need of hospitalization; and
5   development of specific living facilities for psychiatric patients who cannot live any longer in their home context.

Psychiatric care in Belgium is progressively moving toward implementing this new framework.

PMH nursing in Belgium

Federal law regulates the profession of health care providers (Belgian Bulletin, 1967) and the executive decree for the nursing profession dates from 1995 (Belgian Bulletin, 1995). Since 1995, no one can practice the profession of nursing unless she/he has graduated, received a diploma, and the diploma is registered in 1 of the 10 provincial health commissions where the nurse can practice.

Since 2009, nursing education has been organized into two programs that are labeled according to Spitzer & Perrenoud (2006): (1) associate level; and (2) bachelor level. Associate level is situated in the "higher professional education level," level 5 (European Qualification Framework). The learning outcomes relevant to that level are comprehensive, specialized, practical, and theoretical knowledge within a field of work or study and an awareness of the boundaries of that knowledge. Bachelor level is situated on a "college level," level 6 (European Qualification Framework). The learning outcomes relevant to the bachelor level are advanced knowledge of a field of work or study, involving critical understanding of theories and principles (European Bulletin, 2008). Both levels comprise 3 years of study with an equivalent of 180 European Credits Transfer System or 4,600 hours of study. In both levels there is one generic profile that leads to the nursing diploma. Nursing specialization is organized by federal decrees from 2006 to present and concerns special professional titles and professional abilities in the various nursing care specialties. The specialization of mental health nursing is relatively recent and dates from 2013 (Belgian Bulletin, 2013).

Issues and tensions

In realizing the new framework for PMH care, all existing PMH care facilities must agree on a local level on the care circuit or care network they want to establish. They are charged with developing a project plan for the government in which they indicate the patient population they will provide care for, the type of care, and how that care will be delivered. A commission has been established to evaluate the proposed plans and identify best practices and new methodologies for organizing psychiatric mental health care in Belgium. The commission will be instrumental in proposing new mental health legislation and following up with mental health pilot projects. At present, it is unclear how quickly these pilot projects will be developed and when new legislation will be identified and implemented.

In Belgium there is no system of accreditation or certification of nurses. Consequently, once graduated, a Belgian PMH nurse is responsible for his/her own continuous education. Most care facilities provide opportunities for continuous education, but these programs are not part of official curricula and do not result in a formal diploma. There is no Belgian PMH nursing organization to promote positions or important issues concerning PMH nursing. All nurses graduate with a generic nursing curriculum since the nursing education reform of 2009. Before 2009, PMH nurses followed 2 years of general curriculum and a third year of specialization in psychiatric nursing. At present, some nursing colleges have established a modular curriculum during which a nurse with a special interest in psychiatric nursing can take modules that are oriented towards PMH nursing. This leads to a notation on their diploma "option psychiatric nursing" but is not a full PMH nursing curriculum of 1 year as existed before 2009. However, this type of education is not yet organized and there is no clear or unified requirement of what content should be taught.

These are incredibly prevalent issues and tensions in the Belgian PMH nursing situation. Moreover, the educational system is governed by the regions and thus can differ between Flanders and Wallonia. The lack of a specific set of standards for PMH care results in a broad definition in the Ministerial Decree (Belgian Bulletin, 2013) of the content, knowledge, and skills a psychiatric nurse should possess or attain. Every nursing college can determine its own content in the broadly described areas of study and practice. Further, the lack of research and evidence in the field within Belgium hampers outlining a pathway of unification around the content of PMH nursing with focus on a generic root and more specific branches to guide the practice specialty.

In 2013 a hospitalization accreditation movement started as part of the renewal system for licensing hospitals. As a consequence focus is set on improving quality of care and patient safety also in psychiatric hospitals. Fischer, Spaeth-Rubee, and Pincus (2013) state that the lack of a common framework hinders international comparison of mental health care quality indicators. Unfortunately, research evidence is scarce on the specific contribution of psychiatric nursing care let alone on the quality of that care.

Countrywide, PMH nurses are not organized as a professional group. There exist some organizations and branches of labor unions that encompass nursing. These organizations focus on some aspects of the professional practice of the job such as remuneration and working hours. There is no plan at present for moving forward with development of the profession of PMH nursing or coming to a consensus about practice and professional standards surrounding this specialty.

Most PMH nurses work in residential psychiatric facilities. They are trained to work within the therapeutic frame of reference that is used on their unit. Apart from some specific research projects, Belgian research on psychiatric nursing is practically non-existent. Implementation of evidence-based PMH nursing care is not in the scope of practitioners.

PMH nursing standards of practice

The practice of nursing in Belgium is regulated by different federal laws and can be synthesized as follows. A nurse can perform three types of acts:

(a) acts that encompass observing, registering health status, describing nursing problems, informing and advising patients, etc.;

(b) acts that encompass assessing and monitoring all body systems such as respiratory, circulatory, digestive, urogenital, skin and sense organs, metabolic systems, and acts that relate to medication, feeding and infusion, mobility, hygiene, physical protection and restriction, and related to assisting with diagnosis and cure and assisting with medical procedures, etc.; and

(c) acts (medical) such as the preparation and administration of chemotherapy or radioactive materials, operation of radiology equipment, etc., which a nurse can perform under certain conditions.

Standard nursing care plans and/or nursing procedures are required when performing the (b) and (c) acts. The standard nursing care plan describes the different steps a nurse must take within a particular timeframe and enables the nurse to provide care for the patient in a systematic way. A procedure describes the way of executing a certain nursing or medical technique. In some circumstances the act can be performed on a standing order rather than a prescription. In such cases, the order from the doctor predefines the way the nurse executes the care. Standard nursing care plans, nursing procedures, and standing orders are the only nursing care standards used by Belgian nurses. That is, legislation defines what constitutes a standard nursing care plan, a nursing procedure, and a standing order. However, nurses at each hospital define the content based on care plans to ensure unique applicability to each care setting. No nationwide standards exist at this time. Standards are at the micro level of each hospital and need to be developed by the nurses of each hospital. The list of acts does not contain any specific acts related to psychiatric mental health nursing, as mental health was not the focus. The intent was to give a legal ground for general nursing, with acts for nursing specialties to follow; however this has yet to be initiated.

The structural reform of psychiatric care only affects psychiatric nurses who are part of the care circuit or network. The reform process is still in an experimental phase, led by the Federal Ministry of Public Health and an evaluation commission. However, the reform process has already shed light on the future practice of PMH nursing. Care has become deinstitutionalized, more focused on outreach and diversification, and more demand-driven. How quickly this reform will be implemented or generalized remains unclear. Complete implementation of structural reform will depend on the way that the financing of the care circuit or care network will be arranged.

The structural reform of mental health care will take place at its own pace. The most important and urgent point for the future of PMH nursing in Belgium is the professionalism of the discipline. Without formal professional nursing organizations, changing the practice of the profession comes from structural reform, not from the profession itself. The discipline of PMH nursing should also critically appraise the need for certification of psychiatric nurses during their professional career. The ultimate goal should be to provide up-to-date, evidenced-informed, quality psychiatric nursing care for patients with mental health needs irrespective of where the patient is receiving care.

Denmark

Danish PMH care context: background and history

Historically, PMH care can be traced back to the early 1800s, where public authorities had a greater responsibility for individuals with mental illness. Until this period, the task of caring for or housing people, who were then called "lunatics," was still a private matter for the family (Kragh, 2008). At the end of the nineteenth century, employment of qualified nurses at the large mental asylums in Denmark began, and the asylums were gradually reorganized into hospital settings for treatment and care. The introduction of new and effective antipsychotic medications in the 1950s gradually changed the scope and context of psychiatric nursing in Denmark: from inpatient to outpatient services, from extended admissions to short and intensive admissions, followed up in specialized outpatient units, and from a narrow focus of medical models and mind–body dichotomy, towards a bio-psychosocial approach to mental illness and recovery (Hoof, 2011).

At the heart of the newest recommendations for a more modern and open mental health care system in Denmark, is the notion of inclusion of people with mental health issues in society (Ministry of Health, 2013). However, recently, research has drawn attention to an undesirable effect of reorganizing mental health services in Denmark, which functions as a barrier to inclusion. A review of mental health care institutions in nine European Countries found that the decreasing number of forensic beds, identified mental health slots in supervised and supported housing, and a significant increase in the prison population occurred during this period of reorganization, thus pointing to a potential trend of a new form of institutionalized PMH care in Denmark (Nordentoft, Pedersen, Pedersen, Blinkenberg, & Mortensen, 2012; Priebe *et al.*, 2008).

PMH nursing in Denmark

As a response to the historical development and scope of modern PMH practice, specialty training committed to promoting mental health through the assessment, diagnosis, and treatment of human responses to mental health problems and psychiatric disorders has evolved in Denmark. Since 1996, a 1-year diploma program (60 European Credit Transfer and Accumulation System (ECTS) credits equivalent to 1500–1800 hours of study) of specialized training has been available in three of the five regions of the country. The diploma program is available to all qualified nurses meeting the requirement of two years of work experience within mental health care (Ministry of Health, 1996). The course of training is divided between clinical (60 percent) and theoretical (40 percent) education, within the areas of clinical PMH nursing, quality development, teaching, counseling, coordination and multidisciplinary collaboration (Specialuddannelsen i psykiatrisk sygepleje, 2011).

Specialized PMH nurses deliver free and publicly funded care to individuals in need in a variety of settings across the entire continuum of care (Danish Nurses Organization, 2005). Privatized mental health care options are available, but only to those who may have employment insurance coverage or the financial resources to pay. The free and publicly funded services include inpatient psychiatric facilities, outpatient clinics, acute care emergency rooms, assertive community treatment teams, general practitioner clinics, crisis management services, mental health organizations, addiction services, transcultural teams for traumatized refugees, and services within the criminal justice system and in residential care and supervised housing facilities.

A recent report from the Danish Nurses Organization has documented that only 15 percent of nurses working within mental health care facilities in Denmark are certificated as PMH nurses, despite other intentions and needs. Lack of certified nurses is an issue of great concern due to the broad scope of practice, and it has been stated that 50 percent of nurses working within PMH care must obtain specialty training by 2020 in order to support the national goal of development of high quality care for all (Danish Nurses Organization, 2013).

Issues and tensions

One of the most evident concerns shared within mental health nursing in Denmark, is the growing need for PMH services. Mental disorders account for 25 percent of the total burden of disease in the health care system followed by cancer and circulatory diseases, respectively accounting for 17 percent and 15.2 percent. Mental disorders such as depression, anxiety, and behavioral disorders further account for 50 percent of all long-term sick leave in Denmark and 48 percent of all disability pensions, and when people younger than 30 years of age in Denmark are granted an early retirement pension, four out of five cases are due to a mental disorder (Ministry of Health, 2013). The trend leaves PMH nurses with important tasks throughout the continuum of care in order to develop supportive and engaging health promoting initiatives. However, this work is complicated by stigma, which is the most powerful obstacle to the development of comprehensive mental health care in the Western countries (Beldie *et al.*, 2012).

The extended need of PMH services in concordance with new demands, such as release and implementation of new assessment and treatment guarantees, lack of psychiatrists, and lack of specialized PMH nurses, poses a further serious challenge to the quality of mental health care in Denmark in the future. Recently it was stated that the mental health system needs a transition to meet evident and future challenges. The initial step of transition is a governing vision of user-centered treatment and care (Ministry of Health, 2013). Key to this vision is a service system where values of self-determination and user involvement, user participation, recovery, and inclusion serve as a frame for mental health services, and inform its practices. The vision is grounded in a philosophy of partnerships to promote and develop a more user-centered, engaging, empowering, cost-effective and less stigmatizing health care system (Coulter, 2012; Coulter, 2011; Coulter & Ellins, 2006; Tambuyzer, Pieters, & Van Audenhove, 2011). The vision emphasizes a movement away from the patient as a passive partner in need of care, towards the patient as an active partner on an individual level of care, and patients as valuable partners and important knowledge sources in the process of developing services responsive to needs, problems, preferences, and values of patients (WHO, 2001b).

In Denmark organizational user-involvement projects are on the rise within PMH care development. An example is the SmartCare project where a smartphone application—MindFrame—supportive to everyday living with newly diagnosed schizophrenia, has been co-designed with end-users (Terp *et al.*, 2016). The project emphasizes that involvement should encompass the full range of people's experiences—not just the concerns that workers or planners consider important. The project, which is grounded in a participatory mindset, is one of the first research projects within psychiatric mental health nursing to investigate how individuals with severe mental illness can serve as co-designers of a "modern" mental health service and show that there is room for people with mental health problems to be strong collaborators in mental health service design and development for future care.

PMH nursing standards of practice

In Denmark national standards to guide and evaluate health care within the areas of organization (quality and risk management, data safety, work planning, and competence development), general patient pathways (medication, user-involvement, information and communication, coordination and continuity, health promotion and transition), and disease recognition and management (treatment, care, diagnostics, prevention, and rehabilitation) are seen as key to high-quality care in a patient-centered twenty-first century. Standards have been available since 2009, and are now available in its second version (Danish Institute for Quality and Accreditation in Healthcare (IKAS), 2012). There are no specific standards for PMH nursing practice as the national standards represent a joint model for quality and quality development in health care in Denmark, within all specialties. The governing vision of the standards is to achieve: 1) a consistent and high level of quality across the full range of health care services, from general practitioners to hospital, through pharmacies to home nursing and rehabilitation services; 2) coherence in the patients' experience within the course of care; 3) transparency in relation to the services and benefits of the health care system; and 4) a culture where all employees and institutions engage in ongoing and mutual learning and thereby generate and facilitate quality development.

The national standards serve as a frame for description of good-quality mental health care, which implies patients as collaborative partners in own care. Moving into the future it is clear that standards must be further evaluated and developed in regard to strongest evidence at a national level to improve the quality of care, but also that standards must be adapted and managed at local levels to address target groups and contexts of PMH nursing. There is an immense need to develop transparent and systematic description of best practice within the mental health care domain to guide the practice of PMH nursing, thus to increase the role and visibility of PMH nurses. However, the low number of nurses with academic skills and competences to develop transparent and systematic descriptions of best practice within the mental health care domain, in conjunction with the low number of certificated PMH nurses in Denmark, poses a serious challenge to the development, adaption and management of standards to guide the practice of PMH nursing, and therefore increase the role and visibility of PMH nurses.

Conclusion

PMH nursing standards can offer a necessary guide for nurses to ensure high-quality practice and to "promote competent, safe, and ethical service" (Canadian Nurses Association, 2008, p. 9) to people with mental health care needs. PMH nursing standards should not be static, but rather dynamic documents that are reflective of current issues and tensions within the mental health care system.

The development and implementation of PMH nursing standards are dependent on a variety of factors, and can be discussed in relation to the structure and processes of mental health care and nursing within each country. For each country discussed in this chapter, there is a structure in place for the delivery of mental health care to people with mental health needs. These structures vary from country to country. As these structures continue to evolve, roles for psychiatric nurses also develop. In countries where the mental health care system is in its infancy, it is logical that development and/or implementation of specific mental health nursing standards is currently lacking. For example, in Jordan, where mental health care has been established relatively recently, no psychiatric mental health nursing standards of practice exist at this time. Canada, Jordan, and Denmark have general nursing standards of practice related to professional regulation, standards by which all nurses are legally and professionally bound. Canada, in addition to general nursing standards, has an additional professional and ethical framework specific for psychiatric and mental health nurses. Nationwide nursing standards do not exist in Belgium. Standardization of care is undertaken at the hospital level within the legal framework of standard nursing care plans, procedures, and standing orders.

Based on the limited development of psychiatric and mental health nursing standards of practice within the countries discussed in this chapter, one might question if their existence is advantageous or purposeful. We, the authors of this chapter, propose that specialized standards of practice for PMH nursing are warranted and necessary in attempts to provide high-quality nursing care to this unique population with specific needs. While general nursing standards are applicable to all nursing practice, there are additional, specialized health care and nursing concerns in working within mental health care. We propose that specialty-specific standards of practice should reflect current issues in that practice area and should include clients and their family members as key stakeholders in the development process. We recognize that the development of PMH standards is dependent on several variables, including the country's current state of health care infrastructure, the autonomy and role of the nursing profession, the existence and current state of mental health care infrastructure, the value of clients and their family members at an organizational level, as well as the establishment and role of nursing associations and groups in initiating the development of such standards. This will vary from country to country and will also be shaped by the economic development of the country.

An additional challenge when standards are created is ensuring effective implementation into practice. Therefore, a main challenge is developing standards that focus on the translation of the generally formulated existing standards into practical guidelines in which these standards can be utilized in the individual therapeutic relationship with patients. Acting so can bridge the gap between the theoretical formulation of standards and its practical usage every day by each PMH nurse. Research on the implementation and effectiveness of PMH nursing standards of practice can illuminate implementation issues, challenges, and effectiveness.

Table 8.3 provides a comparison of several factors across all four countries. Factors included are income, number of health care providers, presence of policy and mental health legislation, number of beds within and outside of psychiatric hospitals, and the number of psychiatric nurses per 100,000 in the population. Table 8.4 Provides country profile data.

Table 8.3 Country demographic comparison

Country	World Bank income categories	Health providers per 100,000 people	Presence of MH policy or program	Presence of MH legislation	Total number MH beds per 100,000 people	MH beds outside MH hospitals % of total MH beds	Psychiatric nurses per 100,000 people
Canada	H	1209	Y	Y	19.34	52.95	44
Jordan	LM	527	Y	Y	1.57	10.83	2
Belgium	H	1097	Y	Y	22.1	41.63	unknown
Denmark	H	1351	Y	Y	7.1	unknown	59

Source: Jacob *et al.*, 2007, pp. 1063–1069.

Table 8.4 Country profiles

Country	Government	Location	Population	Official languages
Canada	A constitutional monarchy and federal state with a democratic parliament	Located in the northern part of North America consisting of 10 provinces and 3 territories	Estimated 35 million (Statistics Canada, 2013) with approximately 21% of the population consisting of newcomers (Statistics Canada, 2011). Aboriginal Peoples are comprised of Inuit, Native, and Métis Peoples	English and French
Jordan	Jordan (The Hashemite Kingdom) is a constitutional monarchy with an appointed government	Located in the Middle East and shares borders with Palestine/Israel, Syria, Iraq and Saudi Arabia	Estimated 6.9 million of whom approximately 2 million Palestinian refugees (UNRWA), 597,300 Syrian refugees, and 55,500 Iraqi refugees. Muslims represent 97.2% of the population, Christians 2.2%, and others 0.6% (CIA, 2014)	Arabic
Belgium	A constitutional monarchy, organized as a parliamentary democracy. The country is politically and economically integrated in Europe	Located in the center of Europe consisting of three regions (Flanders, Wallonia, and Brussels) and three communities (Flemish, French and German) with their own language. It shares borders with the Netherlands (north), Germany (east), Luxembourg (south-east), France (south) and the North Sea (west)	Estimated 11 million with 6.5 million residing in Flanders, 3.5 million in Wallonia and 1 million in Brussels (Statistics Belgium, 2015)	Dutch, French, and German
Denmark	A unitary constitutional monarchy, organized as a parliamentary democracy. The country is politically and economically integrated in Europe	Located in Northern Europe: south-west of Sweden, south of Norway and is bordered to the south by Germany. The country has two autonomous constituent countries in the North Atlantic Ocean, the Faroe Islands and Greenland	Estimated 5.5 million with an urban population of 87%. It is home to 600,000 newcomers from more than 200 different countries (Statistics Denmark, 2013)	Danish

References

Beldie, A., den Boer, J.A., Brain, C., Constant, E., Figueira, M.L., Filipcic, I., Gillain, B., Jakovljevic, M., Jarema, M., Jelenova, D., Karamustafalioglu, O., Kores Plesnicar, B., Kovacsova, A., Latalova, K., Marksteiner, J., Palha, F., Pecenak, J., Prasko, J., Prelipceanu, D., Ringen, P.A., Sartorius, N., Seifritz, E., Svestka, J., Tyszkowska, M., & Wancata, J. (2012). Fighting stigma of mental illness in midsize European countries. *Social Psychiatry and Psychiatric Epidemiology*, *47*(Suppl 1), 1–38.

Belgian Bulletin (1967). Royal Decree 78 10/11/1967, *The Belgian Official Journal*. Brussels: Belgian Government.

Belgian Bulletin (1990). Royal Decree 10/07/1990, *The Belgian Official Journal*. Brussels: Belgian Government.

Belgian Bulletin (1995). Law 6/04/1995, *The Belgian Official Journal*. Brussels: Belgian Government.

Belgian Bulletin (2002). Law 14/01/2002, *The Belgian Official Journal*. Brussels: Belgian Government.

Belgian Bulletin (2013). Ministerial Decree 24/04/2013, *The Belgian Official Journal*. Brussels: Belgian Government.

Benbow, S. (2009). Societal abuse in the lives of individuals with mental illness. *Canadian Nurse*, *105*(6), 30–32.

Benbow, S., Forchuk, C., & Ray, S. (2011). Mothers with mental illness experiencing homelessness: A critical analysis. *Journal of Psychiatric and Mental Health Nursing*, *18*(9), 687–695.

Benbow, S., Rudnick, A., Forchuk, C., & Edwards, B. (2014). Using a capabilities approach to understand poverty and social exclusion of psychiatric survivors in Canada. *Disability and Society*, *29*(7), 1046–1060.

Canadian Centre for Substance Abuse. (2009). *Concurrent Disorders: Substance Abuse in Canada*. Retrieved on July 13, 2013 from www.ccsa.ca/2010%20CCSA%20Documents/ccsa-011811–2010.pdf.

Canadian Federation for Mental Health Nurses. (2006). *Canadian Standards for Psychiatric-Mental Health Nursing*. Retrieved on June 1, 2010 from http://cfmhn.ca/sites/cfmhn.ca/files/CFMHN%20standards%201.pdf.

Canadian Federation for Mental Health Nurses (2014). *Canadian Standards for Psychiatric-Mental Health Nursing*. Retrieved on March 1, 2015 from http://cfmhn.ca/sites/cfmhn.ca/files/212922-CFMHN-standards-rv-3a.pdf.

Canadian Nurses Association. (2008). *Code of Ethics for Registered Nurses*. Retrieved on April 25, 2016 from www.cna-aiic.ca/~/media/cna/files/en/codeofethics.pdf.

Canadian Psychiatric Association. (2011). *Psychiatrists Urge Government to Address Worsening Mental Health Problems among Inmates*. Retrieved on July 20, 2013 from www.cpa-apc.org/media.php?mid=1664.

Central Intelligence Agency (CIA) (2014). *The World Factbook 2013–14*. Middle East: Jordan. Washington, DC: CIHI. Retrieved on February 10, 2015 from www.cia.gov/library/publications/the-world-factbook/geos/jo.html.

Coulter, A. (2011). *Engaging Patients in Healthcare*. Milton Keynes, UK: Open University Press.

Coulter, A. (2012). Patient engagement: What works? *The Journal of Ambulatory Care Management*, *35*(2), 80–89.

Coulter, A., & Ellins, J. (2006). *Patient-Focused Interventions: A Review of the Evidence*. London: The Health Foundation.

Danish Institute for Quality and Accreditation in Healthcare, IKAS (2012). Accreditation Standards. Retrieved on February 10, 2014 from www.ikas.dk/IKAS/English/Print-and-download.aspx.

Danish Nurses Organization (2005). Funktionsbeskrivelse for sygeplejesker med specialuddannelse i psykiatrisk sygepleje. Retrieved on February 1, 2014 from http://shop.dsr.dk/product/funktionsbeskrivelse-for-sygeplejersker-med-specialuddannelse-i-psykiatrisk-sygepleje-132/.

Danish Nurses Organization (2013). Vejen mod en bedre psykiatri. Retrieved on February 1, 2014 from www.dsr.dk/Temaer/Sider/Vejen-mod-et-bedre-psykiatri.aspx.

European Bulletin (2008). *European Qualification Framework for Lifelong Learning*. The European Official Journal, Brussels: European Union.

Farkas, M. (2013). Introduction to psychiatric/psychosocial rehabilitation: History and foundations. *Current Psychiatric Reviews*, *9*(3), 177–187.

Fisher, C.E., Spaeth-Rubee, B., & Pincus, H.A. (2013). Developing mental health care quality indicators: Toward a common framework. *International Journal for Quality in Health Care*, *25*(1), 75–80

Forchuk, C., Nelson, G., & Hall, B. (2006). "It's important to be proud of the place you live in": Housing problems and preferences of psychiatric survivors. *Perspectives in Psychiatric Care*, *42*(1), 42–52.

Forchuk, C., Russell, G., Kingston-MacClure, S., Turner, K., & Dill, S. (2006). From psychiatric wards to the streets and shelters. *Journal of Psychiatric and Mental Health Nursing, 13*(3), 301–308.

Greenland, C., Griffin, J.D., & Goffman, B.F. (2001). Psychiatry in Canada from 1951–2001. In M.B. Quentin Rae-Grant (Ed.), *Psychiatry in Canada: 50 years (2nd ed.).* Ottawa: Canadian Psychiatric Association, 1–16.

Hawamdeh, S. (2002). *The Nature of Psychiatric Mental Health Nursing Practices within Arab Culture.* Unpublished PhD thesis. The University of Toronto, Ontario, Canada.

Health Canada. (2010). Canada's health care system. Retrieved on April 30, 2013 from www.hc-sc.gc.ca/hcs-sss/medi-assur/index-eng.php.

Health Commission of Canada. (2009). *Diversity Issues Report Summary.* Retrieved on July 20, 2013 from www.mentalhealthcommission.ca/Diversity_Issues_Options_Report_Summary_Eng-3.pdf.

Hoof, F.V. (2011). *Outpatient Care and Community Support for Persons with Severe Mental Health Problems: A Comparison of National Policies and systems in Denmark, England and the Netherlands.* Utrecht: Netherlands Institute of Mental Health and Addiction.

Jacob, K.S., Sharan, P., Mirza, I., Garrido-Cumbrera, M., Seedat, S., Mari, J.J., Sreenivas, V., & Saxena, S. (2007). Mental health systems in countries: Where are we now? *The Lancet, 370,* 1061–1077.

Jordanian Nursing Council (2006a). *Nursing Scope of Practice.* Amman, Jordan. Retrieved on 1 February 2015 from www.jnc.gov.jo/english/publications/english%20scope%20.pdf.

Jordanian Nursing Council (2006b). *Nursing Professional Standards.* Amman, Jordan. Retrieved on February 1, 2015 from www.jnc.gov.jo/english/publications/professional%20standerd.pdf.

Jordanian Nursing Council (2011). *National Nursing Strategy: Towards Excellence in Nursing Care for All By 2015.* Amman, Jordan. Retrieved on February 1, 2015 from www.jnc.gov.jo.

Jrasat, M., Samawi, O., & Wilson, C. (2005). Belief, attitudes and perceived practice among newly enrolled students at the Jordanian Ministry of health nursing colleges and institutes in 2003. *Education for Health, 18*(2), 145–156.

Kim, M., Swanson, J., Swartz, M., Bradford, D., Mustillo, S., Elbogen, & E. (2007). Health care barriers among severely mentally ill homeless adults: Evidence from the five-site health and risk study. *Administration and Policy in Mental Health, 34*(4), 363–375.

Kragh, J. V. (2008). *Psykiatriens historie i Danmark* (1. udgave ed.). Kbh: Hans Reitzel.Mental

Ministry of Health (1996). Bekendtgørelse om specialuddannelsen for sygeplejersker i psykiatrisk sygepleje. BEK nr. 447. Retrieved on 30 June, 2014 from www.retsinformation.dk/Forms/R0710.aspx?id=81591.

Ministry of Health (2013). En moderne, åben og inkluderende indsats for mennesker med psykiske lidelser. Retrieved on February 1, 2014 from www.sum.dk/Aktuelt/Nyheder/Psykiatri/2013/Oktober/~/media/Filer%20-%20Publikationer_i_pdf/2013/Rapport-psykiatriudvalg-okt-2013/En%20moderne%20åben%20og%20inkluderende%20indsats_hovedrapport.ashx.

Morgan, C., Burns, T., Fitzpatrick, R., Pinfold, V., & Priebe, S. (2007). Social exclusion and mental health: Conceptual and methodological review. *British Journal of Psychiatry, 191,* 477–483.

Nordentoft, M., Pedersen, M.G., Pedersen, C.B., Blinkenberg, S., & Mortensen, P.B. (2012). The new asylums in the community: Severely ill psychiatric patients living in psychiatric supported housing facilities. A Danish register-based study of prognostic factors, use of psychiatric services, and mortality. *Social Psychiatry and Psychiatric Epidemiology, 47*(8), 1251–1261.

Portal Belgium (2012). About Belgium. Portal belguim.be: official information and services. Retrieved on May 1, 2015 from www.belgium.be/en/about_belgium/government/

Priebe, S., Frottier, P., Gaddini, A., Kilian, R., Lauber, C., Martinez-Leal, R., Munk-Jørgensen, P., Walsh, D., Wiersma, D., & Wright, D. (2008). Mental health care institutions in 9 European countries, 2002 to 2006. *Psychiatric Services (Washington, DC), 59*(5), 570–573.

Specialuddannelesen i psykiatrisk sygepleje (2011). Uddannelsesordning, specialuddannelsen for sygeplejersker i psykiatrisk sygepleje. Retrieved on June 1, 2014 from www.specpsyksygeplejerske.dk/files/Psykiatri%20og%20Social/Spec%20udd%20sygepl/INFO/Gældende_24%20april%202014_Uddannelsesordning.pdf.

Spitzer, A. & Perrenoud, B. (2006). Reform in nursing education across Western Europe: Implementation processes and current status. *Journal of Professional Nursing, 22*(3), 162–171.

Statistics Belgium (2015). *Bevolking—Cijfers bevolking 2010–2014.* Retrieved on February 10, 2015 from http://statbel.fgov.be/nl/statistieken/cijfers/.

Statistics Canada (2011). *Immigration and Ethno-Cultural Diversity in Canada.* Retrieved on January 1, 2014 from www12.statcan.gc.ca/nhs-enm/2011/as-sa/99-010-x/99-010-x2011001-eng.cfm.

Statistics Canada (2013). *Latest Indicators.* Retrieved on January 1, 2014 from www.statcan.gc.ca/start-debut-eng.html.

Statistics Denmark (2013). *Nordic Statistical Yearbook.* Retrieved on February 1, 2014 from www.dst.dk/en.

Stuart, H. (2008). Fighting the stigma caused by mental disorders: Past perspectives, present activities, and future directions. *World Psychiatry, 7*(3), 185–188

Tambuyzer, E., Pieters, G., & Van Audenhove, C. (2011). Patient involvement in mental health care: One size does not fit all. *Health Expectation: An International Journal of Public Participation in Health Care and Health Policy, 17,* 138–150.

Terp, M., Lauersen, B.S., Jørgensen, R., Mainz, J., Bjørnes, C.D. (2016). A room for design: Through participatory design young adults with schizophrenia become strong collaborators. *International Journal of Mental Health Nursing.* [Epub ahead of print].

Tipliski V. 2002. *Parting at the Crossroads: The Development of Education for Psychiatric Nursing in Three Canadian Provinces, 1909–1955.* PhD thesis, University of Manitoba.

World Health Organization. (2001a). *Solving mental health problems.* Retrieved on April 17, 2013 from www.who.int/whr/2001/en/whr01_ch3_en.pdf.

World Health Organization. (2001b). *Community Participation in Local Health and Sustainable Development: Approaches and Techniques.* Development and Health Series: 4. Copenhagen: WHO Regional Office for Europe 2001.

World Health Organization. (2011). *WHO–Aims Report on Mental Health System in Jordan. A Report of the Assessment of the Mental Health System in Jordan Using the World Health Organization: Assessment Instrument for Mental Health Systems (WHO–AIMS).* Amman, Jordan: WHO & Ministry of Health.

9

TRANSFORMATIONAL LEADERSHIP TO PROMOTE WELL-BEING

Angela Barron McBride

Comprehensive mental health not only encompasses the treatment of a range of behavioral and mental disorders, but it presupposes preventive efforts directed at vulnerable populations and the ability to promote a well-being that enables individuals to maximize their abilities, cope with stresses, enjoy satisfying family and work relationships, and actively participate in the life of their communities. Practitioners who would implement and realize such a broad and full professional agenda must see themselves as leaders getting better over time and able to orchestrate their careers for maximum effect. Not only must they be capable of best practices themselves, but they must mentor the less educated and less experienced, and work across disciplinary barriers to move forward initiatives that no one profession can manage by itself. Realizing this complex professional agenda is further complicated by the fact that many of the commonplace mental disorders are associated with co-morbidities, from HIV/AIDS to poverty, which are challenging to address.

On May 27, 2013, the sixty-sixth World Health Assembly adopted a *Comprehensive Mental Health Action Plan 2013–2020* (World Health Organization (WHO), 2013), which had as one of its major objectives strengthening effective leadership. The idea behind this recommendation is that you can only achieve all of the clinical goals with effective leadership. While the focus of the action plan was on governance within government and non-governmental organizations, the called-for updating of policies and plans presupposes a workforce prepared to exert leadership at both micro (what is going on within an individual or family) and macro (what is going on within a community, country or globally) levels. But are twenty-first-century health care professionals, particularly nurses, prepared to exert that kind of more transformational leadership? Not really, because most of today's providers were educated to focus on developing the provider–patient relationship rather than being taught (and expected) to redesign the delivery system in light of changing realities. Historically, health professional education emphasized informative learning (acquiring facts), but now the emphasis is additionally on formative learning (developing professional ethics) and transformative learning (developing leadership attributes), because the individual is expected to become not only an expert but a values-driven professional who can act as a change agent (Frenk *et al.*, 2010). The emphasis in behavioral/ mental health treatment has historically been on "giving therapy" to the patient or family rather than on the system issues that limit how therapeutic health care professionals can actually be, e.g., the actual services provided by an agency. Transformational leadership is not easy to achieve because it implies a formidable assignment—moving away from a focus on transitory, isolated performance improvements by individuals to an emphasis on creating sustained, integrated, comprehensive system change (Bass, 1985).

Moreover, the lifecycle perspective in this action plan also suggests that health care professionals be inculcated with a lifespan perspective about their own careers, and that hasn't been the orientation of most nurses. Health care professionals have largely been educated to obtain licensure in their discipline and board certification in a specialty, but relatively few have been expected to exert over time the leadership needed to be transformative. If they accomplish such transformation, they are regarded as exceptional because that wasn't a normative expectation. Nurses have been socialized to demonstrate high-level individual performance and productive teamwork, but few of them have been prepared to exact higher performance in others and create enduring excellence, which are higher-level leadership goals (Collins, 2005).

If the developmental emphasis is placed on the competencies that professionals are supposed to demonstrate when initially licensed or board certified, then little attention is paid to how each health professional changes over time and orchestrates a full career. Specifically, the many functional roles associated with leadership responsibilities—becoming a preceptor or mentor, a committee chair, an administrator, an author, an editor, a researcher, a community organizer, a spokesperson, a consultant, an officer of a professional or community association, a fund raiser, a grants manager, a board member, a planner, policy analyst, and the like—are given short shrift.

Since there is some evidence that mental health professionals are less likely to experience burnout if they have a sense of personal accomplishment and a positive self-image (Jeanneau & Amelius, 2001), lifespan career development should also include some mastery of the strategies thought to sustain optimism over the course of a career. Staying engaged and seeing opportunities are not mainly a matter of luck or of what others do to be supportive, but of how you explain your situation and think about matters. To address all of these career issues, this chapter: (a) defines leadership in terms of transformative expectations; (b) describes five career stages and the mentoring needed at each stage to reflect how the nurse develops a larger sphere of influence over time; and (c) ends with a listing of what nurses can do to sustain their professional optimism over time.

Leadership defined

In the twentieth century, nurses were more likely to be described in the media as handmaidens or helpers rather than as leaders or doers (Kalisch & Kalisch, 1987). Nursing has traditionally been seen as more technical than professional, and without career advancement. If anything, nurses were reproached, whenever they assumed leadership responsibilities that limited their time at the bedside, as having left the profession. Nurses who obtained a doctorate or became administrators were chided as "not real nurses" because their responsibilities involved data analysis and strategic planning rather than hands-on care. Perceptions of a career in nursing have been described as different from those for an "ideal career" with regard to respect, autonomy, compensation, and "busyness," with the profession being seen as evoking less of the first three and more of the last (Cohen, Palumbo, Rambur, & Mongeon, 2004). Even in recent times, middle-school children have tended to describe nursing as boring, doing the same job year after year (Sherman, 2000).

Views of leadership have also long been gendered, and that has consequences for a profession still largely peopled by women. Dominance and self-assurance, more likely to be regarded as men's traits, have generally been equated with leadership more than being responsible and responsive, leadership qualities more associated with women. Leaders have been depicted historically as strong, heroic figures—the scientist works alone to find the cure; the captain single-handedly lands the crippled plane—the antithesis of what nurses do on a day-to-day basis as team members (Northouse, 2004). Because nurses collectively take 24-hour responsibility for their patients, what anyone does as an individual, no matter how innovative, may be relatively invisible. It goes against the "center stage" expectations we have of leaders to read that some nurse leaders even describe humility as an important aspect of their effectiveness (Houser & Player, 2004).

However, the model for what qualities and competencies leaders should possess is changing. The rigid command-and-control models of leadership that once held sway in military and monastic settings are thought to be counterproductive in settings that place a premium on collaboration (Eagly, 2007). A survey of 64,000 people in 13 countries demonstrated that women and men both prefer leaders with more "feminine" leadership styles, for example, leaders who build consensus in order to move the organization forward (Gerzema & D'Antonia, 2013). A team-oriented approach has increasingly been found to have a positive impact on quality in hospital settings (Gittell *et al.*, 2000). The more complex an organization is—with diverse programs, stakeholders, and professional backgrounds—the more leadership needs to *enable* organizational effectiveness as opposed to *deciding* that effectiveness (Marion & Uhl-Bien, 2001). Interestingly, a meta-analysis of 45 studies of different leadership styles found that women leaders were more transformational in their approach than their male counterparts (Eagly, Johannesen-Schmidt, & von Engen, 2003). Women managers were more likely to motivate their colleagues to feel pride and respect because of their association with them, to convey optimism about future goals, and they were more attuned to their colleagues' developmental needs (Eagly & Johannesen-Schmidt, 2002).

It is not surprising that views of health care leadership are changing to emphasize a more transformational—as opposed to a transactional—approach, because there has been increased demand for comprehensive system change. Over the last eight decades, there have emerged three major views of leadership. Early attempts at defining leadership emphasized the qualities all leaders are expected to possess, with "know thyself" being regarded as the key to leadership since Socratic times. But this *leadership as personal* view, though never discounted, was eventually criticized as incomplete because someone can be charming even charismatic, but fail miserably in accomplishing organizational goals. Are you much of a leader if you are repeatedly ineffective in achieving institutional mission? That questioning gave rise to a new view of *leadership as achieving organizational goals*, which emphasized the importance of various instrumental abilities so necessary to the achievement of institutional mission—problem definition and solution, interpersonal and communication effectiveness, team building, performance management, sense making, resource development (human and otherwise), evaluation of outcomes, and an appreciation of diversity.

Achieving organizational goals was itself ultimately judged to be insufficiently dynamic in a quickly changing world. Can you claim to be a leader if you are content to keep doing what has always been done and don't do anything to get your practice or your organization ready for the future? That is why the leadership literature began to emphasize *leadership as transformational*. This view acknowledges that work in general, and particularly in health care, has changed in recent decades. For example, nurses have to act more as leaders than managers (Surakkat, 2008), because they must increasingly demonstrate a global perspective, expert decision-making skills, political savvy, and team-building abilities, so they can create culture change and proactively adapt to changing circumstances (Huston, 2008; Sorensen, Iedema, &

Severinsson, 2008). It is not enough to be able to meet your country's current national standards; you must increasingly develop the multidisciplinary and multinational perspectives essential for successful strategic planning. Networking these days must be across borders, otherwise you are not likely to be thinking boldly enough to envision the opportunities and address the challenges of this period of time (Thompson & Hyrkas, 2014). When individuals are living longer and the fastest growing demographic group is those individuals aged 85 and older, it no longer makes sense to treat everyone over 60 or 65 as having the same mental health needs. At a time of constrained resources, not every contact between patient and provider must or should take place in person, nor do all caregiving activities have to be carried out by a registered nurse.

What is needed in the twenty-first century is a view of leadership that blends all three views of leadership because each perspective adds to the description of what successful performance entails, and complex organizations need professionals with personal abilities who know how to keep addressing the achievement of institutional mission even as the context for providing care is constantly changing. Accordingly, leadership in this chapter is defined as *inspiring and catalyzing others to realize shared mission and goals in an environment that is constantly changing and requiring us to design new ways of achieving our long-held values* (McBride, 2011, 2014). Values do not change with the times, but how they are to be realized inevitably does. The advantage of this definition is that it does not equate leadership with administration. You hope that individuals with organizational responsibilities and administrative titles exert leadership, but you do not need to be on the organizational chart to exert leadership. This definition of leadership emphasizes team work and systems change, not just the masterfulness of the individual health care professional. But in order to develop such leaders we need to prepare a professional workforce who expect to change over the course of their careers, are mentored to exert leadership at each career stage, and who mentor others along the way.

Leadership at each career stage

The advantage of a career framework, complete with multiple stages, is that no one need start out expecting to be fully developed upon graduation. Benner's 1984 work on the customary progress of clinicians from novice to expert was the first nursing study to elaborate on the learning that must be part of life after graduation as the individual moves in abilities from fledgling to competence to authority. In the ensuing decades, it has become even more commonplace for practice environments to be described as "continuously learning" systems because changing circumstances—reimbursement policies, technologic developments, regulatory requirements, climate change, economic situation, infectious outbreaks and the like—demand that health professionals be committed to lifelong learning, and not just because accumulating continuing education units fulfills some country's regulatory expectation (Davie & Nutley, 2000; Hazer, Russell, & Fletcher, 2008; Institute of Medicine (IOM), 2013). This notion of continuous transformation isn't confined to industrialized countries (Bass, 1997). A Health Leadership Development Model is being used in Africa that emphasizes leadership as effecting organizational change (Daniels *et al.*, 2014). The International Council of Nurses (ICN) has developed a Leadership for Change™ programme aimed at providing nurses around the world with an understanding of trends in health reform, a vision of how health and nursing services may develop in their countries, the ability to plan strategically for and manage change, and the wherewithal to be proactive in challenging and stressful environments (ICN, 2013). Nurses cannot be content to just know the content that was taught when they graduated 15 years ago, but must constantly strive to keep up with what is now being taught in that program.

What is more, course work can never fully prepare practitioners for the intricacies of patient-provider relationships and the subtleties of work environments. To learn how to "read between the lines," you need socialization and mentoring experiences. Mentoring—defined as the broad range of developmental relationships whereby more senior individuals work to promote the careers of more junior individuals—is not just needed at the beginning of a career but is important in every career transition (Hargreaves & Fullan, 2000). Since mentoring is important to professional development, every nurse also incurs the obligation to mentor the less educated and less experienced.

To maximize their impact on the health care system, mental health nurses must orchestrate full careers. A career is a long-term commitment to provide services that address societal needs, but doing so with some expectation of being changed for the good in the process (Care, 1984; Pellegrino, 2002). This notion of personal development over time is in contrast to what it means to hold a job whereby you may become more efficient over time, but without an expanded sphere of influence or a driving passion to develop new insights into what is entailed in "being therapeutic." Getting prepared to make contributions isn't enough if you don't subsequently improve health care, your home setting, and your profession in the process, because part of being professional is leaving settings and systems better than you found them. Building on Dalton, Thompson, and Price's 1977 article on stages of a professional career, five career stages are elucidated along with the mentoring needed at each transition. This stage model is like other such developmental frameworks (e.g., Erikson's stages of ego development or Kohlberg's stages of moral development) in that it is primarily meant to be a heuristic device for conceptualizing how the major career themes shift over time in an enlarged direction. The model isn't meant to categorize exactly where you are, but to point broadly to developmental markers ahead.

In the *preparation stage*, the focus is on hardwiring the values, knowledge base, and skills important to the practice of nursing and mental health care. There is no substitute for formal education—BSN, MSN/DNP—to learn core competencies and what is the latest in specialty practice. The PhD and postdoctoral training are important if your career is going to focus on building the knowledge base for improved future practice, because that level of education provides the tools necessary to design studies, obtain needed resources, collect data, analyze trends, disseminate findings, and consider whether the results have policy consequences. Socialization experiences—clinical rotations, internships, residencies, human relations training, group work, workshops, committee assignments, and assistantships—are a necessary complement to course work because they enable the learner to function in real-life situations that don't always proceed as the text suggests. Work as a research assistant on a funded project, and you will soon understand how many things don't go quite as described in the original grant application, and that problem solving is a major scientific activity. Work with a dysfunctional family, and you soon learn that some children can demonstrate a surprising resilience in the face of difficulties that would overwhelm others.

Part of preparation is achieving licensure, thus demonstrating a grasp of fundamentals; specialty knowledge is typically confirmed by certification. It is in this first career stage that one also does certain other groundwork—figuring out personal strengths and limitations; understanding the basics of time management; learning self-presentation (e.g., creating a Curriculum Vitae and/or personal website); figuring out how to connect with likeminded colleagues at professional meetings; deciding which nursing, community and/or inter-professional organizations to join. A nursing shortage in some industrialized countries has complicated this career stage as the number of international migrants continues to increase fueled by lack of opportunities in the home country and incentives in the recruiting country (Kingma, 2007). It is in the hope of addressing some of these resource issues that the ICN has sought to create a collaborative and stimulating learning culture by harnessing the expertise of international faculty (Benton, 2012).

At this career stage, you need mentors who can model values and practices, provide graded challenges that test abilities without overwhelming, help you get over your inevitably stereotyped thinking about the profession, set short-term and career goals, and who will welcome you to the profession as a budding health care leader. But even in this stage, you can mentor the less educated and the less experienced, for example, serving as a big brother or big sister to a beginning nursing student or sharing a successful small-grant application with a graduate student putting the first proposal together.

Once prepared, the focus in the *independent contributions stage* is on moving from novice to competence while working independently and interdependently with nursing colleagues, other professionals, a myriad of staff and other personnel. Building teams, both intra-professional and inter-professional, is a requirement every health professional must assume—learning how to give away tasks and monitor their completion while developing a sense of collaboratively pursuing shared goals; using those who know more than you do as consultants to shore up your inexperience; making good use of peers with skills you do not possess; figuring out how secretarial and non-nurse professional staff can help you achieve your nursing goals. If you are embarking at this point on a faculty role, then one of your biggest concerns is likely to be learning how to be an effective teacher to nursing students at different levels or an assortment of lay partners, such as health navigators and other peer-support personnel.

Whether you are orchestrating a career in academia, service, government, industry, or the military, there is a great deal of tacit knowledge to learn about how to operate within the home setting (Eraut, 2000; Sternberg & Horvath, 1999). What are the unwritten rules of the organization? What are the resources in place for what the institution values? Your practice is shaped by the standards, history, policies, resources, and mores of the group(s) in which you work and the settings that you frequent. That is why the mentoring that is needed at this stage is largely geared to helping navigate the inner workings of institutions and professions—opening doors of opportunity, directing to resources (human and otherwise), facilitating networking, and keeping the focus on meeting professional and institutional benchmarks of success while understanding how difficult "being new" can be. Even though this is the stage when you are still getting established, it is also a time when you may be asked to preceptor students in their clinical practicums or mentor them in a research project, and coaching them encourages you to have new thoughts about your own practice, so there is a reciprocal relationship between helping someone learn something new and getting fresh insights into the situation.

As practitioners and educators come to realize the extent to which the context of care hinders or supports personal efforts, they are likely to be drawn into governance matters, getting increasingly involved in how the structure can be improved. That realization "If I were in charge, I bet that I could do better than what we now have" frequently propels individuals to consider taking on additional responsibilities, which moves them into the next career stage. But the historic emphasis in Western countries on independent practice has left many mental health professionals ill or insufficiently prepared for the systems involvement being demanded these days by the move for hospitals (and all clinical facilities) to become accountable and affordable care organizations—integrated delivery systems that align financial incentives with team-based care to provide cost-effective, non-fragmented care. There are many opportunities in today's changing circumstances for mental health nurses to insinuate their ideas and services into growing expectations for care coordination and comprehensive case management (Mechanic, 2011). Previously non-reimbursable health services, such as transition care and behavioral coaching, are likely to be in greater demand once the focus is on keeping patients out of expensive acute and emergency care.

By the third career stage, *development of home setting*, the mental health nurse is learning how to be more of a boundary spanner and how to juggle additional responsibilities and projects. In assuming more responsibility for committee work and the development of the home setting, the practitioner is in a position to think about and implement needed changes that might improve services. In assuming more responsibility for the development of those less experienced and less educated, the person at this stage, not only can mentor others struggling to handle changing job expectations, but this investment in coaching drives the person to new depths of understanding, thus propelling her or him to move from competence to expertise. Where before, the focus was on what could be personally accomplished with a particular roster of patients or class of students; now the emphasis switches to what she or he can get done within the home institution. This broadened sense of responsibility involves knowledge of strategic planning for the future, which requires a tolerance for ambiguity and political savvy.

Though we sometimes forget this fundamental truth, no new plan starts out with a detailed blueprint, hence the need to learn how to proceed forward in the face of vagueness. Practitioners, thankfully, like to practice, but that action-oriented stance can be counterproductive at this career stage if the discussions about how to greet the future have left the practitioner wanting action before some clear buy-in has been reached for a new or enhanced direction. At this stage, you have to learn not to get frustrated by seeming inaction because a certain amount of uncertainty is necessary to the weighing of options and possibilities. But even when you and others have a good sense of next steps, you have to remember that personal certainty about a course of action is not the same thing as getting what needs doing done, hence the need to be politically astute. Heretofore, the person's focus may have been largely on learning and applying that knowledge to care of one's own patients or students. Now the issue becomes how to get buy-in from others for needed environmental changes when others either don't yet understand the need for them or may even be opposed to anything new.

At this third career stage, the kind of mentoring needed changes to emphasize feedback regarding strategy, particularly how you facilitate junior colleagues who aren't like you, and tips for making the best use of others. Because most people have some difficulty in using others well when they are used to doing things themselves, a mentor can be useful at this point to prevent the burnout that inevitably follows when an individual keeps taking on additional responsibilities either without the needed resources or without giving up assignments that a less experienced person can learn to handle with some direction and encouragement. As the person's expertise builds, a mentor can also be useful in discussing whether one's authority is at a level to merit some honor or external recognition. Obviously being recognized by one's peers is personally gratifying, but in many ways the biggest advantage of any such public acknowledgment is the fact that the award serves to confirm the award-winning nature of nursing within that setting, an authority that can be an advantage as one seeks increasingly to make a difference beyond the confines of one's home setting. Sigma Theta Tau International (n.d.), the honor society of nursing, has made a major commitment to creating awards locally, regionally, nationally, and internationally for the full range of nursing excellence, because that organization values the importance of reputational recognition to changing stereotyped thinking.

By the fourth career stage, *development of field/health care*, the nurse takes a more active role beyond the home setting in shaping psychiatric-mental health nursing and mental health care. By this time, the individual has earned credibility at home and increasingly uses that developing sense of authority to improve the future. Given personal success as a mental health professional, the individual is increasingly asked to serve as a consultant to efforts and organizations interested in moving forward in that same area of expertise. Any speaking or writing that the person did in the past would have focused largely on personal experience, for example, cases you have managed or programs developed. Now the nurse is likely to be invited to speak more broadly about what we know and what we don't know, and to articulate a practice or research agenda for the future that will set new directions. For example, Hanrahan, Delaney, and Stuart (2012) demonstrated the kind of futuristic thinking expected at this career stage when they published a blueprint for development of the advanced psychiatric nurse workforce.

As you chair a committee of a specialty organization—e.g., the American Psychiatric Nurses Association (APNA), International Society of Psychiatric-Mental Health Nurses (ISPN), International Nurses Society on Addictions (INSA)—you are forced to analyze anew where the specialty now stands, and these reflections often propel your thinking to another level of conceptual complexity. This career stage may be a time for getting more involved in global matters (American International Health Alliance, 2014; Florence Nightingale International Foundation, 2014).

In going elsewhere to consult on what you have done for your home setting, you will see what that institution is doing and may have new insights into needed next steps back home. Even though you are in greater demand as a resource to *other* organizations—serving as a journal editor or grant reviewer and as an officer in an inter-professional or consumer organization—you still need some mentoring. For example, you will need someone who can provide tips on effective board behavior when you are appointed or elected to some group such as the local chapter of the National Alliance for the Mentally Ill (NAMI) or the state chapter of the Mental Health Association (MHA), then later to national or international organizations such as the Substance Abuse and Mental Health Services Administration (SAMHSA) or the International Mental Health Research Organization (IMRHO).

The fifth career stage, *the gadfly period*, is when you continue to shape mental health care and your specialty, but are no longer employed full time by an institution. While the gadfly is now mainly thought of as a pest, Socrates described the gadfly as one who asks the questions that stir others into life (Jowett, 1937), and that kind of creative questioning may be more possible at this stage when the experienced individual is less concerned with institutional obligations or specific achievements. Because you no longer worry about being invited back if you ask a difficult question, you can be more outspoken, more of a truth teller who helps others to confront what they might prefer to ignore, but need to tackle for the sake of either the greater good or a deeper meaning. At this stage, when your personal opinions can no longer be mistaken for the institutional position you once held, the nurse may be able to voice views that might have once embarrassed an employer. Free of formal organizational obligations, you can be more direct in tackling sensitive subjects. In Western countries, former executives may be asked to be available for confidential, wide-ranging discussions with the current leadership (Friel & Duboff, 2009). In Asia where the age of retirement is typically 60, rather than 65 or older, professionals are often expected to give up their full-time positions so younger people can assume them, but then to spend the next few years in part-time work as a consultant. The nature of that work will, of course, be influenced by cultural values and current socioeconomic trends (Pang, Senaratana, Kunaviktikul, Klunkin, & McElmurry, 2009).

The gadfly period need not be a time of retirement but of "preferment," doing what you most prefer, whether that is consulting or taking on special assignments. This stage offers new opportunities to demonstrate compassion and search for meaning (Bateson, 2011; Bennis, 2004). At this point in time, the individual usually has a stronger sense than ever before that the best answers really depend on posing the best questions (Riegel, 1973, 1975). But even at this stage, some mentoring is likely to be needed in envisioning post "retirement" opportunities, because ours is a world that continues to think that professional contributions and being chronologically gifted are mutually exclusive categories.

If you look at the progression from stage to stage, you may have noted three possible tensions over the course of one's developmental journey. First, there is the seeming opposition between *attention to detail* and *being innovative*. At the beginning of a career, you are consumed with learning the thousand and one details associated with professional responsibilities. The focus is on learning best practices and how to execute protocols carefully, but once basics are mastered, then the emphasis is increasingly on innovation—how do you redesign processes for a better result? The same person who once worried about giving the right medication to the right person at the right time has to become playful enough to imagine new possibilities for promoting medication safety, but after years of learning to respect existing standards this isn't always an easy transition.

The second seeming conflict is between *doing things yourself and getting things done through others*. You learn in a practice profession by doing, but the more effective you become, the more you will be asked to mentor and facilitate others, and as responsibilities geometrically increase, you have to figure out new ways of accomplishing goals through the efforts of others. Since being personally effective doesn't necessarily mean you intuitively know how to get others to do the same, the learning curve can be steep, and sometimes you cling to doing it yourself because it seems easier than motivating and shaping the behavior of others. But if you go in that direction, you cannot sustain the pile-up of tasks and burnout is a real probability.

The third seeming strain is between *building your authoritative voice and giving voice to others*. When you are new to a profession, you often feel inadequate and can be hesitant in what you say and how you act. Clance and Imes (1978) coined the phrase "imposter phenomenon" to describe how individuals still unsure of their abilities might think of themselves as pretenders or frauds because there is a gap between how they see themselves and are seen by others. Arena and Page (1992) have documented that phenomenon in some nurses new to the Clinical Nurse Specialist (CNS) role. With support and experience you grow to know your own mind, and have confidence in your judgments, but that very sureness that took years to build may then get in the way of appreciating how important it is to get feedback from people who don't think the way you do because they are different in gender, race, education, sexual preference, religion, socioeconomic status, and a host of other factors. Yet if you don't learn to ask for broad feedback on major plans or projects, the chances are that any final product will be incomplete.

The choice in each area of tension isn't mutually exclusive, but it can feel that way. The nurse who is meticulous and conscientious, two very good qualities, will need to be encouraged to brainstorm new ideas, but those ideas may be particularly helpful because that kind of person fully understands existing processes. Nurses used to doing things themselves are the mainstays of organizations, but their opportunities will be truncated if they don't learn to make appropriate use of others as their responsibilities increase. If it took you some time to take yourself and your authority as a nurse seriously, it may take you even more time to listen to those who see matters differently, but you have to be able to do that if you are going to be effective in diverse forums and on assorted boards.

Exerting twenty-first-century leadership presupposes that each mental health professional is prepared to have a full career, moving over time from promise to momentum to harvest (Shirey, 2009). While some nurses will always choose just to hold a job—good at what they do but what they do doesn't change over time—rather than a career, the high-level practice increasingly required of each professional in the twenty-first century mandates that normative expectations be shifted in a careerist direction whereby each nurse is expected to work as a valued team member at the top of her/his license and abilities, and simultaneously be prepared to redesign systems to address the challenges and opportunities of tomorrow.

Sustaining career optimism

Career development presupposes that individuals remain optimistic over time—about their leadership, their work, and their ability to deal with changing circumstances. To be able to sustain this level of engagement in caregiving, the individual must see self-care as a crucial aspect of being a caregiver (Hem, Halvorsen, & Nortvedt, 2014; Pettersen, 2012). The level of leadership expected of nurses in the twenty-first century is impossible if they don't take seriously that high-level caregiving must include self-care plans. In one way, there's little disagreement about this message because nurses already preach that message to family caregivers, but historically self-care was the lowest priority of busy nurses, particularly women with substantial family responsibilities.

Nurses must take seriously all of the advice that they have long been giving their patients about the importance of diet, exercise, sleep, recreation, meditation, and social support. Being able to get by with 4–5 hours of sleep for days on end isn't a mark of executive ability. All it does is increase your risk for obesity and diabetes (Knutson & Van Cauter, 2008). Health professionals need to get good at "body listening" so they can proactively read the cues that indicate they may be close to a breaking point (e.g., feeling a bit paranoid about co-workers), because "losing it" is a good way to sabotage your authority with colleagues. Nurses are not the highest paid professionals, but they increasingly make decent salaries proportionate to their country's national average, so starting a career with a financial plan regarding repayment of student loans and investments for the future is yet another important aspect of self-care (Worldsalaries, 2008).

Most mental health nurses are familiar with cognitive-behavioral therapy and its proven effectiveness with unipolar depression, generalized anxiety disorder, panic disorder, social phobias, posttraumatic stress disorder and the like (Butler, Chapman, Forman, & Beck, 2006). Those therapeutic techniques can be equally effective in monitoring how you as a leader think. For example, you don't want to overgeneralize—"I'm a lousy writer"—when what you really mean is that you haven't made the progress you want in a particular assignment; overgeneralizing just makes the task seem unachievable. You don't want to ruminate focusing only on the negative, ignoring the neutral (most of everyday life) and discounting the positive; otherwise you will be depressed a good deal of the time. You want to confront your irrational beliefs—wanting to be loved by everyone, wanting to be perfect, wanting a problem-free life—because such thinking is normal but those are unattainable expectations. You want to reframe your experience when appropriate, for example, reframing some problems as developmental challenges. Having a problem sounds grim, but experiencing a developmental challenge sounds normal and even interesting.

Learning to manage anger constructively is another aspect of learned optimism (Seligman, 1991). Thomas (2001, 2005, 2008) has studied women/nurses and anger, and found that powerlessness (not being listened to) and injustice (being treated unfairly) are the themes behind most anger-producing situations. She is quick to say that anger in and of itself is not negative, and offers tips for harnessing that emotion on behalf of some greater good. For example, she suggests calling a HALT to acting poorly when **h**ungry, **a**ngry, **l**onely, and/or **t**ired. She recommends engaging others in tackling a shared issue, and encourages being properly assertive— describing what happened factually without accusing anyone else of bad faith, then saying how that made you feel, and specifying what you hope will happen next.

The intention of this discussion is not to list every strategy for sustaining career optimism, for there are many more, from counting your blessings regularly to triaging daily and always striving to focus on what is strategically most important. The point of this section is that many of the strategies that mental health nurses employ with their patients to help them cope with their frustrations and stresses can be applied to career disappointments and irritations. You cannot orchestrate a career for leadership without feeling regularly overwhelmed, and what you need to do is see yourself as an executive deserving to be sustained physically, emotionally, mentally, and spiritually so you can then be there for others. And that sustenance begins with an appreciation of the relationship between leadership and self-care.

In summary

The demand for nurse leadership has never been greater than it is today, nor have the opportunities and challenges. To deliver comprehensive mental health, nurses in this specialty area must all see themselves as leaders who will enlarge their spans of influence over the course of their careers, knowing full well that their aspirational goals are so big and broad that they also must take concrete steps along the way to sustain their engagement over time. Worldwide, they cannot be content merely to run organizations, but must now be prepare to set directions (Kumar, Adhish, & Deoki, 2014).

References

American International Health Alliance. (2014). Nursing. Retrieved on April 23, 2016 from www.aiha. com/technical-areas/nursing.

Arena, D.M., & Page, N.E. (1992). The imposter phenomenon in the clinical nurse specialist role. *Image: The Journal of Nursing Scholarship, 24*, 121–125.

Bass, B.M. (1985). *Leadership and performance beyond expectations*. New York: Free Press.

Bass, B.M. (1997). Does the transactional-transformational leadership paradigm transcend organizational and national boundaries? *American Psychologist, 52*, 130–139.

Bateson, M.C. (2011). *Composing a further life: The age of active wisdom*. New York: Vintage Books.

Benner, P. (1984). *From novice to expert: Excellence and power in clinical nursing practice*. Menlo Park, CA: Addison-Wesley.

Bennis, W.G. (2004). The seven ages of the leader. *Harvard Business Review, 82*, 46–53, 112.

Benton, D. (2012). Advocating globally to shape policy and strengthen nursing's influence. *The Online Journal of Issues in Nursing, 17*. Retrieved on April 23, 2016 from www.nursingworld.org/MainMenu Categories/ANAMarketplace/ANAPeriodicals/OJIN/TableofContents/Vol-17-2012/No1-Jan-2012/Advocating-Globally-to-Shape-Policy.html.

Butler, A.C., Chapman, J.E., Forman, E.M., & Beck, A.T. (2006). The empirical status of cognitive-behavioral therapy: A review of meta-analyses. *Clinical Psychology Review, 26*, 17–31.

Care, N. (1984). Career choice. *Ethics, 94*, 283–302.

Clance, P.R., & Imes, S.A. (1978). The imposter phenomenon in high achieving women: Dynamics and therapeutic intervention. *Psychotherapy: Theory, Research & Practice, 15*, 241–247.

Cohen, J.A., Palumbo, M.V., Rambur, B., & Mongeon, J. (2004). Middle-school students' perceptions of an ideal career and a career in nursing. *Journal of Professional Nursing, 20*, 202–210.

Collins, J.C. (2005). *Good to great and the social sectors*. New York: Harper Collins.

Dalton, G.W., Thompson, P.H., & Price, R.L. (1977). The four stages of professional careers: A new look at performance by professionals. *Organizational Dynamics, 6*, 19–42.

Daniels, J., Farquhar, C., Nathanson, N., Mashalla, Y., Petracca, F., Desmond, M., Green, W., Davies, L., & O'Malley, G. (2014). Training tomorrow's global health leaders: Applying a transtheoretical model to identify behavior change strategies within an intervention for leadership development. *Global Health Promotion, 21*(4), 24–34.

Davie, T.O., & Nutley, S.M. (2000). Developing learning organizations in the new NHS. *British Journal of Medicine, 320*, 998.

Eagly, A.H. (2007). Female leadership advantage and disadvantage: Resolving the contradictions. *Psychology of Women Quarterly, 31*, 1–12.

Eagly, A.H., & Johannesen-Schmidt, M.C. (2002). The leadership styles of women and men. *Journal of Social Issues, 57*, 781–797.

Eagly, A.H., Johannesen-Schmidt, M.C., & von Engen, M.L. (2003). Transformational, transactional, and laissez-faire leadership styles: A meta-analysis comparing women and men. *Psychological Bulletin, 129,* 569–591.

Eraut, M. (2000). Non-formal learning and tacit knowledge in professional work. *British Journal of Educational Psychology, 70,* 113–136.

Florence Nightingale International Foundation. (2014). The global nursing review initiative. Retrieved on April 23, 2016 from www.fnif.org/global.htm.

Frenk, J., Chen, L., Bhutta, Z.A., Cohen, J., Crisp, N., Evans, T., Fineberg, H., Garcia, P., Yang, K., Kelley, P., Kistnasamy, B., Meleis, A., Naylor, D., Pablos-Mendez, A., Reddy, S., Scrinshaw, S., Sepulveda, J., Servadda, D., & Zurayk, H. (2010). Health professionals for a new century: Transforming education to strengthen health systems in an interdependent world. *The Lancet, 376,* 1923–1968.

Friel, T.J., & Duboff, R.S. (2009). The last act of a great CEO. *Harvard Business Review, 87,* 82–89, 118.

Gerzema, J., & D'Antonio, M. (2013). *The Athena doctrine: How women (and the men who think like them) will rule the future.* San Francisco, CA: Jossey-Bass.

Gittell, J.H., Fairfield, K.M., Bierbaum, B., Head, W., Jackson, R., Kelly, M., Laskin, R., Lipson, S., Siliski, J., Thornhill, T., & Zuckerman, J. (2000). Impact of relational coordination on quality of care, postoperative pain, and functioning, and length of stay: A nine-hospital study of surgical patients. *Medical Care, 38,* 807–819.

Hanrahan, N.P., Delaney, K.R., & Stuart, G.W. (2012). Blueprint for development of the advanced practice psychiatric nurse workforce. *Nursing Outlook, 60,* 91–104.

Hargreaves, A., & Fullan, M. (2000). Mentoring in the new millennium. *Theory into practice, 39*(1), 50–56.

Hazer, M., Russell, S., & Fletcher, S.W. (Eds.). (2008). *Continuing education in the health professions: Improving health care through lifelong learning.* New York: Josiah Macy, Jr. Foundation.

Hem, M.H., Halvorsen, K., & Nortvedt, P. (2014). Altruism and mature care: Some rival considerations in care ethics. *Nursing Ethics, 21,* 1–9.

Houser, B.P., & Player, K.N. (2004). *Pivotal moments in nursing: Leaders who changed the path of a profession.* Indianapolis, IN: Sigma Theta Tau International.

Huston, C. (2008). Preparing nurse leaders for 2020. *Journal of Nursing Management, 16,* 905–911.

Institute of Medicine. (2013). *Best care at lower cost: The path to continuously learning health care in America.* Washington, DC: The National Academies Press.

International Council of Nurses. (March 2013). *Leadership for Change™.* Retrieved on April 23, 2016 from www.icn.ch/pillarsprograms/leadership-for-change/.

Jeanneau, M., & Amelius, K. (2001). Self-image and burnout in psychiatric staff. *Journal of Psychiatric and Mental Health Nursing, 7,* 399–406.

Jowett, M.A., trans. (1937). *The dialogues of Plato,* vol 1. New York: Random House.

Kalisch, P.A., & Kalisch, B.J. (1987). *The changing image of the nurse.* Menlo Park, CA: Addison-Wesley.

Kingma, M. (2007). Nurses on the move: A global overview. *Health Services Research, 42,* 1281–1298.

Knutson, K.L., & Van Cauter, E. (2008). Associations between sleep loss and increased risk of obesity and diabetes. *Annals of the New York Academy of Sciences, 1129,* 287–304.

Kumar, S., Adhish, V.S., & Deoki, N. (2014). Introduction to strategic management and leadership for health professionals. *Indian Journal of Community Medicine, 39,* 13–16.

McBride, A.B. (2011). *The growth and development of nurse leaders.* New York: Springer.

McBride, A.B. (2014). Leadership and the journey toward wisdom. In P. Plews-Ogan & G. Beyt (Ed.), *Wisdom Leadership in academic health science centers. Leading positive change.* Oxford: Radcliffe Publishing, 193–210.

Marion, R., & Uhl-Bien, M. (2001). Leadership in complex organizations. *The Leadership Quarterly, 12,* 389–418.

Mechanic, D. (2011). Seizing opportunities in the Affordable Care Act for transforming the mental and behavioral health system. *Health Affairs, 31,* 376–382.

Northouse, P.G. (2004). *Leadership: Theory and practice* (3rd ed.). Thousand Oaks, CA: Sage.

Pang, D., Senaratana, W., Kunaviktikul, W., Klunkin, A., & McElmurry, B.J. (2009). Nursing values in China: The expectations of registered nurses. *Nursing and Health Sciences, 11*(3), 312–317.

Pellegrino, E.D. (2002). Professionalism, profession and the virtues of the good physician. *Mount Sinai Journal of Medicine, 69,* 378–384.

Pettersen, T. (2012). Conceptions of care: Altruism, feminism, and mature care. *Hypatia, 27,* 366–389.

Riegel, K.F. (1973). Dialectic operations: The final period of cognitive development. *Human Development, 16,* 346–370.

Riegel, K.F. (1975). Toward a dialectical theory of development. *Human Development, 18,* 50–64.

Seligman, M.E.P. (1991). *Learned optimism.* New York: A.A. Knopf.

Sherman, G. (2000). *Nurses for a healthier tomorrow coalition members.* Retrieved on April 23, 2016 from www.truthaboutnursing.org/research/lit/jwt_memo1.html.

Shirey, M.R. (2009). Building an extraordinary career in nursing: Promise, momentum and harvest. *Journal of Continuing Education in Nursing, 40,* 394–400.

Sigma Theta Tau International. (n.d.). Awards. Retrieved on April 23, 2016 from www.nursingsociety.org/Awards/Pages/awards.aspx.

Sorensen, R., Iedema, R., & Severinsson, E. (2008). Beyond profession: Nursing leadership in contemporary health care. *Journal of Nursing Management, 16,* 535–544.

Sternberg, R.J., & Horvath, J.A. (Eds.). (1999). *Tacit knowledge in professional practice: Researcher and practitioner perspectives.* Mahwah, NJ: Lawrence Erlbaum.

Surakkat, T. (2008). The nurse manager's work in the hospital environment during the 1990s and 2000s: Responsibility, accountability and expertise in nursing leadership. *Journal of Nursing Management, 16,* 525–534.

Thomas, S.P. (2001). Teaching healthy anger management. *Perspectives in Psychiatric Care, 37,* 41–48.

Thomas, S.P. (2005). Women's anger, aggression, and violence. *Health Care for Women International, 26,* 504–522.

Thomas, S.P. (2008). *Transforming nurses' anger and pain: Steps toward healing* (3rd ed.). New York: Springer.

Thompson, P., & Hyrkas, K. (2014). Global nursing leadership. *Journal of Nursing Management, 22*(1), 1–3.

World Health Organization. (2013). Comprehensive mental health action plan 2013–2020. Retrieved 23 April, 2016 from www.who.int/mental_health/action_plan_2013/en/.

Worldsalaries. (2008). Professional nurse salaries—international comparison. Retrieved on April 23, 2016 from www.worldsalaries.org/professionalnurse.shtml.

PART II

Promoting mental health nursing within social and cultural contexts

Research, best practices and clinical perspectives

10

RECOGNIZING AND MANAGING STRESS

Catherine Batscha and Jessica Gill

What is important is to live so that one's distress is converted into eustress.

(Selye, 1976, p. 55)

Introduction

In 1932, Hans Selye introduced the concept of stress as a syndrome that occurs as organisms attempt to adapt to various "noxious" substances (Szabo, Tache, & Somogyi, 2012). Within 40 years, more than 100,000 papers had been published on the topics of stress and stress response indicating its importance as a topic of investigation (Selye, 1976). In any discussion of mental health and illness, stress is an important and universal concept. All people will experience it during their lives. The way in which stressors are perceived and interpreted can determine whether stress functions as a motivator for change or a cause of distress or illness. It is imperative that nurses understand the nature of stress, factors that facilitate or hinder an individual's ability to cope with stressors, and specific interventions that are effective for the management of stress or disorders associated with stress. This chapter will focus primarily on chronic stress and variables that affect its management by individuals, families, communities and societies.

Central concepts related to stress

Stress and stressors

Stress is most precisely defined as the nonspecific response of an organism or person to any demand (Selye, 1976). These demands are characterized as stressors and range from mild discomforts or challenges to physiological or psychological traumas. Stressors can be acute or chronic in nature. In the literature, the stress response and the stressors causing this response are often described as if they were the same phenomenon. This can be a source of confusion in the study of stress and stress-related disorders. Stress can be positive if it motivates positive change or growth. However, excessive stressors, either chronic or acute, or the inability to cope successfully with stressors can lead to adverse physical and psychological health outcomes.

Trauma

In their most extreme form, stressors are considered to be traumatic. Trauma is described as experiencing an event in which death or violence is witnessed or expected. The experience of a traumatic event is common among the general public with most people experiencing at least one traumatic event in their lifetime (Kilpatrick *et al.*, 2013). Acute stress disorder is characterized by the development within 1 month after a trauma of intrusive thoughts, avoidance, and hyperarousal. Post-traumatic stress disorder (PTSD) is a chronic, pervasive illness that can develop after experiencing a trauma, although most people exposed to a traumatic event do not develop PTSD. Repeated exposure to trauma increases the likelihood that PTSD will occur. People experiencing more than four traumatic events are significantly more likely to develop this disorder (Karam *et al.*, 2014). Living in a high-income country does not necessarily lead to a lower likelihood of PTSD. For example, incidence of PTSD in 11 countries surveyed was lowest in three countries identified as upper- or lower-middle income: the People's Republic of China (0.2 percent), Colombia (0.3 percent), Mexico (0.3 percent); and highest in three high-income countries: Northern Ireland (3.8 percent), the United States (2.5 percent), and New Zealand (2.3 percent) (Karam *et al.*, 2014). The likelihood of developing PTSD is increased in people who are victims of war or victims of crime (Burri & Maercker, 2014) and the incidence of PTSD in conflict areas is reported to be much higher than in other areas. Interpersonal violence may increase the risk of PTSD. According to the World Health Organization, childhood sexual abuse is implicated in 1/3 of women and 1/5 of men who develop PTSD (World Health Organization, 2009).

Children may experience violence or trauma in the family or community, the effects of which can persist into adult life. Childhood trauma interferes with learning and development because there is relative overdevelopment of parts of the brain related to anxiety and fear at the expense of other parts of the brain (Butchart, Harvey, Mian, & Furniss, 2006). Adverse childhood events have been associated with mental disorders such as anxiety, depression, suicidality, and psychosis and with physical illnesses including heart, lung, and autoimmune disorders, sleep disturbances, obesity, and headaches. Despite this association, health care providers do not routinely ask patients about occurrence of childhood adverse events (Kalmakis & Chandler, 2015).

Nada es verdad ni es mentira; todo es según el color del cristal con que se mira.
(There is neither truth nor lies, but the lens through which one looks.)

(Campoamor, 1903, p. 88)

Attribution

Psychological response to stressors will be determined, in part, by the way in which the person experiencing it interprets the situation. Cognitive behavioral therapy (CBT) is one theoretical framework that focuses on changing personal, unhelpful responses to a stimulus. For example, in CBT a person might be encouraged to change thoughts that predict catastrophe as a way of managing the initial phases of a panic reaction to something that is feared. Meditation, as practiced by Buddhists, is another way of reducing distress through its focus on increasing acceptance and mindfulness. In the words of Thich Nhat Hanh, "The ocean of suffering is immense, but if you turn around you can see the land" (Hanh, 1999, p. 3). This view illustrates both the universality of suffering and the possibility of transcending suffering.

Culture

Culture is an additional variable that must be considered when examining which stressors people encounter, the ways in which stressors and trauma are viewed, and coping preferences. Two common worldviews are individualist, frequently found in Western culture, and collectivist, frequently found in Asian or African cultures. Individualists and collectivists may prefer different methods of coping with stressors and may have different expectations of what successful coping will look like. Table 10.1 summarizes these two world views in regard to stress and coping. It is imperative for the nurse to determine what kind of worldview a person has and consequently how stressors are explained and preferred methods of coping.

Access to resources

The amount of work done in small companies or families in developing nations is growing (Kortum, Leka, & Cox, 2010). Although this brings opportunities for increased income, it also brings increased psychological stressors, worries about job instability and physical stress responses such as increases in blood pressure and cardiac events. The resources available for mitigating work-related exposures to toxins and psychological and physiologic stresses at work are not as readily available in these decentralized work environments. Expert knowledge about work-related stressors exists in developing countires, but this knowledge may not be disseminated widely to workers in need of it (Kortum *et al.*, 2010). Nurses in the community can educate people about work-related issues that may impact physical or mental health and can teach ways of preventing, recognizing, and responding to stressors that occur in a work environment. One important area will be working with families to identify ways in which work and family responsibilities can be balanced (Houtman, Jettinghoff, & Cedillo, 2007).

Table 10.1 Individualist and collectivist worldviews

World View	Stressors	Preferred locus of control	Preferred coping mechanisms	Examples of coping mechanisms	Outcome of successful coping
Individualist	Events that disrupt independence and self-development are most disruptive	internal	Confront and modify external stressor	Problem focused Behavioral Approach oriented	Reduction of stress or distress
Collectivist	Events that disrupt social harmony, security and sense of consistency are most disruptive	external	Modifying oneself	Cognitive avoidance Emotion-focused coping	Optimal social and relational consequences Ingroup harmony preserved Social obligations fulfilled Mutual interdependence enhanced

Source: From Kuo (2013)

Resilience

Not all people who experience significant adversity will become ill or develop stress-related disorders. Resilience is defined as "the capacity to adapt successfully in the presence of risk and adversity" (Meichenbaum, 2012, p. 3) and is currently being studied to determine factors that may decrease susceptibility to the effects of life stressors. The society-to-cells model of resilience formulated by Szanton and Gill (2010) describes three types of resilient response to stressors: resistance, recovery, and rebounding. Resistance occurs when people who are exposed to trauma do not develop psychiatric illness. Recovery is seen when individuals return to previous levels of functioning following exposure to trauma. Rebounding responses result in attainment of a higher level of achievement than was present before the challenge faced by the person.

The concept of being able to grow and recover after adversity is found in many cultures. Victor Frankl, who survived Auschwitz, viewed finding meaning in life as a central purpose saying; "Once an individual's search for meaning is successful, it not only renders him happy but also gives him the capability to cope with suffering" (Frankl, 2006, p. 139). Women among the 50,000 survivors of the 250,000 women who were raped during the Rwandan genocide described the necessity to withstand, to live after disaster, and to find willingness and motivation to live as personally helpful in reclaiming life after severe trauma (Zraly & Nyirazinyoye, 2010). The ability to display resilience in the face of adversity is affected by psychological and biological factors in the individual exposed to trauma. In the following section, adaptation to stress will be examined in more detail.

General adaptation syndrome

The physiology of the general adaptation syndrome is not dependent on the nature of the stressor, but rather on the magnitude and the length of time that the stressor continues to affect the individual. Homeostasis or physiologic balance is the tendency of the body to try to maintain equilibrium, even when faced with challenges. The general adaptation response occurs when stress is prolonged and has three stages: alarm, resistance, and exhaustion.

Alarm

The alarm stage is the first stage of the stress response and occurs when a stressor is perceived. Catecholamines, neurotransmitters, and hormones are released in response to a stressor preparing an individual to fight or flee from a danger (Tank & Wong, 2015). Sympathetic nervous system activation results in increased pulse, blood pressure, respiration, and increased neuronal activity in the amygdala, the portion of the brain involved in fear reactions. These changes increase focus and energy available to muscles in the short term. During the alarm stage, the hypo-thalamic-pituitary-adrenal (HPA) axis is activated, resulting in increased production of cortisol. The HPA axis influences biological functions related to mood, growth, immune function, metabolism, and regulation of biological systems on a circadian rhythm (Spiers, Chen, Sernia, & Lavidis, 2014).

Resistance

The second stage is resistance, in which the body responds over time to a continuing stressor and tries to maintain a state of homeostasis. Increased activity of the HPA axis further intensifies the body's systemic response by increasing glucose, fat, and amino acid/protein concentrations in the blood (Reader *et al.*, 2015). This means that as stressors become chronic, initial reactions geared towards survival can result in the development of hypertension, cardiovascular disease, and metabolic syndrome and diabetes (Gill & Szanton, 2011). The body begins to use energy stores and resources are gradually depleted (Spiers *et al.*, 2014), which can increase susceptibility to infection and illness.

There are also biological changes that can mitigate these risks. For example, high levels of neuropeptide Y reduce anxiety symptoms in soldiers undergoing high stress training (Morgan *et al.*, 2002), and high levels of brain-derived neurotrophic factor mitigate stress-induced neuronal changes that increase the risk for psychiatric symptoms. Serotonin has stress-mitigating properties and increases in its activity improve depression, pain, and health perception (Cooke, Grover, & Spangler, 2009).

Exhaustion

Exhaustion is the final stage of the stress response, a stage in which coping mechanisms no longer work and health is compromised. The stage of exhaustion is most commonly reached in individuals who are exposed to chronic and/or severe stressors. Such stress can result in changes in the structure or functions of neurons as they respond to excess cortisol or glutamate. Cortisol increases the consolidation of relevant memories making traumatic memories even more firmly established. Cortisol also contributes to kindling, a phenomenon where decreasing levels of stimuli provoke increasingly strong physiological and psychological responses. Glutamate increases connections between synapses serving to strengthen traumatic memories (Weiss, 2007). Development of PTSD after trauma is linked to genetic and environmental factors with presence of a psychiatric history, child abuse, and family psychiatric history being associated with development of PTSD (Afifi, Asmundson, Taylor, & Jang, 2010). Twin studies indicate that genetic factors and the number of traumas both contribute to the development of PTSD following traumatic experiences (Afifi *et al.*, 2010). Thus, exposure to trauma may have different results in people with different susceptibility to PTSD.

In summary, although the stress response is effective as a response to acute stressors, it can cause morbidity if stress is prolonged or if a person does not have the ability to cope effectively with life stressors. An important nursing role is mitigating the effects of acute and chronic stress so that the risk of stress-related illness is reduced. Approaches to reduce stress and increase coping abilities will be discussed in the next section.

Evidence-based prevention and mental health promotion strategies

While not all traumas are preventable, the most efficient way to prevent trauma-related illnesses is to reduce the number of people exposed to trauma. A wide variety of interventions can be used by nurses and other community leaders, from advocating for seatbelt use, thereby preventing serious injury from motor vehicle accidents, to providing assistance to communities in setting up programs to reduce community or domestic violence, to advocating as strongly as possible against the use of torture. Successful efforts can decrease the number of people susceptible to developing PTSD who will be exposed to events that could cause it. This kind of primary prevention is most important since some traumas, like PTSD following torture, have not been shown to be easily responsive to treatment of any kind (Patel, Kellezi, & Williams, 2014).

Interventions targeting stress should focus on promoting resilience and preventing or decreasing disability. Stress, particularly acute, may be most appropriately treated with non-pharmacologic approaches, which is ideal in circumstances such as poverty or disaster where the ability to access or pay for medications may be limited. An additional justification for non-pharmacologic approaches to stress responses immediately after trauma, is that the presence of acute stress disorder does not adequately predict who will develop post-traumatic stress disorder (Bryant, 2011). The question of who should deliver non-pharmacologic treatment is important for lower-income countries, which often lack adequate numbers of psychiatric practitioners to provide services to people who have been traumatized or impacted by war or disaster. In response to these concerns, WHO has developed guidelines for use by non-specialist health care providers in places where mental health specialists are not available. A summary of these recommendations for adults and children with acute stress disorder and post-traumatic stress disorder is included in Table 10.2. These recommendations are most helpful in providing information about what to avoid. Recommendations for interventions that help people who have been traumatized are not as clearly delineated, often because there is insufficient evidence to know what will work. An Agency for Healthcare Research and Quality (AHRQ) comparative effectiveness review of interventions (debriefing, cognitive behavioral therapy with or without hypnosis, prolonged exposure therapy, psychoeducation self-help, supportive counseling, and collaborative care) offers little guidance as to which interventions might prevent PTSD, saying that the few existing studies have methodological problems that make it difficult to evaluate effectiveness. They did find that collaborative care may be effective in reducing the severity of symptoms and that critical incident debriefing has not demonstrated effectiveness in preventing PTSD (Gartlehner, Forneris, & Brownley, 2013).

Cognitive Behavioral Therapy (CBT) does demonstrate some effectiveness in relieving symptoms of acute stress disorder in adults (Gartlehner *et al.*, 2013; Roberts, Kitchiner, Kenardy, & Bisson, 2010). Trauma-focused CBT (TF-CBT) is used to reduce symptoms of trauma in children, to increase mastery and to teach individuals to cope more effectively with stressors. CBT techniques will differ for children and adults, with an emphasis on involving parents in the case of a traumatized child. Components of CBT after trauma include (Child Sexual Abuse Task Force and Research and Practice Core, 2004; Israel Trauma Center for Victims of Terror and War, n.d.):

(a) *Psychoeducation about effects of trauma:* this can be helpful in allowing individuals to link changes to trauma. For parents of children, linking problems such as enuresis to trauma helps them to adopt non-punitive approaches to trauma-related problems.

Table 10.2 Recommendations for adults and children with acute stress disorder or post-traumatic stress disorder

Population/disorder	Trauma-focused CBT	Benzodiazepines	Antidepressants within first month
Acute stress disorder			
Adults	Yes	Not within first month	Not within first month
Children	Insufficient data for recommendations	Not within first month	Not within first month
Post-traumatic stress disorder			
Adults	Individual or group	No	If other treatments do not work
Children	Individual or group	No	No

Source: World Health Organization (2013).

(b) *Teaching relaxation skills*: enables individuals to develop specific techniques for responding to symptoms of fear and anxiety, and empowers the individual to decrease such symptoms. Skills include progressive muscle relaxation, and slow deep breathing.

(c) *Affect expression and regulation skills*: these skills help children and parents to identify and cope with distressing emotions.

(d) *Cognitive coping skills*: people who have experienced trauma may have thoughts that are inaccurate, exaggerate the amount of present danger, or blame themselves for common reactions to traumatic events. Modifying such thoughts can increase a person's ability to live life the way that they prefer.

(e) *Exposure*: avoidance is often a response to trauma as someone avoids things that are re-minders of the event. Exposure can be imagined or actual and can involve writing or telling accounts of the traumatic event in an effort to decrease distress that is experienced when remembering the event.

It is not possible for nurses to wait until perfectly effective interventions are identified when faced with people who need assistance. The existing literature describes factors that are associated with developing or maintaining resilience. This literature, despite its limitations, can identify nursing interventions useful in collaborating with persons to identify self-care practices or thinking styles that promote or interfere with resilience. The next section of this chapter will focus on strategies that are aimed at building resilience and the ability to cope with stressors to prevent development of stress-related illnesses. Chapter 12 contains additional information regarding specific approaches to people with anxiety disorders.

Building mastery

Mastery refers to the degree to which people perceive that they can control stressors that influence their life. Lack of control in a situation is a defining characteristic of trauma and one of the challenges for nurses is to help individuals to begin to recognize the areas in their lives where they are able to exert control and mastery. Mastery increases quality of life and well-being, and lowers mortality risk related to cardiovascular disease (Surtees *et al.*, 2010). Effective coping with stressors is linked to the onset of fewer anxiety and depression symptoms in stressed individuals (Ben-Zur, 2008; Potter *et al.*, 2013; Rodriguez *et al.*, 2008). By facilitating the ability to recognize stressors and effective ways to cope with them, nurses help individuals to achieve mastery.

Social support

The importance of social support in predicting psychological well-being has been shown over decades of research (White-Williams *et al.*, 2013). Social support networks have been identified as helping people to build resilience after trauma. Moreover, impaired social support is one of the most powerful risk factors for anxiety disorders across sample populations (Steinert, Hofmann, Leichsenring, & Kruse, 2015). Children who have experienced trauma can use social support networks to express feelings and learn ways to cope with life stressors (Garcia-Dia, DiNapoli, Garcia-Ona, Jakubowski, & O'Flaherty, 2013). Effective social support by others who have similar experiences can help decrease isolation that can occur following trauma. Support can promote help-seeking behaviors and can help individuals learn and practice adaptive coping strategies. Sources of support can include family, community members, or people with shared experiences or religious affiliations. Nurses should work with individuals to identify relevant sources of positive support and strategies to access this support when needed.

Mindfulness

Mindfulness is a meditative practice that encourages a person to be aware of experiences in the present moment while maintaining an openness and non-judgmental attitude towards the current experience. Emotional difficulties in this framework may be reframed as either "opportunities to meet challenges" or a "reflection of universal characteristics of existing" (Brensilver, 2011). Mindfulness-based cognitive therapy and mindfulness-based stress reduction have both been used to help people to cope with pain, anxiety and depression (Sharma & Rush, 2014). Mindfulness has been associated with decreased symptoms in people with anxiety disorders. This effect was larger in Western countries than in Eastern. Mindfulness practice also demonstrated some reduction in depressive symptoms, although not significantly more than treatment as usual. Mindfulness can lower blood pressure and pulse, and induce changes in brain activity consistent with relaxation. However, mindfulness has not been demonstrated to reduce symptoms of PTSD (Chiesa & Serretti, 2010). Therefore, mindfulness may be most useful in people as part of a combination of strategies to reduce stress and increase functioning.

Sleep

Sleep is a necessary human function. When sleep duration or quality is disrupted, benefits of sleep, such as muscle repair, memory consolidation, and neuronal repair are disrupted as well. Even slight sleep deprivation can negatively affect memory, judgment, and mood, and can contribute to anxiety symptoms. Chronic sleep deprivation contributes to health problems, ranging from obesity and high blood pressure to safety risks (Irish, Kline, Gunn, Buysse, & Hall, 2014). Because disrupted sleep increases stress and anxiety (Abazyan *et al.*, 2010; Powell *et al.*, 2009; Wohleb *et al.*, 2011), helping individuals to improve sleep may decrease these symptoms.

Insomnia is a frequent complaint of people with acute or chronic responses to trauma. One contributor to insomnia is nightmares that may be related to the traumatic experience. An approach for coping with nightmares is called imagery retraining. Meichenbaum (2012) describes this approach as having the person write down the nightmare, change it in anyway desired, and then to write down the altered version. In this process the ending can be changed, the person can add protective features, or view events from a distance. The person mentally rehearses the changed dream twice a day for about 10 minutes. This exposure helps to increase feelings of control. Pharmacological treatments may be used to reduce nightmares in PTSD and will be discussed further in Chapter 11.

Sleep problems can become chronic in people with trauma histories. Individuals may spend much time in bed at night worrying about whether they will get to sleep and whether they will get enough sleep. This type of worry further interferes with the ability to sleep. Sleep hygiene measures are often more useful in the long term than medications for insomnia. Such measures include (National Center for Chronic Disease Prevention and Health Promotion, 2012; National Sleep Foundation, 2015):

1   Establish regular sleep routines, particularly times for awakening. Part of a sleep routine should be relaxing activities that promote restfulness. These can include reading, listening to music, or other soothing activities.
2   Keep TVs or computers out of the bedroom.
3   Avoid caffeine, nicotine, stimulants that may interfere with sleep, and avoid alcohol or over-the-counter sleep remedies.
4   Use relaxation techniques, guided imagery, and mindfulness routines to promote sleep. Smart phone apps and CDs are available with short exercises to help with this. A sample of a

relaxation exercise is available through the National Sleep Foundation (National Sleep Foundation, 2014).

5 Avoid exercise right before bed. However, exercise earlier is helpful in getting to sleep.
6 Get out of bed if awake for more than 20 minutes or if worried.
7 Avoid naps during the day.

Such interventions are most easily achieved if people have adequate privacy and security to promote a quiet, restful environment that promotes sleep. In some situations, such as crowded living conditions, displacement, environmental instability, or continuing physical danger, typical sleep hygiene measures are less likely to be sufficient. People can be helped by use of earplugs or sleep masks that cover the eyes if it is only light and noise that interfere with sleep. However, if a person does not feel safe in a particular environment, as after an earthquake or in a place where violence or gunshots is a possibility, the nurse must approach each situation individually. It is helpful in such cases to help an individual to implement sleep routines that are personally acceptable while working to reduce sources of continuing stimulation or danger. Having somewhere designated as the sleeping area is useful, even if this involves establishing this area nightly when preparing to go to sleep. Additional measures may be simple as establishing a family "quiet time" in crowded living quarters, or more complex as establishing "watch" schedules to guard group safety when sleeping on the streets or in shelters. The nurse will work at an individual level to help people to implement measures that will improve sleep but will also need to work at a community level to address environmental causes of sleep deprivation that impact the community more broadly.

Summary

In summary, stress is a universal phenomenon and traumatic experiences are common. Prolonged or severe stress can adversely affect physical and mental health in individuals. Although most people who are exposed to trauma do not develop trauma-related psychological disorders, some people will require short- or long-term assistance to cope with stressors. Appropriate nursing interventions include a thorough assessment, support, referrals to appropriate treatment resources, and addressing societal problems that cause chronic stress and trauma. Nurses should also be aware of and support strategies that promote individual, group, and community resilience and flourishing.

Available resources

World Health Organization literature—WHO.int

World Health Organization, War Trauma Foundation and World Vision International (2011). *Psychological First Aid: Guide for Field Workers* is available for download in multiple languages. It was developed as a resource for use in low- and middle-income countries where adequate resources are scarce.

Building Back Better—this pamphlet discusses ways in which to build improved sustainable mental health service delivery systems and discusses 10 diverse countries' experience in doing this.

The Melissa Institute for Violence Prevention and Treatment www.melissainstitute.org Donald Meichenbaum is research director of the Institute and materials include downloadable information on resilience as well as violence prevention.

Trauma-informed care

www.nasmhpd.org/TA/nctic.aspx

This site contains downloadable materials on assessment of trauma, components of treatment and using women as peer supports in trauma-informed care.

www.theannainstitute.org

Additional trauma informed resources are available through links to the Anna Institute

https://depts.washington.edu/hcsats/PDF/TF-%20CBT/pages/Theoretical%20Perspective/
TF-CBT%20Components,%20Rationale,%20&%20Methods%20Worksheet.pdf
www.nctsnet.org/nctsn_assets/pdfs/TF-CBT_Implementation_Manual.pdf

The preceding two sites include information on conducting trauma-focused CBT.

http://tfcbt.musc.edu/

This site offers a free on-line training in conducting trauma-focused CBT with children. A master's degree in a mental health discipline or enrollment in a graduate program is required to take the course.

References

Abazyan, B., Nomura, J., Kannan, G., Ishizuka, K., Tamashiro, K. L., Nucifora, F., Pogorelov, V., Ladenheim, B., Yang, C., Krasnova, I.N., Cadet, J.L., Pardo, C., Mori, S., Kamiya, A., Vogel, M.W., Sawa, A., Ross, C.A., & Pletnikov, M.V. (2010). Prenatal interaction of mutant DISC1 and immune activation produces adult psychopathology. *Biological Psychiatry, 68*(12), 1172–1181.

Afifi, T.O., Asmundson, G.J., Taylor, S., & Jang, K.L. (2010). The role of genes and environment on trauma exposure and posttraumatic stress disorder symptoms: a review of twin studies. *Clinical Psychology Review, 30*(1), 101–112.

Ben-Zur, H. (2008). Personal resources of mastery-optimism, and communal support beliefs, as predictors of posttraumatic stress in uprooted Israelis. *Anxiety Stress Coping, 21*(3), 295–307.

Brensilver, M. (2011). Letter to the editor: response to "a systematic review of neurobiological and clinical features of mindfulness meditations." *Psychological Medicine, 41*(3), 666–668.

Bryant, R.A. (2011). Acute stress disorder as a predictor of posttraumatic stress disorder: a systematic review. *Journal of Clinical Psychiatry, 72*(2), 233–239.

Burri, A., & Maercker, A. (2014). Differences in prevalence rates of PTSD in various European countries explained by war exposure, other trauma and cultural value orientation. *BMC Research Notes, 7*(1), 407.

Butchart, A., Harvey, A.P., Mian, M., & Furniss, T. (2006). Preventing child maltreatment: a guide to taking action and generating evidence. World Health Organization. Retrieved April 13, 2015 from from www.who.int/violence_injury_prevention/publications/violence/child_maltreatment/en/#.

Campoamor, R. (1903). *Obras poéticas completas.* Barcelona: L. Tasso. Retrieved April 13, 2015 from http://babel.hathitrust.org/cgi/pt?id=mdp.39015062904670;view=1up;seq=7.

Chiesa, A., & Serretti, A. (2010). A systematic review of neurobiological and clinical features of mindfulness meditations. *Psychological Medicine, 40*(8), 1239–1252.

Child Sexual Abuse Task Force and Research and Practice Core, N.C.T.S.N. (2004). *How to implement trauma-focused cognitive behavioral therapy (TF-CBT).* Durham, NC and Los Angeles, CA: National Center for Child Traumatic Stress.

Cooke, J.D., Grover, L.M., & Spangler, P.R. (2009). Venlafaxine treatment stimulates expression of brain-derived neurotrophic factor protein in frontal cortex and inhibits long-term potentiation in hippocampus. *Neuroscience, 162*(4), 1411–1419.

Frankl, V. (2006) *Man's search for meaning.* Boston, MA: Beacon Press.

Garcia-Dia, M.J., DiNapoli, J.M., Garcia-Ona, L., Jakubowski, R., & O'Flaherty, D. (2013). Concept analysis: resilience. *Archives of psychiatric nursing, 27*(6), 264–270.

Gartlehner, G., Forneris, C., & Brownley, K. (2013). Interventions for the prevention of posttraumatic stress disorder (PTSD) in adults after exposure to psychological trauma. Retrieved April 15, 2015 from www.ncbi.nlm.nih.gov.echo.louisville.edu/books/NBK133344/pdf/Bookshelf_NBK133344. pdf

Gill, J M., & Szanton, S. (2011). Inflammation and traumatic stress: the society to cells resiliency model to support integrative interventions. *Journal of the American Psychiatric Nurses Association, 17*(6), 404–416.

Hanh, T. N. (1999). *The heart of Buddha's teaching: Transforming suffering into peace, joy and liberation* (S.A. Laity, Trans.). New York: Broadway Books.

Houtman, I., Jettinghoff, K., & Cedillo, L. (2007). Protecting workers' health series no. 6: raising awareness of stress at work in developing countries: a modern hazard in a traditional working environment: advice to employers and worker representatives. Geneva: World Health Organization.

Irish, L.A., Kline, C.E., Gunn, H.E., Buysse, D.J., & Hall, M.H. (2014). The role of sleep hygiene in promoting public health: a review of empirical evidence. *Sleep Medicine Reviews, 22,* 23–36.

Israel Trauma Center for Victims of Terror and War. (n.d.). Retrieved May 3, 2015, from www.natal. org.il/english/?CategoryID=229&ArticleID=200.

Kalmakis, K.A., & Chandler, G.E. (2015). Health consequences of adverse childhood experiences: a systematic review. *Journal of the American Association of Nurse Practitioners, 27*(8), 457–465.

Karam, E.G., Friedman, M.J., Hill, E.D., Kessler, R.C., McLaughlin, K.A., Petukhova, M., Sampson, L., Shahly, V., Angermeyer, M.C., Bromet, E.J., & Bromet, E.J. (2014). Cumulative traumas and risk thresholds: 12-month PTSD in the World Mental Health (WMH) surveys. *Depression and Anxiety, 31*(2), 130–142.

Kilpatrick, D.G., Resnick, H.S., Milanak, M.E., Miller, M.W., Keyes, K.M., & Friedman, M.J. (2013). National estimates of exposure to traumatic events and PTSD prevalence using DSM-IV and DSM-5 criteria. *Journal of Traumatic Stress, 26*(5), 537–547.

Kortum, E., Leka, S., & Cox, T. (2010). Psychosocial risks and work-related stress in developing countries: health impact, priorities, barriers and solutions. *International Journal of Occupational Medicine and Environmental Health, 23*(3), 225–238.

Kuo, B.C. (2013). Collectivism and coping: current theories, evidence, and measurements of collective coping. *International Journal of Psychology 48*(3), 374–388.

Meichenbaum, D. (2012). *Roadmap to resilience: A guide for military, trauma victims and their families.* Clearwater, FL: Institute Press.

Morgan, C.A., Rasmusson, A.M., Wang, S., Hoyt, G., Hauger, R.L., & Hazlett, G. (2002). Neuropeptide-Y, cortisol, and subjective distress in humans exposed to acute stress: replication and extension of previous report. *Biological Psychiatry, 52*(2), 136–142.

National Center for Chronic Disease Prevention and Health Promotion (2012). Sleep hygiene tips. Retrieved June 1, 2015 from www.cdc.gov/sleep/about_sleep/sleep_hygiene.htm.

National Sleep Foundation. (2014). Relaxation exercise. Retrieved May 1, 2015, from http://sleep foundation.org/insomnia/content/relaxation-exercise.

National Sleep Foundation. (2015). Sleep hygiene. Retrieved May 1, 2015 from http://sleepfoundation. org/ask-the-expert/sleep-hygiene/page/0/1.

Patel, N., Kellezi, B., & Williams, A.C. (2014). Psychological, social and welfare interventions for psychological health and well-being of torture survivors. *Cochrane Database of Systematic Reviews, 11.* Retrieved May 1, 2015 from http://irep.ntu.ac.uk/26172/1/PubSub3016_Kellezi.pdf.

Potter, C.M., Kaiser, A.P., King, L.A., King, D.W., Davison, E.H., Seligowski, A.V., Brady, C.B., & Spiro, A. (2013). Distinguishing late-onset stress symptomatology from posttraumatic stress disorder in older combat veterans. *Aging Mental Health, 17*(2), 173–179.

Powell, N.D., Bailey, M.T., Mays, J.W., Stiner-Jones, L.M., Hanke, M.L., Padgett, D.A., & Sheridan, J.F. (2009). Repeated social defeat activates dendritic cells and enhances toll-like receptor dependent cytokine secretion. *Brain, Behavior, and Immunity, 23*(2), 225–231.

Reader, B.F., Jarrett, B.L., McKim, D.B., Wohleb, E.S., Godbout, J.P., & Sheridan, J.F. (2015). Peripheral and central effects of repeated social defeat stress: monocyte trafficking, microglial activation, and anxiety. *Neuroscience, 289C,* 429–442.

Roberts, N.P., Kitchiner, N.J., Kenardy, J., & Bisson, J.I. (2010). Early psychological interventions to treat acute traumatic stress symptoms. *Cochrane Database of Systematic Reviews, 3.* Retrieved May 1, 2015 from www.researchgate.net/profile/Justin_Kennardy/publication/42256390_Early_psychological_ interventions_to_treat_acute_traumatic_stress_symptoms/links/09e415100761e442e5000000.pdf.

Rodriguez, M.A., Heilemann, M.V., Fielder, E., Ang, A., Nevarez, F., & Mangione, C.M. (2008). Intimate partner violence, depression, and PTSD among pregnant Latina women. *Annals of Family Medicine, 6*(1), 44–52.

Selye, H. (1976). Forty years of stress research: principal remaining problems and misconceptions. *Canadian Medical Association Journal, 115*(1), 53.

Sharma, M., & Rush, S.E. (2014). Mindfulness-based stress reduction as a stress management intervention for healthy individuals: a systematic review. *Journal of Evidence-Based Complementary & Alternative Medicine, 19*(4), 271–286.

Spiers, J.G., Chen, H.J., Sernia, C., & Lavidis, N.A. (2014). Activation of the hypothalamic-pituitary-adrenal stress axis induces cellular oxidative stress. *Frontiers in Neuroscience, 8,* 456.

Steinert, C., Hofmann, M., Leichsenring, F., & Kruse, J. (2015). The course of PTSD in naturalistic long-term studies: high variability of outcomes. A systematic review. *Nordic Journal of Psychiatry,* 1–14.

Surtees, P.G., Wainwright, N.W., Luben, R., Wareham, N.J., Bingham, S.A., & Khaw, K.T. (2010). Mastery is associated with cardiovascular disease mortality in men and women at apparently low risk. *Health Psychology, 29*(4), 412–420.

Szabo, S., Tache, Y., & Somogyi, A. (2012). The legacy of Hans Selye and the origins of stress research: a retrospective 75 years after his landmark brief "Letter" to the Editor of Nature. *Stress, 15*(5), 472–478.

Szanton, S.L., & Gill, J.M. (2010). Facilitating resilience using a society-to-cells framework: a theory of nursing essentials applied to research and practice. *Advances in Nursing Science, 33*(4), 329–343.

Tank, A.W., & D. Lee Wong. (2015). Peripheral and central effects of circulating catecholamines. *Comprehensive Physiology, 5*(1), 1–15.

Weiss, S.J. (2007). Neurobiological alterations associated with traumatic stress. *Perspectives in Psychiatric Care, 43*(3), 114–122.

White-Williams, C., Grady, K.L., Myers, S., Naftel, D.C., Wang, E., Bourge, R. C., & Rybarczyk, B. (2013). The relationships among satisfaction with social support, quality of life, and survival 5 to 10 years after heart transplantation. *Journal of Cardiovascular Nursing, 28*(5), 407–416.

Wohleb, E.S., Hanke, M.L., Corona, A.W., Powell, N.D., Stiner, L.M., Bailey, M.T., Nelson, R.J., Godbout, J.P., & Sheridan, J.F. (2011). Beta-adrenergic receptor antagonism prevents anxiety-like behavior and microglial reactivity induced by repeated social defeat. *Journal of Neuroscience, 31*(17), 6277–6288.

World Health Organization. (2009). Global health risks: mortality and burden of disease attributable to selected major risks. Retrieved April 13, 2015 from www.who.int/healthinfo/global_burden_disease/GlobalHealthRisks_report_full.pdf?ua=1.

Zraly, M., & Nyirazinyoye, L. (2010). Don't let the suffering make you fade away: an ethnographic study of resilience among survivors of genocide-rape in southern Rwanda. *Social Science Medicine, 70*(10), 1656–1664.

11

STRATEGIES FOR HEALTH PROMOTION IN INDIVIDUALS EXPERIENCING ANXIETY OR ANXIETY DISORDERS

Deborah V. Thomas and Magdala Habib Farid Maximos

Introduction

Generally, the words anxiety and stress are often used interchangeably, however, they are not the same. For the purpose of this chapter, stress (which is discussed in Chapter 10), is defined as a biochemical and adaptive response to threat in a variety of situations. Conversely, anxiety will be defined as an emotional and behavioral reaction resulting from acute or chronic stress. Anxiety is often described as excessive and ongoing fear, apprehension, dread, worry, or overall uneasiness occurring as a result of a real or perceived threat, the actual source of which is not identifiable. The focus of this anxiety can be driven by internal or external stimuli.

Anxiety is a common, normal emotion and it is critical to distinguish between normal levels of anxiety and pathological levels of anxiety. The easiest way to think of this is simply by evaluating if the symptoms are bad enough to interfere with any major domain of daily living and functioning. Anxiety disorders most often involve some physical or somatic complaint, which is not the case with normal anxiety levels.

Anxiety disorders or illnesses have features of fear and anxiety along with a variety of behavioral manifestations that will be briefly discussed in the context of various anxiety disorders. Anxiety disorders are likely the most missed and misdiagnosed disorders in individuals of all ages (Katzman, *et al.*, 2014). Frequently anxiety is misdiagnosed as depression and while anxiety and depression are frequently co-occurring disorders, they are not the same. Anxiety is a common feature of other psychiatric disorders such as depression, bipolar disorder, PTSD, OCD, and many others. While it is important to note these common comorbidities, it is beyond the scope of this chapter to cover these other disorders.

This chapter will provide an overview of anxiety and commonly occurring anxiety disorders, discuss incidence and prevalence, screening or testing, health promotion and intervention strategies, and other issues of clinical importance. There will be a concise description of the recent changes in the *Diagnostic and Statistical Manual of Mental Disorders*, fifth edition's (DSM-5) (APA, 2013) list of anxiety disorders noting the code sets for both ICD-9 and ICD-10. A "real world" clinical picture of anxiety and several common anxiety disorders with two case vignettes will be presented along with cultural variations and manifestations of anxiety and anxiety disorders.

An interview with a health care provider from Jordan will be included to provide a snapshot of a particular cultural perspective or difference in interpretation and meaning of anxiety and how it is approached through mental health promotion strategies and evidence-based interventions. A range of available interventions including pharmacotherapy, and complementary and alternative therapy options will be provided. Concluding this chapter will be recommendations for future research, additional readings, resources for patients and health care providers and a list of treatment guidelines from various countries addressing specific disorders.

General etiology of anxiety

According to current research, anxiety disorders have several possible causes. It is likely that most anxiety disorders result from combined influences of neurobiological vulnerabilities, developmental stages, and psychosocial stress. Anxiety disorders develop when the sympathetic response chronically fires off in the absence of threat. The dysregulation of noradrenergic neurotransmission may contribute to the dysregulated arousal states associated with a variety of anxiety and stress related disorders (Berridge, 2008).

The release of hormones such as epinephrine and cortisol can cause physiological effects that are beneficial for short-term stress such as increased heart rate, elevated blood pressure, increased respiration, muscle contraction, and decreased digestion. Additionally, the response lowers the immune system in order to give a person more energy in the present moment. When cortisol is released in the brain, the amygdala or "fear center" of the brain, increases in responsiveness and grows new connections. Additionally, high levels of stress actually cause cell death in the hippocampus, which helps with logic, context, relaxation, and controls anxiety. The combination of these two effects unfortunately is why panic and anxiety can take over one's life (Harrington, 2011).

Hereditary predisposition or genetic loading contributes to the development of anxiety disorders (NIMH Genetics Workgroup, 1998). Biologic vulnerability to certain anxiety disorders varies. In individuals who have a family history of panic disorder, evidence suggests that their heritable neuronal state may generate a lower threshold for their response to incidents that might generate anxiety. In other words, they are predisposed to a more intense response to emergencies and thus are more likely to experience anxiety (Benarroch, 2009).

Levels of anxiety

- *Mild anxiety* can be understood as a response to the routine tensions of everyday life. Mild anxiety can have positive effects. It can motivate, produce growth, enhance creativity and increase learning because at this level, you are alert and perception is increased.
- *Moderate anxiety* may cause the individual to lose sight of the broader picture and focus only on the cause of the anxiety. It may be difficult to pay attention as usual, and even though the perceptual field is narrowed, the individual is still able to solve a problem and learn. Mild and moderate levels of anxiety are considered normal and often helpful.
- *Severe anxiety* can be explained as a strong pervasive feeling that something bad is about to happen. The individual experiencing severe anxiety will likely find it very difficult or impossible to solve problems. The individual may feel their focus

is completely scattered. The person experiencing severe anxiety may feel at a loss about what to do without external direction because the awareness of their surroundings is significantly narrowed.

• *Panic level anxiety* is the highest level of anxiety and is associated with dread, terror and a sense of impending doom. You may not be able to communicate, function or concentrate because you are unable to think rationally. You may become immobilized or conversely start uncontrollably pacing and become increasingly active without a focused purpose.

(Hutchinson, 2015)

Neurobiological theories of anxiety

Maxmen, Ward, and Kilgus (2009) present three factors that support a neurobiological model for anxiety including the production of norepinephrine at the locus ceruleus—an area that incites a sense of anxiety when stimulated—the presence of benzodiazepine receptors and how benzodiazepines facilitate gamma amino-butyric acid (an inhibitory neurotransmitter) improving anxiety, and the influence of efficacious serotonin agonists to treat anxiety. Clearly, the experience of anxiety involves a complex chemical and structural interplay that requires additional research to optimize treatments (Benarroch, 2009).

Recent research demonstrates a neurobiological basis for anxiety disorders that could contribute to treatment and management of the diagnosis, thus the continued emphasis on research. Creating the concept of the Westphal paradigm, (Wittman *et al.*, 2011) pictures were generated signifying agoraphobic events, and magnetic resonance imaging (MRI) of the head of subjects who reviewed these pictures was studied, along with anxiety scale measurements. The authors hypothesized that in patients affected by anxiety there would be brain activation at the fear circuit and in brain structures that anticipate worrisome stimuli.

Magnetic resonance imaging results demonstrated 16 patients with panic disorder and agoraphobia had activation in areas associated with the fear circuit including the amygdala, insula and hippocampal areas. This particular study was very helpful in the development and validation of the Westphal paradigm. A limitation of the study was that there was no control group for the MRI evaluation. Subsequently, Wittman *et al.* (2014) compared neural activations by presenting specified agoraphobic stimulus sets to 72 patients with panic disorder with agoraphobia and 72 control patients. The patients with panic disorder with agoraphobia had stronger activation responses in the bilateral ventral striatum and left insula.

The authors concluded that there were stronger region-specific activations in patients suffering from this diagnosis in anticipation of agoraphobic-specific stimuli. Patients seem to process these stimuli more intensively based on individual salience. The authors conclude that knowledge of this neural activity as related to anticipation and cognitive processing for affected patients could be beneficial to optimize therapeutic measures.

Pharmacogenetics is another growing area of research addressing the neurobiology of anxiety disorders. Tiwari, Souza and Muller (2009) introduced the concept that patients with the same mental health disorder may not have a comparable therapeutic response to the same psychiatric medications. For example, a third of patients with anxiety will not respond to anti-depressants. The authors address areas of ongoing research involving the serotonin transporter and receptor genes, and the tryptophan hydroxylase gene and how gene activity affects drug efficacy for individuals.

Importantly, the cytochrome P450 (CYP450) variants are being studied to understand how patients may differ in metabolizing medications that could assist the prescriber with more specific information about effective medications for the individual patient. Similarly, there is also the relatively new concept of "therapygenetics" where genomic makeup could influence therapy efficacy. Knuts *et al.* (2014) presented 99 patients with panic disorder with agoraphobia who participated in a week-long therapy program and had their DNA analyzed for the 5 hydroxy tryptamine (serotonin) transport gene linked polymorphic region (5-HTTLPR) and related allele categories. This gene has been implicated in emotional status, for example, in populations who have experienced child abuse and anxiety. The authors report that the low expression 5-HTTLPR type gene responded more favorably to the therapy and concluded this result suggests serotonin plays a part in a patient's response to therapy. This means that medications used to create more circulating serotonin are likely to be first-line medication interventions for anxiety disorders. Most importantly, this new understanding can help nurses better educate others regarding why some individuals respond differently when prescribed the same medication.

Overview of incidence and prevalence

Anxiety disorders are common throughout our global society. These disorders are the sixth leading cause of disability in high-, low-, and middle-income countries. In 2006, the best estimates of 1-year and lifetime prevalence for total anxiety disorders world-wide based on analysis of 39 studies was 10.6 percent and 16.6 percent respectively (Somers, Goldner, Waraich, & Hsu, 2006). The disorders accounted for 390 disability-adjusted life years per 100,000 persons in 2010. Females accounted for 65 percent of these disability-adjusted life years, with the highest burden in both males and females experienced by those aged between 15 and 34 years (Baxter, Vos, Scott, Ferrari, & Whiteford, 2014).

According to the CDC (2011), anxiety disorders, which included panic disorder, generalized anxiety disorder, post-traumatic stress disorder, phobias, and separation anxiety disorder, are the most common class of mental disorders present in the general population. The estimated lifetime prevalence of any anxiety disorder is over 15 percent, while the 12-month prevalence is more than 10 percent. Prevalence estimates of anxiety disorders are generally higher in developed countries than in developing countries.

Most anxiety disorders are more prevalent in women than in men. One study estimated the annual cost of anxiety disorders in the United States to be approximately $42.3 billion in the 1990s, a majority of which was due to non-psychiatric medical treatment costs. This estimate focused on short-term effects and did not include the effect of outcomes such as the increased risk of other disorders (CDC, 2011). Gender differentiality is noted to have an influence relative to the power and control both men and women have over some socioeconomic determinants as well as their access to available resources, status, roles, options and treatment in their particular culture and living environment (WHO, n.d.).

The World Health Organization conducted a World Mental Health Survey between 2002 and 2005 that included Belgium, Colombia, France, Germany, Israel, Italy, Japan, Lebanon, Mexico, Netherlands, New Zealand, Nigeria, People's Republic of China, South Africa, Spain, Ukraine, and the United States. The authors note that interpretation of prevalence of anxiety disorders may be more complicated than with many other disorders. This was primarily due to the age of onset distributions that fell into two distinct categories. Phobias and separation anxiety disorder had early age of onset with a median range of ages at 7–14. However, generalized anxiety disorder and panic disorder showed a median age of onset between 24–50, with a much wider cross-national variation (WHO World Mental Health Survey Consortium, 2007).

It is noted that there may be some biases that may have led to under-estimating prevalence. This includes the notion that many people with mental illnesses or disorders may be less likely to participate in surveys. There can also be a reluctance to admit to a mental illness, which may be especially likely in less developed countries (WHO Mental Health Survey Consortium, 2007). It is imperative to be mindful of other culture's definitions, interpretations and management strategies for various anxiety disorders.

Cultural variations and manifestations of anxiety and anxiety disorders

Culture influences the source of anxiety, the form of illness experience, symptomatology, the interpretation of symptoms, modes of coping with distress, help-seeking, and the social response to distress and disability. Each of these ways in which culture may influence the regulation of emotion has potential implications for the expression of dysphoric affect in clinical settings. In many cultures anxiety and anxiety disorders are not viewed as mental health problems but as social or moral problems. Cultural ideologies of emotion also govern developmental experiences as well as coping strategies that may influence the course of anxiety and its disorders.

There are often culture-related diagnostic issues. For example, in relationship to children tolerating separation, there is a variation among cultures regarding the age in which children should leave the home and become independent. It is important to be mindful of immigrated families where the spoken and unspoken language is different, thus our interpretations cannot be single-minded.

According to the DSM-5 (APA, 2013) there are significantly lower rates of specific phobias among Americans, Asians, and Latinos when compared to non-Latino whites, African Americans, and Native Americans. Immigrant status is associated with significantly lower rates of social anxiety in both Latino and non-Latino white groups. Actual prevalence rates may not reflect the self-reported social anxiety levels in the same culture, especially in cultures with a strong collectivistic orientation that may report high levels of social anxiety but have a low prevalence of social anxiety disorder.

Clearly there are varied cultural conceptualizations of distress related to the continuum of anxiety and anxiety disorders. It is critical to utilize a framework for gathering information about the individuals' social and cultural context and history. The DSM-5 (APA, 2013) includes a comprehensive outline for using the Cultural Formulation Interview (CFI), which is a set of 16 questions. The benefit in using the CFI or a similar assessment framework lies in the core goals of mental health intervention. Simply stated, these goals are to improve overall patient-desired outcomes, increase quality of life in all domains, and decrease pain and suffering. Included in the DSM-5's appendix entitled "Glossary of cultural concepts of distress," there are examples of well-studied concepts illustrative of cultural information critical for diagnosis. The interrelationships among cultural syndromes, idioms of distress, and causal explanations are also discussed (APA, 2013).

Anxiety disorders in DSM-5, ICD-9 and ICD-10

To better communicate globally regarding anxiety and other mental health conditions, a diagnostic coding system has been developed and used. However, as with many other areas of mental health and mental health care, this system is not uniform worldwide. Within this multinational mental health environment, the International Classification of Diseases (ICD) and *Diagnostic and Statistical Manual* (DSM) systems are used. The DSM-5 (APA, 2013) is organized using a developmental and lifespan framework. It is important to note that providers in all countries do not use the DSM. The World Health Organization's International Classification of Diseases and Related Health Problems is more widely used in many countries. To facilitate a global understanding of the classification of anxiety disorders the DSM-5 codes are the same as the ICD-9 codes. Current ICD-10 codes are noted for each disorder. The framework for discussion of anxiety disorders in this chapter will follow the same developmental format for ease of reading and convenience in facilitating cohesion with the DSM-5 and ICD-10. The reader is encouraged to refer to the DSM-5 or the appropriate ICD-code set for a thorough list of diagnostic criteria and specifiers appropriate for coding a particular anxiety disorder and symptom specifier, if appropriate.

Currently the United States lags behind the rest of the world in using the most up-to-date International Classification of Diseases commonly referred to as the ICD-10. On July 31, 2014 the US Department of Health and Human Services issued a final rule finalizing October 1, 2015 as the new compliance date for the US to transition to the ICD-10 code sets. According to the World Health Organization's (WHO) Fact sheet and classifications page, the ICD-11 is scheduled for release in 2017 (WHO, 2015).

All anxiety disorders may occur co-morbidly with other mental health disorders, especially depression, as well as physiologic illnesses or disorders. It is always imperative to review differential diagnosis possibilities to provide the most optimal outcomes for the patient. Notably, all experiences of anxiety do not constitute a "disorder." It is important to note whether the particular symptoms of the disorder impair one's abilities in a major domain of functioning such as academic, work, personal and/or social relationships.

Table 11.1 lists the 11 anxiety disorders and a panic specifier delineated in the most current DSM (APA, 2013), which is organized to be harmonious with the planned ICD-11. Notably, many currently available references related to these diagnoses still include discussion of PTSD, and OCD under anxiety disorders which were in former iterations of the DSM.

Table 11.1 Anxiety disorders: DSM and ICD codes

Anxiety disorder name	DSM and ICD-9 code	ICD-10 code
Separation anxiety disorder	309.21	F93.0
Selective mutism	312.23	F94.0
Specific phobia	300.29	Will vary by specific phobia EX. F40.218 (fear of specific animal); F40.230 (fear of blood); F40.231 (fear of injections or transfusions
Social anxiety disorder (SAD)	300.23	F40.10
Panic disorder	300.01	F41.0
Agorophobia	300.22	F40.00
Generalized anxiety disorder (GAD)	300.02	F41.1
Substance/medication induced anxiety disorder	Same as ICD-10	Coding is specific to the substance with the appropriate specifier of onset or severity
Anxiety due to another medical condition	293.84	F06.4
Other specified anxiety disorder	300.09	F41.8
Unspecified anxiety disorder	300.00	F41.9

Note: Under panic disorder there is a panic attack specifier that refers to the symptoms present for the purpose of identifying a panic attack. However, according to the DSM-5 (APA, 2013) a panic attack itself is not a mental disorder and cannot be coded.

Separation anxiety disorder

Separation anxiety disorder refers to excessive developmentally inappropriate fear or anxiety about leaving or being away from home or the primary attachment figure. The worry is persistent and excessive and often involves fear that something such as a car accident or some other illness or injury will occur, thus harming the caregiver. Often, there will be a partial or total inability to go to school, based on unwarranted fear of school and/or inappropriate anxiety about leaving home. Additionally, children will often fear being home alone, going to friends' houses for any extended period of time (especially spending the night), school trips, and other events requiring separation from the caregiver.

Complaints are often physical and most frequently include stomachaches, headaches, nausea, and vomiting. Bedtime is especially difficult for these children because going to sleep is the quintessential act of "voluntarily going unconscious" and not knowing what might happen. The worry keeps them awake. Nightmares are frequent and often the content is very disturbing to the child and family. All ages are affected, but two peaks of incidence, ages 6–7 at the start of school life, and ages 12–15 at the start of middle school or high school; boys and girls are equally affected and the youngest child in family is most likely to be affected.

Incidence/prevalence

Approximately 1–2 percent of school-age children suffer from school refusal while 3–4 percent are absent on grounds of truancy. Likely risk factors can be especially problematic after time away from school (such as new school year, after vacations, after prolonged illness, change of school). Associated conditions include mood disorder, especially depression. There is often an increased incidence of anxiety and mood disorders in the family. Pathogenesis suggests some children may have inborn vulnerability or predisposition for development of emotional disturbances, including school refusal, which is also known as separation anxiety disorder.

There is no specific testing necessary (unless warranted by specific findings on history and exam). Treatment for separation anxiety should specifically involve reassuring parents that their child is not physically ill and obtaining parental support for treatment. There should be an immediate return to school and parents must help their child face a distressing experience to overcome their anxiety about the event (APA, 2013).

Selective mutism

Selective mutism is a consistent pattern of inability to speak due to extreme fear and anxiety. This should not be confused with an oppositional "refusal" to speak. The individual is often extremely shy and is afraid of social embarrassment. They are often socially isolating and appear to have some oppositional behavior, which may be secondary to other co-morbid disorders of communication, anxiety, and other neurodevelopmental or psychotic disorders. This behavior is driven by anxiety. The disorder itself is rare and according to DSM-5 (APA, 2013) has not been included as a diagnostic category in epidemiological studies of prevalence of childhood disorders.

Specific phobia

Specific phobia usually involves a fear or anxiety of at least three different objects or situations. The DSM-5 (APA, 2013) requires each specific phobia to have its own code. The fear or anxiety is disproportionate to the actual danger the object or situation can present. Specific phobia may develop in response to an experienced or witnessed traumatic event.

Social anxiety disorder (social phobia or SAD)

Social anxiety disorder (social phobia or SAD) can be described as an intense fear of being in any social situation in which the individual may be judged. The degree and the type of fear and anxiety may vary depending on the situation. For example, some individuals may have a panic attack before giving a speech and will avoid doing so as much as possible. Some individuals only have a performance type of social anxiety and do not fear or avoid nonperformance activities or social situations.

Again, the fear or anxiety about being judged is disproportionate to the reality of being judged or to the negative consequences, which may occur as a result (such as in giving a speech at school). Catastrophic thinking often accompanies such intense social anxiety and fear. Due to the nature of SAD related to a fear of being judged, there is a direct link to the social standards and role expectations, which are culture dependent (Hofmann, Asnaani, & Hinton, 2010).

Incidence/prevalence

Interestingly, data from the National Comorbidity Survey (NCS) (Kessler, 2005a; 2005b) show that the 12-month prevalence rate of SAD among US adults is 7.1–7.9 percent, with similar rates found in other cultural groups such as 6.4 percent in Chile and 9.1 percent in Brazil. However, the 12-month prevalence rate of SAD from East Asian surveys, while less studied, reports much lower ranges such as 0.4 percent in Taiwan, 0.2–0.6 percent in Korea, 0.2 percent in China, and 0.8 percent in Japan. Similar low prevalence rates were shown in epidemiological surveys of Mexico, Nigeria, South Africa, and Europe (Kessler *et al.*, 2009). Clearly a consideration of factors that influence a disorder must be examined further and it appears a cultural perspective is essential to also explore and understand.

Panic disorder

Panic disorder refers to recurrent and unexpected panic attacks. A panic attack can be described as an abrupt, "out of the blue" onset of intense psychological and physiological discomfort. It may arise from a calm or an anxious state and usually only lasts for several minutes. Panic attacks often present with symptoms of palpitations, sweating, numbness and tingling, abdominal distress, difficulty catching one's breath, dizziness, or light-headedness. Individuals who experience panic attacks will often appear in the emergency room feeling and believing they are having a heart attack.

The physiological and psychological symptoms can be quite frightening. The fact that the surge of symptoms only lasts for a few minutes is of little comfort to the individual experiencing those symptoms. Understandably, one feature of panic attack is the "fear of the next one." Due to the abrupt and insidious onset, the individual cannot "be prepared." Being caught off guard often results in hypervigilance and avoidance of the same activity or being in the same place where a previous attack occurred.

For example, if an individual experienced a panic attack at a certain restaurant, they may avoid going to that restaurant again for some period of time. Consequently, if they go to another restaurant and have a panic attack it can begin what is known as "the stimulus generalization response" (Watson & Raynor, 1920). This can result in a ripple effect and create a path of avoidance, which can grow and make the individual's world smaller and smaller. The most common onset of panic disorder is during late adolescence to early adulthood, usually prior to 35 years old and is more common among women than men (APA, 2013).

Incidence/prevalence

The lifetime prevalence of panic disorder alone is approximately 5 percent in the United States. There is a 5.1 percent lifetime prevalence of panic disorder and 2.1 percent 1-year prevalence of panic disorder in United States. Risk factors associated with risk of panic disorder include family history and genetic predisposition. Evidence-based prevention and screening can include use of the self-reported Patient Health Questionnaire that appears helpful for diagnosis of panic disorder in primary care populations (Herr, Williams, Benjamin, & McDuffie, 2014). The Autonomic Nervous System (ANS) two-item questionnaire may be useful as a primary care screening tool to rule out patients needing further evaluation for panic disorder. The reference standard was the confirmatory diagnostic interview from the World Health Organization's Composite International Diagnostic Interview panic attack/panic disorder module.

Agoraphobia

Agoraphobia refers to an intense fear or anxiety triggered by the real or anticipated exposure to a multitude of situations or places. Some examples of situations causing agoraphobic fear include public transportation, open spaces (for example, parking lots or bridges), being in stores or theaters, standing in line or being in a crowd, being outside of the home alone (World Health Organization, 1992). Avoidance often accompanies agoraphobia and in the extreme may result in an individual being afraid to leave their home. Agoraphobia often occurs with panic attacks and panic disorders often occur before and/or with agoraphobia. The course of the disorder is usually persistent and chronic with initial onset before the age of 35, and occurs more commonly in women than men. Screening and prevention is not directly to applicable agoraphobia (APA, 2013).

Incidence/prevalence

Differences in definitions from DSM-IV-TR, DSM-5, and ICD-10 may produce different estimates of incidence or prevalence.

Generalized anxiety disorder (GAD)

Generalized anxiety disorder (GAD) is essentially excessive and persistent worry and apprehension about many things or anything. The experience of worry or anxiety can be viewed in terms of intensity, duration, frequency and severity. A combination of genetics and environmental influence may play a role in symptom manifestation. It is difficult for the individual to manage the worrisome thoughts, which tend to spill over into many aspects of their life and can cause considerable distress and a lack of enjoyment of life. Often there is a fear that if they do not worry something will happen.

You can delineate generalized anxiety disorder from the expected worries of daily life by considering the degree in which the anxiety or worries interfere with overall psychosocial functioning. This should be examined in the context of the pervasive, intense, frequent and long lasting nature of generalized anxiety disorder and the distress it brings. It is a chronic disorder, which may have exacerbations, but is usually "percolating" at some level. It requires a good deal of energy to worry and often the individual also experiences feeling "wound up" or "on edge" and often experiences difficulties with sleeping.

It appears that the age of onset is bimodal and typically occurs between the ages of 10–14 in children and adolescents and a median age of 31 in adults (Katzman *et al.*, 2014). It is more common in women, Caucasians, older adults and those who are widowed, separated, or divorced (Weisberg, 2009). As noted above, the course is usually chronic, with lower likelihood of remission in those with comorbid psychological conditions and poor family support. GAD is associated with increased mortality and suicidal behavior.

There are several anxiety scales commonly used to help clarify the diagnostic construct of GAD. They include the Hamilton Rating Scale for Anxiety (HAM-A), which scores 14 features of anxiety from not present (0 points) to disabling (4 points), with total score range 0–56; and the 7-item generalized anxiety disorder scale (GAD-7), which is useful for specific diagnosis of generalized anxiety disorder (Hamilton, 1959). Also helpful is the Clinical Global Impressions (CGI) scale, which quantifies clinician's experience-based assessment of the severity of a patient's mental condition (total score range 1–7) and/or assessment of the change in a patient's condition from one week before the start of treatment (total score range 1–7) to the current state (Busner & Targum, 2007).

Incidence/prevalence

There is a 4–7 percent lifetime prevalence and 1–4 percent annual incidence reported with 0.3 percent estimated 12-month prevalence in children aged 8–15 years in the United States from 2001 to 2004 (Tyrer & Baldwin, 2006).

Prevention

Brief parental intervention in anxious and behaviorally inhibited preschool-aged children is associated with decreased development of anxiety disorders at middle childhood (*level 2 (mid-level) evidence*). School-based group cognitive behavior therapy may prevent development of anxiety disorder in children with anxious or depressive symptoms (*level 2 (mid-level) evidence*) (Tyrer & Baldwin 2006).

Substance/medication-induced anxiety disorder

Substance/medication-induced anxiety disorder is one in which the manifestations or symptoms look like an anxiety disorder, or often a panic attack. However, a drug or substance, which can be alcohol, caffeine, cannabis, phencyclidine, hallucinogens, inhalants, opioids, sedatives, cocaine, amphetamines, or other drugs or substances drive the symptoms. Importantly, the substance or medication may be one that is prescribed or non-prescribed. Diagnostically, the symptoms must have developed while or soon after a substance was introduced or withdrawn. According to the DSM-5 (APA, 2013) this diagnosis should not be given if panic or anxiety symptoms preceded use of the substance or if symptoms remain longer than a month. It is important to note this may be a result of prescribed or non-prescribed medications or substances.

DSM-5, ICD-9, and ICD-10 codes

Coding is specific to the substance with the appropriate specifier of onset or severity. *Anxiety disorder due to another medical condition* is best described as anxiety that is caused by a medical condition such as hyperthyroidism, pheochromocytoma, hypoglycemia, congestive heart failure, asthma, and multiple others. To determine an accurate diagnosis in this instance it is critical that the clinician first determines if there is a medical condition. It should be established that the anxiety symptoms have a physiological etiology. A thorough physical exam and blood tests, if available can be most helpful to the provider in determining appropriate interventions (APA, 2013).

Other specified anxiety disorder applies to presentations in which symptoms of an anxiety disorder exist, but do not meet full DSM-5 criteria.

Unspecified anxiety disorder applies to presentations in which symptoms of anxiety disorders predominate but do not meet full criteria for any of the anxiety disorders. According to the DSM-5 this is used when there is insufficient information to make a more specific diagnosis such as in an emergency room.

Notably, the DSM-5 no longer includes obsessive-compulsive disorder, post-traumatic stress disorder or adjustment disorder in the category of anxiety disorders. Some past specifiers related to age and length of time for symptom presence are no longer indicated.

Clinical picture

There are a number of empirically tested anxiety rating scales available. Commonly used are The Generalized Anxiety Scale GAD-7 (Spitzer, Kroenke, Williams, & Lowe, 2006), the Hamilton Anxiety Rating Scale (Hamilton, 1959) and The Zung Self-rating Anxiety Scale (Zung, 1971). These are available electronically or as a hard copy, and are simple to score and interpret. These and other measures have been translated into other languages.

The following two vignettes are real clinical cases and will endeavor to describe what anxiety looks, sounds, and feels like from the patient's point of view.

Vignette 1

Lia is a 52 year-old female who reports a lifelong history of general pervasive anxiety and panic attacks. She reports recently having an increasingly difficult time leaving her home to go to the market, visit with friends and/or family, or go to her part-time job as a high-school math teacher. Lia reports that once she is at her destination she sometimes feels OK and her anxiety seems to dissipate.

However, she reports more often it seems her symptoms become more intense and disconcerting to the point of having a panic attack. She describes this feeling as "horrifying," a sensation of feeling outside herself, as if she were watching the events going on but she herself is not really present. She describes an overwhelming sense of fear and impending doom and truly feels she may die or go crazy.

She reports feeling dizzy, having palpitations, difficulty swallowing, sweaty palms, and feeling nauseous. Recently these symptoms have occurred at least 3–4 times a week. She can not name any event that she feels or believes has influenced or caused this recent exacerbation of symptoms. Lia does not have a strong social support system other than her husband and a sister. She has two grown-up children who do not live nearby. She does not have many friends, in part, she says, because of her lack of desire or ability to socialize.

Past interventions

Lia had been prescribed antidepressants and benzodiazepines in the past but had negative side effects to several medications, which made her more apprehensive about trying other medications. She prefers non-medication interventions if possible. She had not engaged in any type of non-psychopharmacological intervention in the past. She reports that she thought therapy would not help and didn't want people to think she was weak.

Current intervention

Lia completed a 12-week program of CBT for panic and anxiety and continues to participate in a church support group for women. She has started attending a yoga and meditation class to help her stay calm and centered. She reports having a broader social support system as a result. She occasionally experiences increase in anxiety but has learned to stop the symptom progression before a panic attack ensues. She reports that what works well is using the technique of counting backwards from 100 to zero by three's until the symptoms subside.

Vignette 2

Josiah is a 7-year-old male who has recently experienced increased difficulty in attending school. Once he is at school he complains of stomachaches, headaches, and episodes of nausea and vomiting. His mother reports he has experienced some of these symptoms since he began kindergarten but in the past few months it has gotten so bad the school has had to report Josiah's absences to authorities. This resulted in Josiah's hospitalization for several weeks.

Past interventions

None, other than being forced to go to school. In the past few months his mother has gone to school where she sits outside his classroom door, reporting, "it makes him feel better." The school did not support this but gave in to see if it would be a short-term solution and hoped Josiah would learn to stay on his own. However, whenever his mother would get up and leave for any short period of time to make a phone call or tend to other business he would get more anxious and became inconsolable. His behavior in class had reportedly gotten worse.

Current intervention

Josiah's family engaged in family therapy. His parents are attending parenting classes and understand part of Josiah's separation anxiety, which manifested as school refusal, is a result of his mother's fear of not being there to watch over him and manage everything in his world on a daily basis. Therefore, Josiah had become dependent on her to feel safe in the world and when she was not there he felt anxious and scared to the point of being sick.

His mother had nothing but good intentions and now understands it was her own anxiety that was out of control and caused her son this level of anxiety. After three months of parenting classes, support, and play and art therapy for Josiah, he now looks forward to school and seeing his friends. Josiah's mom has learned to manage her individual anxiety with the use of an anti-depressant for anxiety and cognitive behavioral therapy (CBT).

Interventions and cultural point of view

An interview with a 45-year-old male health care provider from Jordan, F. Alaloul (personal communication, April 20, 2015) was conducted and provides a different perspective on anxiety and various anxiety illnesses and disorders. He was born, raised, and completed his undergraduate degree in nursing in Jordan. He came to the United States to complete his Master's Degree and his PhD. He then returned to Jordan for several years before returning to the US where he is now a professor in nursing. When asked to describe what he saw as the difference in anxiety and anxiety disorders in the US and Jordan, he immediately notes "life is very busy here, always a lot to do . . . it is hard to relax . . . there is no time to just be . . . it feels like there is no time to just stop and think here."

He describes a much less harried lifestyle in Jordan with a great deal more extended family and neighbors to be of support. Also of importance is his commentary on religion and prayer, which he emphasizes helps in "relieving stress and anxiety." He points out the gender differences saying men especially did not like to have anxiety, were not prone to cry and thus internalized and held everything in. He articulated the great importance the sense of "community" gave to the women and children. "It provides them with an outlet to vent or process what is going on in their life." Some things were to be kept in the family only and other things were acceptable to talk about with neighbors and friends.

When asked why he felt there was more anxiety here in the US than in Jordan he reported observations of differences in how anxiety is perceived. In Jordan "it is integrated as part of your life . . . it is just the way it is . . . not a separate issue." He also points out that mostly in the Middle East, people do not generally like to talk about mental health. He notes that when people go to the doctor they don't talk about mental health issues because of a fear of distracting the doctor from doing the physical exam. His final comments were related to issues of confidentiality. He said there are no (patient confidentiality regulations in Jordan), so people really try to hide any psychiatric mental health issues. The physician's first line of communication is talking with the family not the patient. He suggested stigma and lack of confidentiality are significant reasons there are very few statistics on mental health or psychiatric mental health studies done in the Middle East. This interview provides insight into best practice and the importance of cultural context in patient care.

Mental health promotion and evidence-based intervention strategies

Health promotion strategies are common across all anxiety disorders and non-disordered anxiety states. Collaboration with patients for agreed-upon healthy behaviors will yield the most optimal results. Some of these more common strategies include a focus on exercise, healthy diet, adequate fluid intake, good sleep hygiene, and decreased use of caffeine, tobacco, alcohol, and other potentially harmful substances. There are a number of evidence-based psychotherapeutic interventions listed in Table 11.2.

Complementary and alternative (CAM) strategies listed in Table 11.3 should be offered to patients as another option in managing anxiety. YOGA, Tai Chi, Qigong (Abbott & Lavretsky, 2013), mindfulness meditation, praying and other self-reflective health behaviors are significant to the emotional regulation in clients with various anxiety disorders. It is important to support the patients' choices between pharmacotherapy, psychotherapy and psychosocial treatment and also explain from an evidence-based perspective what may have the best outcome for their specific situation and set of symptoms.

There is a collective professional responsibility to be mindful that every patient, health care provider, and country will not have readily available resources to resolve the symptoms and distress that might accompany various anxiety disorders occurring in patients across the lifespan. Because many anxiety states and disorders utilize the same treatment intervention strategies they

Table 11.2 Psychotherapeutic interventions

Psychodynamic psychotherapy
Cognitive behavioral therapy (CBT)
Exposure or de-sensitization therapy
Parent-led CBT
Group CBT
Internet or computer-assisted CBT

Table 11.3 Complementary and alternative strategies

YOGA
Tai Chi and Qigong
Mindfulness meditation
Praying

Table 11.4 Psychopharmacological interventions

Antidepressants, specifically SSRIs such as sertraline, fluoxetine, and paroxetine and some SNRIs such as venlafaxine
Benzodiazepines such as clonazepam, diazepam, lorazepam, and alprazolam
Non-benzodiazepine anxiolytics such as buspirone, hydroxyzine, and diphenhydramine
Beta-blockers such as propranolol
Antiepileptic medications such as lamotrogine, pregabalin, and Neurontin

will be listed below. Information on many of these interventions is readily available electronically or in hard copy format. A list of international clinical guidelines and resources are included as well as those from the United States, United Kingdom, Europe, Australia, New Zealand, and Canada. Psychopharmacological interventions as well as complementary and alternative therapy interventions are considered.

Psychopharmacological interventions

Table 11.4 provides a list of generic psychotropic medications listed as choices that may be less expensive and more readily available in some areas of the world. According to Buoli, Caldiroli, Caletti, Paoli, & Altamura (2013), selective serotonin reuptake inhibitors (SSRIs) and serotonin and norepinephrine reuptake inhibitors (SNRIs) together with pregabalin are considered by international guidelines as the first-line choice for generalized anxiety disorder (GAD) treatment. They note however, that 50 percent of GAD patients have poor response to these first-line treatments.

Alternative medications such as atypical antipsychotics and antiepileptic medications are often used "off label" to treat this condition. Mula, Pini, and Cassano (2007) reviewed the evidence related to the efficacy of antiepileptic drugs (AEDs) and found the strongest evidence for use of pregabalin in social phobia and generalized anxiety disorder, and gabapentin for social anxiety. The data for gabapentin in panic disorder is mixed and requires further research. This may be helpful for individuals who are partial responders or non-responders to conventional pharmacotherapy.

Herbal remedies

The use of herbal remedies is often the choice of the patient, especially if it is more acceptable and available in their culture and their environment. The herbal remedies listed have an evidenced based recommendation of at least "suggested benefit" unless otherwise noted according to the DYNAMED Plus system for review of evidence and the Canadian guidelines for evidence-based interventions. Kava is listed because of the commonality in which it has been used in the past and the current caution related to the use of Kava.

Lavender oil has evidence for efficacy (level 2 (mid-level) evidence). Lavender oil gel caps reduce anxiety symptoms in patients with generalized anxiety disorder with outcomes comparable to the benzodiazepine lorazepam (Kasper *et al.*, 2014).

Evidence suggests effectiveness of Galphimia glauca extract for generalized anxiety disorder (level 2 (mid-level) evidence). Galphimia glauca extract appears to reduce anxiety as much as lorazepam in adults with generalized anxiety disorder (Herrera-Arellano, *et al.*, 2007).

Kava originally appeared as effective as buspirone or opipramol for treating generalized anxiety disorder and reducing anxiety symptoms in patients with anxiety disorders with mild, transient, and infrequent adverse events reported. However, Kava is now considered unsafe due to hepato-toxicity with 25 cases of liver toxicity reported with products (dietary supplements) containing herbal extracts of kava (US Food and Drug Administration, 2001). Additional FDA warnings were issued to consumers about rare hepatic failure associated with use of kava-containing products (US Food and Drug Administration, 2002). Centers for Disease Control and Prevention reports 10 cases of fulminant hepatic failure requiring liver transplant associated with kava (CDC, 2002). Kava has high potential for drug interactions through inhibition of cytochrome P450 enzymes (Mathews, Etheridge, & Black, 2002).

There was minimal evidence found assessing efficacy of herbal remedies as adjunctive treatment for patients with anxiety disorders (Ravindran & da Silva 2013). There is insufficient evidence regarding valerian for anxiety (Miyasaka, Atallah, & Soares, 2006) or for the use of passiflora (passionflower extract) for anxiety disorders (Miyasaka, Atallah, & Soares, 2007).

Rhodiola rosea (roseroot) had been reported to reduce anxiety symptoms, however, studies did not support this (level 3 (lacking direct) evidence) (Bystritsky, Kerwin, & Feusner, 2008). This is supported by Mental Health America (2013).

Naturopathic care plus ashwagandha (Withania somnifera) may reduce anxiety in patients with moderate-to-severe anxiety (level 2 (mid-level) evidence) (Cooley, *et al.*, 2009).

Manasamitra Vataka with or without dripping of medicated oil over the forehead is associated with similar improvement in symptoms compared with clonazepam in adults with generalized anxiety disorder and comorbid social phobia (level 2 (mid-level) evidence) (Tubaki *et al.*, 2012).

There are many botanical and nutritional supplements that anecdotally appear to be effective for many people. While there have been a number of studies on various herbal remedies and supplements, there need to be more RCT studies to provide practitioners and consumers with evidence in which to base practice decisions. Mental Health America (2013), notes that while many natural remedies are safe they are not risk free. Thus, informed decisions regarding use of CAM treatments must include reviewing evidence of effectiveness, risks versus benefits, and other treatment options. This can often be difficult because of many varying claims regarding safety and efficacy of some CAM treatments.

Recommendations

While there have been many studies on anxiety and the various anxiety disorders it appears it would be most helpful to move toward a research agenda that looks at the various interpretations and experiences of anxiety. In order for this research to be meaningful it must be done in the context of the appropriate cultural considerations. More research is needed in the field of the neurosciences to better understand all of the neurobiological possibilities not limited to genetic loading, pharmacotherapy, and neurocircuitry.

Sarris, Glick, Hoenders, Duffy, & Lake (2013) note several primary areas of research needed for implementing an integrative mental health approach. These include pharmacogenomics, epigenetics, and neuroimaging to determine mechanisms of action of the intervention strategies. Research related to the impact of exercise, diet, and stress management as both preventive measures and intervention strategies for anxiety and anxiety disorders are needed. Integrative mental health care will hopefully provide for the establishment of clinical guidelines to determine safe and effective assessment and intervention strategies based on the evidence for both conventional and CAM therapies.

A comprehensive research agenda that moves toward innovative intervention models, and novel prevention and intervention strategies will ground us as we move toward health and wellness. A more open and intentional understanding of anxiety and anxiety disorders from the individual's perspective is necessary to achieve our global goals of mental health. Achieving these goals will require a great deal of education for communities of patients, families, health care providers, and researchers.

Summary

Anxiety is a common, normal emotion and it is critical to distinguish between normal levels of anxiety and pathological levels of anxiety. It is likely that most anxiety disorders result from a combination of neurobiological vulnerabilities, developmental stages, and psychosocial stress. There are a number of anxiety disorders identified in the DSM-5 and the ICD-10. While the categorizations of disorders serve a purpose for insurance, billing and practicality, it also allows for mental health providers to talk to each other using a shared framework.

However, these diagnostic constructs must be utilized in concert with an appropriate cultural interview and an awareness of the various perceptions and interpretations that might influence any particular diagnosis. Strategies for managing anxiety and anxiety disorders range from focused breath-work, yoga, meditation and prayer, to exercise, therapy, medications, herbal remedies, and a whole cadre of other things and techniques. Providers need to be aware that some individuals use remedies and intervention strategies dictated by their culture, their financial means, and their access to care.

Guidelines and resources for anxiety disorders

International guidelines

World Federation of Biological Psychiatry (WFSBP) guideline on pharmacological treatment of anxiety disorders, obsessive-compulsive disorder, and posttraumatic stress disorder in primary care can be found in *International Journal of Psychiatric Clinical Practice* 2012 June; 16(2): 77.

United States guidelines

Work Loss Data Institute (WLDI) guideline on mental illness and stress can be found at *National Guideline Clearinghouse* 2011 May 19: 25703.

American Psychiatric Association (APA) guideline on treatment of patients with panic disorder can be found at APA 2009 January PDF. http://psychiatryonline.org/pb/assets/raw/sitewide/practice_guidelines/guidelines/panicdisorder.pdf

Expert guideline on pharmacotherapy of panic disorder can be found in *Journal of the American Board of Family Practice* 1998 July–August; 11(4): 282. Commentary can be found in *Journal of the American Board of Family Practice* 1999 January–February; 12(1): 102.

New York State Department of Health guideline on anxiety disorders in patients with HIV/AIDS can be found at 2006 March full-text. www.hivguidelines.org/clinical-guidelines/hiv-and-mental-health/anxiety-disorders-in-patients-with-hivaids/

United Kingdom guidelines

National Collaborating Centre for Mental Health. Common mental health disorders. Identification and pathways to care. London (UK): National Institute for Health and Clinical Excellence (NICE), 2011 May, 61 pp. (Clinical guideline no. 123).

National Institute for Health and Care Excellence (NICE) guideline on generalized anxiety disorder and panic disorder (with or without agoraphobia) in adults can be found at *NICE* 2011 January: CG113 PDF or at *National Guideline Clearinghouse* 2012 February 6: 34280. Summary can be found in *BMJ* 2011 January 26; 342: c7460 full-text. www.nice.org.uk/guidance/cg113

British Association for Psychopharmacology (BAP) evidence-based guidelines on pharmacological treatment of anxiety disorders, post-traumatic stress disorder, and obsessive-compulsive disorder can be found in *Journal of Psychopharmacology*, 2014 May; 28(5): 403 or at BAP 2014 PDF. http://docplayer.net/704846-1-introduction-bap-guidelines.html

European guidelines

Health Technology Assessment Unit, Laín Entralgo Agency clinical practice guideline on treatment of patients with anxiety disorders in primary care can be found at 2008 PDF or at *National Guideline Clearinghouse* 2013 February 25: 38981. www.guideline.gov/browse/by-organization.aspx?orgid=2399

Australian and New Zealand guidelines

Australian and New Zealand clinical guideline on treatment of panic disorder and agoraphobia can be found in *Australian and New Zealand Journal of Psychiatry* 2003 December; 37(6): 641.

Beyond Blue Australian clinical practice guidelines on depression and related disorders (anxiety, bipolar disorder, and puerperal psychosis) in perinatal period can be found at *National Guideline Clearinghouse* 2013 August 12: 43862.

Canadian guidelines

Anxiety Disorders Association of Canada (Association Canadienne des Troubles Anxieux [ADAC/ACTA])/McGill University clinical practice guidelines on management of anxiety, posttraumatic stress, and obsessive-compulsive disorders can be found in *BMC Psychiatry* 2014 July 2; 14(Suppl 1): S1 full-text.

British Columbia Medical Services Commission (MSC) guideline on diagnosis and treatment of anxiety and depression in children and youth can be found at *MSC* 2010 January PDF or at *National Guideline Clearinghouse* 2013 May 13: 38904. www2.gov.bc.ca/gov/content/health/practitioner-professional-resources/bc-guidelines/anxiety-and-depression-in-youth

Additional suggested references for pharmacotherapy

Review of new pharmacological management of generalized anxiety disorder can be found in *Expert Opinion in Pharmacotherapy* 2013 February; 14(2): 175.

Review of pharmacological management of generalized anxiety disorder can be found in *BMJ* 2011 March 11; 342: d1199 full-text. Editorial can be found in *BMJ* 2011 Mar 11; 342: d1216. www.apa.org/pi/families/resources/child-medications.pdf

Review of adjunctive use of atypical antipsychotics for treatment-resistant generalized anxiety disorder can be found in *Pharmacotherapy* 2010 September; 30(9): 942.

Review of psychopharmacological, psychosocial, and combined interventions for childhood disorders can be found at *American Psychological Association Working group on Psychotropic Medications for Children and Adolescents* 2006 August PDF.

Additional suggested references for anxiety disorders

Review of diagnosis of anxiety disorders in primary care can be found in *American Family Physician* 2008 August 15; 78(4): 501.

Best Treatments review and commentary can be found in *BMJ* 2003 March 29; 326(7391): 700 full-text, editorial can be found in *BMJ* 2003 March 29; 326(7391): 700.

Review of anxiety in late life can be found in *Annals of Long-Term Care* 2004 August; 12(8): 28.

Review of anxiety disorders in children can be found in *Current Opinions in Pediatrics* 2008 October; 20(5): 538.

Review of treatment of anxiety disorders in children can be found in *Annals of the New York Academy of Sciences*, 2013 November; 1304: 52.

Review of brief intervention for anxiety in primary care patients can be found in *Journal of the American Board of Family Medicine* 2009 March–April; 22(2): 175 full-text.

Review of excessive worry disorders can be found in *American Family Physician* 2006 March 15; 73(6): 1049 full-text.

Review of exercise, yoga, and meditation for depressive and anxiety disorders can be found in *American Family Physician* 2010 April 15; 81(8): 981 full-text.

Review of herbal and dietary supplements for treatment of anxiety disorders can be found in *American Family Physician* 2007 August 15; 76(4): 549 full-text. Commentary can be found in *American Family Physician* 2008 August 15; 78(4): 433.

Review of epidemiology and prognosis of sub-threshold generalized anxiety disorder can be found in *BMC Psychiatry* 2014 May 1; 14: 128 full-text.

Review of non-psychotic mental disorders in perinatal period can be found in *The Lancet* 2014 November 15; 384(9956): 1775.

Review of applied relaxation techniques for generalized anxiety disorder can be found in

Review of treatment-resistant panic disorder can be found in *CNS Spectrum* 2004 October; 9(10): 725.

Case report of panic attacks can be found in *The Lancet* 2014 July 19; 384(9939): 280.

Handouts and other resources for patients and providers

Handout on panic disorder—*National Institute of Mental Health*

Handout on panic disorder —*JAMA Patient Page*

Handout on anxiety and panic—*American Academy of Family Physicians* available in English or in Spanish

Handout on cognitive behavior therapy with contact info for British therapists from *Mind Publications PDF*

Handout on controlled breathing—*Patient UK PDF*

Anxiety and Depression Association of America (ADAA.org)—Free handouts and videos are available

Handout on general anxiety disorder—*American Academy of Family Physicians* available in English and Spanish

Handout on general anxiety disorder—*Mayo Clinic*

Handout on general anxiety disorder—*Patient UK PDF*

Handout on anxiety disorders—*American Psychiatric Association*

Handout on anxiety disorders—*TeensHealth* available in English or in Spanish

Handout on living with anxiety disorders—*National Institute of Health*

The Anxiety and Phobia Workbook by Edmund Bourne, 2005

The Line Between Anxiety and Depression. HealthyPlace.com. www.healthyplace.com/anxiety-panic/articles/line-between-anxiety-and-depression/(accessed July 5; 2012).

References

Abbott, R., & Lavretsky, H. (2013). Tai Chi and Qigong for the treatment and prevention of mental disorders. *Psychiatric Clinics of North America*, 36(1), 109–119.

American Psychiatric Association. (2013). *Diagnostic and Statistical Manual of Mental Disorders* (5th ed.). Washington, DC: American Psychiatric Association.

Baxter, A., Vos, T., Scott, K., Ferrari, A., & Whiteford, H. (2014). The global burden of anxiety disorders in 2010. *Psychological Medicine*, 44, 2363–2374.

Benarroch, E.E. (2009). The locus ceruleus norepinephrine system: functional organization and potential significance. *Neurology*, 73(20), 1699–1704.

Berridge, C.W. (2008). Noradrenergic modulation of arousal. *Brain Research Review*, 58(1), 1–17.

Buoli, M., Caldiroli, A., Caletti, E., Paoli, R.A., & Altamura, A.C. (2013). New approaches to the pharmacological management of generalized anxiety disorder. *Expert Opinion on Pharmacotherapy*, 14(2), 175–184.

Busner, J., & Targum, S.D. (2007). The clinical global impressions scale: applying a research tool in clinical practice. *Psychiatry*, 4(7), 28–37.

Bystritsky, A., Kerwin, L., & Feusner, J.D. (2008). A pilot study of Rhodiola rosea (Rhodax) for generalized anxiety disorder (GAD). *Journal of Alternative and Complementary Medicine*, 14(2), 175–180.

Centers for Disease Control and Prvention (CDC). (2002). Hepatic toxicity possibly associated with kava-containing products—United States, Germany, and Switzerland, 1999–2002. *Morbidity and Mortality Weekly Report*, 51(47), 1065–1067.

Centers for Disease Control (CDC 2011), Reeves, W.C., Strine, T.W., Pratt, W.T., Ahluwalia, I., Dhingra, S.S., McKnight-Fily, L.R., & Safran, M.A. (2011). Mental illness surveillance among adults in the United States. Retrieved May 17, 2016 from www.cdc.gov/mmwr/preview/mmwrhtml/su6003a1.htm.

Centers for Disease Control (CDC). (2013). Burden of mental illness. Retrieved December 6, 2015 from www.cdc.gov/mentalhealth/basics/buden.htm

Cooley, K., Szczurko, O., Perri, D., Mills, E. J., Bernhardt, B., Zhou, Q., Seely, D. (2009). Naturopathic care for anxiety: a randomized controlled trial ISRCTN78958974. *PLoS One*, 4(8), e6628.

Hamilton, M. (1959). The assessment of anxiety states by rating. *British Journal of Medical Psychology*, 32(1), 502–555.

Harrington, H. (2011). The neurobiology of panic attacks and anxiety. Retrieved December 6, 2015 from http://ezinearticles.com/?The-Neurobiology-of-Panic-Attacks-and-Anxiety&id=6070366.

Hayes-Skelton, S.A. & Roemer, L. (2013). A contemporary view of applied relaxation for generalized anxiety disorder. *Cognitive Behavioral Therapy*, 42(4).

Herr, R., Williams, J. W., Benjamin, S., & McDuffie, J. (2014). Does this patient have generalized anxiety or panic disorder? The rational clinical examination system. *Journal of the American Medical Association*, 312(1), 78.

Herrera-Arellano, A., Jiménez-Ferrer, E., Zamilpa, A., Morales-Valdéz, M., García-Valencia, C.E., & Tortoriello J. (2007). Efficacy and tolerability of a standardized herbal product from Galphimia glauca on generalized anxiety disorder: a randomized, double-blind clinical trial controlled with lorazepam. *Planta Medica*, 73(8), 713–717. Epub 2007, June 11.

Hofman, S.G., Asnaani, A., & Hinton, D.E. (2010). Cultural aspects in social anxiety and social anxiety disorder. *Depression and Anxiety*, 27(12), 1117–1127.

Hutchinson, K. (2015). *Psychiatric Mental Health Nursing Review and Resource Manual, 5th Edition*. Silver Springs, MD: American Nurses Association.

Kasper, S., Gastpar, M., Müller, W.E., Volz, H.P., Möller, H.J., Schläfke, S., & Dienel, A. (2014). Lavender oil preparation Silexan is effective in generalized anxiety disorder: a randomized, double-blind comparison to placebo and paroxetine. *International Journal of Neuropsychopharmacology*, 17(6), 859–869.

Katzman, M.A., Bleau, P., Blier, P., Chokka, P., Kjernisted, K., & Van Ameringen, M. (2014). Canadian Anxiety Guidelines Initiative Group on behalf of the Anxiety Disorders Association of Canada/Association Canadienne des troubles anxieux and McGill University. Canadian Clinical practice guidelines for the management of anxiety, posttraumatic stress and obsessive-compulsive disorders. *BMC Psychiatry*, 14, Supplement 1, S1. Doi: 10.1186/1471–244X-14-S1-S1.

Kessler, R.C., Chin, W.T., Merikangas, K.R., Demler, O., & Walters, E.E. (2005a). Prevalence, severity, and comorbidity of 12-month DSM-IV disorders in the National Comorbidity Survey Replication. *Archives of General Psychiatry*, 62, 617–627.

Kessler R.,C., Berglund, P., Demler O., Jin, R., Merikangas K.R., & Walters, E.E. (2005b). Lifetime prevalence and age-of-onset distributions of DSM-IV Disorders in the National Comorbidity Survey replication. *Archives of General Psychiatry*, 62(6), 593–602.

Kessler, R.C., Aguilar-Gaxiola, S., Alonso, J., Chatterji, S., Lee, S., Ormel, J., Ustün, T.B., & Wang, P.S. (2009). The global burden of mental disorders: an update from the WHO World Mental Health (WMH) surveys. *Epidemiologia e Psichiatria Sociale*, 18(1), 23–33.

Knuts, I., Esquivel, G., Kenis, G., Overbeek, T., Leibold, N., Goossens, L., & Schruers, K. (2014). Therapygeneticss: 5-HTTLPR genotype predicts the response to exposure therapy for agoraphobia. *European Neuropsychopharmacology*, 24(8), 1222–1228.

Mathews, J.M., Etheridge, A.S., & Black, S.R. (2002). Inhibition of human cytochrome P450 activities by kava extract and kavalactones. *Drug Metabolism and Disposition* November; 30(11), 1153–1157.

Maxmen, J.S., Ward, N.G., & Kilgus, M. (2009). *Essential Psychopathology and its Treatments* (3rd ed.). New York: Norton.

Mental Health America (2013). *Mental Health Complementary and Alternative Medicine*. Retrieved from www.mentalhealthamerica.net/sites/default/files/MHA_CAM.pdf.

Miyasaka, L.S., Atallah, A.N., & Soares, B.G., (2006). Valerian for anxiety disorders. *Cochrane Database of Systematic Reviews*, October 18; (4), CD004515.

Miyasaka, L.S., Atallah, A.N., & Soares, B.G., (2007). Passiflora for anxiety disorder. *Cochrane Database of Systematic Reviews*, January 24; (1), CD004518.

Mula, M., Pini, S., & Cassano, G. (2007). The role of anticonvulsant drugs in anxiety disorders: a critical review of the evidence. *Journal of Clinical Psychopharmacology*, 27(3), 263–272.

National Institute of Mental Health (NIMH) Genetics Workgroup. (1998). *Genetics and Mental Disorders* (NIH Publication No. 98–4268). Rockville, MD: Author

Ravindran, A.V., & da Silva, T.L. (2013). Complementary and alternative therapies as add-on to pharmacotherapy for mood and anxiety disorders: a systematic review. *Journal of Affective Disorders*, 150(3), 707–719.

Sarris, J., Glick, R., Hoenders, R., Duffy, J., & Lake, J. (2013). Integrative mental health care White Paper: establishing a new paradigm through research, education and clinical guidelines. *Advances in Integrative Medicine*, 1(1), 9–16.

Spitzer, R.L., Kroenke, K., Williams, J.B.W., & Lowe, B. (2006). A brief measure for assessing generalized anxiety disorder. *Archives of Internal Medicine*, 166, 1092–1097.

Somers, J., Goldner, E., Waraich, P., & Hsu, L. (2006). Prevalence and incidence studies of anxiety disorders: a systematic review of the literature. *Candian Journal of Psychiatry*, 1(2), 100–113.

Tiwari, A., Souza, R., & Muller, D. (2009). Pharmacogenetics of anxiolytic drugs. *Journal of Neural Transmission*, 116, 667–677.

Tubaki, B.R., Chandrashekar C.R., Sudhakar, D., Prabha, T.N., Lavekar, GS., & Kutty, B.M. (2012). Clinical efficacy of Manasamitra Vataka (an Ayurveda medication) on generalized anxiety disorder with comorbid generalized social phobia: a randomized controlled study. *Journal of Alternative and Complementary Medicine*, 18(6), 612–621.

Tyrer, P., & Baldwin, D. (2006). Generalised anxiety disorder. *The Lancet*, 368(9553), 2156–2166.

US Food and Drug Administration. (2001). *MedWatch: Safety – Kava (Piper Methysticum)*. Retrieved May 17, 2016 from www.fda.gov/Safety/MedWatch/SafetyInformation/SafetyAlertsforHumanMedical Products/ucm172818.htm.

US Food and Drug Administration. (2002). *MedWatch: Consumer Advisory – Kava Containing Dietary Supplements may be Associated with Severe Liver Injury*. Retrieved May 17, 2016 from www.fda.gov/food/recallsoutbreaksemergencies/safetyalertsadvisories/ucm085482.htm.

Watson, J.B., & Raynor, R. (1920). Conditioned emotional reactions. *Journal of Experimental Psychology*, 3(1), 1–14.

Weisberg, R.B. (2009). Overview of generalized anxiety disorder: epidemiology, presentation, and course. *Journal of Clinical Psychiatry*, 70, Supplement 2, 4–9.

Wittman, A., Schlagenhauf, F., John, T., Guhn, A., Rehbein, H., Siegmund, F., Stoy, M., Held, D., Schulz, I., Fehm, L., Fydrich, T., Heinz, A., Bruhn, H., & Strohle, A. (2011). A new paradigm (Westphal paradigm) to study the neural correlates of panic disorder with agoraphobia. *European Archives of Psychiatry and Clinical Neuroscience*, 261(3), 185–194.

Wittman, A., Schlagenhauf, F., Guhn, A., Leuken, U., Gaehlsdorf, C., Stoy, M., Bermpohl, F., Fydrich, T., Pfleiderer, B., Bruhn, H., Gerlach, A.L., Kircher, T., Straube, B., Wittchen, H.U., Arolt, V., Heinz, A., & Strohle, A. (2014). Anticipating agoraphobic situations: the neural correlates of panic disorder with Agoraphobia. *Psychological Medicine*, 44, 2385–2396.

World Health Organization. (n.d.). *Gender and Women's Mental Health: Gender Disparities and Mental Health: The Facts.* Retrieved May 16, 2016 from World Health Organization www.who.int/mental_health/prevention/genderwomen/en/.

World Health Organization (1992). *The ICD-10 Classification of Mental and Behavioural Disorder: Clinical Descriptions and Diagnostic Guidelines.* Geneva: World Health Organization.

World Health Organization. (2015). *External Review of ICD-11 Revision Report.* Retrieved May 17, 2016 from www.who.int/classifications/icd/externalreview/en/.

World Health Organization World Mental Health Survey Consortium. (2007). Lifetime prevalence and age-of-onset distribution of mental disorders in the World Health Organization's World Mental Health Survey Initiative. *World Psychiatry*, 6, 168–176.

Zung, W.W.K. (1971). A rating instrument for anxiety disorders. *Psychometrics*, 12, 371–379.

12

SUICIDE AND OTHER DELIBERATE SELF-HARM BEHAVIORS

Promoting prevention

Edilma L. Yearwood

Introduction

Suicide, referred to as a preventable public health crisis, is responsible for between 850,000–1,0000,00 deaths worldwide annually (Hawton & van Heeringen, 2009; WHO, 2014). These rates are likely an underestimation due to religious taboos about suicide, cultures that consider suicide illegal or a criminal offense, variability across countries as to who conducts the examination, how the death is classified and potential assigning of the death to the category of mortality due to injury rather than suicide (Fisher, Herman, de Mello, & Chandra, 2014; Hawton & van Heeringen, 2009). While suicide is the tenth leading cause of overall deaths, it is frequently cited as the second or third cause of death among adolescents and young adults ages 15–29 (Phillips & Cheng, 2012; WHO, 2014), and has consistently been a driver of deaths in older adults over the age of 70, with rates higher in low- and middle-income countries, rural areas, the unemployed and those with a psychiatric disorder (Carlson & Ong, 2014; Hawton & van Heeringen, 2009; WHO, 2014). When mental, neurological, and substance use burden was added to the 2010 Global Burden of Disease estimates, the burden associated with suicide from these disorders shifted the mental health GBD from fifth to third worldwide (Ferrari *et al.*, 2014). Completed suicides are higher in men when compared to women, primarily due to the use of high lethal methods including firearms, hanging, jumping, and pesticide poisoning (Phillips & Cheng, 2012; Schlebusch, n.d.). Risk factors have been associated with disorders of mood, substance use, schizophrenia, prior attempt, chronic stress, and living in poorly resourced, crowded, and violent environments. Highest suicide rates are found in Asia (China, South Korea, Sri Lanka, India, and Russia), Africa (South Africa, Mozambique, and Tanzania), and Europe (Lithuania, Latvia, Finland) with lowest rates found in Greece, Islamic countries (Saudi Arabia, Kuwait, Oman), Mexico, Spain, and Caribbean countries such as Barbados and Jamaica (Hawton & van Heeringen, 2009; WHO, 2012). For every completed suicide, it is estimated that there are 10 or more unsuccessful attempts, making suicide a daunting and pervasive societal issue. Therefore, universal screening for self-harm intent is a recommended prevention activity that should be incorporated in all health care visits and taught to non-specialist health workers who provide community-based interventions. Of note, risky behaviors such as reckless driving that results in death may actually be an intended suicide that was classified as an injury-related automobile accident in the absence of definitive suicide evidence, such as a note. Additional hazardous behaviors involving unprotected sex, polysubstance use, certain eating disorders, and frequent risk-taking actions can be viewed as self-harm behaviors with high potential for death.

This chapter will examine the global trends in non-suicidal self injury (NSSI) and suicide, describe etiological theories associated with self injuring behaviors, identify risk-factors for self-harm, present evidence-based global prevention and treatment interventions, and describe the role nurses can take when treating individuals at-risk for or post-engagement in self injuring behaviors across all income global communities. The term NSSI is used interchangeably with self-harm and self-injurious behaviors.

Non-suicidal self-injury (NSSI)

NSSI has been defined as deliberate self-inflicted injury to body tissue where there is no overt suicidal intent and the action is not socially sanctioned (such as in body piercing and tattooing behaviors) (Favazza, 1998, 2009; Klonsky, 2007; Muelhenkamp *et al.*, 2012). Types of NSSI include head banging, cutting, burning, skin picking, self-biting and embedding of objects either under the skin or internally through swallowing. Extreme acts of NSSI can result in infections, mutilation, scarring or functional loss of the affected part.

Self-initiated NSSI behaviors can be found in individuals across the lifespan and is addressed in the *Diagnostic and Statistical Manual of Psychiatric Disorders* (DSM-5) (APA, 2013) as one of the conditions needing additional research for possible inclusion as a stand-alone disorder in the next iteration of the DSM. NSSI criterion includes frequency of occurrence, reason for engaging in the activity, and associated feelings. Previously, NSSI had primarily been associated with border-line personality disorder and characterized as impulsive reactivity to overwhelming emotions. However, NSSI is now understood to be a mechanism that is sometimes used for affect regulation to help the individual manage overwhelming emotions, relieve negative thoughts and solve inter-personal problems. The individual may have frequent urges to self-harm, can be preoccupied with the act, and may see no other plausible action to take to relieve the flood of emotions experienced. Other reasons offered for engaging in NSSI include self-punishment, to prevent initiation of a dissociative episode, to prevent suicide, to influence others, to experience a particular sensation, to avoid a consequence or reactive to bullying (van Geel, Goemans, & Vedder, 2015).

Two self-report tools used to assess NSSI are the Inventory of Statements About Self-Injury (ISAS) (Klonsky, 2007), and the Functional Assessment of Self-Injury (FASM) (Lloyd, Kelley, & Hope, 1997; Nock & Prinstein, 2004). A comparison of both tools is found in Table 12.1. The tools reflect a variety of factors typically associated with NSSI behaviors with completion of the self-report indicating that there are usually multiple reasons leading to the self-harm sequence. When tested in a clinical sample of adolescents and adults, the intrapersonal elements of NSSI (i.e. affect regulation, distress relief, or self-punishment) are more strongly associated with clinical severity than the social elements (i.e. to fit in or gain attention from others) (Klonsky, Glenn, Styer, Olino, & Washburn, 2015).

Deliberate self-harm behaviors can be viewed as existing on a trajectory, illustrated below from non-fatal intent to fatal intent. Engaging in the behavior may result in feelings ranging from need to self-punish via the experience of pain, to attempts to trigger a feeling state in the absence of feelings, to self-regulation, to adrenalin surge excitation, or ultimately, to death.

Table 12.1 A comparison of ISAS and FASM self-report tools

	Inventory of Statements About Self-Injury (ISAS)	Functional Assessment of Self-Mutilation (FASM)
Number of items on the measure	39	22
Sample of precipitating factors for NSSI behavior	Affect regulation Distress Peer bonding/solidarity Toughness Achieve interpersonal influence (attention) Prevent dissociation and suicide Form of self-punishment	Relieves numbness Attention-seeking Avoid unpleasant actions, punishment, or being with others To feel (even if it's pain) Self-punishment To prompt an action/reaction in others To stop bad feelings To be part of a group (fit in) To feel relaxed (after self-harm)

Source: Adapted from Klonsky *et al.*, 2015.

Non-suicidal self injury (no suicide intent) → Risky behaviors (ambivalent outcomes) → Suicide (intent)

Cultural rituals causing body injury, on the other hand, are formal activities usually conducted by adults usually on children, and passed from generation to generation. The subsequent body modification serves to endorse beliefs or traditions viewed as valuable to the culture (Favazza, 2009). These activities can include female genital mutilation, branding, scarring, or other types of physical alteration. While these actions do not involve intent to kill, the psychological consequences especially to children can be significant and long-standing.

Treatment of non-suicidal self-harm

The health care provider should approach individuals who engage in suicidal and non-suicidal self-harm behaviors with empathy and support rather than rejection, anger, or disappointment. Individuals who engage in these behaviors are frequently experiencing isolation, rejection, and possibly discrimination and bias, and do not need to be re-traumatized or admonished for their behavior by the health care provider.

There are several effective pharmacological and non-pharmacological interventions used to treat non-suicidal self-injuring behaviors. Pharmacological interventions include antidepressants such as fluoxetine (Prozac), which targets effective regulation of the serotonergic system, atypical antipsychotics such as ziprasidone (Geodon) and aripiprazole (Abilify), which target the neurotransmitter dopamine, or the opioid antagonist naltrexone (ReVia) that regulates the opioid system. Non-pharmacological interventions that are effective focus on emotion regulation skills through short-term and focused group therapy, dialectic behavioral therapy, or manual assisted cognitive behavioral therapy (Turner, Austin, & Chapman, 2014).

Suicide risk and protective factors

Suicide, an unnatural cause of death, is defined as an act of self-harm with the intent of dying. Additional terminology associated with the range of related behaviors include suicidal ideation, plan, threat, and attempt. Suicidal ideation refers to thoughts of engaging in behavior(s) intended to end one's life (thinking about what it would be like to die). Suicidal plan is having a specific idea of actions (method) to take to end one's life (thinking about killing oneself by jumping from a specific bridge). Suicidal threat is an overt or covert communication forecasting a desire to self-harm with the intent of killing oneself (a teen impulsively stating, "I'm going to kill myself if I don't get to go to the party"). Lastly, suicidal attempt is engaging in a specific self-harm action with clear intent to die (ingesting a lethal dose of tricyclic antidepressants combined with alcohol) (Schlebusch, n.d.).

Risk factors for suicide are experiences, vulnerabilities, or characteristics that put someone at risk for engaging in self-harm with the intent to end their life. Protective factors, on the other hand, are elements that serve to buffer the individual from engaging in intentional actions aimed at ending their life. Table 12.2 contains specific risk and protective factors for suicide.

While suicide prevention is not guaranteed, there are behaviors that the suicidal individual, who may be ambivalent, exhibits and which should not be ignored but further assessed. Talking with someone who is suicidal will not provoke a suicidal gesture. It will, however, indicate

Table 12.2 Specific risk and protective factors for suicide

Risk factors	Protective factors
Depression	Sense of social integration/connection
Substance use disorder	Strong religious or spiritual grounding
Schizophrenia	Sense of attachment
Bipolar disorder	Sense of purpose and worth
★Age (adolescents and older adults)	Access to care and treatment
★Gender (males more successful)	Good coping and problem-solving skills
Family history	Lack of access to means to commit suicide
★Previous attempt	Moral objection to suicide/self-harm
★Impulsivity	Employment
★Having access to means	Social support
Isolation	
Unemployment	
Illness	
Poor or no access to treatment	
Victim of bullying or stigma	
Sense of hopelessness	
History of trauma (including child maltreatment and domestic violence)	
Significant loss (people, relationships, things, self-worth)	
Living in chronically violent and conflict-ridden environments	
Personality disorders characterized by poor emotion regulation	
Chronic stress	

Note: ★ Indicates significant factors

Source: Adapted from CDC, (n.d.); National Suicide Prevention Lifeline. (n.d.); Nock, *et al.* (2008).

Table 12.3 Warning signs of possible impending suicidal intent

---

Extreme mood swings or significant changes in personality
Changes in eating and sleeping habits (such as sleeping too little or all the time)
A heightened fixation with death or violence
Expressing feelings of hopelessness or no reason to live
Engaging in self-destructive or risky behavior
Withdrawal from loved ones, friends, and community (isolating behaviors)
Announcing a plan to kill one's self
Talking about or writing about hurting one's self, wanting to die or kill oneself
Giving away prized possessions
Obtaining a weapon or some other means of hurting oneself
Increased use of alcohol or drugs
Telling people he or she is "going away"
Loss of interest in things one used to care about
Being a victim of bullying, sexual abuse, violence
For youth, a sudden worsening of school performance
For youth, indications that the teen is in some form of an abusive relationship
Verbalized disappointment or anger with God/religious/spiritual object of worship
Putting affairs in order
Saying goodbyes to friends and loved ones
Taking significant risks that could result in death
Making comments such as:
  "I wish I were dead."
  "Things will be better soon."
  "You would be better off without me."
  "What's the point of living?"
  "What's my purpose?"
  "Soon you won't have to worry about me."
  "Who cares if I'm dead, anyway?"

Source: Adapted from: National Institute of Mental Health (NIMH) (n.d.); The Samaritans (n.d.).

caring and concern, and provide the individual with a sense that they are not alone. Behavioral cues that someone may be contemplating suicide are found in Table 12.3.

Etiology of suicide

Neurobiological

Suicidal behaviors are complex and usually involve factors across neurobiological, psychological, and social categories. Family history and therefore genetic vulnerability, and exposure to self-harm behavior in formative developmental years are risk factors for suicide in youth and adults. The experience of chronic stress can also be a co-morbid or stand-alone catalyst for a suicide gesture.

Postmortem studies of brain and tissue samples after successful suicides point to low levels of the neurotransmitter serotonin in the pre-frontal cortex, impaired serotonin neurotransmitter system and an increase in pro-inflammatory cytokine markers (Courtet *et al.*, 2015; van Heeringer & Mann, 2014). Associated symptoms include mood lability, pessimism, over-reactivity, depressive symptoms, and suicidal behaviors.

Psychological

Psychological factors pose risk to overall well-being and can contribute to suicidal ideation, intent, and attempts. Psychological features refer to having psychiatric symptoms with a possible DSM-5 or ICD-10 diagnosis, or traumatic experiences that contribute to psychological vulnerabilities. Mood dysregulation disorders (depression, hypomania, and mania) are considered the most significant group of disorders associated with suicidal behaviors. Other contributing psychiatric conditions include anxiety disorders, schizophrenia, and substance use. Associated traumatic experiences can include childhood sexual or physical abuse, family dysfunction, bullying, and exposure to chronic environmental violence such as war.

Social

Social contributors to suicidal behavior include engagement in mass or cluster suicide as a group phenomenon, mimicking the suicidal act of someone who is idealized, or adhering to an external or internal directive to commit suicide. More recently, access to social messaging urging involvement in and providing instructions on self-harm can be found, and is easily accessible to young, impressionable, and vulnerable individuals.

Age

Suicide in adolescence and young adults, ages 15–29 has consistently been the second or third cause of death in this age group (McLoughlin, Gould, & Malone, 2015; WHO, 2014). Data examined from 81 countries in 10–14-year-olds shows a higher rate of completed suicides in boys as compared to girls; however, in the last two decades, the rate in girls is increasing (Kolves & DeLeo, 2014). In addition, suicide in adults over the age of 70 remains a significant global concern impacting all world regions and all socio-economic groups (WHO, 2014).

Sexual orientation in sexual minorities

Members of the LGBTQ community are also at-risk for engaging in fatal and non-fatal self-harm behaviors. Risk factors in this group include "coming out" or disclosing, age (adolescents are at higher risk), bullying victimization, self-stigma/self-hatred, confusion, lack of social support, impulsivity, discrimination, gender nonconformity, substance use, sensation seeking, and poor mental health status. Protective factors include social support from trusted family members and significant adults such as teachers or coaches, peer acceptance, self-acceptance, and high self-esteem (GLEN, 2015; King *et al.*, 2008; Liu & Mustanski, 2012; Skerret, Kolves, & DeLeo, 2012).

WHO regional data

In 2012, WHO provided a summary by world region of their suicide profile data.

In the African region, the suicide rates increased nearly 40 percent between 2000 and 2012, however, given the extreme poverty in some African countries and difficulty around collecting accurate data, these estimates may be informed by poor or missing data. In addition, high un-employment, poor literacy, compromised food sources as a result of frequent drought, and lack of water have all been implicated in a view that life is not worth living (*tedium vitae*) and contribute to risk for suicide (Jenkins *et al.*, 2015). Additional studies indicate that personal characteristics including interpersonal difficulties, mental ill health, substance use disorders, and poverty also contributed significantly to risk for suicide (Botha, 2012; Mars, Burrows, Hjelmeland, & Gunnell, 2014). In the *region of the Americas*, the country with the highest global suicide rate is Guyana. However, the region in which Guyana is found has the lowest overall global rate. Youth and elderly males have the highest prevalence rate and high lethal methods of hanging and firearms are used frequently. In the *Eastern Mediterranean region*, young women, women over age 60 and men between 15 and 29 years of age constitute those at high risk for fatal self-harm. The *European region* has 6 of the top 20 countries with the highest global suicide rates and has developed evidence-based suicide prevention strategies in response to this public health concern. The *Southeast Asian region* has a high suicide rate with India identified as the country with the highest rate in the region (Jordan *et al.*, 2014). The most frequent method used is pesticide poisoning (Joshi, Guggilla, Praveen, & Maulik, 2015) with significant success rates in youth and the elderly. Lastly, the suicide rate in the *Western Pacific region* of the world is high in the elderly with Korea and China contributing significantly to the overall high regional rate (Dong, Chang, Zeng, & Simon, 2015). In this region, deaths in females are higher when compared to males, the only place globally where this demographic exists (WHO, 2012). One fifth of all suicides world-wide are in older Chinese individuals, with rates higher than other racial groups in the United States and higher than the general population in China. In older Chinese living outside of China, contributing factors include cultural and linguistic barriers, isolation, and decreased acculturation. Other associated factors include living in rural areas, being female, experiencing depressive symptoms, previous attempts, negative life events, perceiving oneself as being a burden, and medical complications. Protective factors include living with children, high involvement in community, and activities of daily living and social support (Dong *et al.*, 2015).

Methods

Suicide methods are categorized as high and low lethality. High lethal methods are those that have a high probability of success and include use of firearms to strategic areas of the body (head, chest), hanging, jumping, drowning, and suffocation. Lower lethality methods, or those with lower probability of success, include taking a limited number of pills, superficial cutting, piercing, and poisoning (Huang, Wu, Chen, & Wang, 2014). Intentional pesticide poisoning as a method is gaining popularity in low- and middle-income countries particularly in females because of its ready availability in agricultural societies and overall effectiveness (Banerjee, Chowdhury, Schelling, & Weis, 2013; Gunnell, Phillips, & Konradeson, 2007).

Reducing ready access to pesticides, proper and safe storage strategies, and available quality treatment post ingestion have been identified as case fatality prevention methods (Gunnell *et al.*, 2007).

Suicide screening

All health care providers and non-specialist community workers globally should be trained and prepared to screen for self-harm ideation and behaviors, and be prepared to provide initial management when a screen is positive. All formal and informal medical and psychiatric assessments should include questions about potential self-harm ideation and practices and should be asked of all children, adolescents, adults and older adults routinely, and whenever there are behavioral cues warranting follow-up. Direct questions such as, "Have you ever (or recently) thought about hurting or killing yourself?" should be asked. Indirect/non-specific questions about self-harm should be avoided. Screening tools such as the Columbia-Suicide

Severity Rating Scale (C-SSRS), which is a 6-item screen, the Ask-Suicide-Screening Questions (ASQ), a 7-item screen and the Nursing Best Practice Guidelines from the Registered Nurses' Association of Ontario (2009) are easy to administer. While these tools provide more structure to the assessment, it is important to pay close attention to the specific verbal and non-verbal behaviors of the potentially suicidal individual and gear the assessment process to their specific unique presentation.

The National Institute of Mental Health *ASQ* includes seven questions:

1 In the past few weeks, have you wished you were dead?
2 In the past few weeks, have you felt that you or your family would be better off if you were dead?
3 In the past week, have you been having thoughts about killing yourself?
4 Have you ever tried to kill yourself?
5 If yes, how (assessment of lethality)
6 When?
7 If there is a positive response to questions 1–6, ask if the individual is currently having thoughts about killing himself/herself.

(ASQ n.d.)

Additional interview questions for assessment of suicidal ideation and plan

A general question about the person's thoughts and feelings about living is frequently a recommended way to begin the assessment. Questions can include (modified from RNAO 2008; 2009):

• Sometimes people feel that life is not worth living. Can you tell me how you feel about your own life?
• What are some of the aspects of your life that make it worth living?
• Do you find yourself wishing for a permanent escape from life?
• How would that happen for you?
• Do you ever think about your own death or about dying?
• Have you ever thought of harming yourself or trying to take your own life?
• Do you think or feel this way presently?

If the person expresses thoughts of self-harm, and/or suicide, or even if he/she seems ambivalent, continue with these questions:

• When did you begin to experience these thoughts and feelings?
• How frequently have you had these thoughts and feelings?
• Can you stop yourself from having them by distracting yourself with an activity or other more positive thoughts?
• Have you ever acted upon these thoughts?
• What might help you from acting on them?
• If you did take your own life, what do you imagine would happen after you die to those people who are important to you?
• Do you have a plan to harm yourself or take your own life? If so, describe your plan.
• Do you have those methods available to you to take your life, such as over-the-counter pills, prescription pills, knives or proximity to a balcony, bridge or subway?

If a person has attempted suicide or engaged in self-harm behavior(s), ask additional questions to assess circumstances surrounding the event(s):

- What happened in your previous attempts to self-harm or take your life? What led up to it? Were you using alcohol or other substances? What method did you use? Sometimes people have many reasons for harming themselves in addition to wanting to die. What might have been some of your reasons for self-harm or suicide? How severe were your injuries?
- What were your thoughts just before you harmed yourself?
- What did you anticipate would be the outcome of your self-harm or suicide attempt? Did you think you would die? What did you think would be the response of others to your self-harm or suicide?
- How did you feel after your attempt? Did you feel relief or regret at being alive?
- Did you receive treatment after your attempt?

For individuals with repeated suicidal thoughts or attempts, these additional questions can be asked:

- How many times have you tried to harm yourself, or tried to take your life?
- When was the most recent time?
- What were your thoughts and feelings at the time that you were most serious about suicide?
- When was your most serious attempt at harming or taking your life?
- What happened just before you did this, and what happened after?

It would also be important to assess reasons for living or protective factors involved such as

- How do you feel about your own future?
- What would help you to feel or think more positively, optimistically or hopefully about your future?
- What would make it more (or less) likely that you would try to take your own life?
- If you began to have thoughts of harming or killing yourself again, what would you do to prevent them?

Evidence-based prevention strategies

Effective prevention of suicide involves a comprehensive approach with involvement of multiple stakeholders across different community environments. To begin with, there has to be a national suicide prevention strategy that establishes basic policies for all. According to the WHO, there are only 28 countries globally that have a national strategy. Essential components should include a plan for surveillance, attention to means restriction, healthy, clear and informative messages from the media, a stigma reduction and public awareness plan, training for health workers, police, educators and other key stakeholders, crisis hotline and intervention supports, treatment services, support for families and friends after a completed suicide, and resources to support all levels of prevention (Hoven, Wasserman, Wasserman, & Mandell, 2009; WHO, 2014). On the practice/intervention side, training health care and non-specialist community workers about suicide risk and management, screening and treatment; pharmacotherapy; self-help groups; use of treatment versus jail after a non-fatal suicidal gesture and scaling up of successful treatment approaches is recommended (Mann *et al.*, 2005). The use of brief intervention and

Table 12.4 Recommendations for nurses from assessment and care of adults at risk for suicidal ideation and behavior

Practice recommendation	Type of evidence
1 The nurse will take seriously all statements made by the client that indicate, directly or indirectly, a wish to die by suicide, and/or all available information that indicates a risk for suicide	III
2 The nurse works toward establishing a therapeutic relationship with clients at risk for suicidal ideation and behaviour	IV
3 The nurse works with the client to minimize the feelings of shame, guilt and stigma that may be associated with suicidality, mental illness, and addictions	III
4 The nurse provides care in keeping with the principles of cultural safety/cultural competence	III
5 The nurse assesses and manages factors that may impact the physical safety of both the client and the interdisciplinary team	IV
6 a) The nurse recognizes key indicators that put an individual at risk for suicidal behaviour, even in the absence of expressed suicidality. For individuals who exhibit risk indicators, the nurse conducts and documents an assessment of suicidal ideation and plan.	IV
b) The nurse assesses for protective factors associated with suicide prevention	IV
c) The nurse obtains collateral information from all available sources: family, friends, community supports, medical records and mental health professionals	
7 The nurse mobilizes resources based upon the client's assessed level of suicide risk and associated needs	IV
8 The nurse ensures that observation and therapeutic engagement reflects the client's changing suicide risk	IV
9 The nurse works collaboratively with the client to understand his/her perspective and meet his/her needs	IV
10 The nurse uses a mutual (client nurse) problem-solving approach to facilitate the client's understanding of how they perceive his/her own problems and generate solutions	IV
11 The nurse fosters hope with the suicidal client	IV
12 The nurse is aware of current treatments to provide advocacy, referral, monitoring, and health teaching interventions, as appropriate	IV
13 a) The nurse identifies persons affected by suicide that may benefit from resources and supports, and refers as required	IV
b) The nurse may initiate and participate in a debriefing process with other health care team members as per organizational protocol	
14 The nurse seeks support through clinical supervision when working with adults at risk for suicidal ideation and behaviour to become aware of the emotional impact to the nurse and enhance clinical practice	IV

Source: Reprinted with permission from *Assessment and Care of Adults at Risk for Suicidal Ideation and Behaviours Practice Guidelines*, Registered Nurses' Association of Ontario (2008).

supportive contact (BIC) after a suicide gesture has been shown to be supportive, cost effective, and requires less training than other forms of therapies like cognitive behavioral or interpersonal therapy (Fleischmann *et al.*, 2008).

Because of the complexity surrounding suicide, additional research is needed across the lifespan and in all income countries. With global suicide rates continuing to rise, there is a need to uncover additional strategies to treat this troubling phenomenon. Country- and culture-specific data on self-harm and suicide will assist with development of best practices that can then be scaled up to meet existing local needs. The National Action Alliance for Suicide Prevention of the National Institute of Mental Health in the United States developed a suicide research prioritization plan that identifies the six key areas of research that are needed along with aspirational goals associated with each question. These questions include: 1) Why do people become suicidal? 2) How can we more optimally detect and predict risk? 3) What interventions prevent individuals from engaging in suicidal behavior? 4) What services are most effective for treating the suicidal person and preventing suicidal behaviors? 5) What other types of prevention interventions (external to the health care setting) reduce suicidal risk? and 6) What new and existing research infrastructure is needed to reduce suicidal behavior? (National Action Alliance for Suicide Prevention, 2014).

Figure 12.1. depicts suicide risk factors and universal, selective, and indicated prevention interventions to address risks (WHO, 2014). Universal strategies focus on providing an intervention that is applied to all. Examples include public awareness campaigns and providing health education to all, such as all third graders throughout a school system. Selective strategies target at-risk groups or individuals within the population and include actions such as screening, targeted support, crisis supports, and training key individuals. Indicated strategies are provided to high-risk individuals and include situation-specific coping strategies (skill building), treatment, and case management (Nordentoft, 2011).

Roles for nurses in suicide prevention

As trusted health care providers operating in hospitals, primary care, community treatment services, and in schools, among other sites, nurses globally have a unique opportunity to work within the three levels of prevention categories to positively impact the public health crisis surrounding self-harm and suicide. As part of the nursing process, nurses are particularly skilled at assessment, developing and implementing a plan of care, and working to ensure patient safety. All nurses must intentionally include self-harm and suicide assessment questions in their routine nursing assessment tools. In addition, we must increase awareness in the public about the suicide epidemic, provide information about risk factors for self-harm, and teach skills to assist vulnerable individuals to appropriately manage their emotional states. As a protective factor for suicide is social support and a sense of worth/purpose, nurses can work with schools, families, and community stakeholders to help establish and facilitate healthy and positive relationships/connections between the self-harming individual and caring community resources (people and places). Nurses can also develop and conduct supportive groups centered on prevention, treatment, and skill building. Lastly, as has been mentioned, nurses can and should conduct research at local levels, using a variety of methodologies to arrive at culture-specific strategies to help reduce self-harm behaviors in all age groups. In addition, nurses can and should vigorously engage in suicide prevention policy development and enforcement, assess and advocate for resources to implement interventions, recommend strategies to support access for all, and actions to increase public awareness.

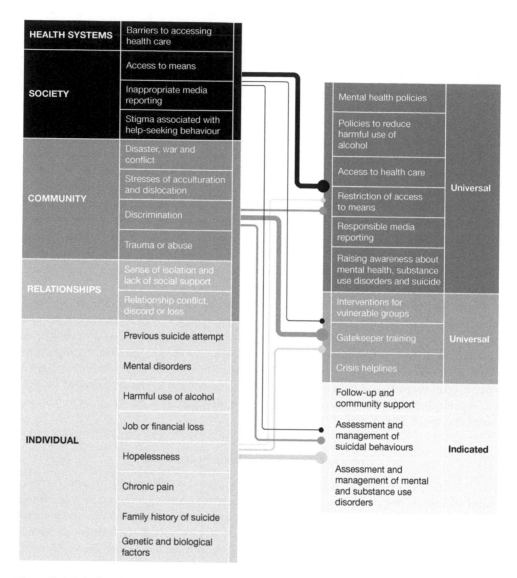

Figure 12.1 Suicide risk factors and associated universal, selective, and intended prevention strategies

Source: Image from World Health Organization (2014). Preventing suicide: A global imperative. Geneva, Switzerland http://apps.who.int/iris/handle/10665/131056.

Conclusion

Self-harm behaviors, including suicide, are a significant public health crisis in all six WHO global regions and impact all age groups. While prevalence rates are highest in adolescence and young adults, ages 15–29 and in older adults over the age of 70, the effect of global burden of disease, on families and communities, along with the sobering loss of nearly one million individuals yearly cannot be underestimated. All health care providers, including nurses, are in a unique position to identify at-risk individuals early through use of universal screening and to provide support, treatment, and referral as needed to prevent self-harm and suicidal behaviors from resulting in a fatality. Activities that reduce stigma associated with self-harm, that increase public awareness and knowledge of factors contributing to suicide, and the availability of policies and resources to reduce suicide risk and offer treatment are needed across all countries, socioeconomic levels and age groups. In addition, basic mental health education of all health care providers and non-specialist community workers must be incorporated into prevention policies across all countries with stipulations that care providers must participate in periodic skills renewal focused on self-harm assessment and suicide prevention management strategies informed by the latest evidence in this area.

References

American Psychiatric Association (APA). (2013). *Diagnostic and statistical manual of psychiatric disorders*, 5th ed. Arlington, VA: American Psychiatric Association.

Ask Suicide-Screening Questions (ASQ). (n.d.) Available at www.nimh.nih.gov/news/science-news/ask-suicide-screening-asq.shtml (accessed May 17, 2016).

Banerjee, S., Chowdhury, A., Schelling, E., & Weis, M. (2013). Household survey of pesticide practice, deliberate self-harm, and suicide in the Sundardan region of West Bengal, India. *BioMed Research International, 2013*. Available at http://dx.doi.org/10.1155/2013/949076 (accessed May 24, 2016).

Botha, F. (2012). The economics of suicide in South Africa. *South African Journal of Economics, 80*(4), 526–552.

Carlson, W.L., & Ong, T.D. (2014). Suicide in later life: Failed treatment or rational choice? *Clinical Geriatric Medicine, 30*(3), 553–576.

Centers for Disease Control (CDC). (n.d.). Suicide: Risk and protective factors. Available at www.cdc.gov/violenceprevention/suicide/riskprotectivefactors.html (accessed May 24, 2016).

Courtet, P., Giner, L., Seneque, M., Guillaume, S., Olie, E., & Ducasse, D. (2015). Neuroinflammation in suicide: Toward a comprehensive model. *World Journal of Biological Psychiatry, 30*, 1–23.

Dong, X., Chang, E.S., Zeng, P., & Simon, M. (2015). Suicide in the global Chinese aging population: A review of risk and protective factors, consequences, and interventions. *Aging and Disease, 6*(2), 121–130.

Favazza, A. (1998). The coming of age of self-mutilation. *Journal of Nervous & Mental Disease, 186*(5), 259–268.

Favazza, A. (2009). A cultural understanding of nonsuicidal self-injury. In M. Nock (Ed.). *Understanding nonsuicidal self-injury*. Washington, DC: American Psychological Association, pp. 19–35.

Ferrari, A., Norman, R., Freedman, G., Baxter, A., Pirkis, J., Harris, M., Page, A., Carnaham, E., Degenhardt, L., Vos, T., & Whiteford, H. (2014). The burden attributable to mental and substance use disorders as risk factors for suicide: Findings from the global burden of disease study 2010. *PLOSOne, 9*(4), e91936.

Fisher, J., Herrman, H., de Mello, M., & Chandra, P. (2014). Women's mental health. In V. Patel, H. Minas, A. Cohen, & M. Prince. *Global Mental Health*. New York: Oxford University Press, pp. 354–383.

Fleischmann, A., Bertolote, J., Wasserman, D., De Leo, D., Bolhari, J., Botega, N., Page, A., Carnahan, E., Degenhardt, L., Vos, T., & Thanh, H. (2008). Effectiveness of brief intervention and contact for suicide attempters: A randomized controlled trial in five countries. *Bulletin of the World Health Organization, 86*(9), 703–709.

Gay and Lesbian Equality Network (GLEN). (2015). LGBT self-harm & suicidality: An overview of national & international research findings. Available at www.glen.ie/mentalhealth (accessed May 24, 2016).

Gunnell, D., Eddleston, M., Phillips, M., & Konradsen, F. (2007). The global distribution of fatal pesticide self-poisoning: Systematic review. *BMC Public Health, 7*, 357.

Hawton, K., & van Heeringen, K. (2009). Suicide. *The Lancet, 373*, 1372–1381.

Hoven, C., Wasserman, D., Wasserman, C., & Mandell, D. (2009). Awareness in nine countries: A public health approach to suicide prevention. *Legal Medicine, 11*, S13–S17.

Huang, J.C., Wu, Y.W., Chen, C.K., & Wang, L.J. (2014). Methods of suicide predict the risks and method switching of subsequent suicide attempts: A community cohort study in Taiwan. *Neuropsychiatric Disease and Treatment, 10*, 711–718.

Jenkins, R., Othieno, C., Omollo, R., Ongeri, L., Sifuna, P., Ongecha, M., & Ogutu, B. (2015). Tedium vitae, death wishes, suicidal ideation and attempts in Kenya: Prevalence and risk factors. *BMC Public Health, 15*, 759.

Jordan, M., Kaufman, A., Brenman, N., Adhikari, R., Luitel, N., Tol, W., & Komproe, I. (2014). Suicide in South Asia: A scoping review. *BMC Psychiatry*, *14*, 358.

Joshi, R., Guggilla, R., Praveen, D., & Maulik, P. (2015). Suicide deaths in rural Andhra Pradesh: A cause for global health action. *Tropical Medicine and International Health*, *20*(2), 188–193.

King, M., Semlyen, J., Tai, S., Killaspy, H., Osborn, D., Popelyuk, D., & Nazareth, I. (2008). A systematic review of mental disorder, suicide, and deliberate self harm in lesbian, gay and bisexual people. *BMC Psychiatry*, *8*, 70.

Klonsky, E.D. (2007). The functions of deliberate self-injury: A review of the evidence. *Clinical Psychology Review*, *27*, 226–239.

Klonsky, E.D, Glenn, C.R., Styer, D.M., Olino, T.M., & Washburn, J.J. (2015). The functions of nonsuicidal self-injury: Converging evidence for a two-factor structure. *Child and Adolescent Psychiatry and Mental Health*, *9*, 44.

Kolves, K. & DeLeo, D. (2014). Suicide rates in children aged 10–14 years worldwide: Changes in the past two decades. *British Journal of Psychiatry*, *205*, 283–285.

Liu, R. & Mustanski, B. (2012). Suicidal ideation and self-harm in lesbian, gay, bisexual, and transgender youth. *American Journal of Preventive Medicine*, *42*(3), 221–228.

Lloyd, E., Kelley, M., & Hope, T. (1997). Self mutilation in a community sample of adolescents: Descriptive characteristics and provisional prevalence rates. Poster presentation at the Society for Behavioral Medicine. New Orleans, LA.

McLoughlin, A., Gould, M., & Malone, K. (2015). Global trends in teenage suicide: 2003–2014. *QJM*, *108*(10), 765–780.

Mann, J., Apter, A., Bertolote, J., Beautrais, A., Currier, D., Haas, A., Hegerl, U., & Hendin, H. (2005). Suicide prevention strategies: A systematic review, *JAMA*, *294*(16), 2064–2074.

Mars, B., Burrows, S., Hjelmeland, H., & Gunnell, D. (2014). Suicidal behavior across the African continent: A review of the literature. *BMC Public Health*, *14*, 606.

Muehlenkamp, J.J., Claes, L., Havertape, L., & Plener, P.L. (2012). International prevalence of adolescents non-suicidal self-injury and deliberate self-harm. *Child and Adolescent Psychiatry and Mental Health*, *6*, 10.

National Action Alliance for Suicide Prevention: Research Prioritization Task Force. (2014). *A prioritized research agenda for suicide prevention: An action plan to save lives*. Rockville, MD: National Institute of Mental Health and the Research Prioritization Task Force.

National Institute of Mental Health (NIMH). (n.d.). Warning signs of suicide. Available at www.nimh.-nih.gov/health/topics/suicide-prevention-studies/warning-signs-of-suicide.shtml (accessed May 24, 2016).

National Suicide Prevention Lifeline. (n.d.). Risk factors. Available at www.suicidepreventionlifeline.org/learn/riskfactors.aspx (accessed May 24, 2016).

Nock, M. & Prinstein, M. (2004). A functional approach to the assessment of self-mutilative behavior. *Journal of Consulting Clinical Psychology*, *72*(5), 885–890.

Nock, M., Borges, G., Bromet, E., Cha, C., Kessler, R., & Lee, S. (2008). Suicide and suicidal behavior. *Epidemiol Review*, *30*(1), 133–154.

Nordentoft, M. (2011). Crucial elements in suicide prevention strategies. *Progress in Neuro-Psychopharmacology & Biological Psychiatry*, *35*, 848–853.

Phillips, M.R. & Cheng, H.G. (2012). The changing global face of suicide. *The Lancet*, *379*, 2318–2319.

Registered Nurses' Association of Ontario (2008). *Assessment and care of adults at risk for suicidal ideation and behaviour*. Toronto, Canada: Registered Nurses' Association of Ontario. Available at http://rnao.ca/sites/rnao-ca/files/Assessment_and_Care_of_Adults_at_Risk_for_Suicidal_Ideation_and_Behaviour.pdf (accessed December 20, 2015).

Registered Nurses' Association of Ontario (RNAO). (2009). *Assessment and care of adults at risk for suicidal ideation and behaviours*. Toronto, Canada: Registered Nurses' Association of Ontario. Available at rnao.ca/bpg/guidelines/assessment-and-care-adults-risk-suicidal-ideation-and-behaviour. (accessed May 24, 2016).

The Samaritans (n.d.). Know the warning signs. Available at samaritansnyc.org/know-the-warning-signs (accessed April 22, 2016).

Schlebusch, L. (n.d.). Suicidal behavior. (Chapter 13). Available at www.yumpu.com/en/chapter-13-sa-medical-research-council (accessed May 24, 2016).

Skerrett, D., Kolves, K., & DeLeo, D. (2012). *Suicidal behaviours in LGB populations: A literature review of research trends*. Brisbane, Australia: Australian Institute for Suicide Research and Prevention.

Turner, B., Austin, S., & Chapman, A. (2014). Treating nonsuicidal self-injury: A systematic review of psychosocial and pharmacological interventions. *Canadian Journal of Psychiatry, 59*(11), 576–585.

Van Geel, M., Goemans, A., & Vedder, P. (2015). A meta-analysis on the relation between peer victimization and adolescent non-suicidal self-injury. *Psychiatry Research, 230*(2), 364–368.

van Heeringen, K. & Mann, J.J. (2014). The neurobiology of suicide. *Lancet Psychiatry, 1*(1), 63–72.

World Health Organization (WHO). (2012). *Suicide rates data by country*. Geneva: WHO.

World Health Organization (WHO). (2014). *Preventing suicide: A global imperative*. Geneva: WHO.

13

STRATEGIES FOR HEALTH PROMOTION IN INDIVIDUALS EXPERIENCING DEPRESSION

Kunsook S. Bernstein

Introduction

Depressive disorders were reported to be the second leading cause of disability and the eleventh leading cause of global burden (or disability-adjusted life years [DALYs]) in 2010, and major depressive disorder (MDD) accounted for 8.2(5.9–1 percent 0.8 percent) of global years lived with disability (YLDs) (Ferrari *et al.*, 2013). Although direct information on the prevalence of depression does not exist for most countries, particularly low- to middle-income countries, major depressive disorder (MDD) currently affects an estimated 350 million people worldwide (WHO, 2012). Furthermore, depression at its most severe case can lead to suicide and has been responsible for 850,000 deaths every year (BioMed Central, 2011). MDD is also reported to be a contributor of burden allocated to 16 million suicides related to DALYs and to almost 4 million ischemic heart disease related to DALYs. These findings emphasize the importance of including depressive disorders as a public-health priority and implementing cost-effective interventions to reduce its burden (Ferrari *et al.*, 2013). In conjunction with the WHO's report, World Mental Health (WMH) Survey Initiative, researchers in 18 different countries conducted the study of cross-national epidemiology of major depressive episode (MDE) and collected data from over 89,000 people (Bromet *et al.*, 2011). The results of the study showed that the average lifetime and 12-month prevalence estimates of MDE were; 14.6 percent and 5.5 percent in the 10 high-income countries (Belgium, France, Germany, Israel, Italy, Japan, Netherlands, New Zealand, Spain, and United States) and 11.1 percent and 5.9 percent in the eight low- to middle-income countries (Brazil, Colombia, India, Lebanon, Mexico, South Africa, Ukraine, and China). The Centers for Disease Control and Prevention (CDC) (2010) also reports that depression is a major mental health problem across all ethnic groups in the United States. This chapter will cover global mental health issues and strategies for mental health promotion in individuals experiencing depression.

What is depression?

Depression is a prevalent, chronic and recurrent disorder and its impact on a person's life cannot be overestimated (Buchanan, 2012) and can be costly. The personal and societal costs of depression are significant, with severe costs for the individual, including impaired social and occupational functioning, ill health, increased mortality and suicide (Wulsin *et al.*, 1999), and major economic costs for society (Üstün, Ayuso-Mateos, Chatterji, Mathers, & Murray, 2004).

First, direct and indirect workplace costs related to depression are estimated to be over $34 billion per year (National Alliance Mental Illness (NAMI), 2013b). Major depression is associated with more annual sick days and higher rates of short-term disability than other chronic diseases. People suffering from depression have high rates of absenteeism (in some cases, three times more sick days than non-depressed workers) and are less productive at work. They include higher rates of death, serious complications for chronic disease patients, significantly higher health care costs for employers, added family caregiver burden and associated substance abuse problems (NAMI, 2013b). In a study comparing depression treatment costs to lost productivity costs, 45 to 98 percent of treatment costs were offset by increased productivity. Depressed employees may cost US employers an estimated $44 billion annually, compared with only $13 billion for non-depressed individuals (Stewart, Ricci, Chee, Hahn & Morganstein, 2003). Findings from an additional study estimated the total economic burden at $83.1 billion in 2000 for treating depression in the US population (Greenberg *et al.*, 2003). Depression also can generate detrimental effects on all family members. The caregiver burden associated with depression can affect workplace performance, and children of mothers who suffer from chronic depression are more likely to have behavioral problems at school (Greenberg, *et al.*, 2003).

Second, studies show that depression is associated with higher mortality rates in all age groups. Depression's impact is clear in the case of suicide, which is a risk of untreated depression. Suicide is the eleventh leading cause of death in the US, accounting for 30,000 deaths each year (Xu, Kochanek, Murphy, & Tejada-Vera, 2010) and is reportedly the cause of between 850,000 to one million deaths per year globally (Glover, 2011).

Over 15 percent of depressed people take their own lives. The suicide rate is six times higher among men aged 85 and over than it is for the general population (NAMI, 2013a). The new findings from Substance Abuse and Mental Health Services Administration (SAMHSA) (2013) also found that 9 million American adults aged 18 and older (3.9 percent) had serious thoughts of suicide in the past year—2.7 million (1.1 percent) made suicide plans and 1.3 million (0.6 percent) attempted suicide. In 2012, 6.9 percent of adults aged 18 or older (16.0 million people) had at least one MDE in the past year. The percentage of adults who had a past year MDE remained stable between 2005 (6.6 percent) and 2012 (6.9 percent).

Third, depression with medical morbidity often negatively affects the course of chronic diseases. For example, depressed heart disease patients are much more likely to die after a heart attack than heart disease patients who are not depressed. For those who have suffered a stroke or heart disease, diabetes, cancer, Parkinson's disease, and/or HIV/AIDS are at a much greater risk for depression than the overall population. Annual prevalence estimates of depression for these groups range from 10 percent to 65 percent (NAMI, 2013a). Depression can interfere with the ability of patients to follow medication and dietary regimens and has recently been linked to increased bone loss in women. Another medical comorbidity with depression is its association to substance abuse problems. Rates of undetected depression among drug and alcohol users are estimated to be as high as 30 percent. In 2001, a federal government survey reported that adults who used illicit drugs were twice as likely to report suffering from serious mental illness, such as depression, as adults who did not use drugs. Due to the substantial co-morbidity of substance use and depressive disorders, restricting services is likely to result in movement to another part of the system, such as jails and emergency departments (NAMI, 2013b).

Lastly, impact of depression on a person's quality of life can render his/her ability to perform daily activities poorly such as taking care of family as parents, workplace performance, and schoolwork. Depressed individuals may present with confusion, poor concentration and attention span, and thought blocking, poor judgment, and poor decision-making abilities because they cannot assess their situation objectively and tend to perceive themselves as in worse condition than those with a physical chronic health diagnosis (Cornwell, 2003), which can further impact the individual's quality of life.

Main contributing factors to depression across cultures were reported to be gender and loss of a significant other. For example, females were twice as likely to suffer depression as males, and the loss of a partner, whether from death, divorce or separation was linked to depressive episodes. However the contribution of age varied from country to country and the findings showed that age of onset of depression was almost 2 years earlier in low-income countries, compared to people from high-income countries (Bromet *et al.*, 2011).

Depressive disorders are a global health priority when setting global health objectives. It is not only important to understand variations in burden by disorder, country, region, age, sex, and year but also estimating the burden attributable to MDD as a risk factor for other health outcomes, which allows for a more accurate estimate of burden and reinforces the importance of implementing cost-effectiveness interventions to reduce its ubiquitous burden (Ferrari, *et al.*, 2013). The National Institute of Mental Health (NIMH) recommends that interventions be designed to prevent the onset of clinical depression in at-risk groups such as women, non-Hispanic whites, adolescents (13- to 18-year-olds) and older adults (85 and older) (NIMH, 2013a). Understanding the patterns and causes of depression can help inform global initiatives in order to reduce the impact of depression on individual lives and in reducing the burden to society (Bromet *et al.*, 2011).

Clinical presentation of depression

Characteristics of Depression

Depressive disorder has been categorized by the *Diagnostic and Statistical Manual of Mental Disorders*, 5th edition (DSM-5) into eight different types: 1) disruptive mood dysregulation disorder; 2) major depressive disorder; 3) persistent depressive disorder (Dysthymia); 4) premenstrual dysphoric disorder; 5) substance/medication induced depressive disorder; 6) depressive disorder due to another medical condition (e.g., hypothyroidism); 7) other specified depressive disorder (e.g., short-duration depressive episode); and 8) unspecified depressive disorder. Each category has its own diagnostic criteria. The common feature of all of these depressive disorders is the presence of sad, empty, or irritable mood, accompanied by somatic and cognitive changes that significantly affect the individual's capacity to function (APA, 2013). Among eight different categories of depressive disorder, major depressive disorder has highest 12-month prevalence (7 percent) in the United States (APA, 2013), and is often represented as a general term of depression in several studies (Bromet *et al.*, 2011; Buchanan, 2012). This chapter is mainly focused on major depressive disorder, which will be referred to as depression throughout the chapter. Depression is characterized by discrete episodes of at least two weeks' duration involving a significant change in the person's affect, cognition, and neuro-vegetative functions and inter-episode remissions. A diagnosis of depression is made based on the criteria that a person experiences five or more of the following symptom criteria during the same two-week period with presence of at least one symptom to include either depressed mood or loss of pleasure. The five symptom criteria listed are disturbed sleep or appetite, psychomotor agitation or retardation, fatigue, feelings of worthlessness or excessive guilt, poor concentration, and recurrent thoughts of death and suicidal ideation (APA, 2013; BioMed Central, 2011). Depression is associated with high mortality mostly accounted for by suicide, and presentation of other symptoms such as tearfulness, irritability, brooding, obsessive rumination, anxiety, phobias, and excessive worry over physical health (APA, 2013).

In the United States (US), the average 12-month prevalence of major depressive disorder is estimated to be 6.7 percent of the US adult population and 30.4 percent of these cases (i.e., 2.0 percent of the US adult population) are classified as "severe" (Kessler, Chiu, Demler, & Walters, 2005). Socio-demographic reports of the lifetime prevalence of depression in the US are: 1) women are 70 percent more likely than men to experience depression during their lifetime; 2) non-Hispanic blacks are 40 percent less likely than non-Hispanic whites to experience depression during their lifetime; 3) the age group of 18–29-year-olds are 200 percent more likely than those aged 60+, and 30–44-year-olds are 80 percent more likely to have experienced depression (Kessler *et al.*, 2003). According to the SAMHSA (2013) News Release, 2.2 million youth aged 12 to 17 (9.1 percent of this population) experienced a MDE in 2012, and were more than three times as likely to have a substance use disorder (16.0 percent) than their counterparts who had not experienced a major depressive episode (5.1 percent).

Etiology of depression

The specific cause of major depressive disorder is not known. The etiology of depression as an illness has been conceptualized to have a number of interacting biological, psychological, and social components. As with most psychiatric disorders, depression appears to be a multifactorial and heterogeneous group of disorders involving genetic, neuro-endocrinological, and environmental factors including social determinants and cultural influences.

Genetic factors

Genetic factors may play an important role in the development of major depression. Studies have been done to determine how a person's genes play a role in the development of depression. Sullivan and colleagues (2000) conducted a review of meta-analysis of genetic epidemiology of major depression and reported that depression is a familial disorder and its familial factors mostly or entirely result from genetic influences. Evidence from twin studies suggests that major depression has a concordance of 40–50 percent. First-degree relatives of depressed individuals are about three times as likely to develop depression as the general population. However, depression can occur in people without family histories of depression, as well (National Institute of Mental Health (NIMH), 2014). In a national twin study of lifetime major depression in Sweden, the researchers reported that the genetic risk factors for major depression were moderately correlated in the study group, but there were no significant differences found in the etiologic roles of genetic and environmental factors in depression among members of this sample (Kendler, Gatz, Gardner, & Pedersen, 2006).

Neuro-endocrinological factors

Studies of neuro-endocrinological abnormality in relation to depression have found that hypothalamic-pituitary-adrenocortical (HPA) axis hyperactivity is associated with depression (Stetler & Miller, 2011). Depressed patients show a variety of alterations in HPA system regulation, which is reflected by increased pituitary-adrenocortical hormone secretion at baseline and a number of aberrant neuroendocrine function tests. Neuroendocrine studies of depressive illness support the hypothesis that there is defective noradrenergic function in the brains of some patients with depressive illness. Neuroendocrine tests are now available for studying monoamine function in the brains of patients with depression (Duval *et al.*, 2005).

Functional magnetic resonance imaging studies also provided evidence for functional abnormalities in specific neural systems supporting emotion processing, reward seeking, and emotion regulation in adults with depression (Ebmeier, Rose, & Steele, 2006). However, the neuro-endocrinological factors are still in need of further investigation to fully understand their relation to the etiology of depression.

Social determinant factors

Variations in social factors are determinate influences on variations in health, including mental health, and health inequity is associated with social inequity, a problem needing policy responses and action (WHO, 2010a). There has been a relative dearth of past research on the social determinants of health (SDH) and mental health. A study by Liang and colleagues (2012) explored the relationship between SDH and depression in China and provided initial evidence of the importance of SDH in depression. Three variables of SDH were socioeconomic status (years of schooling and self-reported economic status of family), social cohesion, and negative life events. Subramanian and colleagues (2005) conducted a study analyzing multivariate and multilevel individuals and communities in the United States to determine the socioeconomic determinants of self-related health using social influences on depression. The researchers reported that there was significant correlation between social factors such as child abuse, dysfunctional family, stressful life events, and depression. The finding of these studies consistently report that SDH is closely associated with depression. Consequently, social inequity and the role of policy action emphasized by SDH should be considered high priorities when addressing the issue of depression.

Cultural factors

Culture is one of many factors within human societies that has a bearing on the epidemiology of depression, and other factors such as gender and income inequality are also identified as major risk factors for depression (Patel, 2001). One cannot fully assess the nature of depression without addressing the context (cultural, communal, familial) within which it occurs, and the growth of the phenomenon (incidence and prevalence) of depression without understanding the culture of the society within which this phenomenon exists (Hedaya, 2009). Culture-related diagnostic issues in relation to depression are important for clinicians to be aware of. In most countries the majority of cases of depression go unrecognized in primary care settings and in many cultures, somatic symptoms are very likely to constitute the presenting complaint (APA, 2013). Culturally appropriate terminology for depression can be identified and their use may improve levels of recognition and treatment compliance. Examples of culturally shaped terminologies used in relation to depression or similar symptom categories are listed below (Flaskerud, 2000).

1 **Chronic fatigue syndrome:**
   a) *Principal population*: North America women and men.
   b) *Features*: somatic, anxious, depressive.
   c) *Symptoms*: exhaustion, muscle weakness, irritability, depression, and anxiety, memory and concentration problems, family or work problems.
2 **Neurasthenia (Shinkeisuijaku):**
   a) *Principal population*: Asia (Japan), women and men.
   b) *Features*: somatic, depressive anxious, social distress.

   c) *Symptoms*: exhaustion, muscle weakness, irritability, depression, anxiety, memory and concentration problems, family or work problems.

3 **Ataque de nervios:**
   a) *Principal population*: Latin America, women and men;
   b) *Features*: somatic, anxious, dissociative;
   c) *Symptoms*: convulsions, shaking, palpitations, dyspnea, dizziness.

4 **Susto:**
   a) *Principal population*: Hispanic, Old and New World women and men.
   b) *Features:* somatic, anxious, depressive, dissociative,
   c) *Symptoms*: anorexia, vomiting, diarrhea, tachycardia, sweating, insomnia, anxiety, depression, irritability.

5 **Hwa-byung:**
   a) *Principal population*: Koreans and Korean Americans, women and men.
   b) *Features*: somatic, anxious, depressive, social distress.
   c) *Symptoms*: epigastric pain, burning, feeing hot, anxiety, depression, tiredness, insomnia.

6 **Voodoo:**
   a) *Principal population*: Hex Blacks and Latinos from United States and Caribbean.
   b) *Features*: somatic, anxious.
   c) *Symptoms*: malaise, dyspnea, chest pain, syncope, anxiety and fear.

Pathophysiology of depression

The underlying pathophysiology of major depressive disorder has not been clearly understood. Current evidence points to a complex interaction between neurotransmitter availability and receptor regulation and sensitivity underlying the affective symptoms. Neurotransmitters, which are implicated in depression, include serotonin (5-HT), norepinephrine (NE), dopamine (DA), glutamate, and brain-derived neurotrophic factor (BDNF). For example, the role of serotonin (5-HT) activity in the pathophysiology of major depressive disorder is suggested by the therapeutic efficacy of antidepressants such as selective serotonin reuptake inhibitors (SSRIs). Serotonin activities include neuronal receptor regulation, intracellular signaling, and gene expression over time, in addition to enhanced neurotransmitter availability (Stahl, 2013).

Evidence-based prevention and mental health promotion strategies

Evidence-based mental illness prevention and health promotion are vital to meet not only the needs of persons with defined mental disorders including depression, but also to protect and promote the mental well-being of all citizens. However, global health systems have not yet adequately responded to the burden of mental disorders including depression to reduce the gap between the need for treatment and its provision of evidence-based illness prevention and health promotion. In low-income and middle-income countries, a majority (range between 76 percent and 85 percent) of people with severe mental disorders receive no treatment for their disorder, and the corresponding range for high-income countries falls between 35 percent and 50 percent, which further compounds the problem of the poor quality of care for those receiving treatment (WHO, 2013). WHO's *Mental Health Atlas 2011* (2011) reports that resources within countries to meet mental health needs are scarce and also use of the existing resources is reported to be inefficient and inequitable in its distribution. For example, annual spending on mental health is less than US$ 2 per person in high-income countries and less than US$ 0.25 per person in low-income countries. Out of these financial resources, 67 percent are allocated to psychiatric hospitals despite their association with poor health outcomes and human rights violations (WHO, 2013). In the context of national efforts to develop and implement health policies and programs to implement strategies for promotion and prevention in mental health, the US President's fiscal year 2014 budget proposed new enhanced demonstration authority under social security administration's disability programs to test promising, research-based interventions (Office of Management and Budget, 2013). This proposal allows early intervention efforts aimed at preserving the well-being and work ability of individuals most at risk of becoming severely impaired. Since mental health evolves throughout the life cycle, building early interventions for mental health services could provide better access to treatment and structured support services for individuals struggling with severe mental illness. Also, governments have an important role in using information on risk and protective factors for mental health to put in place actions to prevent mental disorders, and to protect and promote mental health at all stages of life focusing on prevention and intervention for all disorders, including depression.

Broad strategies for mental health promotion and prevention targeting depression may focus on prevention using education to promote public knowledge of depression as a disease process and early intervention through identification, prevention and treatment of depression. Early intervention can be implemented through evidence-based psychosocial, and psychotherapeutic and pharmacological interventions.

Early intervention and treatment of depression

Early intervention: consumer education to promote individual well-being

Early intervention including early identification and treatment for depressed individuals can prevent the loss in productivity and reduce high medical costs, as well as the associated burdens on family members and caregivers (Santoro & Murphy, 2010). Early intervention includes early identification of illness, and reducing duration of untreated mental illness including depression through community education of mental illness (WHO, 2004). Over the long term, patients may also become aware of signs of relapse and may seek treatment early before deterioration. Patients should be educated to increase their awareness of the rationale behind the choice of treatment, potential adverse effects, and expected results, and be encouraged to be actively involved in their treatment plan, which can enhance medication and overall compliance. Family members also need education about the nature of depression and may benefit from supportive interactions. Engaging family can be a critical component of the treatment plan, especially for pediatric and late-onset depression. Family members are helpful informants, can promote medication compliance, and can encourage patients to change behaviors that perpetuate depression (e.g., inactivity). The following websites are valuable resources for patient and family education about depression: National Institute of Mental Health (www.nimh.nih.gov/health/topics/depression); Depression, Medline Plus (www.nlm.nih.gov/medlineplus/depression.html); Depression, and FamilyDoctor.org (http://familydoctor.org/familydoctor/en/diseases-conditions/depression) Depression (Halverson, 2013). Educating individuals suffering with depression as consumers in the health care field can enhance their attained knowledge to empower themselves on how to promote self-care to reach maximum well-being. Education about depression as a disease process, and its available treatment options including psychotherapies and medications as well as expected therapeutic effects and side effects of treatment is an important factor contributing to treatment adherence (Bernstein, 2007; Mitchell, 2006). Lastly, educating depressed individuals on how to cope with their illness by using a problem–solving process such as exploring possible options, examining the consequences of each alternative, selecting and implementing an alternative, and evaluating the result, could help individuals in recovery from their depression. There is evidence of the effective treatment and intervention for depression in low-income and middle-income countries with low-cost antidepressants and/or psychological interventions (such as cognitive-behavior therapy and interpersonal therapies). In these countries, cost-effective depression treatment and prevention of depression can be delivered in primary care and community-based rehabilitation programs providing low-cost integrative care for children and adults with chronic mental disabilities (Patel *et al.*, 2007). Depression is a disorder that can be reliably diagnosed and treated in primary care with referable treatment options as outlined in the WHO mhGAP Intervention Guide (WHO, 2010b). Those options consist of basic psychosocial support combined with antidepressant medication or psychological interventions (Andrews, Cuijpers, Craske, McEvoy, & Titov, 2010). A study of depression treatment by family physicians (Van *et al.*, 2005) has found that patients are more likely to improve if their primary care providers are not only prescribing adequate medication but also being good communicators. Maintaining a good rapport and trusting relationship with their patients when treating depressive disorder is an important aspect of treatment intervention. Jacobs (2005) states that attaining treatment adherence is dependent on how well the alliances between clinicians and patients are built through interactive and interpersonal processes.

Suicide prevention is also an important priority. Helplines have been increasingly recognized as vital components of a suicide prevention strategy. Their effectiveness lies in the offer of accessible (by phone), convenient (often 24/7 delivery) and confidential (no names) support to people who are in crisis. Many helplines worldwide use volunteers and non-professional workforces in their delivery to harness community resources towards suicide prevention. Accordingly, helplines can attract suicidal persons to reach out for help at a critical time, thereby enabling a compassionate response to be provided and the potential for life saving intervention towards safety and continuing support (International Association for Suicide Prevention, 2015). Unfortunately, suicide rates tend to be underreported owing to weak surveillance systems, a misattribution of suicide to accidental deaths, as well as its criminalization in some countries. As there are many risk factors associated with suicide beyond mental disorder, such as chronic pain or acute emotional distress, actions to prevent suicide must not only come from the health sector, but also from other sectors simultaneously. For example, reducing access to means to self-harm and commit suicide (including firearms, pesticides and availability of toxic medicines that can be used in overdoses), responsible reporting by the media, protecting persons at high risk of suicide, and early identification and management of mental disorder and of suicidal behaviors can be effective (WHO, 2013).

Pharmacological treatment of depression

Antidepressant treatment for depression is available and successful with a full recovery in some cases and a partial symptom relief in others. Currently the treatment of major depressive disorder has developed to the point that effective antidepressant medication and depression-specific brief psychotherapies have become the standard treatment (NAMI, 2013a). For nearly 20 years, the selective serotonin reuptake inhibitors (SSRIs) have been the primary pharmacological agents to treat depression. These antidepressants: fluoxetine (Prozac), sertraline (Zoloft), paroxetine (Paxil), Fluvoxamine (Luvox), citalopram (Celexa), and escitalopram (Lexapro), are among the world's most widely prescribed medications (Harvard Medical School, 2005). They are effective and considerably safer compared to the older antidepressants such as tricyclic

Table 13.1 Sample of commonly used antidepressants and dose range

Selective serotonin reuptake inhibitors (SSRIs)	Dose range (mg)	Tricyclic antidepressants (TCAs)	Dose range (mg)	Other antidepressants	Dose range (mg)
Fluoxetine (Prozac)	20–80	Imipramine (Tofranil)	100–300	Bupropion (Wellbutrin)	150–450
Sertraline (Zoloft)	50–200	Desipramine (Norpramin)	100–300	Mirtazapine (Remeron)	7.5–45
Paroxetine (Paxil)	20–50	Doxepin (Sinequan)	100–300	Duloxetine (Cymbalta)	20–60
Fluvoxamine (Luvox)	100–200	Nortriptyline (Pamelor)	75–150	Trazodone (Desyrel)	150–600
Venlafaxine (Effexor)	75–225	Amitriptyline (Elavil)	100–300	Venlafaxine (Effexor)	75–225
Citalopram (Celexa)	20–60				
Esocitalopram (Lexapro)	10–20				

antidepressants (TCAs): desipramine (Norpramin), nortriptyline (Pamelor), doxepin (Sinequan), amitriptyline (Elavil), imipramine (Tofranil), and Monoamine oxidase inhibitors (MAOIs). The range of the use of SSRIs has expanded from depression to anxiety, obsessive-compulsive disorder, eating disorders, and many other psychiatric conditions. Lately, side effects of these drugs, from sexual dysfunction to suicidal behavior, have received more attention, especially when treating the child and adolescent population. Other types of antidepressants commonly used are: the selective serotonin and norepinephrine reuptake inhibitors (SNRIs)—venlafaxine (Effexor XR) and duloxitine (Cymbalta); atypical antidepressants—mirtazapine (Remeron), bupropione (Wellbutrin), and nefazodone (Serzone). These medications are included in Table 13.1.

When treating clients who suffer from depression, measuring the risk and benefit of each drug should be the standard practice, which should be the same as any other drug treatments by health care professionals (Bernstein, 2007). The American Psychiatric Association (APA) 2010 practice guidelines for the treatment of major depressive disorders in adults stated that the effectiveness of antidepressants is generally comparable between classes and within classes of medications. Therefore the initial selection of an antidepressant medication will largely be based on anticipated side effects, safety or tolerability of these side effects for individual patients, patient preference, quantity and quality of clinical trial data regarding the medication, and its cost (APA, 2010).

Non-pharmacological depression treatment

Several different types of depression-prevention interventions were found in the randomized control trials, which included cognitive-behavioral therapy and interpersonal-process therapy among other interventions (Buchanan, 2012), which are most commonly practiced in so called, "Talk therapy" or psychotherapy for depression. Cognitive behavioral therapy (CBT) has gained recognition to be an effective treatment for major depression. CBT focuses on identifying and challenging pessimistic or self-critical thinking, and emphasizes increasing involvement in rewarding activities (Bernstein, 2007), and advocates guided discovery of one's own problem solving approach (Freeman & Freeman, 2005). Several studies that included sufficient numbers of individuals from different cultural backgrounds have found support for the efficacy of cognitive behavioral therapy (CBT) as a form of depression treatment with Latinos and African Americans (Miranda, Azocar, Organista, Dwyer, & Arean, 2014; Foster, 2007). The efficacy of CBT was reported in studies with depressed Latino adults and adolescents (Rosselló, Bernal, & Rivera-Medina, 2012), African American women (Kohn, Oden, Muñoz, Robinson, & Leavitt, 2002), and elderly Chinese Americans (Chen & Davenport, 2005). There also exists some support for the efficacy of CBT in the prevention of depressive symptoms among Latino adolescents (Cardemil, Reivich, Beevers, Seligman, & James, 2007) and adults (Le, Zmuda, Perry, & Muñoz, 2010). Despite the evidence of efficacy of CBT, the research base for the CBT treatment and prevention of depression is significantly more limited for Asian Americans (one study of CBT for Chinese Americans), and is almost nonexistent for individuals from other cultural groups. There are studies (Arnow & Constantino, 2003; Griffiths, Ravindran, Merali, & Anisman, 2000; Whooley & Simon, 2000) reporting that combined treatment of CBT and antidepressants demonstrated significant superiority over CBT or antidepressants alone in treatment of chronic major depression.

Interpersonal therapy (IPT) is another therapeutic model to treat depression. The treatment addresses the four types of interpersonal problems; interpersonal disputes, role transitions, grief, and interpersonal deficits (Wheeler, 2013). A study with Latinos and African Americans in the treatment and prevention of depression using IPT found its efficacy, the majority of which has been found with perinatal depression among Latina women (Spinelli & Endicott, 2003). Other therapeutic modality for depression intervention studies targeting low-income and African American women (Crockett, Zlotnick, Davis, Payne, & Washington, 2008), Puerto Rican adolescents (Rosselló *et al.*, 2012), and low-income, Latina and African American adolescents (Miller, Gur, Shanok, & Weissman, 2008) reported the similar positive outcomes of IPT.

Other types of non-pharmacological interventions beside psychotherapy in caring for depressed individuals include health promotion and maintenance such as on-going evaluation, assisting with self-care, implementing health teaching, counseling and crisis interventions, psychiatric rehabilitation, and psychoeducation. WHO's (2010b) Mental Health Gap (mhGAP) Intervention Guide for mental, neurological and substance use disorders in non-specialized health settings describes depression intervention detailing psychosocial/non-pharmacological treatment and advice, which includes: 1) psychoeducation for the person and his or her family; 2) addressing current psychosocial stressors; 3) reactivating social networks; 4) structured physical activity programs as adjunct treatment options for moderate-severe depression; and 5) offering regular follow-up. Furthermore, the use of complementary and alternative treatments for depression is increasingly common, and some of those studied for treatment benefits include St John's Wort, S-adenosyl methionine (SAMe), Omega-3 fatty acids, and Folate with modest evidence for antidepressant efficacy; however, they deserve further study and an understanding of potential interactions with other medications used. Other depression treatment modalities known to the public for the treatment of depression are light therapy and acupuncture, which show limited evidence of treatment efficacy for depression (APA, 2010). The ultimate goal of caring for the depressed person is to focus on global function improvement, illness prevention, medication maintenance, social function, and health maintenance.

Recommendation

WHO (2003) published the *Mental Health Policy and Service Guidance Package* on advocacy for mental health in general and defined advocacy as a means of raising awareness on mental health issues and ensuring that mental health is on the national agenda of governments. Advocacy was further elaborated in its importance to improvements in policy, legislation, and service development as it aimed to improve the knowledge, understanding, and acceptance of mental disorders in the general population so that people can recognize them and ask for treatment as early as possible. Depression as a form of mental illness is important and methods that can be used to raise depression awareness advocacy will be addressed here.

General strategies for supporting advocacy activities to raise depression awareness with the general population through public events and the distribution of educational materials such as brochures, pamphlets, posters, and videos, as well as utilizing media by raising of depression awareness has been recommended by WHO (2003). Through these advocacy activities, the needs of persons suffering from depression could be better understood and their rights could be better protected. They could receive services of improved quality and could participate actively in their planning, development, monitoring, and evaluation. Families could be supported in their role as caretakers, and the public could gain an improved understanding of depression as a treatable illness. The National Institute of Mental Health (NIMH) recommends how to help oneself and loved ones who suffer from depression by recognizing depression and seeking treatment early, and staying in treatment (NIMH, 2014). In most parts of the world, mental disorders including depression are not regarded with the same importance as physical health and have been largely ignored or neglected (WHO, 2003). Many communities are faced with factors that present risks to depression and barriers to mental health services since many of them become targets of stigma and discrimination. Table 13.2 includes WHO (2003) proposed strategies of how to combat mental health stigma.

Summary

In summary, depression is a prevalent, chronic and recurrent disorder and can significantly impact individuals and overall community functioning and quality. However, depression is treatable

Table 13.2 WHO recommendations to combat mental health stigma

1   Community education on mental disorders (prevalence, causes, symptoms, treatment, myths and prejudices)
2   Anti-stigma training for teachers and health workers
3   Psychoeducation for consumers and families on how to live with persons who have mental disorders
4   Empowerment of consumer and family organizations (as described in this module)
5   Improvement of mental health services (quality, access, deinstitutionalization, community care)
6   Legislation on the rights of persons with mental disorders
7   Education of persons working in the mass media, aimed at changing stereotypes and misconceptions about mental disorders
8   Development of demonstration areas with community care and social integration for persons with mental disorders

Since there is no one set of recommendations that can be applied worldwide because of the diversity of social, economic, cultural and other realities, each country and each community need to adopt the fundamental concepts of advocacy strategies that are applicable to own culture and society

Source: WHO 2003, p. 11.

and a person with depression can recover from the illness and function with the assistance of early interventions and relapse-prevention strategies. Since many countries are still faced with factors that present risks to depression and barriers to mental health services, it is imperative that each government engages all stakeholders in advocacy to raise awareness of the magnitude of burden of disease associated with depression, and the availability of effective intervention strategies for mental health promotion in general, prevention of depression and its treatment, care, and recovery of individuals suffering from depression.

References

American Psychiatric Association (APA) (2010). Practice guideline for the treatment of patients with major depressive disorders. Retrieved March 7, 2015 from www.psychiatryonline.com/pracGuide/pracGuideTopic_7.aspx.

American Psychiatric Association (APA) (2013). *Diagnostic and statistical manual of mental disorders (DSM-5)* (5th ed.). Washington DC: APA.

Andrews, G., Cuijpers, P., Craske, M. G., McEvoy, P., & Titov, N. (2010). Computer therapy for the anxiety and depressive disorders is effective, acceptable and practical health care: a meta-analysis. *PLoS One*, 5(10), e13196.

Arnow, B.A. & Constantino, M.J. (2003). Effectiveness of psychotherapy and combination treatment for chronic depression. *Journal of Clinical Psychology*, 59(8), 893–905

Bernstein, K.S. (2007). Clinical assessment of depression and its management. *Journal of Adult Health – MEDSUR Nursing*, 15(6), 333–342.

BioMed Central (2011, July 26). Global depression statistics. *Science Daily*. Retrieved August 31, 2013, from www.sciencedaily.com_/releases/2011/07/110725202240.htm.

Bromet, E., Andrade, H.A., Hwang, I., Sampson, N.A., Alonso, J., Girolamo, G., Ron de Graaf, R., Williams, D., & Kessler, R.C. (2011). Cross-national epidemiology of DSM-IV major depressive episode. *BMC Medicine*, 90(9), 1–16.

Buchanan, J. (2012). Prevention of depression in the college student population: a review of the literature. *Archives of Psychiatric Nursing*, 26(1), 21–42.

Cardemil, E.V., Reivich, K.J., Beevers, C.G., Seligman, M.E.P., & James, J. (2007). The prevention of depressive symptoms in low-income, minority children: two-year follow-up. *Behaviour Research and Therapy*, 45, 313–327.

Center for Disease Control (CDC) and Prevention (2010). Current depression among adults: United States, 2006 and 2008. *Morbidity and Mortality Weekly Report* 59(38), 1229–1235.

Chen, S.W. & Davenport, D.S. (2005). Cognitive-behavioral therapy with Chinese American clients: cautions and modifications. *Psychotherapy: Theory, Research, Practice, Training*, 42(1), 101–110.

Cornwell, B. (2003). The dynamic properties of social support: decay, growth, and staticity, and their effects on adolescent depression. *Social Forces*, 81(3), 953–978.

Crockett, K., Zlotnick, C., Davis, M., Payne, N., & Washington, R. (2008). A depression preventive intervention for rural low-income African-American pregnant women at risk for postpartum depression. *Archives of Women's Mental Health*, 11(5–6), 319–325.

Duval, F., Mokrani, M.-C., Monreal Ortiz, J.A., Schulz, P., Champeval, C., & Macher, J.-P. (2005). Neuroendocrine predictors of the evolution of depression. *Dialogues in Clinical Neuroscience*, 7(3), 273–282.

Ebmeier, K., Rose, E., & Steele, D. (2006). Cognitive impairment and fMRI in major depression. *Neurotoxicity Research* 10(2), 87–92.

Ferrari, A.J., Charlson, F.J., Norman, R.E., Patten, S.B., Freedman, G., Murray, C.J., Vos, T., & Whiteford, H.V. (2013). Burden of depressive disorders by country, sex, age, and year: findings from The Global Burden of Disease Study 2010. *PLOS Medicine*. Doi: 10.1371/journal.pmed.1001547. Retrieved June 5, 2015, from www.plosmedicine.org/article/info%3Adoi%2F10.1371%2Fjournal.pmed.1001547.

Flaskerud, J. H. (2000). Ethnicity, culture, and neuropsychiatry. *Mental Health Nursing*, 1, 5–29.

Foster, R.P. (2007), Treating depression in vulnerable urban women: a feasibility study of clinical outcomes in community service settings. *American Journal of Orthopsychiatry*, 77, 443–453.

Freeman, S.M. & Freeman, A. (2005). *Cognitive behavior therapy in nursing practice*. New York: Springer.

Glover, H. (2011). *Global depression statistics*. BioMed Central: The Open Access Publisher. Retrieved on June 5, 2015, from www.biomedcentral.com/presscenter/pressreleases/20110722.

Greenberg, P.E., Kessler, R.C., Birnbaum, H.G., Leong, S.A., Lowe, S.W., Berglund, P. A., & Corey-Lisle, P.K. (2003). The economic burden of depression in the United States: how did it change between 1990 and 2000? *Journal of Clinical Psychiatry, 64*(12), 1465–1475.

Griffiths, J., Ravindran, A.V., Merali, Z., & Anisman, H. (2000). Dysthymia: a review of pharmacological and behavioral factors. *Molecular Psychiatry, 5*(3), 242–261.

Halverson, J. L. (2013). Depression. Retrieved on May 17, 2014, from http://emedicine.medscape.com/article/286759-overview#aw2aab6b2b7.

Harvard Medical School (2005). What are the real risks of antidepressants? *Harvard Mental Health Letter,* May; *21*(11).

Hedaya, R. (2009). The cultural context of depression. *Psychology Today.* Retrieved on May 5, 2014, from www.psychologytoday.com/blog/health-matters/200901/the-cultural-context-depression.

International Association for Suicide Prevention (IASP) (2015). IASP SPECIAL INTEREST GROUP on Helplines Best. Retrieved on June 6, 2015 from www.iasp.info/helplines_best_practices.php.

Jacobs, J. (2005). Treatment of depressive disorders in split versus integrated therapy and comparisons of prescriptive practices of psychiatrists and advance practice registered nurses. *Archives of Psychiatric Nursing, 19*(6), 256–263.

Kendler, K.S., Gatz, M., Gardner, C O., & Pedersen, N.L. (2006). A Swedish national twin study of lifetime major depression. *American Journal of Psychiatry, 163*(1), 109–14.

Kessler, R.C., Chiu, W.T., Demler, O., Walters, E.E. (2005). Prevalence, severity, and comorbidity of 12-month DSM-IV disorders in the National Comorbidity Survey Replication (NCS-R). *Archives of General Psychiatry, 62*(6), 617–627.

Kessler, R.C., Berglund, P., Demler, O., Jin, R., Koretz, D., Merikangas, K.R., Rush, A J., Walters, E.E., & Wang, P.S. (2003). The epidemiology of major depressive disorder: results from the National Comorbidity Survey Replication (NCS-R). *Journal of the American Medical Association, 289*(23), 3095–3105.

Kohn, L.P., Oden, T., Munoz, R.F., Robinson, A., & Leavitt, D. (2002). Adapted cognitive behavioral group therapy for depressed low-income African American women. *Community Mental Health Journal, 38,* 497–504.

Le, H.N., Zmuda, J., Perry, D.F., & Muñoz, R.F. (2010). Transforming an evidence-based intervention to prevent perinatal depression for low-income Latina immigrants. *American Journal of Orthopsychiatry, 80*(1), 34.

Liang, Y., Gong, Y-H., Wen, X-P., Guan, C-P., Li, M-C., & Wang, Y.P. (2012). Social determinants of health and depression: a preliminary investigation from rural China. *PLoS ONE 7*(1), e30553.

Miller, L., Gur, M., Shanok, A., & Weissman, M. (2008). Interpersonal psychotherapy with pregnant adolescents: two pilot studies. *Journal of Child Psychology and Psychiatry, 49*(7), 733–742.

Miranda, J., Azocar, F., Organista, K.C., Dwyer, E., & Areane, P. (2014). Treatment of depression among impoverished primary care patients from ethnic minority groups. *Psychiatric Services, 54*(2), 219–225.

Mitchell, A.J. (2006). Depressed patients and treatment adherence. *The Lancet, 367*(9528), 2041–2043.

National Alliance of Mental Illness (NAMI, 2013a). Understanding depression. Retrieved on June 6, 2015, from www2.nami.org/Template.cfm?Section=Depression&template=contentmanagement/content display.cfm&ContentID=67727.

National Alliance of Mental Illness (NAMI, 2013b). The impact and cost of mental illness: the case of depression. Retrieved on June 6, 2015, from www.nami.org/Template.cfm?Section=Policymakers_Toolkit&Template=/ContentManagement/ContentDisplay.cfm&ContentID=19043.

National Institute of Mental Health (NIMH, 2014). Transforming the understanding and treatment of mental illnesses: depression. Retrieved on June 6, 2015, from www.nimh.nih.gov/health/topics/depression/index.shtml.

Office of Management and Budget (2013). Improving mental health prevention and treatment services. Retrieved on December 20, 2013, from www.whitehouse.gov/omb/budget/factsheet/improving-mental-health-prevention-and-treatment-services.

Patel, V. (2001). Cultural factors and international epidemiology. *British Medical Bulletin. 57*(1), 33–45.

Patel, V., Araya, R., Chatterjee, S., Chisholm, D., Cohen, A., De Silva, M., Rojas, G., & van Ommeren, M. (2007). Treatment and prevention of mental disorders in low-income and middle-income countries. *The Lancet, 370*(9591), 991–1005.

Rosselló, J., Bernal, G., & Rivera-Medina, C. (2012). Individual and group CBT and IPT for Puerto Rican adolescents with depressive symptoms. *Journal of Latina/o Psychology, 1*(S), August, 36–51.

Santoro, K. & Murphy, B., (2010). Improving early identification and treatment of adolescent depression: considerations and strategies for health plans. NIHCM Issue Brief February 2010. NIHCM Foundation. Retrieved January 6, 2014, from www.nihcm.org/pdf/Adol_MH_Issue_Brief_FINAL.pdf.

Spinelli, M. G., & Endicott, J. (2003). Controlled clinical trial of interpersonal psychotherapy versus parenting education program for depressed pregnant women. *American Journal of Psychiatry, 160*(3), 555–562.

Stahl, S.M. (2013). *Essential psychopharmacology: neuroscientific basis and practical Application* (4th ed.). New York: Cambridge University Press.

Stewart, W.F., Ricci, J.A., Chee, E, Hahn, S.R., & Morganstein, D. (2003). Cost of lost productive work time among US workers with depression. *JAMA, 289*(23), 3135–3144.

Stetler, C. & Miller, G E. (2011). Depression and hypothalamic-pituitary-adrenal activation: a quantitative summary of four decades of research. *Psychosomatic Medicine, 73*(2), 114–126.

Substance Abuse and Mental Health Services Administration (SAMHSA) (2013). SAMHSA News Release December 19, 2013. Retrieved January 6, 2014, from www.icpsr.umich.edu/icpsrweb/SAMHDA/support/announcements/2013/12/2012-national-survey-on-drug-use.

Subramanian, S.V., Kim, D., & Kawachi, I. (2005). Covariation in the socioeconomic determinants of self-rated health and happiness: a multivariate multilevel analysis of individuals and communities in the USA. *Journal of Epidemiology and Community Health, 59*(8), 664–669.

Sullivan, P.F., Neale, M.C., Kendler, K.S. (2000). Genetic epidemiology of major depression: review and meta-analysis. *American Journal of Psychiatry*, 157, 1552–1562.

Üstün, T.B., Ayuso-Mateos, J.L., Chatterji, S., Mathers, C., & Murray, C.J. (2004). Global burden of depressive disorders in the year 2000. *British Journal of Psychiatry, 184*, 386–392.

Van Os, T.W., Van den, B.R., Tiemens, B.G., Jenner, J.A., Van der, M.K., & Ormel, J. (2005). Communicative skills of general practitioners augment the effectiveness of guideline-based depression treatment. *Journal of Affective Disorder, 84*(1), 43–51.

Wheeler, K. (Ed.). (2013). *Psychotherapy for the advanced practice psychiatric nurse: a how-to guide for evidence-based practice.* New York: Springer.

Whooley, M.A., and Simon, G.E. (2000). Managing depression in medical outpatients. *New England Journal of Medicine, 343*(26), 1942–1949.

World Health Organization (WHO) (2003). *Advocacy for mental health. (Mental health policy and service guidance package).* WHO Library Cataloguing-in-Publication Data.

World Health Organization (WHO) (2004). *Prevention of mental disorders: effective interventions and policy options. Summary report.* Retrieved January 6, 2014, from www.who.int/mental_health/evidence/en/prevention_of_mental_disorders_sr.pdf.

World Health Organization (WHO) (2010a). *A conceptual framework for action on the social determinants of health.* Retrieved January 6, 2014, from http://whqlibdoc.who.int/publications/2010/9789241500852_eng.pdf.

World Health Organization (WHO) (2010b). *mhGAP Intervention Guide for mental, neurological and substance use disorders in non-specialized health settings.* Retrieved January 6, 2014, from www.who.int/mental_health/publications/mhGAP_intervention_guide/en/.

World Health Organization (WHO) (2011). *Mental health atlas 2011.* Retrieved January 6, 2014, from www.who.int/mental_health/publications/mental_health_atlas_2011/en/.

World Health Organization (WHO) (2012). *Depression: a global public health concern.* Developed by M. Marcus, M.T. Yasamy, M. van Ommeren, D. Chisholm, & S. Saxena. WHO Department of Mental Health and Substance Abuse. Retrieved January 6, 2014, from www.who.int/mental_health/management/depression/who_paper_depression_wfm h_2012.pdf.

World Health Organization (WHO) (2013). *Comprehensive mental health action plan 2013–2020* (sixty-sixth World Health Assembly, agenda item 13.3). Retrieved January 6, 2014, from http://apps.who.int/gb/ebwha/pdf_files/WHA66/A66_R8-en.pdf.

Wulsin, L.R., Vaillant, G.E., & Wells, V.E. (1999). A systematic review of the mortality of depression. *Psychosomatic Medicine, 61*(1), 6–17.

Xu, J., Kochanek, K.D., Murphy, S.L., & Tejada-Vera, B. (2010). *Deaths: final data for 2007.* Hyattsville, MD: US Department of Health and Human Services, CDC, National Center for Health Statistics.

14

STRATEGIES FOR HEALTH PROMOTION IN INDIVIDUALS EXPERIENCING BIPOLAR SYMPTOMS AND ILLNESS

Victoria Soltis-Jarrett

Introduction

This chapter will focus on bipolar disorder with a global perspective and will consider the social and cultural concepts that shape how nurses practice. It will endeavor to deconstruct some of the misconceptions that are buried beneath centuries of mythical rubble and will allow each reader to rebuild a practice of nursing that is culturally sensitive and clinically competent wherever they may live and/or work. A historical overview of the spectrum of bipolarity will provide a background for understanding how stigma and misconceptions have led to the marginalization of individuals and their families as well as suggestions for how to approach assessment, management and the potential referral of the individual who presents with the disorder's signs and symptoms with a focus on strategies in low- and middle-income countries.

Historical overview of bipolar disorder

The diagnosis of bipolar disorder has a complex narrative of signs, symptoms, and illness behaviors, which are fraught with multiple meanings that are rooted in ancient history. Some have asserted that its meaning and definition, like most psychiatric diagnoses, have been traditionally defined through the eyes and standards of one's own restricted social, cultural and gender experiences (Bartholomew, 1990; Soltis-Jarrett, 2003). Suffering from a mood disorder was derived from the notion of opposites or extremes: with depressive symptoms on one "pole" and mania on the other "pole." Those who suffered from both "poles" were labeled as "bipolar" or previously known as being a "manic-depressive," a term coined by Emil Kraepelin (1919) from his conceptual framework at the turn of the century, now known as the Kraepelinian dichotomy. Kraepelinian views were further expanded upon in the twentieth century as a spectrum or division of the symptomatology that included melancholia and psychosis, then manic-depression and subsequently manic-depressive disorder. Kraepelin may have drawn his knowledge from the Ancient Greek physicians who first described and documented an individual's shifts between two mood states. Pre-Hippocratic Greek physicians conceptualized their ideas from humoral theories speculating that disease and illness originated from the interaction between body liquids (in particular bile) and the brain (Angst, 2001):

> melancholia is the beginning and a part of mania . . . The development of a mania is really a worsening of the disease (melancholia) rather than a change into another disease . . . In most of them (melancholics), the sadness became better after various lengths of time and changed into happiness; the patients then developed a mania.
>
> *(Aretaeus of Cappadocia, 150 AD)*

Melancholia ("melas" means black, and "chole" means bile) described the symptoms of depression, while mania was less understood and began to take on a more mythical meaning such as Homer in his Iliad describing a reaction to an event with the meaning of rage, anger or excitation (Angst, 2001).

Over time, and depending upon the worldview, those individuals who were reported to suffer from "mood swings, " "manic-depression" or in some cultures, "a curse"; were believed to be afflicted from demonic possession, epilepsy, the bite of a tarantula, ergot poisoning, and even social adversity (Bartholomew, 1990). It has also been speculated that many of the women burned at the stake "as witches" during the Middle Ages were suffering from depression, mania or both. This scrutiny of "witches" also included those individuals who participated in medieval flagellation, dancing mania, lycanthropy (turning into a wolf) and demonology (Bootzin & Acocella, 1980; Duke & Nowicki, 1986; Meyer & Salmon, 1988). Philippe Pinel (1745–1826) used the terms "melancholic or maniac" to define the mood swings that he observed in his patients and documented in his seminal paper entitled "Memoir on Madness" in 1794 (Weiner, 1992). In the mid-1800s, Rudolf Virchow developed an influential theory that mental illnesses were a result of social and cultural maladjustment (Rosen, 1968). Many of these threads of value-laden beliefs continued to inform Western culture well into the twentieth century. In the fullness of time, they became twisted and skewed into other concepts, diagnoses and labels including hysteria, somatization (Soltis-Jarrett, 2003) and even being equated to being a "conscientious objector"; an individual (often women) who refuse to conform to social, legal and religious mores (Soltis-Jarrett, 2011). The modern term of "bipolar disorder" was reborn in 1966 from two separate landmark studies in Europe clarifying that manic-depressive illness is not homogenous with melancholia, and that unipolar depression differs significantly from the bipolar disorders in multiple ways including genetics, gender, course and pre-morbid personality (Angst, 2001). The focus on manic-depressive illness and the treatment of the symptoms were already in full force with the use of electroconvulsive therapy (Berrios, 1997) and the seminal work of John Cade in Australia in 1949, who tested the use of lithium citrate to treat and manage the mood instability (Cole, 2012).

By the twenty-first century, health care has also evolved and is more aligned as "illness care" with the relative morbidity increasing as a consequence of the improvement in general health indicators and longevity especially in middle- to low-income countries (Mari, 2013). The health care system in the USA is better known as an industry that continues to view the symptoms and signs of any psychiatric diagnosis with uncertainty and fear, which perpetuates stigma and silences those who do not have a voice. Health care in the USA also lags behind even though biological research has fast-forwarded the idea and conceptual model that mental health problems, symptoms, and illnesses are brain diseases, requiring sophisticated brain mapping and scanning, pharmaceutical applications, and indications for treatment. One could argue that it is much better than believing that mental health problems originate from a curse, a demonic possession and/or tarantula bite. The twenty-first century has taken a more civilized world view to mental illness, but still it appears to maintain the same oppressive linguistic meanings, just using a different name and a more manufactured approach to how it is translated into Eastern and Western culture, society, health and illness.

In summary, rather than focusing on a disease and illness model, mental health nurses globally need to maintain their belief of "wholism": that individuals are more than a sum of their parts (Aristotle, Metaphysica in Ross, 1924) and that nursing epistemologically focuses on care rather than cure; health promotion rather than illness treatment. This chapter will present the phenomenon of bipolar illness as it is known in medicine and psychiatry, and to reframe it to focus on the individual's experience and center on nursing care within a social and cultural context and with consideration of nurses that may live and work in low- to middle-income countries.

Clinical picture

The characteristics of bipolar disorder (BD) have been defined in a variety of ways globally using two different methods of classification, the *Diagnostic and Statistical Manual for Mental Disorders* (DSM) and the *International Classification of Disease* (ICD). The major difference between these two resources is that the ICD-10 does not discriminate between the classifications of bipolar I and II that are used in the DSM-5 (Phillips, 2013). Whether using either of the classification manuals, the term disorder or illness, both equate to significant suffering and often, a lifetime of disabling and chronic symptoms. Trends have suggested that bipolar illness is "over-diagnosed" in the US, yet the prevalence of this disorder is remarkably similar internationally, with a few notable differences between countries (Merikangas, Jin, He, Kessler, & Lee, 2011). In this particular international study, researchers focused on 11 countries and determined that the Cross-National Lifetime and 12-month Prevalence of Bipolar Disorder Sub-threshold (BPS) was calculated to be the highest for the United States (4.4 percent and 2.8 percent respectively) and the lowest for India, (0.1 percent and 0.1 percent respectively). This particular difference suggests that perhaps there are social and cultural variables that lend to how an illness is understood and managed in the context of the culture. For example, behaviors are determined to be normal or abnormal within a society's mores and cultural beliefs. It is therefore important for health care providers to consider this difference in the context of the individual's culture, community, and belief system.

When one considers the cultural context of any psychiatric illness (bipolar disorder in this instance), and uses the manuals and criteria that assign a diagnosis, both the DSM-5 and ICD-10 identify that the central characteristic of bipolar disorder is that of mood and behavioral changes that are marked by severe mood swings (manic or depressive episodes) and a tendency toward remission and recurrence (APA, 2013; WHO, 2010a). The changes in mood are conceptualized as being on a spectrum ranging from severe mania to severe depression as well as experiencing mixed and primarily depressive episodes. Other behavioral changes include: talking very fast, jumping from one idea to another, being "over restless," having little sleep and high energy, unrealistic beliefs in one's abilities, impulsivity to low mood, poor sleep with low energy, hopelessness, and low motivation. Although the lifetime prevalence of bipolar disorder in the USA and other Western cultures of similar social mores was also reported to be at 2.8 percent (Kessler, Ormel, Petukhova, & McLaughlin, 2011), it remains questionable whether the manuals (DSM and ICD) are being used to diagnose within the cultural context of the individual at hand, or if the manuals are being used as defined by the culture of those who authored the manuals. Outside of the USA, the *Diagnostic and Statistical Manual for Mental Disorders* is not necessarily the favored source for diagnostic guidance. Previous versions of the DSM have had years of criticism for its lack of cultural feasibility, acceptability and clinical utility related to patient-clinician communication despite its attempt to address cross-cultural issues as part of the psychiatric interview (Aggarwal, Desilva, Nicasio, Boller, & Lewis-Fernandez, 2015).

The Cultural Formulation Interview (CFI) is a cross-cultural assessment tool that was developed as part of the most recent version of the *Diagnostic and Statistical Manual* (DSM-5) and was specifically created to address the shortcomings from the DSM-IV Outline for Cultural Formulation (OCF) (Aggarwal *et al.*, 2015). Interview questions were created to consider the cross-cultural differences between the clinician and the patient. An example includes questions such as: "Is there anything about your background, for example your culture, race, ethnicity, religion or geographical origin that is causing problems for you in your current life situation? In what way?" (Aggarwal *et al.*, 2015). These questions are important for any clinician to consider and use when interviewing or caring for individuals of color and ethnicity as well as individuals of different sexual orientation, gender, and/or economic stratification (class, status, power).

Approximately four million people suffer from bipolar disorder in the USA and 60 million people worldwide (Substance Abuse and Mental Health Services Administration, 2012; WHO, 2010b). This chronic illness and potentially fatal disorder is also associated with a higher occurrence of attempted suicide than most other psychiatric disorders (Kessler, Chui, Demler, Merikangas, & Walters, 2005). Even by conservative standards, 82.9 percent of the four million cases in the USA are classified as "severe," with 48.8 percent of those receiving some form of health care treatment (Kessler, 2005). However, in low- and middle-income countries, many individuals with bipolar illness are inadequately treated, because of lack of access to treatment, lack of response to medications prescribed to decrease and manage the distressing symptoms, and/or lack of providers who can evaluate and manage the symptoms (Merikangas *et al.*, 2011). Overall, those individuals who suffer from manic or hypomanic episodes are socially and functionally impaired; and many also suffer from multiple comorbidities associated with poor health outcomes, particularly in low- and middle-income countries (Kessler *et al.*, 2011). Individuals who suffer from this chronic illnesses are likely to have a reduction of 9.2 years in life expectancy, and as many as 20 percent of individuals with bipolar disorder complete suicide (Kessler *et al.*, 2011).

Bipolar disorder can be divided into three specific symptom clusters as well as a mixed state of two or more: mania, hypomania and depression (APA, 2013). The severity of the symptom clusters varies extensively among those who suffer from this disorder and the prognosis is equally unpredictable. The majority (54 percent) of those individuals diagnosed with bipolar disorder over the span of their lifetime, reported presenting as "depressed" in their first episode of the illness (Baldessarini, 2014). To this end, nurses and clinicians need to be aware that a first presentation of depression needs to be assessed thoroughly and managed with caution. A comprehensive psychiatric evaluation and consideration of differential diagnoses need to be at the forefront, especially when medications are first initiated and titrated up to a higher dose. The danger and incidence of creating an iatrogenic illness is possible when using some classes of antidepressants (such as Selected Serotonin Reuptake Inhibitors: SSRIs) with individuals who have a family history of bipolar illness, a previous history of hypomania or mania and/or multiple trials of antidepressants (Goldberg, 2003).

Etiology

The etiology of bipolar disorders is not clearly known or understood. And some researchers have stated that from a neurobiological perspective, there is no such thing as bipolar disorder (Maletic, 2014). However, despite these "unknowns," researchers have proposed that its insidious symptoms and natural history may more likely involve a synergy of biological, psychological, and social factors.

Family studies (including twin and to a lesser extent, adoption) have revealed that genetic influences may be involved in the pathogenesis of what is called bipolarity (Barnett, 2009) and that there may be several common polymorphisms that affect susceptibility to its development in families. Examples of this model included variants within the genes CACNA1C, ODZ4, and NCAN and studies that demonstrate identical-twin concordance rates ranging from 40 percent to 70 percent, with the estimated heritability reaching as high as 90 percent in the most recent reports (Craddock, 2013). There is a paucity of information cross-culturally comparing genetic influences especially in low-income countries where access to assessment, treatment, and services were poor and/or lacking (Merikangas *et al.*, 2011).

However, it is known from previous studies published a few decades ago, that a first-degree relative of an individual with bipolar disorder is actually more likely to meet diagnostic criteria for recurrent unipolar depression than for any other diagnosis, including bipolar disorder (McGuffin, 1989). This has led clinicians to the assumption that for individuals with an established bipolar illness presentation, a family history of mood or psychotic illness is common among other members of a family and has extended to other generations. This model now asserts that there is a significant relationship between bipolar illness and schizophrenia and that bipolar disorder is genetically more closely related to schizophrenia than major depressive disorder (Lee, 2013; Smoller, 2013). Regardless of the similarities between diagnoses, a family history of bipolar disorder and/or schizophrenia is an important clinical predictor of the course of the illness and frequently an individual will present with one or more episodes of depression even before their first episode of psychosis, mood elevation, hypomania, or mania (Craddock, 2013).

Probably the most exciting and innovative work in the twenty-first century has focused on the notion of bipolarity as a neurodevelopmental disorder that begins at the cellular level (Maletic, 2014); and with the concurrence of psychological abuse (stress diathesis model) and social discordance, will progress, looking differently at each stage, across the lifespan. In this etiological model, Maletic (2014) asserts that the combination of brain changes, the interaction between multiple genetic factors and life adversities may begin to explain the neurogenesis of the disease and the hope for new treatment to manage its debilitating symptoms.

Introduction to evidence-based prevention and mental health promotion strategies

Mental health nurses are in a unique position to use their knowledge of caring, health promotion, and disease prevention to implement strategies in their practice and their communities. What are the strategies that parallel the epistemology of nursing and in particular the specialty knowledge of psychiatric-mental health nurses in the twenty-first century?

Probably first and foremost, it is the assertion that nurses provide "care" rather than a "cure." It is well known that illnesses such as bipolar disorder are chronic and debilitating, often beginning in childhood and worsening over adolescence and adulthood. It is also known that comorbidities are common among those who suffer from chronic illnesses, shortening their lives after years of functional and social disability. Individuals with bipolar disorder have an increased prevalence of cardio- and cerebrovascular disease, metabolic, and endocrine disorders (Post *et al.*, 2014). With this knowledge at hand, it is important to consider strategies that are focused on *prevention and health promotion* as well as treatment and care of the individual's suffering from the symptoms of the illness at hand. Being able to distinguish between hypomania, mania, and depression is the first step to selecting an appropriate evidence-based intervention and then determining the symptom cluster in the current episode is the second step. The following section will focus on the evidence based strategies that parallel the epistemology of nursing practice, focusing on three specific areas followed by a list of evidence-based practices: (a) promoting health and preventing morbidity; (b) acute phase of treatment; and (c) long-term or sustaining treatments that honor the individual and their families.

Promoting health and preventing morbidity: defining recovery in the twenty-first century

Recovery is a process of change through which individuals improve their health and wellness, live a self-directed life, and strive to reach their full potential (Substance Abuse and Mental Health Services Administration, 2012).

Recovery in its broadest sense is linked to how one's culture defines health and illness. Models in the twenty-first century emphasize that the patient (or consumer) of health care services must be central to the assessment, planning, and evaluation of their recovery and therefore collaboration is crucial between health care providers, individuals with mental health problems, and their families. Reports indicate that only 25 percent of those with bipolar disorder in low-income countries and only one-third of those in middle-income countries seek mental health services, (Merikangas *et al.*, 2011). It is then recommended that mental health nurses consider other options for increasing access to mental health services when there is a lack in health care providers or lack of services (WHO, 2010b). The training of non-mental health nurses and community members to learn to be competent in mental health assessment and basic management skills is a promising strategy for linking individuals suffering from mental health problems within a community/culture to those who are known to them (e.g. nurses). Not only does this promote trust and the potential for improved health care and illness management, it also empowers the community as a whole to learn how to interact with those who are unwell in order to understand their behaviors rather than to marginalize the individual and their family who are suffering.

This is also extremely important because health disparities are borne by an environment that breeds stigma, prejudice, and discrimination among belief systems, cultural mores, and people that are different from the mainstream population. This lack of understanding, and behaviors associated with the abuse of power and blatant disregard for humanity and benevolence among people who are diverse, bears witness to many of the atrocities that have accumulated both historically and currently in the twenty-first century. The mayhem occurs in countries where inequities, bias and preconceived notions abound across the socioeconomic spectrum. Cultural sensitivity and psychoeducation provides a light to shine in the darkness that perpetuates the dissonance and lack of parity among many populations. The next section addresses several evidence-based strategies and practices that may be useful for nurses working in low- to middle-income countries to use when working with individuals who present as having a bipolar disorder.

Evidence-based practice 1: cultural sensitivity is at the core of any local or global health care strategy focusing on bipolar disorder

Nurses must ensure that the cultural context of the individual, their family, and/or any community they serve is at the core of, and provides the foundation for, any health care strategy, intervention, or plan. As well, nurses must have the willingness, knowledge and skills to work within that cultural context. Acknowledging your own values, bias and judgments is paramount to caring for any individual, family, or global community. Recognizing one's own limitations and strengths is also part of any evidence-based practice.

In the context of bipolar disorder, nurses need to take time to elicit the individual's (and their family's) understanding and meaning of their illness. In many cultures, having a psychiatric illness is abhorrent and often shunned. As previously stated, mental health and illness in general has historical roots laden with bias, values, and preconceived judgments. This is best illustrated in an article articulated by a Chinese woman with bipolar disorder, who migrated to Canada from Hong Kong (Kwok, 2014). In her own words, the author speaks of the need for individuals to be empowered to learn self-management skills, such as being able to identify the triggers of illness, the signs of decline and the resources to remain healthy and well. Through the use of social support, a meaningful occupation, and the foundation of spiritual fulfillment, Kwok (2014) was able to express her *raisons d'être* in the world and more importantly, the limitations of a traditional clinical model of recovery for her.

Evidence-based practice 2: using mhGAP as a screening tool and guide for initiating basic management strategies

The mhGAP Intervention Guide for Mental, Neurological and Substance Use Disorders in Non-Specialized Health Settings (WHO, 2010b) is a standardized assessment and guide for management of several common mental health problems. Designed for use by non-psychiatric nurses and clinicians, this WHO guide focuses on providing clear steps towards providing excellent, safe and culturally sensitive mental health care. The section on bipolar disorders offers an algorithm for screening, brief interventions and referral. The WHO asserts that expensive treatments are not always the best, nor the preferred choice for individuals and their families, rather, having choices is the key component to empowerment and the promotion of health, wellness, and recovery.

The most important aspects of bipolar disorder are addressed and used as screening measures in order to assist the health care provider to determine the severity of the illness episode.

Examples of screening questions to differentiate the likelihood of bipolar disorder are:

• Is the person in a manic state?
• Does the person have a known prior episode of mania but now has depression?

Strategies for management using the mhGAP for bipolar disorders reflect the current international best practices for bipolar disorder including using medications (e.g. mood stabilizers such as valproate acid for mania or benzodiazepines such as diazepam for agitation) that are affordable and often available due to their use for other illness states such as epilepsy. Highlighting the importance of discontinuing and/or not initiating an anti-depressant medication is clearly indicated as it is contraindicated for use in those with mania and can potentially worsen their symptoms and illness presentation.

Comorbidities are also important to address, as well as planning ahead using anticipatory guidance and prevention of another episode of illness. Nurses can consider questions such as: Is the individual not currently manic or depressed but has a history of mania? If so, then the guide offers the opportunity for initiating a mood stabilizer as a means for preventing another episode. Finally, the algorithm also specifically addressed the notion of whether the individual is in a special group: elderly, adolescent or pregnant/breast-feeding. Indications for referral are highlighted, yet strategies for management can empower any health care provider to initiate treatment with confidence.

Evidence-based practice 3: using psychoeducation as a means for empowerment

Knowledge is power, and teaching basic skills to individuals and their families in the area of self-care management is a best practice. Nurses are ideally poised to provide psychoeducation in their communities with a focus on self-care. Identifying a community's unique needs is necessary for developing this particular type of program so that the objectives are focused on strategies that not only teach and empower the individuals that are suffering from bipolar disorder, but also consider the needs of their families, friends, and the communities where they live and interact. One nursing study out of the Netherlands surveyed individuals diagnosed with bipolar disorder (*n* = 157) using a Need for Care Questionnaire (NCQ). The results highlighted that the individuals (with bipolar disorder) identified needing education and support focused on social functioning, activities of daily living, and financial and administrative skills (Goossens, Knoppert-Van Der Klein, Kroon, & Van Achterberg, 2007). Issues such as "clarification of problems," "discovery of what you want in life," and "gaining more confidence" were highly ranked as important and desired needs for that particular population, in the community that was surveyed.

Nurses in low- and middle-income countries without resources for implementing formal needs assessments may want to consider holding focus groups with individuals diagnosed with bipolar disorder (and their families) as a means for gathering information about their community's specific learning needs, as well as providing a venue for social support among both individuals and their families/friends. Reactivating social networks is a strategy recommended by WHO to promote individuals to seek out "direct or indirect psychosocial support" such as attending family gatherings, agreeing to see friends, visiting neighbors, and attending social activities such as sports and/or community events (WHO, 2010b, p. 27).

Evidence-based practice 4: advanced pharmaceutical management of mania in the acute and maintenance phases of illness

There is no doubt that the discovery and use of pharmacological agents such as Lithium Carbonate have had a major impact on the health and well-being of those individuals (and their families) who suffer from the symptoms of bipolar disorder. Just in the past few decades, the notion of having two distinct forms of the illness (bipolar, manic and bipolar, depressed) have surfaced, again positively and negatively impacting the prognosis over the individual's lifespan. The assessment and diagnosis of bipolar disorder according to the DSM-5 (APA, 2013) continues to be debated and challenging even to the most skilled clinicians (Phillips, 2013). For the purposes of this section, it will be important to delineate between the evidence in terms of acute phase and long-term management of bipolar symptoms, including episodes of primarily depression and those primarily of mania or hypomania.

As previously mentioned, the mhGAP (WHO, 2010b) is an ideal tool to use for non-mental health nurses and clinicians. However, there are additional algorithms that can be used to manage the severe and persistent symptoms of the disorders especially in countries where generic medications may be available and nurses are able to practice at an advanced level.

Algorithms and/or clinical practice guidelines for using psychotropic medications as one intervention for the acute and maintenance phases of bipolar disorder is well documented (Fountoulakisa *et al.*, 2005; Maletic, 2014; Nivoli, 2011; Saddichha, 2014). Mood stabilizers are ideally the first line of treatment indicated for both the acute and long-term phases of treatment. Studies dating back to the mid-twentieth century were able to illuminate the possibility of providing stabilization and calming of the manic and depressive mood swings reported in the disorder (versus the experimental use of lithium in the treatment of gout) (Malhi, 2014). However, its efficacious response is yet to be explained in terms of mechanisms of action (Burrows, 1999). There are approximately 10–12 different sources of information guiding clinicians to using psychotropic medications for the acute and long-term management of bipolar illness spectrum globally (Saddichha, 2014). Algorithms for the acute to long-term phases of treatment are available and cover a wide range of international expertise (Fountoulakisa *et al.*, 2005).

Overall, Lithium Carbonate is still considered to be the drug of choice for a first, second or third episode of acute mania and if not well tolerated, then use of valproate and/or carbamazepine is recommended. Valproate and carbamazepine, used for treatment of seizure disorders are thought to work in a similar manner, "calming the irritable brain" symptoms that occur during a manic phase of bipolar disorder. Other algorithms have suggested that atypical antipsychotics such as olanzapine or risperidone be used as first line treatments for mania (Nivoli, 2011; Saddichha, 2014). In low- and middle-income countries where atypical antipsychotics may not be available, haloperidol is an excellent option for symptoms of acute mania (Mari, 2013).

There does seem to be some consensus among clinicians and researchers that severity of the symptoms of the disorder need to determine the long-term treatment regimen (Phillips, 2013; Saddichha, 2014) and it is critical to determine whether medications are needed for the symptoms of hypomania (the less severe symptom cluster related to mania). Evidence of suicidal or homicidal ideation or behaviors, aggression, psychosis (e.g. delusions or hallucinations), and/or poor judgment that places the individual at risk for being harmed (e.g. having unprotected multiple sexual partners, driving recklessly) have been identified as a starting place for determining severity and are frequently related to an episode of mania. The combined use of substances (such as alcohol or other illicit drugs) with severe risk-taking behaviors, add to the seriousness and often lethal nature of the episode and disorder overall and have guided clinicians to choose psychotropic medication precipitously.

In countries where available, long-lasting injectables have also been a consideration when adherence to the treatment regimen is difficult or unpredictable. Some expert clinicians have recommended that global, unified guidelines need to be developed for all psychiatric illnesses to lessen the confusion and improve health care outcomes (Saddichha, 2014). Table 14.1 includes some of the other psychotropic medications that have been approved for use in the USA as well as globally for the acute and long-term phases of mania.

Evidence-based practice 5: advanced pharmaceutical management of depression in bipolar disorder

The treatment of depressive episodes as part of the bipolar spectrum creates another variable in an already difficult treatment regimen. Frequently, an antidepressant used in combination with a mood stabilizer (lithium carbonate and/or lamotrigine) is the first-line choice although recent studies have indicated that a combination of olanzapine and fluoxetine is also efficacious (Brown, 2009; Frank, 1991). In low- to middle-income countries where this combination is not available, fluoxetine is the first line of treatment along with the adjunctive treatment of a mood stabilizer also prescribed to manage the risk of the adverse effects of switching the individual into a manic phase (Mari, 2013).

Randomized trials of second generation atypical antipsychotic medications (i.e. quetiapine, lurasidone, and olanzapine) have also been shown to be efficacious as a first-line choice (Brown, 2009; Chiesa, 2012; Loebel, 2014). However, the Federal Drug Administration in the USA has only approved two (quetiapine and the combination of fluoxetine/olanzapine) for the treatment of bipolar disorder, depressed (Gutman, 2007).

Table 14.1 Medications used in the treatment of bipolar disorder and acute mania

Mood stabilizers	First generation antipsychotic medications	Second generation antipsychotic medications	Combination medications
Lithium Divalproex, divalproex ER Carbamazepine ER Lamotrigine	Haloperidol	Olanzapine Risperidone Quetiapine, quetiapine XR Ziprasidone Aripiprazole Asenapine Paliperidone ER	Olanzapine fluoxetine

Evidence-based practice 6: psychotherapy as a primary or adjunctive treatment for individuals and their families

Psychotherapy for the treatment of mood disorders has gained a great deal of momentum over the past 50 years (Picardi, 2014) and strong empirical evidence suggests that cognitive behavioral therapy (CBT), interpersonal psychotherapy (IPT) as well as brief psychodynamic psychotherapy are useful in the treatment of the acute and chronic phases of illness associated with mood disorders (Guidi, 2011; Scott, 2006). CBT and IPT have been shown to be as efficacious as the use of medications, such as antidepressants, in the treatment of major depressive disorder (Hollon, 2010), and in many cases, the success of psychotherapy begins with educating the individual and their family about the illness and prognosis (Deckersbach, 2000). Family psychoeducational groups have also been effective and empirically tested for assisting family members to better understand the symptoms, treatments and long-term needs of individuals with mood disorders and have been instrumental in providing the social support and empathy needed to learn to live with a chronic and often debilitating disease (Bond, 2015).

Interpersonal and social rhythm therapy (IPSRT) is a type of individual psychotherapy treatment that is specifically designed for individuals diagnosed with bipolar disorder (Frank, 2000) and has been empirically tested over the past 15 years. IPSRT fundamentally asserts that in order to teach individuals how to manage the chaos of their illness: irregular sleep–wake cycles, symptom/mood instability and a clinical course that is often unpredictable and rarely static, treatment needs to address the psycho-chronobiological theory of the mood disorder. It combines the notion of the biopsychosocial dimensions of the illness, considering the genetic components, the chaotic, often unpredictable emotional and physical symptoms with the potential for stressful life events (Frank, 2000). The balancing of three types of treatments, over time, assists the individual and their social support (family) to learn how to recognize, plan, and self-manage the symptoms of bipolar disorder. IPSRT is a manual-based psychotherapy with an entire website devoted to its mission and goals (see www.ipsrt.org/).

In low- to middle-income countries with limited resources, the focus is to engage the individual and their family first and foremost (Mari, 2013). Psychoeducation as an intervention is an essential part of nursing care and is considered supportive psychotherapy. Explaining the signs and symptoms of the illness as well as the risk factors and when to seek professional help are key to promoting health and wellness. Nurses are ideally poised to offer the individual and their family support, alone or in groups of families in the communities where they live and work. Way to demystify the illness and explaining the importance of health-promotion strategies

Table 14.2 Summary of nursing strategies for health promotion in individuals experiencing bipolar symptoms and illness in low- to middle-income countries

Nursing strategies	Individual	Family	Multi-family
Engage and develop trust, empathy and compassion	X	X	X
Demystify the illness: it is not a "curse"	X	X	X
Teach signs and symptoms of bipolar disorder: mania, hypomania, depression	X	X	X
Encourage self-care for the individual: sleep, diet and support	X		
Teach when to ask for help from family	X		
Teach how to calm the irritability		X	X
Review what to do if the symptoms worsen		X	X
Teach adverse effects of medications and what to do	X	X	X
Discuss risk factors with families related to be aware of suicidal and homicidal ideation		X	X

are listed in Table 14.2 and can be used as a guide for individual or family education sessions. If trained professionals are available, cognitive behavioral therapy (CBT) is an excellent intervention for assisting both the individual and their family with techniques for managing milder symptoms and also for periods of stability and maintenance.

Summary

The evidence demonstrating best practices for the assessment and management of the symptoms of bipolar disorder are well documented and point to the need to consider the biopsychosocial and cultural facets of individuals, families, and communities that are suffering from psychiatric illnesses. In this chapter, the importance of cultural sensitivity cannot be emphasized enough, as often the social determinants of health weigh heavily on the health outcomes of individuals and their families. The first (and in many cases, most important) step in ascertaining the promotion of health and prevention of bipolar illness is to consider the culture and community where the individual comes from, lives, and thrives. Understanding the health beliefs, practices, cultural and linguistic needs of diverse individuals and communities at any point in the nursing process impacts the trust, respect and interpersonal relationship that nurses have with those that they care for and serve. Using this knowledge and promoting cultural sensitivity guide best practice in nursing and for all health care delivery.

References

Aggarwal, N., Desilva, R., Nicasio, A., Boller, M., & Lewis-Fernandez, R. (2015). Does the Cultural Formulation Interview for the fifth revision of the *Diagnostic and Statistical Manual or Mental Disorders* affect medical communication? *Ethnicity and Health*, 20(1), 1–28.

Angst, J.M. (2001). Bipolarity from ancient to modern times. *Journal of Affective Disorders*, 671–3), 3–19.

American Psychiatric Association. (2013). *Diagnostic and Statistical Manual of Mental Disorders*, 5th edition. Washington, DC: APA.

Baldessarini, R.J. (2014). First-episode types in bipolar disorder: predictive associations with later illness. *Acta Psychiatrica Scandinavica*, 129(5), 383–392.

Barnett, J.H. (2009). The genetics of bipolar disorder. *Neuroscience*, 14(4), 331–343.

Bartholomew, R. (1990). Ethnocentricity and the social construction of mass hysteria. *Culture, Medicine and Psychiatry*, 14(4), 455–494.

Berrios, G. (1997). The scientific origins of electroconvulsive therapy: a conceptual history. *History Psychiatry*, 18(29), 105–119.

Bond, K. (2015). Psychoeducation for relapse prevention in bipolar disorder: a systematic review of efficacy in randomized controlled trials. *Bipolar Disorder*, 17(4), 349–362.

Bootzin, R.R. & Acocella, J.R. (1980). *Abnormal Psychology: Current Perspectives*. New York: Random House.

Brown E. (2009). Olanzapine/fluoxetine combination vs. lamotrigine in the 6-month treatment of bipolar I depression. *International Journal of Neuropsychopharmacology*, 12(6), 773–782.

Burrows, G.T. (1999). Cade's observation of the antimanic effect of lithium and early Australian research. *Australian and New Zealand Journal of Psychiatry*, 33 Suppl, S27–S31.

Chiesa A. (2012). Quetiapine for bipolar depression: a systematic review and meta-analysis. *International Clinical Psychopharmacology*, 27(2), 76–90.

Cole, B. (2012). Cade's identification of lithium for manaic-depressive illness: the prospector who found a gold nugget. *Nervous and Mental Disease*, 200(12), 1101–1104.

Craddock N. (2013). Genetics of bipolar disorder. *The Lancet*, 381(9878), 1654–1662.

Deckersbach T. (2000). Cognitive-behavioral therapy for depression: applications and outcome. *Psychiatric Clinics of North America*, 23(4), 795–809.

Duke, M. & Nowicki, S. (1986). *Abnormal Psychology: A New Look*. New York: Holt, Rinehart & Winston.

Fountoulakisa, E., Vietab, E., Sanchez-Morenob, J., Kaprinisa, S., Goikoleab, J., & Kaprinis, G. (2005). Treatment guidelines for bipolar disorder: A critical review. *Journal of Affective Disorders*, 86(1), 1–10.

Frank E. (1991). Conceptualization and rationale for consensus definitions of terms in major depressive disorder: remission, recovery, relapse, and recurrence. *Archives of General Psychiatry*, 48(9), 851–855.

Frank, E.S. (2000). Interpersonal and social rhythm therapy: managing the chaos of bipolar disorder. *Biological Psychiatry*, 48(6), 593–604.

Goldberg, J.F. (2003). Antidepressant-induced mania: an overview of current controversies. *Bipolar Disorders*, 14(6), 407–420.

Goossens, P., Knoppert-Van Der Klein, E., Kroon, H., & Van Achterberg, T. (2007). Self-reported care needs of outpatients with a bipolar disorder in the Netherlands. *Journal of Psychiatric and Mental Health Nursing*, 14(6), 549–557.

Guidi, J. (2011). Efficacy of the sequential integration of psychotherapy and pharmacotherapy in major depressive disorder: a preliminary meta-analysis. *Psychological Medicine*, 41(2), 321–331.

Gutman, D.N. (2007). *Medscape Education*. Retrieved March 12, 2015, from atypical antipsychotics in bipolar disorder: www.medscape.org/viewarticle/554128.

Hollon, S.D. (2010). A review of empirically supported psychological therapies for mood disorders in adults. *Depression and Anxiety*, 27(10), 891–932.

Kessler, R.C., Chill, W.T., Demler, O., Merikangas, K.R., & Walters, E.E. (2005). Prevalence, severity, and comorbidity of 12-month DSM-IV disorders in the National Comorbidity Survey Replication (NCS-R). *Archives of General Psychiatry*, 62(6), 617–627.

Kessler, R.C., Ormel, J., Petukhova, M., & McLaughlin, K. (2011). Development of lifetime comorbidity in the World Health Organization World Mental Health Surveys. *Archives of General Psychiatry*, 68(1), 90–100.

Kraepelin, E. (1919). *Manic-Depressive Insanity and Paranoia*. (trans. R.M. Barclay). Edinburgh, UK: Livingstone.

Kwok, C. (2014). Beyond the clinical model of recovery: recovery of a Chinese immigrant woman with bipolar disorder. *East Asian Archives of Psychiatry*, 24(3), 129–133.

Lee, S.R. (2013). Genetic relationship between five psychiatric disorders estimated from genome-wide SNPs. *Nature Genetics*, 45(9), 984–994.

Loebel, A. (2014). Lurasidone monotherapy in the treatment of bipolar I depression: a randomized, double-blind, placebo-controlled study. *American Journal of Psychiatry*, 17(2), 160–168.

McGuffin, P.K.R. (1989). The genetics of depression and manic-depressive disorder. *British Journal of Psychiatry*, 155, 294–304.

Maletic, V. (2014). Integrated neurobiology of bipolar disorder. *Frontiers in Psychiatry*, 25(5), 98.

Malhi, G. (2014). Cade's lithium: an extraordinary experiment with a not-so-ordinary element. *Medical Journal of Australia*, 201(1), 24–25.

Mari, J.T. (2013). Pharmacological and psychosocial management of mental, neurological and substance use disorders in low- and middle-income countries: issues and current strategies. *Drugs*, 73(14), 1549–1568.

Merikangas, K., Jin, R., He, J., Kessler, R., & Lee, S. (2011). Prevalence and correlates of bipolar spectrum disorder in the world mental health organization survey initiative. *Archives of General Psychiatry*, 68(3), 241–251.

Meyer, R.G. & Salmon, P. (1988). *Abnormal Psychology*. Boston, MA: Allyn & Bacon.

Nivoli, A.C. (2011). New treatment guidelines for acute bipolar depression: a systematic review. *Journal of Affective Disorders*, 129(1–3), 14–26.

Phillips, M.K. (2013). Bipolar disorder diagnosis: challenges and future directions. *The Lancet*, 381(9878), 1663–1671.

Picardi, A. (2014). Psychotherapy of mood disorders. *Clinical Practice & Epidemiolgy in Mental Health*, 26(10), 140–158.

Post, R., Altschuler, L., Leverich, G., Frye, M., Suppes, T., McElroy, S., & Keck, P.E. (2014). More medical comorbities in patients with bipolar disorder in the United States than in the Netherlands and Germany. *Journal of Nervous and Mental Disorders*, 202(4), 265–270.

Rosen, G. (1968). *Madness in Society: Chapters in the Historical Sociology of Mental Illness*. London: Routledge & Kegan Paul.

Ross, W.D. (1923). *Aristotle*. London: Methuen & Co.

Saddichha, S.C. (2014). Clinical practice guidelines in psychiatry: more confusion than clarity? A critical review and recommendation of a unified guideline. *ISRN Psychiatry*, March 31, 828917. Doi: 10.1155/2014/828917.

Scott, J. (2006). Psychotherapy for bipolar disorders: efficacy and effectiveness. *Journal of Psychopharmacolgy*, 20(2 Suppl), 46–50.

Seedat S. (2009). Cross-national associations between gender and mental disorders in the World Health Organization World Mental Health Surveys. *Archives of General Psychiatry*, 66(7), 785–795.

Smoller, J.C. (2013). Identification of risk loci with shared effects on five major psychiatric disorders: a genome-wide analysis. *The Lancet*, 381(9875), 1371–1379.

Soltis-Jarrett, V. (2003). *Finding the Health in Illness: Challenging the Concept of Somatization in Women*. Adelaide, South Australia: Flinders University of South Australia.

Soltis-Jarrett, V. (2011, October). His-story or her-story: deconstruction of the concepts of somatization towards a new approach in advanced nursing practice care. *Perspectives in Psychiatric Care*, 47(4), 183–193.

Substance Abuse and Mental Health Services Administration. (2014, August 29). *Behavioral Health Equity*. Retrieved January 15, 2015, from Substance Abuse and Mental Health Services Administration: www.samhsa.gov/behavioral-health-equity.

Weiner, A. (1992). *Inalienable Possessions: The Paradox of Keeping-While-Giving*. Berkeley, CA: University of California Press.

World Health Organization. (2010a). *International Statistical Classification of Diseases and Related Health Problems, 10th Revision*. Geneva: WHO.

World Health Organization. (2010b). *mhGAP Intervention Guide for Mental, Neurological and Substance Use Disorders in Non-Specialized Health Setting: Mental Health Gap Action Programme (mhGAP)*. Geneva: WHO.

15

SCHIZOPHRENIA

Fostering understanding and facilitating health promotion

Ann J. Sheridan

Introduction

According to the World Health Organisation (WHO) determinants of mental health and mental disorders extend far beyond the ability of individuals to manage their personal thoughts and emotions, behaviours and interactions with others. Determinants of mental health and mental disorder are critically located within social, cultural, economic and political factors as well as environmental factors such as national policies, social protection, living standards, working conditions and community social supports (WHO, 2013).

Schizophrenia and schizophrenia spectrum diseases are a leading worldwide public health problem, which impact at personal, family, community and economic levels. Due to the extensiveness of the associated deficits and lifetime course, schizophrenia is considered to be among the top 10 leading causes of disease related disability in the world (WHO, 2001). Found in all sections of society and geographic locations, schizophrenia is frequently described as a disease of variable but severely disruptive psychopathology that involves, cognition, emotions, perception and other aspects of behaviour, the expression of which varies across patients and over time, but effects of this disease are generally considered to be severe and long lasting.

The purpose of this chapter is to provide an overview of the current state of evidence-based knowledge relating to schizophrenia as a serious mental health concern as well as the key areas where health promotion interventions can be addressed. The first half of the chapter presents an overview of the incidence and prevalence of schizophrenia along with a very brief review of the genesis of the concept of schizophrenia. The pathogenesis, features, course and consequences of this illness are then presented. The second half of the chapter examines some of the core issues identified as amenable to health-promoting interventions in schizophrenia and identifies some of the key intervention areas where nurses can act to promote good mental health among people with schizophrenia, their families and the communities in which they live.

Incidence and prevalence

According to Baxter, Patton, Scott, Degenhardt and Whiteford (2013) one quarter of high-income countries and 1 in 14 low- and middle-income countries provide data on schizophrenia.

While estimates of the incidence and prevalence rates of health-related disorders including schizophrenia assist in providing a global picture of the condition, a degree of caution is required in utilising these estimates as the vast majority of the data used in calculation of rates for schizophrenia emanate from high-income countries, particularly in Western Europe and North America (Baxter *et al.*, 2013). While it has long been assumed that rates of schizophrenia are uniform across all regions and populations, there is evidence that variation in the incidence of schizophrenia exists, with male gender, migration and urbanicity associated with a higher risk of developing the disease (MacDonald & Schulz, 2009; McGrath *et al.*, 2004). Risks associated with urbanicity appear to be related to several factors including being born and reared in an urban area up to the age of 15 years; higher rates of cannabis and other substance use in urban areas; poverty, social stress, social disconnectedness and migration; environmental toxins, infections and vitamin deficiency (Tandon, Keshavan, & Nasrallah, 2008). Personal and family history of migration has also been identified as a significant risk factor in schizophrenia (Cantor-Graae & Selten 2005; Tandon *et al.*, 2008) with social adversity including isolation, racism and discrimination cited as major contributors in migration (Cooper *et al.*, 2008). The lifetime risk of developing schizophrenia differs for males and females, with males up to four times more likely to develop the disease (MacDonald & Schluz, 2009; Tandon *et al.*, 2008; Tandon, Shah, Keshavan, & Tandon, 2012). However, Xiang *et al.* (2008) identified that while prevalence rates for schizophrenia were largely similar to those of other countries, women in both urban and rural areas of Beijing were more likely to be diagnosed with schizophrenia. This difference may, according to Xiang *et al.* (2008), be associated with the level of discrimination and increased household and financial burdens experienced by women. The existing evidence identifies that schizophrenia is a disease that persists over prolonged periods with an affected person living with the disease for approximately 30 years. Median point prevalence or the prevalence of schizophrenia that exists in a population over a defined time period is estimated at 4.6 per 1000, while the lifetime prevalence of schizophrenia is estimated at 4.0 per 1000 (Saha, Change, Welhan, & McGrath, 2005).

Pathogenesis of schizophrenia

Schizophrenia has been studied as a major disease entity for over a century. However, despite this, the origins and development of schizophrenia as a disease remain obscure. Over the past century scientists and clinicians worldwide have endeavoured to locate and understand the causes of schizophrenia and in attempting to do so, a wide range of theories and hypothesis have been proposed and investigated. While significant progress has been made in understanding the pathogenesis of schizophrenia, the identification of definitive causes or combination of causative factors remains some way off.

Since the early years of the twentieth century it has been recognised that structural alterations were identifiable in the brains of people with schizophrenia. Initially, such explorations were only possible using invasive techniques on living subjects, but were identified more frequently on post-mortem examination. Developments in diagnostic tools and technologies now facilitate examination of brain structures and processes in non-invasive ways. These investigations have confirmed that within the brain of people with schizophrenia the total volume of grey matter is reduced while ventricular volume is increased (Lawrie, McIntosh, Hall, Owens & Johnstone, 2008; Sun *et al.*, 2008). Volumetric reductions in the brain are also evident in the temporal lobe structures including hippocampus and amygdala; the pre-frontal cortex, thalamus and corpus callosum (Lawrie *et al.*, 2008; Sun *et al.*, 2008). Whether these changes are causative or result from schizophrenia remains unclear. While it is recognised that schizophrenia and its treatment, particularly typical antipsychotic medications, may be instrumental in some of these changes, there is some evidence of the pre-existence of structural alterations at illness onset, at first episode psychosis and in treatment of naïve patients (Gur *et al.*, 2007; Vita *et al.*, 2006). Volumetric reductions in white brain matter have also been reported in schizophrenia and these changes appear to be correlated with cognitive impairments. Evidence is also accumulating, which suggests that an active disease process may be taking place in high-risk individuals who subsequently transition to psychosis when compared to those who do not transition (Sun *et al.*, 2008). Figures 15.1 and 15.2 illustrate areas of the brain impacted by the disease process of schizophrenia.

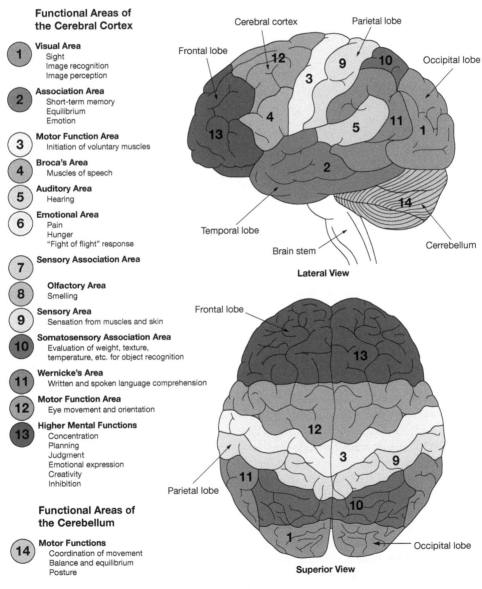

Figure 15.1 Anatomy and functional areas of the brain

Source: Texila University found at http://blog.tauedu.org/anatomy-and-functional-areas-of-the-brain

Ann J. Sheridan

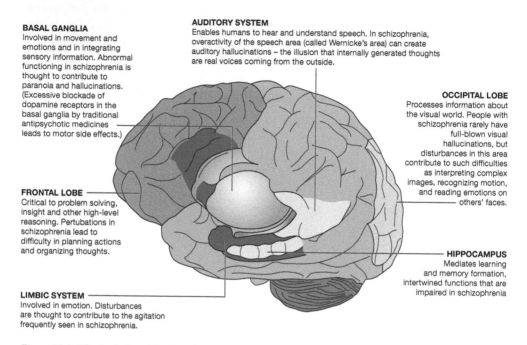

THE BRAIN IN SCHIZOPHRENIA

MANY BRAIN REGIONS and systems operate abnormally in schizophrenia, including those highlighted below. Imbalances in the neurotransmitter dopamine were once thought to be the prime cause of schizophrenia. But new findings suggest that improverished signaling by the more pervasive neurotransmitter glutamate – or, more specifically, by one of glutamate's key targets on neurons (the NMDA receptor) – better explains the wide range of symptoms in this disorder.

BASAL GANGLIA
Involved in movement and emotions and in integrating sensory information. Abnormal functioning in schizophrenia is thought to contribute to paranoia and hallucinations. (Excessive blockade of dopamine receptors in the basal ganglia by traditional antipsychotic medicines leads to motor side effects.)

AUDITORY SYSTEM
Enables humans to hear and understand speech. In schizophrenia, overactivity of the speech area (called Wernicke's area) can create auditory hallucinations – the illusion that internally generated thoughts are real voices coming from the outside.

OCCIPITAL LOBE
Processes information about the visual world. People with schizophrenia rarely have full-blown visual hallucinations, but disturbances in this area contribute to such difficulties as interpreting complex images, recognizing motion, and reading emotions on others' faces.

FRONTAL LOBE
Critical to problem solving, insight and other high-level reasoning. Pertubations in schizophrenia lead to difficulty in planning actions and organizing thoughts.

HIPPOCAMPUS
Mediates learning and memory formation, intertwined functions that are impaired in schizophrenia

LIMBIC SYSTEM
Involved in emotion. Disturbances are thought to contribute to the agitation frequently seen in schizophrenia.

Figure 15.2 The brain in schizophrenia

Source: Javitt, D.C. & Coyle, J.T. (2004). Decoding schizophrenia. *Scientific American*, found at http://schizophrenia.com/schizpictures.html#

Evidence exists indicating that structural changes continue to evolve over the course of the illness. However, caution is required when attempting to link these changes in structure to diagnosis. Structural brain alterations are not exclusive to schizophrenia and similar changes are seen in other diagnostic groups including bi-polar disorder. Therefore, difficulty remains in attempting to identify the diagnostic relevance of these changes and it may be that such changes are common to patients with psychotic features across a range of diagnostic groups rather than being specific to schizophrenia (Keshavan, Tandon, Boutros & Nasrallah, 2008; MacDonald & Schulz, 2009). A substantial literature also exists relating to alterations in brain function and physiology. Impairment in functioning of the pre-frontal cortex has been identified in the early stages of schizophrenia and has been associated with inefficiency in information processing and disorganisation. However, altered pre-frontal function appears to exist in other disorders but does appear to relate specifically to context processing only in early stage schizophrenia.

A relationship between decreased pre-frontal function and genetic factors in schizophrenia has also been identified and is linked to increased activity of dopamine in the striatum region of the brain, which has a role in voluntary movement, eye movement and cognition as well as links to reward pathways in addictive behaviours (Keshavan *et al.*, 2008; MacDonald & Schulz, 2009).

As with identification of structural brain changes, it has long been recognised that schizophrenia has a tendency to occur in families and the closer the genetic relationship, the greater the risk.

The general population risk of developing schizophrenia is approximately 0.7 per cent, whereas first-degree relatives have a 10–15 times greater risk. However, heritability does not account for all cases and it is estimated that over two-thirds of cases are isolated (Tandon *et al.*, 2008). Over the decades confirmation of heritability of schizophrenia has been studied in a variety of ways including adoption and twin studies. These studies have clearly linked the degree of relationship, presence of the illness in the biological rather than the adoptive parent, as being related to risk of developing schizophrenia. Likewise twin studies have consistently identified a greater concordance rate, approximately a threefold risk, for developing schizophrenia among identical/monozygotic twins in comparison to non-identical/dizygotic twins. As identical twins share 100 per cent of their genetic material, if one of the pair develops schizophrenia, the second twin has a 40–50 per cent risk compared to a 10–15 per cent risk in non-identical twins, the same as for other first-degree relatives (MacDonald & Schulz, 2009; Tandon *et al.*, 2012; Tandon *et al.*, 2008). Over the past decade considerable resources have been invested in attempting to identify the genetic basis of schizophrenia. While chromosomal abnormalities have been identified and attempts are being made to understand how schizophrenia is inherited and how the condition is expressed in terms of how the individual experiences the condition, further work is required to provide a fuller understanding of the combination of factors and the part that each individual factor contributes to the disorder (Lichtermann, Karbe & Maier, 2000; Tandon *et al.*, 2008).

Despite the high rate of heritability, what is also clear is that other factors contribute to development of the illness. Whether these environmental factors, both biological and psychological, contribute to causation or act to mediate other pre-existing factors remains unclear. Environmental factors considered significant in schizophrenia include maternal infection during pre- and perinatal periods (Brown *et al.*, 2001; Brown, Schaefer & Queensberry, 2002; Fatemi & Folson, 2009); severe nutritional deficiency and other adverse life events during the first trimester (St Clair *et al.*, 2005; Yuii, 2007), obstetric and perinatal complications associated with foetal hypoxia (Byrne *et al.*, 2007); season of birth, winter and early spring birth, parental age at conception (Byrne *et al.*, 2003; Davies *et al.*, 2003; Torrey, Miller, Rawlings & Yolken, 1997) and childhood trauma and head injury during childhood (David & Prince, 2005; Morgan & Fisher, 2007).

A significant and enduring hypothesis that has influenced thinking about and treatment of schizophrenia over the past five decades has been the dopamine hypothesis. The initial focus of this hypothesis was on dopamine receptors and the ability of certain drugs, primarily antipsychotics to effectively blockade transmissions at these receptor sites. This hypothesis was subsequently generalised as a means to understand schizophrenia as a disease entity (Howes & Kapur, 2009). However it is highly unlikely that one biological factor could explain a disease entity as complex as schizophrenia. Like developments in examination and investigation of structural and functional brain changes, understanding the role of dopamine in psychosis and schizophrenia has evolved over the past two decades. The current evidence suggests that although dopamine abnormalities are present in people with schizophrenia, abnormalities are also seen in those who are psychotic or at risk of developing psychosis. Importantly, what is becoming clear is that dopamine abnormalities are associated not just with alterations in brain structure but are influenced by environmental factors including social isolation, stress and cannabis use. Dopamine elevation appears to be more related to psychosis generally and not just psychosis in schizophrenia. Current thinking on the nature of the dopamine abnormality now focuses on faulty regulation at pre-synaptic neuron and suggests that existing antipsychotic treatments may in fact be resulting in worsening the problem by causing a compensatory increase in dopamine release (Howes & Kapur, 2009).

Figure 15.3 provides an illustration of the synapse where signalling between neurons occurs and is site of neurotransmitter activity.

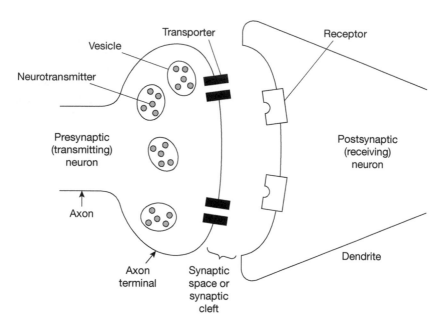

Figure 15.3 Image from *The Brain: Understanding Neurobiology Through the Study of Addiction*

Evidence is increasing of the association between the use of illicit drugs, particularly cannabis and cannabinoids, and the development of psychosis and subsequently schizophrenia. The issue of cannabis and cannabinoids use, while relevant in most cultures, has particular relevance for cultures where its usage is deeply embedded in the social and religious mores of the community. While cannabis and other herbs have been used in an entheogenic context in many countries and traditions throughout history, in more recent times the spiritual use of cannabis has been promoted in some cultures including those across the Caribbean with Rastafari culture being particularly associated with cannabis use. It is well recognised that the use of cannabis can produce acute, transient effects; acute, persistent effects; and delayed, persistent effects (Radhakrishnan, Wilkinson & D'Souza, 2014). Acute transient effects include paranoid ideation, depersonalisation, alterations in perception as well as alterations in mood. Acute episodes of psychosis, which arise as a result of cannabis use and outlast intoxication are also reported (Radhakrishnan *et al.*, 2014). The widespread use of cannabis among certain populations may result in those populations being at an increased risk for psychosis and presents additional challenges for prevention, early detection and interventions in first episode psychosis and schizophrenia. However, it may be that other factors including indicators of social disadvantage, such as unemployment, lone parent status, lower social class, low perceived social support and poverty as well as having a primary social support group of fewer than three close others may contribute more substantially to increased risk of psychosis in these groups (Brugha *et al.*, 2004) The importance of these factors as contributory to higher diagnostic rates is further strengthened by findings that Asian and other immigrant groups composed of people mainly from the Middle East, North Africa, China, Vietnam and Japan are also raised albeit not to the same extent (Fearon *et al.*, 2006). Furthermore Brugha and colleagues (2004) identified that adjusting for these factors modestly attenuated the risk of psychosis in these groups.

Features of schizophrenia

Schizophrenia and schizophrenia spectrum disorders are characterised by a diverse spectrum of signs and symptoms. Central to these conditions are distortions of perception and thinking; impairment in cognition and motor abnormalities, apathy and avolition or a lack of drive or motivation. Symptoms are generally clustered in broad categories including positive symptoms, negative symptoms, cognitive symptoms, social symptoms and mood and motor symptoms. Table 15.1 provides additional information associated with these symptoms.

Onset and course of schizophrenia

Schizophrenia typically emerges during later adolescence and early adulthood with onset in males at an earlier age than females. There is also a recognised course or trajectory of onset, which tends to be sequential in nature and includes a pre-morbid period; a prodromal phase; first psychotic episode and first decade of illness during which repeated episodes of illness occur and finally a plateau or stable period (Tandon, Nashrallah & Keshavan, 2009). The pre-morbid phase is associated with a wide range of subtle and non-specific symptoms, which may or may not progress to the prodromal period. While Welham, Isohanni, Jones and McGrath (2009) in their review of birth cohort studies identified that people who develop schizophrenia have demonstrated a range of behavioural problems during childhood and adolescence, such behaviours had poor predictive value. By contrast, experiencing psychotic symptoms such as hallucinations at an early age was strongly predictive of developing schizophrenia at a later stage indicating the possible continuity of symptoms from childhood to adulthood. As identified previously, people who develop schizophrenia have a range of cognitive deficits and available evidence suggests that these deficits pre-date illness onset. Lower intelligence scores, difficulties with speech development, slower motor development and coordination and reduced school performance have been identified as being more evident in cohorts who later go on to develop schizophrenia (Welham *et al.*, 2009). The prodromal period is considered to include the period from the emergence of the first noticeable symptoms such as alteration in mood, increased levels of anxiety, reduced social engagement and increasing evidence of social isolation and educational or occupational failure, to the appearance of prominent and persistent psychotic symptoms, and can last from weeks to years (Larson, Walker & Compton, 2010; Tandon *et al.*, 2012). Evidence suggests that those with the most severe positive symptoms and greater degree of social impairments are more likely to progress to schizophrenia. However, up to 50 per cent of people who demonstrate symptoms suggestive of schizophrenia do not go on to develop the illness.

The first episode of psychosis is considered to mark the formal onset of schizophrenia. People with an onset prior to the age of 20 years tend to demonstrate more severe pre-morbid functioning, more negative symptoms and have poorer overall prognosis, with men typically having poorer outcomes than women. Following the first episode of psychosis and diagnosis of schizophrenia, the pattern of the illness is variable across individuals but may be episodic and cyclical with patterns of remission, which in some individuals may last for extended periods of time. Over the course of the illness positive symptoms tend to decline with negative symptoms becoming more evident and most of the decline witnessed in functioning happening within the first 5-year period of illness. There is also increasing evidence that the duration of untreated psychosis impacts negatively on functional decline and on longer term outcomes. As time progresses the person may experience a relatively steady state or plateau in which their condition stabilises with no further decline in functioning evident. Alternatively a small number continue to experience decline with their illness becoming persistent in nature.

Table 15.1 Summary of positive, negative, cognitive, social and mood features of schizophrenia

Positive symptoms	Negative symptoms	Cognitive symptoms	Social	Mood
• **Disordered thinking –** generally evident in speech – sudden shifting from one topic to another; lengthy and detailed talking about a subject; responses to questions asked that are irrelevant and unrelated and general lack of speech content unusual or chaotic ways of thinking; difficulty organising and linking their thoughts. • **Impaired reality testing –** include delusions, hallucinations and other distortions of reality. Hallucinations – abnormality in perception in the absence of identifiable external stimulus. Can occur in any of the five senses. Auditory hallucinations, are the most common and involve the hearing of one or more voices speaking to or about the individual. • **Delusions –** abnormality in the content of thought. False beliefs that cannot be explained on the basis of social, educational and cultural background. Beliefs are unfounded, firmly held, and resistant to change and are generally preoccupying, distressing, likely to interfere with social and interpersonal functioning. (Freeman & Garety, 2006).	• **Affective flattening or blunting –** emotional flatness or lack of expression, decreased spontaneous movement; paucity of emotional gestures, poor eye contact, and speech that is brief and devoid of content; inability to start and follow through with activities and a lack of pleasure or interest in life. • **Avolition –** lack of initiative or drive, and apathy, a lack of energy and interest, evident in impersistence at work or school, physical inertia with long periods of time spent inactive, and reduced attention to grooming and personal hygiene. • **Anhedonia –** difficulty in experiencing interest and or pleasure, and asociality, little or no interest in activities. Restricted relationships with friends, reduced ability to feel intimacy or closeness to friends, family or friends and reduced interest in sexual activity. (Freeman & Garety, 2006).	• **Cognitive symptoms** in schizophrenia are considered to be highly prevalent if not universal. • **Deficits** exist at first episode of psychosis and are similar to those identified in patients with long standing illness. • **Impairments** identified in specific areas of episodic memory, processing speed, verbal fluency, attention, executive functioning and working memory. (Tandon et al., 2009). Impairment also appears to persist throughout the course of schizophrenia with modest improvement evident following treatment with anti-psychotic medications (Tandon et al., 2008). These impairments are considered to be the prime driver of the significant disabilities in occupational, social, and economic functioning in patients with schizophrenia (Keefe & Harvey 2012).	• **People** with mental illness often report that they feel excluded from general society. • **Illness-related factors,** including the negative symptoms of schizophrenia, medication and impaired interpersonal and social skills contribute to reduced social networks, a lack of opportunity to meet and engage with people in occupational and other social contexts, along with the absence of intimate partnerships and living in restricted environments such as hostels and supported accommodation, severely restrict opportunities to develop friendships and build social networks (Forrester-Jones et al., 2012; Sheridan et al., 2014). • **The relationships** between persistent or enduring mental health problems such as schizophrenia, social exclusion and stigma are complex, with many elements including housing issues, low income, unemployment and restricted social networks being both a cause and a consequence of living with persistent mental health difficulties (Prince & Gerber, 2005; Repper & Perkins, 2003; Sheridan et al., 2014).	• **Alterations in mood** can often occur in advance of onset of the first episode of psychosis with depression being part of the prodrome, occurring following an acute episode, in between episodes of acute illness and is considered to be more severe in those who have co-existing substance misuse. • **Severity of illness** appears to affect the degree of insight and there is a paradoxical relationship between insight and depression in schizophrenia; as insight improves, mood disimproves.

Consequences of the disorder

The adverse consequences of schizophrenia pervade all aspects of life. In individuals with mental illness, multiple co-morbidities and above average mortality rates are prevalent. Physical health problems, specifically metabolic and cardiovascular co-morbidity, are increasingly being recognised as contributing to the increased risk of premature mortality (De Hert *et al.*, 2011; Mitchell, Delaffon, Vancampfort, Correll & De Hert, 2011). Medical co-morbidity is also associated with more serious psychiatric symptoms and poorer health outcomes (McGrath & Holewa, 2004). Mental illness acts as barrier to accessing and obtaining effective medical care and those diagnosed with schizophrenia live up to 25 years less than the general population. Schizophrenia is also associated with a substantially increase risk for suicide and it is estimated that up to 5 per cent of those with schizophrenia die by suicide. Suicide risk is highest during the early years of the illness and is associated with increased insight, coexisting mood disorders and poor treatment adherence. The co-existence of substance misuse is prevalent among people with schizophrenia and it is likely that this contributes to impulsivity and to suicide. While suicide is responsible for increased mortality rates, it provides only a partial explanation. Overall, the vast majority of the gap in life expectancy between those with mental illness and the general population is accounted for by physical illness (De Hert *et al.*, 2011; Wahlbect, Westman, Nordentoft, Gissler & Laursen, 2011).

Physical health

There is growing recognition that people with mental illness, particularly schizophrenia, are likely to receive less and a poorer quality of physical health care than other population groups. Moreover, the lifespan of people with mental illness is up to 25 years shorter than that of the general population (De Hert, 2011; Mitchell *et al.*, 2011; Nasrallah *et al.*, 2006; Voruganti *et al.*, 2007; Wahlbect *et al.*, 2011). Mental illness is associated with a substantial increase in all causes of mortality and evidence exists to demonstrate that the risks of ischemic health disease, while reducing in the general population, is increasing by up to 40 per cent in women with mental illness (Prince *et al.*, 2007; Wahlbect *et al.*, 2011). For those with diagnosis of schizophrenia, particularly in younger age groups, the prevalence of cardiovascular morbidity and mortality is estimated to be two to three times greater than the general population; 35 per cent to 50 per cent higher in those with bipolar disorders and up to 50 per cent higher in major depression. People with schizophrenia taking antipsychotic medication are reported to be three times more likely to die from sudden cardiac death than the general population. People with mental illness are also less likely to undergo re-vascularisation procedures such as coronary artery by-pass and those with co-morbid mental illness and diabetes who present to the emergency department are less likely to be admitted to hospital for diabetic complications than those with no mental illness (Thornicroft, 2011; Wahlbect *et al.*, 2011). People who experience mental illness also experience additional risk factors for poor health in that they are more likely to be unemployed and dependent on social benefits; live alone or with unrelated others in supported accommodation; be unmarried, have no children and have limited social and family networks. While a proportion of poor physical health in those with mental illness is attributable to modifiable lifestyle choices, structural and systemic health disparities impact access to and utilisation of health care.

Mental illness and obesity overlap to a clinically significant extent, with people with a diagnosis of schizophrenia, schizoaffective disorder and bipolar disorders at greatest risk (De Hert *et al.*, 2011; Mitchell *et al.*, 2011; Nasrallah *et al.*, 2007; Voruganti *et al.*, 2007). Atypical or second generation antipsychotic medication seems to have a stronger diabetic risk than conventional anti-psychotic drugs. The association of obesity and metabolic syndrome with antipsychotic medication, particularly second generation antipsychotic drugs, is well established and it is estimated that this side effect impacts between 15 and 72 per cent of patients taking antipsychotic medication. A hierarchy of weight gain has also been established with the greatest weight gain occurring with Clozapine and Olanazapine, and Amisulpride and Ziparsidone having the least effect on weight (De Hert, 2011; Mitchell *et al.*, 2011; Voruganti *et al.*, 2007). The prevalence of diabetes in people with schizophrenia has consistently been shown to be approximately 15 per cent compared to a community prevalence of about 2–3 per cent (Holt, Busche & Citrome, 2005). While multiple comorbidity is a challenging issue for developed and more affluent countries, recognition is required that the existing evidence relating to these is, to a very large extent, originating from higher-income countries. As yet little evidence exists as to the extent or impact of comorbid physical health issues in low- and middle- income countries. Moreover, it is unlikely that these issues are a priority for low- and middle-income countries.

It is clear from emerging evidence that the challenges facing people with mental illness regarding physical health though multifaceted, could be narrowed down as a starting point for health promotion interventions focusing on health risk behaviours such as lack of exercise, excessive weight gain and smoking; and health protective behaviours such as development of good sleeping patterns, improved nutrition, social engagement, uptake of health screening programmes and adherence to treatment plans. The health challenges associated with physical health issues in people with mental illness require a better understanding of health behaviour and the implementation of interventions using evidence-based practice on the part of all clinical practitioners, particularly psychiatric/mental health nurses (Michie *et al.*, 2005). However, as noted above in low- and middle-income countries, other priorities are almost certain to be evident and of necessity interventions are more likely to focus on extending and improving the mental health care available to communities. Likewise, the absence of mental health/psychiatric nurses in these locations presents a further challenge. In such locations responsibility for health-promoting activities tend to reside within the remit of community-based primary health care workers including nurses. The challenge therefore is to upskill and educate this population of health workers about the particular physical health needs of people with mental health issues and specifically those with schizophrenia.

Reducing risk and promoting health

As outlined previously, biology alone is insufficient in explaining the cause, onset, impact or duration of schizophrenia. Equally, the existence of one or a small number of recognised risk factors is also unlikely to result in serious illness. However, the combination of a range of factors including biological, psychological, social, economic, environmental and interpersonal are all likely to contribute. Protective factors act to mitigate or buffer the effects of risk factors and may reduce the likelihood of schizophrenia developing in the first instance and/or decrease the severity and or duration of the illness. Risks related to schizophrenia are complex and multifaceted and likewise the process of addressing these risks needs to adopt a 'total systems' approach, which takes place across the full spectrum of health, social, economic, employment and educational sectors and at multiple levels including legislative and policy levels as well as at professional, personal and community-based levels.

Promoting positive mental health overlaps with wider concerns about population health and well-being (Barry, 2009). Positive mental health is conceptualised as a subjective feeling of positivity and sense of well-being; possessing a sense of mastery in one's life along with resilience to cope with adversity (WHO, 2004). Mental health is context dependent, is clearly influenced by the culture that defines it and will have different meanings depending on social, economic and political contexts. Recognising the cross-cultural perspective of mental health therefore is fundamental to our understanding of what constitutes positive functioning within particular ethnic and social groups and how these beliefs about health and illness, societal values and norms influence health behaviour. Mental health promotion, while focusing on the positive aspects of mental health, also has relevance across the entire spectrum of mental health interventions, including for people experiencing mental health challenges and disorders (Barry, 2009).

Mental health promotion interventions are directed at reducing risk factors that contribute to poor mental health as well as supporting and enhancing protective factors that contribute to good mental health (Barry & McQueen, 2005; Pollett, 2007). The overview of schizophrenia presented above serves to assist in the identification of particular areas amenable to intervention utilising a risk-reduction and health-promotion approach. Health-promotion intervention strategies and approaches need to address the potential causative and sustaining factors of schizophrenia at societal, population, community and individual levels. In addition such strategies and intervention also need to intervene in a range of areas that, while not exclusively related to illnesses such as schizophrenia, have the ability to influence the possible causation and or triggering of schizophrenia; or which have the ability to act to compound or prolong duration of symptoms or disability. A number of key areas are now identified for further exploration. At a structural level these include prenatal, early childhood and environmental factors, cultural factors and stigma. At the professional, personal and community levels some strategies are identified to assist in reducing structural barriers, strengthening individuals and communities.

Addressing health risks and reducing barriers

Prenatal, early childhood and environmental

Specialised perinatal services are as yet relatively uncommon globally. While it is well established that exposure to depravation and adversity at a young age is an established preventable risk factor for mental disorders, globally, preparation for parenting is not considered a high priority. Likewise women with mental illness and specifically those with schizophrenia are generally underprovided for in terms of readiness for parenting. A number of factors contribute to adversity in childhood with a significant amount of these being amenable to intervention to reduce adverse consequences and to promote positive outcomes. Nutrition deprivation and specifically maternal under-nutrition represents a significant public health challenge globally (McGrath, Brown & St. Clair, 2011). It is estimated that maternal under-nutrition ranges from 10 per cent to 20 per cent in most countries rising to 40 per cent in the most deprived countries in Asia and Africa. In particular, micro nutrients including Vitamin D, Folic Acid and Iron are recognised as being of importance. While nutrition deficiency is well established as a causative factor in neural tube defects, the relationship between maternal nutritional deficiency during pregnancy and schizophrenia is less developed. However, some direct evidence that pre-natal nutritional deficiency is related to schizophrenia does exist and this has been derived from studies of severe famine including the Dutch Hunger Winter of 1944–1945 during the blockade of the Western Netherlands by the Nazis, and the Moa Zedong's Great Leap Forward in 1959–1961. The Dutch study by Susser & Lin (1992) demonstrated that there was a two-fold increase in the risk of schizophrenia coinciding with peak increase in neural tube defects. These findings were replicated in two areas in China by St Clair *et al.* (2005). These studies demonstrate that severe nutritional deficiency has catastrophic effects on the neurodevelopment of babies of women who are nutritionally deprived during pregnancy and that the risk of schizophrenia may also be increased as a result. While more evidence about the linkages and type of associations between nutritional deficiency and schizophrenia is required, intervening to prevent under-nutrition in pregnancy is an action that in most developed societies can be achieved through supplementation and programmes similar to those utilised to reduce neural tube defects. In developing and low-income countries feeding programmes need to be established and supported to include pregnant women as well as children.

Gender

Apart from the nutritional issues highlighted above, women experiencing schizophrenia in developing countries often have an early age of onset of the illness, experience victimisation and violence as well as increased illness burden due to the stigma associated with mental illness. The HIV and sexually transmitted diseases status of these women also needs further consideration. Evidence is also beginning to emerge indicating that metabolic syndrome associated with the use of antipsychotic medications appears to have a higher incidence among women in developing countries (Chandra, Kommu & Rudhran, 2012). Gender discrimination resulting in poverty, limited access to resources including nutrition, education and health care, and circumstances such as migration and exposure to disasters act to both contribute to causation and to compound illness.

Early years and parenting

Good mental health in childhood helps establish adaptive life skills and establishes a foundation for mental health across the life span. Central to assisting children to establish and build good mental health is the role of parents and primary care givers. Parental mental health and illnesses including schizophrenia impact directly and profoundly on the mental health of children. The impact of mental health problems and the disabilities associated with these, particularly those of mothers, have been associated with adverse outcomes in children, including conduct problems and hyperactivity, depression, anxiety and medical problems (Beardslee *et al.*, 1998; Gunlicks & Weissman, 2008; Kramer *et al.*, 1998). The parent's ability to parent effectively or to be responsive to their child's needs may be associated with more irritable and angry parenting and lower parental warmth (Wilson & Durbin, 2010). Factors such as unemployment, poverty and lone parent households, the level of involvement of fathers in childcare and activities with their children and maternal employment outside of the home can also impact on parenting role and on the mental health of children. Therefore, policies that support parents to develop and strengthen their existing coping strategies as well as supporting the development of good parenting skills will support the development of good mental health.

School

As children transition to school, the school becomes increasingly important in promoting good mental health. Schools that promote positive and safe environments, which foster inclusion, support the building of self-esteem and personal competence and emotional control and problem solving strengthen mental health. The development and implementation of programmes to support learning reduce exclusion and bullying also act to reduce anxiety among children. While access to education is taken for granted in high-income countries, children in low- and middle-income countries may be denied access for a variety of reasons including socio-economic, political, gender and geographic inequities. Thus the role that schools can play in promoting positive, inclusive and competency-building environments is not experienced by children. Furthermore, exclusion or lack of access to education has long-term economic social and cultural repercussions and acts to sustain poverty through the limitation of life opportunities. Experiencing a mental health problem is a further barrier to accessing education and school. Children with disabilities frequently experience exclusion and the degree to which they experience this is influenced by the nature of their disability, where in the world they live, their gender and the culture and class they belong to. According to UNICEF (2013) girls and young women with disabilities are 'doubly disabled' in that they confront not only the prejudice and inequities encountered by many persons with disabilities, but are also constrained by traditional gender roles and barriers. Girls with disabilities are also less likely to get an education, receive vocational training or find employment (UNICEF, 2013, p. 1).

While there is increasing awareness of the crucial importance of early interventions in childhood to ensure a good start in life and to prevent mortality and to reduce the possibilities for later morbidity both physical and mental, the availability and implementation of such programmes lag behind the recognition of their importance (Petersen, Bhana, Flisher, Swartz & Richter, 2010). Middle childhood and adolescence is also recognised as a key stage, which can influence mental health in later life. In all stages of childhood the influence of parenting is identified as supporting the development of children and adolescents with regard to positive health and well-being. In low- and middle-income countries particular emphasis relating to health promotion is the building of personal, family and community resources to prevent, minimise or overcome the adverse effect of adversity (Petersen *et al.*, 2010).

Environmental factors

In addition to nutritional, parental and school influences, environmental and social factors also impact mental health and it is recognised that heritability alone cannot fully explain the origins, onset, course and duration of schizophrenia. Increasingly it is being recognised that where people live, the nature of the built environment, as well as ethnicity and use of non-prescription drugs influence both development of good mental health and risk for schizophrenia. Belonging to an ethnic minority and growing up in an urban area, particularly one in which you are recognisable as different, contributes to poor mental health. Minority group position is evident in both first- and second-generation migrants, and the evidence suggests that ethnic density of the geographic areas is the critical factor rather than ethnicity per se. Occupying a minority position may be mediated by social adversity including discrimination, exclusion and marginalisation resulting in social defeat (March *et al.*, 2008; Morgan, Charlambides, Hutchinson & Murray, 2010; Van Os, Kenis & Rutten, 2010). Having a good education, being employed with an income that is above the poverty line, having supportive and close relationships and being socially included are all critical to positive mental health, as is living in adequate housing in an environment with low crime rates and access to social and leisure amenities. Thus there is a need to recognise the need for policy-level interventions that address the social determinants of mental health as well as the more individual-level determinants. The available evidence supports the view that interventions to address competence-enhancing programmes, carried out in collaboration with families, schools and wider communities, as well as social policies that address issues such as poverty reduction, housing and education have the potential to effect multiple positive outcomes in social and personal health domains (Barry, 2009; Jané-Llopis & Barry, 2005).

Cultural issues

As identified previously a personal and family history of migration is identified as a significant risk factor in schizophrenia (Cantor-Graae & Selten, 2005; Tandon *et al.*, 2008) with social adversity including isolation, racism and discrimination cited as major contributors in migration (Cooper *et al.*, 2008). Difficulties with integration into the host culture or low levels of acculturation is a significant factor, which acts as a barrier to seeking mental health services among racial and ethnic minorities and may often transcend gender and social class (Leong & Lau, 2001). People's conceptions of the nature, causes and cures of mental illness are culturally defined and influenced and as a result how they think about help seeking, the nature of treatment and cure is also influenced by culture. Among non-Western populations including Asian, African and Caribbean cultures the belief that mental illness can be treated or overcome through willpower, heroic stoicism and avoidance of morbid thoughts rather than by seeking external, professional psychological help is likely to act as a barrier to seeking help and to accepting treatment and or psychologically directed interventions. The existence of stigma or the desire to 'save face' may also play a significant role in deterring help seeking and the acceptance of interventions, as can the perception that focusing on personal or individual difficulties is a selfish act and one that is not in keeping with the collectivist nature of the cultural group. Physical and structural barriers including poverty, affordability of health services and lack of health insurance; language barriers, lack of knowledge of existing services and lack of time to attend services are all likely to act as barriers to access and service utilisation. Thus rather than importing models of mental health services originating pre-dominantly from a Western perspective, mental health services need to take account of the groups they are designed to serve. They must be culturally sensitive and work in close collaboration with local communities to identify appropriate and acceptable service models and strive to intervene in ways consistent with the predominant values and belief systems.

Stigma

One of the most recognised barriers to participation and inclusion for people with mental health difficulties and with schizophrenia in particular, is the stigma associated with their condition. Stigma is considered to act in two ways, directly to exclude individuals with mental health difficulties from areas of participation, including work, education, travel and decent living conditions; and indirectly, with those experiencing mental illness internalising wider societal attitudes resulting in self-stigmatisation. Cultural factors complicate the stigma associated with mental illness. In Asian cultures, particularly Chinese, the prevailing dominant beliefs about causation of schizophrenia being associated with genetic causation further compound the stigma of schizophrenia given the potential impact of genetic factors across subsequent generations. Evidence also highlights that the rise of the genetic model of mental illness while resulting in a positive effect for depression, has resulted in further entrenchment of the negative views associated with schizophrenia, in particular the association of schizophrenia with unpredictable behaviour and violence against the person (Schnittker, 2008). The outcomes of both processes of stigmatisation are perceived powerlessness, lack of control and loss of hope; lower self-esteem, social isolation and exclusion, depression and anxiety (Boardman, 2011; Mental Health Foundation [MHF], 2000). Stigma and discrimination are closely linked to social exclusion and the resultant marginalisation from wider society is both a cause of stigma and a result of it. The outcome is often a spiral of loneliness and lack of opportunity that people experiencing the impact of illnesses such as schizophrenia must struggle with, alongside the symptoms and other consequences of their mental health difficulty (Sheridan *et al.*, 2014). The effects of stigma and discrimination are pervasive across all aspects of life, education and relationships, and according to Gonzáles-Torres *et al.* (2007), they are akin to a second illness. The emotion of shame, a common response to stigma, leads to secrecy, which, itself, is an obstacle to seeking assistance with mental health difficulties, treatment and recovery (Clement *et al.*, 2014).

Promoting health and wellness

Chronic health conditions such as schizophrenia present a common set of challenges for individuals and their families including dealing with symptoms, disability, emotional impact, complex treatment regimens and lifestyle adjustments. As noted previously, schizophrenia and schizophrenia spectrum disorders are characterised by a diverse spectrum of symptoms and these are generally clustered in broad categories including positive and negative symptoms; cognitive symptoms; social symptoms; and mood and motor symptoms. Intervening in schizophrenia is required across all symptom categories and will to a large extent be contingent upon the needs identified at different points in the person's life. Thus priorities will be determined by the needs of individuals and their families and are likely to vary across the lifespan as people attempt to address the complexity of individual, family and community needs.

While originally it was considered unproductive to discuss symptoms with people with schizophrenia, and the ability of the individual with schizophrenia to collaborate in a working therapeutic relationship was questioned, the contemporary focus of nursing intervention is now clearly focused on adopting approaches that strive to recognise the issues of most concern to the individual and their family, thus enhancing the potential for establishing an effective and trusting relationship directed toward managing symptoms of illness, promoting coping, wellness and autonomy, promoting recovery and ultimately improving quality of life. The success of nursing interventions is due to a combination of effective interpersonal approaches and technical interventions based on best existing evidence that focus on skills acquisition and on developing social competency in which strong helping relationships emerge to promote recovery.

Psychiatric nursing – roles in risk reduction and health promotion

The treatment and care of people with schizophrenia has traditionally relied upon symptom reduction and functional recovery and it is only in recent years that health promotion and illness prevention have been incorporated into mental health services. Mental health promotion is premised upon building individual and community capacity by capitalising and supporting existing ability to achieve and maintain good health as well as reducing or minimising factors that act as barriers to good mental health (WHO, 2008). Mental health promotion includes any activity that actively fosters good mental health. This may be achieved through increasing mental health promotion or protective factors such as meaningful employment, as well as decreasing risk factors identified as injurious to good mental health such as abuse or violence, and activities that promote mental health may also prevent mental illness. Activities include practical assistance to help people overcome the barriers to inclusion as well as support in managing complex relationships and emotional distress (NHS Development Agency, 2005).

Globally, the availability of mental health professionals, particularly psychiatric nurses, is limited and this is most evident in low- and middle-income countries (Mari *et al.*, 2009). Throughout the world, nurses are the primary providers of health care and in a significant majority of countries they are providing up to 90 per cent of care and services (Bruckner, *et al.*, 2011). However, significant variability exists with regard to the educational preparation and training nurses receive with a significant proportion receiving only limited or no preparation to provide care to people with mental illness. The goal of mental health promotion is to strengthen and enhance the ability that already exists for health rather than any attempt to eliminate illness. In this way the role of the psychiatric nurse is focused on supporting consolidation, improved access, uptake and utilisation of existing personal and community resources.

Interpersonal relationships

Interpersonal relationships are the cornerstone of psychiatric nursing and form the basis of all interventions in psychiatric nursing. The central position of the relationship is not a new concept for psychiatric/mental health nurses and the elements of the relationship requirements identified by patients (Borg & Davidson, 2008; Eliacin, Salyers, Kukla & Matthias, 2015) are consistent with the nature of the nurse patient relationship as identified by Travelbee (1971).

Travelbee (1971), viewed nursing as an interpersonal process that assists individuals, families and communities to prevent or cope with illness and suffering with the goal of finding meaning in these experiences. To be a full participant in decision-making about health care, patients and their carers require information and knowledge about their condition and the available options for treatments and interventions. In this regard psychiatric nurses have a central role as educators and facilitators of learning.

In contemporary mental health/psychiatric nursing practice, the concepts identified by Travelbee as central to her theory of nursing – being human, suffering and hope, are echoed today in the values underpinning the recovery-based approach to mental health care (Jones, Fitzpatrick & Rogers, 2012). Shared decision-making, a core component of the recovery model, is fundamental to all elements of health care and is linked to positive health outcomes (Eliacin *et al.*, 2015). At the core of shared decision-making is the relationship between care provider and patient. The central role of nurses in health care provision situates them ideally to promote genuine shared decision-making with patients, their families and wider social networks. To fully participate in care decisions a trusting, honest empathic and equal relationship in which power is equally distributed is required. According to Eilacin *et al.* (2015), shared decision-making is, greater than the process of making a decision; it is shaped by the entire clinical encounter and most notably the patient–provider relationship.

Reducing stigma

Addressing and working to reduce stigma is a core role of psychiatric/mental health nurses globally. Nurses, given their central position in the provision of care are best placed among care professionals to act to reduce stigma. Psychiatric/mental health nurses have a key role in providing education to challenge the stigma associated with mental illness. Central to this activity is the provision of culturally sensitive, factual information based upon best available evidence to challenge inaccurate stereotypes and incorrect information about mental illness. Likewise clear information about illness onset, duration and course along with available treatments and interventions will work to reduce ignorance of conditions such as schizophrenia. The role of the nurse is critical at both the community and personal level. At the personal level the nurse needs to work with individuals to assist with the reduction of self-stigma. Self-stigma is reportedly experienced by up to 50 per cent of people with schizophrenia or other psychotic disorders (Brohan, Gauci, Sartorius & Thornicroft, 2010). Self-stigma occurs when people internalise the attitudes expressed by the public and suffer numerous negative consequences as a result. Self-stigmatisation impacts on the individual in a number of ways, diminishing self-esteem and feelings of self-worth and undermining hope and optimism in achieving goals (Corrigan, Watson & Barr, 2006; Livingston *et al.*, 2011; Watson, Corrigan, Larson & Sells, 2007). At the personal level nurses will be required to work with patients to address self-stigmatisation and in doing so they need to adopt evidence-based strategies to mitigate the effects of self-stigmatisation. According to Corrigan, Roe and Tsang (2011) 'righteous indignation', a process whereby the individual rejects societal concepts of mental illness, acts as an antidote to self-stigma. Righteous indignations appears to be akin to personal empowerment and is related to retaining a sense of personal agency with the hope of future goal achievement. One approach to intervening in self-stigma being developed and tested is cognitive restructuring and narrative enhancement. This approach involves facilitated groups to assist people to challenge inaccurate and/or maladaptive personal beliefs about the self and replace them with more accurate and adaptive ones, thus strengthening personal identity. Likewise the education and support of immediate and wider family and friendship networks is critical in reducing stigma and supporting the inclusion of the person with mental illness. Setting up and facilitation of family support groups focusing on the pragmatics of dealing with the challenges of living with a person with a serious mental illness is a key activity for nurses.

At a community-based level the raising of awareness, provision of culturally appropriate information about schizophrenia and education about the nature and impact of the condition are critical in working to reduce stigma. Psychiatric/mental health nurses must also recognise that other professional groups including health professions also require intervention to address their views about mental illness and schizophrenia. Psychiatric/mental health nurses also recognise that in addition to the psychological and social impact of stigma and discrimination, social exclusion is recognised as an important determinant of physical health and this is of particular importance for people with serious mental illnesses such as schizophrenia. Mental health problems can act as a barrier to accessing and obtaining effective medical care with symptoms of physical illness being misattributed to mental illness. In this regard, nurses must work to advocate for people with schizophrenia to ensure parity of access to physical health care.

However, while provision of education is a core part of all approaches to stigma reduction, by itself it cannot fully address the wide range of issues relating to stigma. Available evidence clearly demonstrates that having contact with a person who experiences mental illness is one of the most effective ways of reducing stigma (Corrigan *et al.*, 2011). Thus nurses need to work to facilitate opportunities for those with mental illness to encounter and share their experiences with members of their families and the families of other patients and with the wider community including other health professions and employers. Employing such approaches will of necessity need to recognise and employ culturally sensitive approaches. Not all people with mental illness or their families will want to be engaged with such programmes and in this regard the wishes and rights of individuals and families need to be respected. While in Western cultures the emergence of peer support and advocacy groups who represent and support mental health service users have become popular, similar approaches may not be appropriate in all cultures. Psychiatric/mental health nurses need to work with individuals, families and local communities to identify and develop programmes that have local and cultural relevance and that enable people to live a life that is satisfying and allows them to achieve their personal goals.

Strengthening families and communities

Psychiatric/mental health nurses have a role to support parenting practices, particularly where a parent is coping with an existing mental illness such as schizophrenia. Intervention programmes that act to assist individual to alter their way of thinking such as the 'Thinking Healthy Programme', which seeks to identify and modify maladaptive thinking styles – e.g. fatalism, inability to act, superstitious explanations and somatisation – and replace them with more adaptive ways of thinking can be utilised, as can programmes that act by targeting parenting interaction with their children indirectly address the building of positive approaches to parenting and health. A study in Jamaica by Baker-Henningham, Powell, Walker and Grantham-McGregor (2005) utilised the adapted Learning Through Play (LTP) programmes originally implemented in Pakistan and northern Uganda. The rationale underpinning this programme was that optimal child development requires the maternal caregiver to engage explicitly in development of the physical, social, emotional and cognitive domains of the child. The interventions aimed to enhance mothers' knowledge about normal child development, improve maternal sensitivity and responsiveness towards infants and through group programmes and to reduce social isolation by means of peer support (Rahman *et al.*, 2013). Given the global shortage of nurses and psychiatric nurses in particular, a key role of professionally prepared nurses will be the education and ongoing supervision of local health workers to deliver some programmes locally. Apart from addressing personnel shortages, the use of local health workers may have further advantages in ensuring cultural relevance of programmes and this is of particular importance where programmes developed in one setting are being modified for implementation in a new setting. Nurses also have a role in supporting the mobilisation of support from other family members, neighbours as well as from voluntary and statutory organisations.

In terms of strengthening community, strategies that maximise the active ownership and participation of people in health promotion initiatives contribute positively to the effectiveness and sustainability of these programmes. To this end psychiatric/mental health nurses have a role in supporting the development of community engagement. Within the health care context nurses can assist communities to engage through practices that enhance knowledge and awareness of illnesses such as schizophrenia and of the resources available to support people in their local community. Awareness raising can be achieved in a number of ways but essentially is achieved through the provision of information and education. Psychiatric nurses can act to bring together individuals and voluntary groups who can assist in the provision of information and support for patients, families and wider community members. The creative use of approaches such as community-based displays, dramatisation, art work, creative writing and storytelling in combination with more traditional presentation and printed media can assist in reaching wide sections of communities. Nurses are also well positioned to act as a source of information about other resources that exist within the community and as a means of referral to these resources.

Strengthening the individual

Psychiatric/mental health nurses are central to the delivery of interventions to assist patients and their carers ameliorate troubling symptoms, manage life demands and to support the establishing and achieving of life goals. While a wide range of intervention strategies exist emanating from a range of disciplines, in recent decades many psychiatric/mental health nurses have become skilled in utilising these approaches to support those with schizophrenia and their families. While it is not possible to provide a comprehensive overview of all approaches in this text, three commonly utilised approaches have been selected for further elaboration. The reader is advised to access more detailed information about approaches elsewhere.

Psychosocial interventions

Among the most popular and effective intervention approaches utilised in people with schizophrenia including first episode psychosis, cognitive behavioural therapy (CBT) has at this point the best evidence to support its usage. Other approaches that are also found to be effective include solution-focussed brief therapy (SFBT), assertive community outreach (ACT), psycho-education (PE), cognitive remediation (CR); chronic disease self-management programme (CDSMP) and wellness recovery action planning (WRAP). All of these approaches share a set of core principles, which are related to empowering the person to manage their symptoms, provide them with skills to promote their future self-management and facilitate them achieving desired life goals.

Cognitive behavioural therapy (CBT)

In its pure form CBT is a structured and time-limited approach to therapy, which is problem focussed and action orientated and works to assist the individual to make connections between their thoughts, behaviours and emotions. It also relies to a significant extent on the patient's ability to engage in, complete and generalise from 'homework'. However, patients with either positive and or negative symptoms of schizophrenia may have difficulty adhering to this rigid structure. Therefore the approach to CBT needs to be adapted to reflect the reality of the patient's ability and to be continually modified as the person's situation changes. As a guide, sessions need to reflect the current reality of the person focusing on immediate concerns rather than relying on homework to connect sessions. Likewise the duration of sessions, which are often up to one hour, will need to be reduced to reflect the ability of the person to engage. While the aims of treatment using CBT are usually directed towards resolution of symptoms, modifications in patients with schizophrenia and psychosis tend to be directed at assisting the individual to improve their ability to learn to manage and cope with symptoms such as troubling thoughts and voices and in so doing improve their quality of life.

Chronic disease self-management programme (CDSMP)

Evidence has accumulated to confirm that undertaking systematic efforts to increase patients' knowledge, skills and confidence in managing their conditions positively impacts well-being and in recent years, 'self-management' has become embedded in approaches to managing chronic health conditions including schizophrenia (Lorig & Holman, 2003; Druss et al., 2010). Self-management is predicated on the construct of self-efficacy and it is the individual's perception of their ability to perform an action, which is an important mediator of their health behaviours. Thus focusing on the individual's beliefs about their illness and their capacity to undertake behaviours is likely to lead to a desired outcome. The overall goal of the CDSMP is to enable people to build self-confidence and become self-managers of their chronic health condition. The central focus of CDSMP is on enhancing self-efficacy in areas including the person's ability to manage symptoms along with the consequences of living with a chronic condition including treatments, physical, social, emotional and lifestyle changes and on maintaining wellness.

Wellness recovery action plan (WRAP)

Originally developed in the United States by Mary Ellen Copeland (2015) based on her personal experience of both her own and her mother's mental health difficulties, this programme incorporates the development of a wellness plan and a contingency plan. The programme consists of seven steps, which assist the individual to gain a deeper insight into the dimension of their wellness and illness and to more clearly identify strategies and actions they and others on their behalf can adopt to support wellness, promote recovery and manage episodes of illness. This programme is used worldwide by people who are dealing with mental health challenges as well as conditions such as diabetes, weight gain, pain management and life issues like addictions, smoking and trauma.

Pharmacological and physical interventions

A mainstay of treatment and intervention in schizophrenia has been and continues to be psychopharmacological therapy. While it is widely recognised that pharmacological therapies alone are insufficient to address the complexity and full spectrum of needs, they continue to prove valuable, particularly in assisting with symptom management during the acute phase of illness and in more recent times with addressing some of the debilitating negative features of the illness. The mainstay of pharmacological therapy continues to be antipsychotic agents. Older or first generation antipsychotic agents tend to be more effectively utilised in reducing acute symptoms such as those associated with disordered thinking and perception. Second generation or atypical antipsychotic agents, while also effective in assisting management of acute symptoms, are now recognised as being particularly useful in reducing the impairments associated with negative symptom clusters such as reduced or lack of motivation, flatness of emotional affect and with the social aspect such as interactional abilities and cognitive aspects including the ability to plan and follow through on activities. A second approach that intervenes on a chemical level is electroconvulsive therapy or ECT. Although its use has significantly diminished over the past 50 years and it is frequently regarded with fear and suspicion, ECT remains an effective, if controversial, treatment in schizophrenia. In particular, those with severe suicidal ideation and behaviours, co-existing depression or catatonic features are most likely to benefit and it is particularly valuable where a rapid response to ameliorating symptoms is required to reduce risk.

Coupled with physical interventions are environmental supports, which act to mitigate the impact particularly of cognitive symptoms. Environmental supports are diverse, overlap physical, psychological, social and cognitive domains and include working with patients and their families to develop strategies to support independent living such as medication reminders, checklists for activities such as preparing and cooking meals, undertaking household activities, shopping and budgeting, and socialising.

Prevention of relapse

A key issue for people who experience schizophrenia is the issue of relapse. In most instances relapse is associated with a core number of features including failure to adhere to prescribed medication and intervention programmes, living in situations where the nature of interaction is characterised by criticism, hostility and emotional over-involvement referred to as expressed emotion. Accumulated evidence clearly identifies that high family levels of expressed emotion are consistently associated with higher rates of relapse in patients with schizophrenia (Amaresha & Venkatasubramanian, 2012).

A significant part of the nurse's role is to assist patients in their efforts to avoid relapse and this can be achieved through the provision of psychoeducation programmes assisting patients and families to identify and recognise their particular patterns of family interactions and to adapt them. Exploring communication and problem-solving skills as well as assisting the patient and family to engage socially and occupationally will also assist in preventing relapse in schizophrenia. Assistance may also be required to maintain existing or develop new social networks. Support with educational and occupations goals are also required and links to employers and educational providers to establish support networks will be required. Providing the education and training to identify and manage impending crises along with the development of resilience and healthy coping strategies will act to further support the individual with schizophrenia to avoid relapse. Continued review and monitoring of the therapeutic and adverse effects of medication will also help patients to manage their condition (Amaresha & Venkatasubramanian, 2012).

The role of nurses in promoting health, including mental health is particularly influential. It centres on the interpersonal relationship focal to nursing coupled with a process of linking individual and communities to reliable information sources and trusted support, which together raise awareness and increase the ability to manage health more confidently. This is complex and multifaceted with a considerable range of activities directed towards the personal, community and structural barriers that influence mental health. Looking specifically at people with schizophrenia, their requirements are in effect a sub-set or specific variant of these processes, which need to take into account the particular mental and physical health challenges associated with their condition and to devise positive strategies to address these.

Summary

Despite the prevalence of mental health problems in society, stigma, social isolation, loneliness and reduced social integration persist among those who experience psychiatric and behavioural difficulties. As clearly identified in this chapter the personal costs of schizophrenia are high, with physical health, family relationships, social networks and employment status all being impacted to a significant extent. However, the majority of the costs associated with mental health problems occur outside of the health sector, for example, lost employment, absenteeism and reduced productivity and reduced contribution to society. While the economic costs can be calculated, the personal costs for the individual and families who experience mental health problems are difficult to estimate. Experiencing a persistent mental health issue such as schizophrenia can seriously disrupt a person's sense of self, that is, in terms of identity and how one relates to others and to the community. Mental health issues can also influence how others, including those personally associated with an individual such as friends and others within the wider community, perceive an individual. This fracturing of personal identity, loss of personal agency and relationships with family, friends and community often have deep and enduring effects on all aspects of life, often spanning many years.

Local communities have a part to play in fostering and supporting positive mental health. Within mental health services, the ultimate goal of recovery is linked to community integration and the ability of people to establish and maintain meaningful, purposeful lives within their local areas through developing social networks, positive relationships and community engagement (National Economic & Social Forum (NESF), 2007). Successful recovery depends less on the ability of mental health professionals to teach specific skills and more on their ability to support individuals to find their place within naturally occurring communities rather than those created to deliver services.

References

Amaresha, A.C. & Venkatasubramanian, G. (2012). Expressed emotion in schizophrenia: an overview. *Indian Journal of Psychological Medicine, 34*, 1 12–20.

Baker-Henningham, H., Powell, C., Walker, S., Grantham-McGregor, S. (2005). The effect of early stimulation on maternal depression: a cluster randomised controlled trial. *Arhcives of Disease in Childhood, 90*, 1230–1234.

Barry, M.M. (2009). Addressing the determinants of positive mental health: concepts, evidence and practice. *International Journal of Mental Health Promotion, 11*(3), 4–17.

Barry, M. & McQueen, D. (2005). The nature of evidence and its use in mental health promotion. In Herman, H., Saxena, S. & Moodie, R. (eds). *Promotion Mental Health Concepts, Emerging Evidence Practice* (pp. 108–118). Geneva: World Health Organization.

Baxter, A.J., Patton. G., Scott, K.M., Degenhardt, L. & Whiteford H.A. (2013). Global epidemiology of mental disorders: what are we missing? *PlosOne, 8*, 6, e65514.

Beardslee, W.R., Versage, E.M. & Gladstone, T.R.G. (1998). Children of affectively ill parents: a review of the past 10 years. *Journal of the American Academy of Child and Adolescent Psychiatry, 37*, 1134–1141.

Boardman, J. (2011). Social exclusion and mental health – how people with mental health problems are disadvantaged: an overview. *Mental Health and Social Inclusion, 15*(3), 112–121.

Borg, M. & Davidson, L., 2008. The nature of recovery as lived in everyday experience. *Journal of Mental Health, 17*(2), 129–140.

Brohan, E., Gauci, D., Sartorius, N. & Thornicroft, G. (2010). Self-stigma, empowerment and perceived discrimination among people with bipolar disorder or depression in 13 European countries: the GAMIAN-Europe study. *Journal of Affective Disorders, 129*, 56–63.

Brown, A.S., Cohen, P., Harkavy-Friedman, J., Babulus, V., Malaspina, D., Gorman, J.M. & Susser, E.S. 2001. Prenatal rubella, premorbid abnormalities and adult schizophrenia. *Biological Psychiatry, 49*, 473–486.

Brown, A.S., Schaefer, C.A. & Quesenberry, C.P., 2002. Maternal exposure to toxoplasmosis and risk of schizophrenia in adult offspring. *American Journal of Psychiatry, 162*, 767–773.

Bruckner, T.A., Scheffler, R. M., Shen, G., Yoon, J., Chisholm, D., Morris, J., Fulton, B.D., Dal, P. & M., Saxena, S. (2011). The mental health workforce gap in low- and middle-income countries: a needs-based approach. *Bulletin of the World Health Organization, 89*, 184–194.

Brugha, T., Jenkins, R., Bebbington, P., Meltzer, H., Lewis, G. & Farrell, M. (2004). Risk factors and the prevalence of neurosis and psychosis in ethnic groups in Great Britain. *Social Psychiatry & Psychiatric Epidemiology, 39*, 939–946.

Byrne, M., Agerbo, E., Ewald, H., Eaton, W.W. & Mortensen, P.B. (2003). Parental age and risk of schizophrenia: a case–control study. *Archives of General Psychiatry, 60*, 673–678.

Byrne, M., Agerbo, E., Bennedsen, B., Eaton, W.W. & Mortensen, P.B. (2007). Obstetric conditions and risk of first admission with schizophrenia: a Danish national register based study. *Schizophrenia Research, 97*, 51–59.

Cantor-Graae, E. & Selten, J.P. (2005). Schizophrenia and migration: a meta-analysis and review. *American Journal of Psychiatry, 162*, 12–24.

Chandra, P., Kommu, J.V.S. & Rudhran, V. (2012). Schizophrenia in women and children: a selective review of the literature from developing countries. *International Review of Psychiatry, 24*(5), 467–482.

Clement, S., Schauman, O., Graham, T., Maggioni, F., Evans-Lacko, S., Bezborodovs, N., Morgan, C., Rüsch, N., Brown, J.S.L. & Thornicroft G. (2014). What is the impact of mental health related stigma on help-seeking? A systematic review of quantitative and qualitative studies. *Psychological Medicine, 45*(1), 11–17.

Cooper, C., Morgan, C., Byrne, M., Dazzan, P., Morgan, K., Hutchington, G., Doody, G.A., Harrison, G., Leff, J., Jones, P., Ismail, K., Murray, R., Bebbington, P.E. & Fearon, P. (2008). Perceptions of disadvantage, ethnicity and psychosis. *British Journal of Psychiatry, 192*, 185–190.

Copeland, M.E. (2015). The WRAP story origins and healing. www.mentalhealthrecovery.com/recovery-resources/articles.php?id=16 (accessed 16 May 2016).

Corrigan, P.W., Watson, A.C. & Barr, L. (2006). Understanding the self-stigma of mental illness. *Journal of Social and Clinical Psychology, 25*, 875–884.

Corrigan, P.W., Roe, D. & Tsang, H.W.H. (2011). *Challenging the Stigma of Mental Illness: Lessons for Therapists and Advocates.* Chichester, UK: Wiley-Blackwell.

David, A.S. & Prince, M. (2005). Psychosis following head injury: a critical review. *Journal of Neurology, Neurosurgery and Psychiatry, 76* (Suppl 1), 453–460.

Davies, G., Welham, J., Chant, D., Torrey, E.F. & McGrath, J. (2003). A systematic review and meta-analysis of northern hemisphere season of birth studies in schizophrenia. *Schizophrenia Bulletin, 29*, 587–593.

De Hert, M., Correll, C.U. Bobes, J. Cetkovich-Bakmas, M., Cohen, D., Asai, I., Detraux, J., Gautam, S., Moller, H.J., Ndetei, D.M., Newcomer, J.W., Uwakwe, R. & Leucht, S. (2011). Physical illness in patients with severe mental disorders: prevalence, impact of medication and disparities in health care. *World Psychiatry, 10*(1), 52–77.

Druss, B.G., Zhao L., von Esenwein, S.A., Bona, J.R., Fricks, L., Jenkins-Tucker S., Sterling, E., diClemente, R. & Lorig K. (2010). The Health and Recovery Peer (HARP) Program: a peer-led intervention to improve medical self-management for persons with serious mental illness. *Schizophrenia, 118*, 264–270.

Eliacin, J., Salyers, M.P., Kukla, M. & Matthias, M.S. (2015). Factors influencing patients' preferences and perceived involvement in shared decision-making in mental health care. *Journal of Mental Health, 24*, 24–28.

Fatemi, S.H. & Folsom, T. (2009). The neurodevelopmental hypothesis of schizophrenia, revisited. *Schizophrenia Bulletin*, *35*(3), 528–548.

Fearon, P., Kirkbride, J.B., Morgan, C., Dazzan, P., Morgan, P., Lloyd, T., Hutchinson, G., Tarrant, J., Fung, W.L.A., Holloways, J., Mallett, R., Harrison, G., Leff, J., Jones, P.B. &. Murray, R.M., on behalf of the AESOP Study Group. (2006). Incidence of schizophrenia and other psychoses in ethnic minority groups: results from the MRC AESOP Study. *Psychological Medicine*, *36*, 1541–1550.

Forrester-Jones, R., Carpenter, J., Coolen-Schrijner, P., Cambridge Tate, P.A., Hallam, A., Beecham, J., Knapp, M., & Wooff, D. (2012). Good friends are hard to find? The social networks of people with mental illness 12 years after deinstitutionalization. *Journal of Mental Health*, 21(1), 4–14.

González-Torres, M.A., Oraa, R., Arístegui, M., Fernández-Rivas, A. & Guimon, J. (2007). Stigma and discrimination towards people with schizophrenia and their family members. *Social Psychiatry and Psychiatric Epidemiology*, *42*(1), 14–23.

Gunlicks, M.L. & Weissman, M.M. (2008). Change in child psychopathology with improvement in parental depression: a systematic review. *Journal of the American Academy of Child and Adolescent Psychiatry*, *47*, 379–389.

Gur, R.E., Keshavan, M.S. & Lawrie, SM. (2007). Deconstructing psychosis with human brain imaging. *Schizophrenia Bulletin*, *33*, 921–931.

Holt, R.I., Busche, C. & Citrome, L. (2005). Diabetes and schizophrenia 2005: are we any closer to understanding the link? *Journal of Psychopharmacology*, *19*, 56–65.

Howes, O. & Kapur, S. (2009). The dopamine hypothesis of schizophrenia: version 111 – the final common pathway. *Schizophrenia Bulletin* *35*(3), 549–562.

Jané-Llopis, E. & Barry, M.M. (2005). What makes mental health promotion effective? *Promotion and Educations Supplement*, *2*, 47–55.

Jones, J.S., Fitzpatrick, J.J. & Rogers, V. (2012). *Psychiatric-Mental Health Nursing: An Interpersonal Approach*. New York: Springer.

Keefe, R.S. & Harvey, P.D. (2012). Cognitive impairment in schizophrenia. *Handbook of experimental Pharmacology*, 213, 11–37.

Keshavan, M., Tandon, R., Boutros, N. & Nasrallah, H.A. (2008). Schizophrenia, 'just the facts': what we know in 2008. *Schizophrenia Research*, *106*, 89–107.

Kramer, R.A., Warner, V., Olfson, M., Ebanks, C.M., Chaput, F. & Weissman, M.M. (1998). General medical problems among the offspring of depressed parents: A 10-year follow-up. *Journal of the American Academy of Child and Adolescent Psychiatry*, *37*, 602–611.

Larson, M.K., Walker, E.F. & Compton, M.T. (2010) Early signs, diagnosis and therapeutics of the prodromal phase of schizophrenia and related psychotic disorders. *Expert Review of Neurotherapeutics*, *10*(8), 1347–1359.

Lawrie, S., McIntosh, A., Hall, J., Owens, D. & Johnstone, E. (2008). Brain structure and function changes during the development of schizophrenia: the evidence from studies of subjects at increased genetic risk. *Schizophrenia Bulletin*, *34*(2), 330–340.

Leong, F.T.L. & Lau, A.S.L. (2001). Barriers to providing effective mental health services to Asian Americans. *Mental Health Services Research*, *3*, 201–214.

Livingston, J.D., Rossiter, K.R., Verdun-Jones, S.N., McMillan, D., Gilbody, S.M. & Beresford E, Neilly L. (2011). 'Forensic' labelling: an empirical assessment of its effects on self-stigma for people with severe mental illness. Can we predict suicide and non-fatal self-harm with the Beck Hopelessness Scale? A meta-analysis. *Psychological Medicine*, *37*, 769–778.

Lorig K.R. & Holman, H. (2003). Self-management education: history, definition, outcomes and mechanisms. *Annals of Behavioural Medicine*, *26*(1), 1–7.

Lichtermann, D., Karbe, E. and Maier, W., 2000. The genetic epidemiology of schizophrenia and of schizophrenia spectrum disorders. *European Archives of Psychiatry and Clinical Neuroscience*, *250*(6), 304–310.

MacDonald, AW. & Schulz, S.C. (2009). What we know: findings that every theory of schizophrenia should explain. *Schizophrenia Bulletin*, *35*(3), 493–508.

McGrath, J., Saha, S., Welham, J., El Saadi O., MacCauley, C. & Chant, D. (2004). A systematic review of the incidence of schizophrenia: the distribution of rates and the influence of sex, urbanicity, migrant status and methodology. *BMC Medicine*, *2*(13), 1–22. doi:10.1186/1741-7015-2-13.

McGrath, J., Brown, A. & St Clair, D. (2011). Prevention and schizophrenia – the role of dietary factors. *Schizophrenia Bulletin*, *37*(2), 272–283.

McGrath, P. & Holewa, H. (2004). Mental health and palliative care: exploring the ideological interface. *International Journal of Psychosocial Rehabilitation*, *9*(1), 107–119.

March, D., Hatch, SL., Morgan, C., Kirkbride, J.B., Bresnahan, M., Fearon, P. & Susser, E. (2008). Psychosis and place. *Epidemiologic Review, 30*, 84–100.

Mental Health Foundation. (2000). Pull yourself together! A survey of the stigma and discrimination faced by people who experience mental distress. www.mentalhealth.org.uk.

Mari, J., Razzouk, D., Thara, R., Eaton, J. & Thornicroft, G. (2009). Packages of care for schizophrenia in low- and middle-income countries. *PLoS Med, 6*(10), e1000165.

Michie, S., Johnston, M., Abraham, C., Lawton, R., Parker, D. & Walker, A. (2005). Making psychological theory useful for implementing evidence based practice: a consensus approach. *Quality and safety in health care*, 14(1), 26–33.

Mitchell, A.J. Delaffon, V., Vancampfort, D., Correll, C.U. & De Hert, M. (2011). Guideline concordant monitoring of metabolic risk in people treated with antipsychotic medication: systematic review and meta-analysis of screening practices. *Psychological Medicine, 42*, 125–147.

Morgan, C. & Fisher, H. (2007). Environmental factors in schizophrenia: childhood trauma – a critical review. *Schizophrenia Bulletin 33*, 3–10.

Morgan, C., Charlambides, M., Hutchinson, G. & Murray, R. (2010). Migration, ethnicity and psychosis: towards a sociodevelopment model. *Schizophrenia Bulletin, 36*(4) 655–664.

Nasrallah, H.A., Meyer, J.M., Goff, D.C., McEvoy, J.P., Davis, S.M., Stroup, T.S. & Lieberman, J.A. (2006). Low rates of treatment for hypertension, dyslipidemia and diabetes in schizophrenia: data from the CATIE schizophrenia trial sample at baseline. *Schizophrenia Research, 86*(1), 15–22.

National Economic and Social Forum. (2007). *Mental Health and Social Inclusion. NESF Report 36*. Dublin: Dublin National Economic and Social Forum.

Petersen, I., Bhana, A., Flisher, A.J., Swartz, L. & Richter, L. (eds). (2010). *Promoting Mental Health in Scarce-resource Contexts*. Cape Town, South Africa: HSRC Press.

Pollett, H. (2007). *Mental Health Promotion: A Literature Review, Prepared for the Mental Health Promotion Working Group of the Provincial Wellness Advisory Council*. Ottawa, ON: Canadian Mental Health Association.

Prince, P.N. & Gerber, G.J. (2005). Subjective well-being and community integration among clients of assertive community treatment. *Qual Life Res*, 14(1), 161–169.

Prince, M., Patel, V., Saxena, S., Maj, M., Maskels, J., Phillips, M. & Rahman, A. (2007). Global mental health 1: no health without mental health. *The Lancet, 370*, 859–77.

Radhakrishnan, R., Wilkinson, S.T. & D'Souza, D.C. (2014). Gone to pot: a review of the association between cannabis and psychosis. *Frontiers in Psychiatry, 5*, 1–24.

Rahman, A., Fisher, J., Bower, P., Luchters, S., Tran, T., Yasamy, M.T., Saxena, S. & Waheed, W. (2013). Interventions for common perinatal mental disorders in women in low- and middle-income countries: a systematic review and meta-analysis. *Bulletin of the World Health Organization, 91*, 593–601.

Repper, J., Perkins, R. & UFM Network. (2006). Looking through user's eyes. *Mental Health Today*, 25–28.

Saha, S. Chant, D., Welhan, J. & McGrath, J. (2005). A systematic review of the prevelance of schizophrenia. *PLoSMed, 2*, 413–433.

St Clair, D., Xu, M., Wang, P., Yu, Y., Fang, Y., Zhang, F., Zheng, X., Gu, N., Feng, G., Sham, P. & He, L. (2005). Rates of adult schizophrenia following prenatal exposure to the Chinese famine of 1959–1961. *JAMA, 294*, 557–562.

Schnittker, J. (2008). An uncertain revolution: why the rise of a genetic model of mental illness has not increased tolerance. *Social Science and Medicine, 67*, 1370–1381.

Sheridan, A., Drennan, J., Coughlan, B., O'Keefe, D., Frazer, K., Alexander, D., Howlin, F., Fahy, A., Kow, V. & O'Callaghan, E. (2014). Improving social functioning and reducing social isolation and loneliness among people with enduring mental illness: report of a randomised controlled trial of supported socialization. *International Journal of Social Psychiatry, 61*(3), 241–250.

Sun, D., Phillips, L., Velakoulis, D., Yung, A., McGorry, P., Wood, S., Cannon, T.D. & Pantelis, C. (2008). Progressive brain structural changes mapped as psychosis develops in 'at risk' individuals. *Schizophrenia Research, 108*(1–3), 85–92.

Susser, E.S. & Lin, S.P. (1992). Schizophrenia after prenatal exposure to the Dutch Hunger Winter 1944–1945. *Archives of General Psychiatry, 49*, 983–988.

Tandon, R., Keshavan, M. & Nasrallah, H.A. (2008). Schizophrenia, 'just the facts': what we know in 2008. *Schizophrenia Research, 102*, 1–18.

Tandon, R., Nasrallah, H.A. & Keshavan, M. (2009.) Schizophrenia, 'just the facts' 4. *Clinical Features and Conceptualizations, 110*, 1–23.

Tandon, N., Shah, J., Keshavan, M. & Tandon R. (2012). Attenuated psychosis and the schizophrenia prodrome: current status of risk identification and psychosis prevention. *Neuropsychiatry (London)*, *2*(4), 345–353.

Thornicroft, G. (2011). Physical health disparities and mental illness: the scandal of premature mortality. *British Journal of Psychiatry*, *199*, 441–442.

Torrey, E.F., Miller, J., Rawlings, R. & Yolken, R.H. (1997). Seasonality of birth in schizophrenia and bipolar disorder: a review of the literature. *Schizophrenia Research*, *28*, 1–38.

Travelbee, J. (1971). *Interpersonal Aspects of Nursing*. Philadelphia, PA: F.A. Davis.

UNICEF. (2013). *The State of the World's Children: Children with Disabilities*. New York: United Nations Children's Fund.

Van Os, J., Kenis, G. & Rutten, B.P.F. (2010). The environment and schizophrenia. *Nature*, *468*, 203–212.

Vita, A., De Peri, L., Silenzi, C. & Dieci, M. (2006). Brain Morphology in first episode schizophrenia: a meta-analysis of quantitative magnetic resonance imaging studies. *Schizophrenia Research*, *82*, 75–88.

Voruganti, L.P., Punthakee, Z., Van Lieshout, R.J., MacCrimmon, D., Parker, G., Awad, A.G. & Gerstein, H.C. (2007). Dysglycemia in a community sample of people treated for schizophrenia: the Diabetes in Schizophrenia in Central-South Ontario (DiSCO) study. *Schizophrenia Research*, *96*(1), 215–222.

Wahlbect, K., Westman, J., Nordentoft, M. Gissler, M. & Laursen, T.M. (2011). Outcomes of Nordic mental health system: life expectancy of patients with mental disorders. *British Journal of Psychiatry*, *199*, 453–458.

Watson, A.C., Corrigan, P.W., Larson, J.E. & Sells, M. (2007). Self-stigma in people with mental illness. *Schizophrenia Bulletin*, *33*, 1312–1318.

Welham. J., Isohanni, M., Jones, P. & McGrath, J. (2009). The antecedents of schizophrenia: a review of birth cohort studies. *Schizophrenia Bulletin*, *35*(3), 603–623.

Wilson, S. & Durbin, C.E. (2010). Effects of paternal depression on fathers' parenting behaviors: a meta-analytic review. *Clinical Psychology Review*, *30*, 167–180.

World Health Organization. (2001). *The World Health Report 2001. Mental Health: New Understanding, New Hope*. Geneva: WHO.

World Health Organization. (2004). *Promoting Mental Health: Concepts, Emerging Evidence, Practice: Summary Report*. Geneva: WHO.

World Health Organization. (2008). *The Global Burden of Disease: 2004 Update*. Geneva: WHO.

World Health Organization. (2013). *Mental Health Action Plan 2013–2020*. Geneva: WHO.

Xiang, Y.T., Ma, X., Ji Cai, Z., Li, S.R., Xiang, Y.Q., Guo, H.L., Hou, Y.Z., Li, Z.B., Li, Z.J., Tao, Y.F., Dang, W.M., Wu, X.M., Deng, J., Lai, K.Y.C. & Ungvari, G.S. (2008). Prevalence and socio-demographic correlates of schizophrenia in Beijing, China. *Schizophrenia Research*, *102*, 270–277.

Yuii, K., Suzuki, M. and Kurachi, M. (2007). Stress sensitization in schizophrenia. *Annals of the New York Academy of Sciences*, *1113*(1), 276–290.

16

HEALTH PROMOTION STRATEGIES FOR SUBSTANCE USE

Madeline A. Naegle

Introduction

The use of substances to alter mental states has existed in almost every culture known to man. Psychoactive drug use, however, has the potential to significantly threaten health at all stages of human development. Substances used have their greatest impact on mental and physical health based on the prevalence of use, the severity of induced addiction and negative economic and societal impact. Worldwide, nurses encounter and care for the mental health problems co-occurring and induced by substance use and its disorders. Pearson (2010) notes that mental health promotion strategies, within the umbrella of health promotion are the purview of all nurses. Based on education and practice setting, nurses must intervene to implement primary, secondary, and tertiary interventions to promote health, reduce harm, and build resilience within populations around the globe.

In recent decades, an abundance of social and basic science research has illuminated the social mechanisms, neurophysiology, and psychological changes precipitated by alcohol, tobacco, and other substance use. The negative consequences of substance use erode health, economies, productivity, and quality of family and community life in developed and developing countries. The extent to which scientific findings are the bases for prevention and intervention for substance use disorders is uneven and depends on the resources, politics and state of the science in low-, middle-, and high-income countries. How substance use is recognized, evaluated and addressed varies widely by culture and region. For example, alcohol and nicotine have only recently been regarded as "drugs" in medical and government classifications, and policy about their use and health outcomes are monitored separately. These parameters are very important to understanding the scope of substance use disorders (SUDs) worldwide and how nurses can address these health issues. This chapter will describe prevalence, etiology, and characteristics of substance use disorders, global and cultural patterns of substance use with associated consequences, and nursing strategies to support primary, secondary, and tertiary levels of substance use prevention.

The global context

The Comprehensive Mental Health Action Plan 2013–2020 describes the influence of individual and social determinants on the "state of well-being" which is mental health (WHO, 2013a).

Vulnerable groups, highlighted as "at high risk" for mental health problems are older adults, those with chronic illnesses and adolescents on first exposure to substance use. In addition, the plan highlights alcohol use as a risk factor for acute and chronic illness and conditions requiring complex services that contribute to the global burden of disease. Overall, 5.1 percent of the global burden of disease, measured in disability-adjusted life years (DALYs) and injuries, are directly attributable to alcohol (WHO, 2014a) but in developed countries, psychoactive substance use accounts for 33.4 percent of all DALYs (WHO, 2014b). Approximately 2 billion people worldwide consume alcoholic beverages and 76.3 million consumers have diagnosable alcohol use disorders. Other psychoactive substance use is estimated to account for 8.9 percent of global disease burden expressed in DALYs (WHO, 2012). Combined, tobacco, alcohol and illicit drugs (ATOD), are responsible for 12.4 percent of all deaths worldwide (WHO, 2014c).

While the global burden of ATOD use varies across WHO regions, with the burden significantly higher in Europe and the Western Pacific than in Africa and the Eastern Mediterranean, all countries face challenges associated with drug use. Substance use and SUDs, unfortunately, are often not viewed as psychiatric disorders by psychiatrists, nurses and other mental health professionals. In many countries, psychiatric and substance abuse services are categorized and funded separately from other medical treatment services and research, as in the USA and the Russian Federation. These are two of several factors that complicate the development of research and dissemination of best practices, limiting the strength of evidence on which to base health practices. The amount of attention given to funding research and services contrasts starkly with the size of the global burden and cost to economies associated with psychoactive substance use. The potential for health professionals including psychiatrists, nurses, pharmacists, dentists, and their professional associations to contribute to reducing this burden is yet to be realized (WHO, 2013a).

Tobacco and alcohol are responsible for 8.1 percent of the disease burden attributable to neuropsychiatric disorders, accounting for close to 40 percent of the 58.3 million DALYs. Alcohol use, for example, is the top risk factor for health in low mortality, developing countries with alcohol posing the largest burden in Africa, the Americas and Western Pacific countries (WHO, 2014b). Tobacco use poses the largest burden in Europe and South-East Asia. Worldwide psychoactive substance use is estimated at 2 billion alcohol users, 1.3 billion smokers and 185 million drug users (WHO, 2014b). These figures do not include the prevalence of co-existing mental health and substance use disorders and fluctuate by international trends. For example, the use of prescription opioids in the US and the prevalence of heroin addiction in Asia have continued to rise since the 1990s. The WHO and its member countries address alcohol, illicit and prescription drugs separately in monitoring, policy development, and actions to deter use. Most organized groups of health care providers recognize the category of "psychoactive drugs" as including all of these.

Figure 16.1 illustrates prevalence of illicit drug use among 15–64-year-olds from 2008–2010 worldwide.

Etiology of substance use disorders

Theories on the etiology of substance use disorders are biologic, psychological, and social, and each contributes reasons why exposure and use of drugs with high abuse potential become problematic for some individuals and societies and not for others. Social traditions and patterns of drug use generally determine what drugs are used, the circumstances under which drug use is acceptable and for whom, and how much drug can be used without creating health and social problems. Certain psychological and personality traits have also been identified as placing the individual at risk for drug experimentation, common in many societies, which then becomes

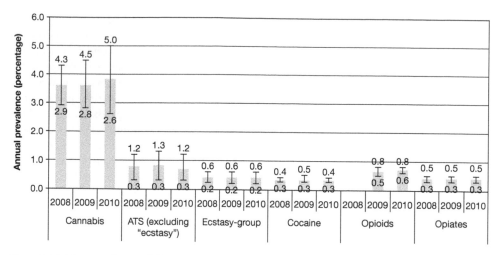

Figure 16.1 The prevalence of illicit drug use among 15–64-year-olds from 2008–2010 worldwide

Source: Reprinted with permission from the *Diagnostic and Statistical Manual of Mental Disorders*, Fifth Edition (Copyright © 2013). American Psychiatric Association. All Rights Reserved.

habitual and extends to compulsive and uncontrolled use of a drug (addiction). Research has consistently supported findings that genetic factors are most influential in the progression from substance use to a substance use disorder.

Research findings demonstrate that the strongest hypothesis for the development of a severe substance use disorder or addiction is neurobiologic. Evidence indicates that addiction to a substance is a dysregulation of reward pathways in the midbrain of the central nervous system. The natural reinforcers of pleasure or reward such as sex, food, or exercise, activate neuro-chemical responses (the neurotransmitters dopamine, serotonin, and GABA among others). Genetic predisposition plays a key role for 40–60 percent of individuals with severe alcohol use disorder, with high prevalence among relatives (APA, 2013). A genetic predisposition implies an inclination to neuroadaptation to chronic drug use, and an increased risk for developing physiologic dependence. This predisposition and familial pattern also exists with individuals with tobacco use disorders and while each of these disorders is linked to a different gene, some overlap exists and supports the co-occurrence of nicotine and alcohol dependence (Grucza & Bierut, 2006). Neurobiologic models of addiction to drugs of abuse have three central phenomena: 1) the drug's property of inducing euphoria i.e. cocaine and amphetamine have high euphorigenicity versus sedative hypnotics; 2) the capacity of the drug to positively re-enforce drug seeking behavior; and 3) the avoidance of aversive feelings, like symptoms of withdrawal or emotional states, which the drug of abuse suppresses (O'Brien & Jaffe, 1992). Euphoria induced by drugs of abuse is the potent re-enforcer of the reward system, evoking a reorganization of the normal reward system. While the pharmacological mechanisms for each class of drug is different, the activation of the reward system is similar for all substances.

At the same time, certain personality traits can be protective inasmuch as they deter the likelihood of developing a severe substance use disorder. These personality traits include positive emotionality, a robust ability to inhibit/control impulses, good executive function in the areas of reasoning, judgment and insight, and a balanced system of reward that considers basic need fulfillment. Learning, behavioral conditioning and good coping skills as well, enhance the ability to manage the frustrations associated with everyday life (Marmot, 2005).

Characteristics of the individual related to their environment, detailed in the WHO social determinants of health report (Marmot, 2005), as well as learning, are major factors in understanding how an individual initially comes to use drugs and continues to be exposed to them (Merikangas & McClair, 2012). Learned patterns of substance use are evident in families and communities where heroin injection and alcohol consumption become a way of life adopted by children and young adults.

The Adverse Childhood Events study (Dube *et al.*, 2003), a longitudinal survey of illness outcomes, correlates the number of adverse events experienced in childhood with physical and mental disorders in adult life; the higher the number of events, the greater the likelihood of developing a range of mental and other medical illnesses (Dube *et al.*, 2003). Among the most prevalent events reported in this American sample of the ACE study is the presence of substance abuse in the household by parents, or other relatives and occupants at 26.9 percent. The identified life events pose challenges to comprehensive health, but in particular, challenge the capacity for adaptation and coping. Life stressors may increase the risk for development of an alcohol use disorder, but stress alone is not considered an etiologic factor for SUDs. Stress more clearly contributes to continuing excess drinking as a learned coping mechanism when an individual already has an alcohol use disorder (Keyes, Hatzenbuehler, Grant, & Hasin, 2012). Examples of the interaction of genetics, learning and family environment were described in a small community in Northern New Mexico (Eckholm, 2008), and in tribes of Native Americans with high rates of alcoholism and fetal alcohol spectrum effects (USDHHS, 2014). Personality, learned patterns of behavior and personal choices all influence the development of maladaptive patterns of drug use (APA, 2013). Research suggests that personality traits such as impulsivity, decreased inhibitions, along with negative emotions (McCue, Slutske, Taylor & Iacono, 1997; Mulder, 2005; Schuckit, 1998; Trull, Waudby, & Sher, 2004) may predispose to substance use and habituation to their psychoactive effects. At the same time, certain personality traits can be protective inasmuch as they deter the likelihood of developing a severe substance use disorder. These personality traits include positive emotionality, a robust ability to inhibit/control impulses, good executive function in the areas of reasoning, judgment and insight, a balanced system of reward that considers basic need fulfillment, and the ability to find meaning and direction in life. Learning, behavioral conditioning and good coping skills as well, enhance the ability to manage the frustrations associated with everyday life (Marmot, 2005). Additional protective factors include living in families, societies and communities as opposed to in isolation, maintaining a positive self-image, and experiencing a sense of social competence (Keyes, 2007; SAMHSA, 2015).

Classification systems

The World Health Organization uses the International *Statistical Classifications of Diseases and Related Health Disorders, 10th edition* (ICD-10) as the standard diagnostic tool for epidemiology, health management and clinical purposes, including substance use disorders. WHO's definition of addiction parallels that of the *Diagnostic and Statistical Manual of Psychological Disorders* (DSM-5) more commonly used in the USA, Canada, and some Western European nations, as well as Latin America. For WHO, the term "harmful use and hazardous use" relates only to effects on health and not to social consequences (APA, 2013; WHO, 2016). Previously "abuse" has referred to non-medical or unsanctioned patterns of use, irrespective of consequences. Similarly, psychoactive substance misuse has referred to use of a substance for purposes not consistent with legal or medical guidelines, as in the non-medical use of prescription medications (WHO, 2016). In the DSM-5 section, "substance-related and addictive disorders" gambling is also addressed, reflecting recent evidence sufficient for the hypothesis that gambling activates reward systems within the brain similar to those activated by psychoactive drugs (Grant & Potenza, 2004). ICD-10 includes gambling as a category of behavioral disorder. The American Psychological Association refers to behavioral patterns or syndromes such as gambling as "behavioral addictions" (APA, 2013). At present, however, there is insufficient evidence to state that these behavior patterns meet criteria and conform to the descriptions necessary to be classified as "addictions." Behavioral addictions include gaming, excessive sexual activity, and compulsive use of the internet. Compulsive use of the internet, for example, has prompted the development of treatment and rehabilitation programs in South Korea, and gambling places many older adults at risk for financial and personal loss. Parallel diagnostic categories exist in the ICD-10.

Table 16.1 illustrates the criteria used to diagnose Alcohol Use Disorder. The reader is referred to the DSM-5 manual for criteria associated with specific substances.

Severity is determined by the number of symptom criteria endorsed, range from mild to severe, and can generally be considered as mild (2–3 symptoms), moderate (5–4 symptoms) and severe, (6 or more) symptoms. Specifiers relate to phases of the illness or disorder, such as early remission, sustained remission, etc. The reader is again referred to the DSM-5 for interpretation and appropriate application (APA, 2013, p. 484).

Trends in international policy related to substance use

Policies, legislation, and social practices can also intentionally or unintentionally create and exacerbate risk and harm for drug users and complicate access for those who need treatment for severe SUDs. Such practices include the criminalization of drug use, stigma and discrimination, failure

Table 16.1 Alcohol Use Disorder

A problematic pattern of alcohol use leading to clinically significant impairment or distress, as manifested by at least two of the following, occurring within a 12-month period:

1 Alcohol is often taken in larger amounts or over a longer period than was intended
2 There is a persistent desire or unsuccessful efforts to cut down or control alcohol use
3 A great deal of time is spent in activities necessary to obtain alcohol, use alcohol, or recover from its effects
4 Craving, or a strong desire or urge to use alcohol
5 Recurrent alcohol use resulting in a failure to fulfill major role obligations at work, school, or home
6 Continued alcohol use despite having persistent or recurrent social or interpersonal problems caused or exacerbated by the effects of alcohol
7 Important social, occupational, or recreational activities are given up or reduced because of alcohol use
8 Recurrent alcohol use in situations in which it is physically hazardous
9 Alcohol use is continued despite knowledge of having a persistent or recurrent physical or psychological problem that is likely to have been caused or exacerbated by alcohol
10 Tolerance, as defined by either of the following:
 a) A need for markedly increased amounts of alcohol to achieve intoxication or desired effect
 b) A markedly diminished effect with continued use of the same amount of alcohol
11 Withdrawal, as manifested by either of the following:
 a) The characteristic withdrawal syndrome for alcohol (refer to Criteria A and B of the criteria set for alcohol withdrawal, pp. 499–500)
 b) Alcohol (or a closely related substance, such as a benzodiazepine) is taken to relieve or avoid withdrawal symptoms

---

Source: Reprinted with permission from the *Diagnostic and Statistical Manual of Mental Disorders*, Fifth Edition, Copyright © 2013. American Psychiatric Association. All Rights Reserved.

to implement policies to restrict accessibility to drugs, abusive and corrupt policing practices, overly restrictive and punitive judicial practices, the absence of harm reduction services, and the denial of life-saving medical care. Social inequities frequently determine access to treatment as evidenced in unemployment, insurance coverage, and inequitable law enforcement. Resources in various regions and countries (social determinants), determine accessibility to SUDs treatment with many areas lacking sufficient treatment resources for persons who develop addiction. These include around 1 in 20 (or approximately 230 million) adults who use an illicit drug annually, and are at risk for a substance use disorder. Only 1.7 beds per 100,000 of the population are available for this kind of treatment (WHO, 2014b).

In 2013, the sixty-sixth World Health Assembly took action to decrease disparities in resources and opportunities for health worldwide (WHO, 2013a). Noting the social determinants of health (place of birth and location of growth, work and aging, as well as resources and systems), they agreed to act to influence economic and environmental policies and politics for better health outcomes. The social determinants of health are particularly relevant to the development of substance use disorders. Tracking substance use around the world reveals patterns by region, age group, gender, and economic status. For example, in countries with the highest income, the disability-adjusted life years (DALYs) due to drug dependence, which increases burden on the economy and raises the human toll of suffering, is almost 20 times higher than in low-income countries (WHO, 2014a).

Influences of stigma, culture, and gender

Addiction is stigmatized throughout the world, but social definitions of addiction vary widely. Even as treatment for SUDs becomes more evidence-based, health ministries are challenged to find public acceptance of formal treatment programs and mutual help organizations such as narcotics and alcoholics anonymous, and other programs (Klingemann & Bergmark, 2006). Treatment enrollment is deterred by stigma, requirements to "register "as an addict e.g. Russia (Boborava *et al.*, 2006), monitoring by law enforcement e.g. China (Lu & Wang, 2008) and absence or limited support services such as childcare and insurance coverage. The lay public often views addiction as a social deviance, or requires evidence of physical pathology before accepting a person's illness. In the US, where addiction specialists have demonstrated the correspondence between addiction's course and recidivism and that of other non-communicable diseases (NCDs), many continue to reject the disease model of addiction. In all societies, men are more likely to use alcohol, tobacco, and other drugs (ATOD) at rates higher than those of women and to drink heavily even into later age (Wilsnack, Wilsnack, Kristjanson, Vogeltanz-Hom, & Gmel, 2009). Gender is a strong factor determining health outcomes of ATOD use and women are disadvantaged by greater stigma, deterrents to seeking treatment, and greater physiologic and biologic vulnerability to the effects of psychoactive drug use. Culturally sensitive approaches to SUD prevention and treatment have yet to be developed and integrated into nursing care in most countries where women, especially pregnant women and older adults do not seek treatment for fear of social consequences and a lack of fit between program design and patient needs. Consequently, there are significant gender differences in the proportion of global deaths attributable to alcohol for men and women. While in 2012, 7.6 percent of deaths among males and 4 percent of deaths among females were attributable to alcohol. Women's vulnerability to serious substance use disorders is evidenced in disproportionately higher tolls on women's health and longevity. In the US, for example, while only 17.4 percent of heavy episodic drinkers are women (men are 30.9 percent), the effects of long-term heavy alcohol use by women makes a higher contribution to their mortality (WHO, 2014a). This is also evident in countries like

Finland, another heavy consuming society, with heavy episodic drinking at 36.5 percent of the population (males 69.8 percent; females 35.4 percent). While alcohol dependence is higher among men, it takes a greater toll on health for women who are heavy drinkers, even though they are fewer in number (WHO, 2014a). The higher vulnerability of women to negative effects of heavy drinking extends to physiologic, social, and psychological outcomes.

Tobacco use disorder

The use of tobacco and tobacco products is linked to the highest mortality and morbidity of any substance, particularly head and neck cancer in men, and lung cancer in women, and cardiovascular disease and chronic respiratory disease, i.e. chronic bronchitis.

Nicotine rapidly induces physical and psychological dependence and rivals cocaine in the tenacity of addiction and challenges of recovery. Its desirable effects are identified as performance enhancement and positive effect on mood (Camí & Farré, 2003). While people of all ages are vulnerable to the negative health outcomes of tobacco use, special concern is reserved for young people, pregnant women, and older adults. Many smokers initiate use before age 18 (as high as 58.8 percent), placing them at risk for many years, and often, a lifetime of nicotine dependence (SAMHSA, 2016). A 2006 national study of students (14,434) and parents (25,697) in mainland China found past-month smoking prevalence to accelerate from middle school (9 percent), and 8 percent among academic high school students, to 26 percent in vocational high school students, 21 percent among college students, and 40 percent among adult patients (Johnson *et al.*, 2006). The projection of rates of tobacco-related disease in Asia indicates the need for widespread prevention to reduce the global burden associated with these illnesses and their human and economic implications. In the US, 25.2 percent of the population uses some form of tobacco and use is broken down to several categories. Within this group, approximately 10 percent of American women (CDC PRAMS, 2011) and Canadian women (Al-Sahab, Saqib, & Tamim, 2010) continue smoking during pregnancy despite evidence that smoking results in fetal risk for lower birth weight and higher risk for infection, respiratory disorders, delayed growth, and learning disabilities (CDC, 2013). Among older adults over age 65, as many as 9 percent continue to smoke, increasing the risks for cardiovascular illness and exacerbating many chronic illnesses, such as cancer and HIV (CDC, 2014).

Smoking tobacco in cigarettes, hookahs, cigars, or exposure to secondary smoke is responsible for 6 million deaths annually worldwide; the smoking rate is 22 percent of the total population. Thirty-one percent of men use some form of tobacco, as do 6 percent of women (WHO, 2014a). Persons aged 8 to 65 smoke, and rates are highest in Southeast Asia and Eastern Europe and lowest in Guinea. Table 16.2 details the prevalence of current smokers in representative countries with some of the highest rates of smoking (Russia and China) as well as some of the lowest rates (many African countries). Data were not reported for several countries in the Middle East.

As cigarette smoking has become more socially acceptable and accessible, the prevalence of lung cancer in women has risen (Torre, Siegel, Ward, & Jemal, 2014) and in some countries prevalence of smoking for men and women varies only slightly as found in Table 16.2.

The practice of hookah smoking, common in Middle Eastern countries is now increasingly common in industrialized nations. Research data suggest that the smoke ingested during one session of waterpipe or "hookah" smoking contains as much "tar" as 20 low tar cigarettes (Shihadeh, 2003 p. 51) and as much smoke as inhaled in cigarettes (Jackson & Aveyard, 2008). Smokers of electronic cigarettes (e-cigarettes) are increasing, with 6 percent of smokers reporting e-cigarette use, double the percent reporting use in 2010 (CDC, 2013). In middle and high school, the use of both e-cigarettes and smoking increased between 2011 and 2012 (CDC, 2013).

Table 16.2 Country smoking rates from high to low rates: regional representation for adults

Country	Percentage of current smokers		WHO Region
	Men (%)	Women (%)	
Argentina	29.4	15.6	PAHO
Albania	44.7	4.2	EURO
China	52.9	2.4	WPRO
Czech Republic	41.3	32.3	EURO
Georgia	55.5	4.8	EURO
Ghana	8.2	0.4	AFRO
Iran	24.58	3.25	EMRO
Japan	32.4	9.7	SEARO
Norway	28	28	EURO
Russian Federation	60.1	15.8	EURO
Spain	32.5	24.6	EURO
United Kingdom and Northern Ireland	21	20	EURO
United States	20.5	15.8	PAHO

Source: WHO (2013b), Appendix XI, Table 11.1: Survey of Adult Tobacco Use in WHO Member States.

While the effects on health of e-cigarettes remain uncertain, cautionary (primary prevention) public health methods focus on the risks of nicotine addiction, the impact of nicotine on the adolescent brain and the risk for progression to conventional cigarette smoking. The value of e-cigarettes as an aide to decreasing cigarette smoking remains widely debated among addictions professionals. Some argue that the vaporized nicotine is far less damaging that inhaling tobacco smoke, and that e-cigarettes can help reduce the overall number of cigarettes used. To date, e-cigarette analysis by the FDA revealed the presence of tobacco impurities in e-cigarettes sampled as well as traces of substances toxic to humans (US Food and Drug Administration, 2014). Nicotine dependence is assessed when the individual reports using over 10 cigarettes daily. This can be done using a quantity/frequency index or the Fagerstrom Test, a 6-item questionnaire (Heatherton, Kozlowski, Frecker, & Fagerström, 1991). Nicotine use disorders are classified as mild, moderate, or severe and best clinical practices include a combination of interpersonal and pharmacotherapies following the US Public Health Service Clinical Practice Guidelines (Fiore *et al.*, 2008). A successful treatment outcome of complete smoking cessation may not occur until the individual has made as many as six quit attempts. Nicotine dependence disorder has high rates of recidivism; most individuals relapsing within 6 months of the first quit (Stead & Lancaster, 2012).

Alcohol use disorders

Comparing drinking patterns and rates for alcohol-related problems across countries is challenging due to the wide variation in measures and study methodologies (WHO, 2000). History and cultural differences are often cited in explaining the worldwide variation in patterns of alcohol consumption. The scope of alcohol problems by country and region is assessed in survey research and limited data are available on the production and consumption of beverages containing alcohol for almost all countries.

Worldwide, about 16.0 percent of drinkers aged 15 years or older are heavy episodic drinkers with high-income countries having the highest alcohol per capita consumption (APC) and the highest prevalence of heavy episodic drinking (WHO, 2014a). Episodic heavy drinking is consumption of 5 or more drinks by men under 65 and 4 or more drinks by women on one occasion. For men and women over 65, heavy drinking is more than 8 drinks a week and more than 4 drinks on one occasion. A pattern of heavy drinking more than once a month is considered binge drinking (CDC, 2014). The global burden related to alcohol consumption and associated morbidity is considerable with mortality, at 3.3 million deaths, or 5.9 percent of all global deaths, attributable to alcohol consumption (WHO, 2014a).

Consequences of regular consumption of alcohol may include health problems, social consequences of intoxication (drunkenness), and alcohol dependence. In addition to chronic diseases that may affect drinkers after many years of heavy use, alcohol contributes to traumatic outcomes that kill or disable at a relatively young age, resulting in the loss of many years of life due to death or disability. Alcohol-induced disorders affect everyone spanning from birth, with fetal alcohol spectrum disorders (FASD), to family life with a parent with a moderate alcohol use disorder, to Wernicke's syndrome with onset after many years of heavy consumption. FASDs are a group of conditions that can occur when mothers drink alcohol during pregnancy. There is no safe level for alcohol consumption during pregnancy, as alcohol's teratogenicity properties are now well known (CDC, 2014). There is increasing evidence that in addition to the volume of alcohol consumed, the pattern of consumption has relevance for health outcomes. There is a causal relationship between harmful alcohol consumption and more than 60 types of diseases, injury, and a range of mental and behavioral disorders. Further, the burden is not equally distributed among countries, with alcohol consumption a leading risk factor for disease burden in low mortality developing countries and the third largest risk factor in developed countries like those in Eastern Europe where high alcohol consumption correlates with lower life expectancy (WHO, 2014a).

Illicit drug use

Internationally, illicit drug use is most prevalent in males, but reliable data on the extent of use, the prevalence of use disorders, and treatment options are not consistently available. World-wide, approximately 158.8 million or 3.8 percent of the population has used illicit drugs in their lifetime (UNODC, 2015). In 2004 the WHO estimated that 0.7 percent of disease burden was attributable to cocaine and opioid use. In addition, the cost of illicit substance use was estimated at roughly 2 percent of the Gross Domestic Product (GDP) when measured (Fogarty International Center, 2011).

Globally, cannabis is the most commonly used substance (129–190 million people), followed by amphetamine-type stimulants, then cocaine and opioids (UNODC, 2015). Opioid and synthetic opioid drug use (codeine, oxycontin, vicodin) now results in the highest mortality rates. While all drug use is highest between the ages of 18 and 26, use of marijuana and misuse/abuse of opioid drugs are now increasingly common in adults over the age of 55 (NIDA, 2016).

Opioid, alcohol, amphetamine, and cocaine dependence are the drugs most frequently linked to suicide. The epidemic proportions of opioid-related deaths among young and late middle-aged adults parallel this worldwide trend. In the US, opioid analgesic use, illicit and prescribed, identified as the cause of death almost quadrupled between 1999 and 2011. In addition, drugs (illicit and prescribed) are now the major cause (90 percent) of poisoning deaths (NIDA, 2014). The use of psychoactive substances causes significant health and social problems for users, their families and communities. The co-morbidities of HIV/AIDs and Hepatitis C are also linked to injection drug use.

Opioid use disorders

Opioid users constitute a large percentage of approximately 15.3 million persons with drug use disorders. Two examples of countries where opioid use has burgeoned in recent years are China and the United States. Opioid addiction in China, dates from the nineteenth century but has been on the rise since the 1990s (Tang & Wao, 2007). Of the 1.6 million drug-dependent persons in China in 2005, at least 75–85 percent were heroin dependent (Liu, Lu, Mu, Lian, & Zhou, 2002). Many of these are young, male and unemployed, corresponding to risk factors delineated by Marmot in the WHO Social Determinants of Health report (Marmot, 2005).

Nursing interventions: promoting global well-being

Nurses and midwives provide 90 percent of the mental health care worldwide (WHO, 2000). Nurse generalists and specialists have roles that can include prevention of SUDs, the treatment of behavioral and substance addictions, and assistance and support for recovery for individuals and families. The role expectations for nurses in all specialties, but particularly in psychiatry and substance disorders treatment, however, are defined by traditions and practices found in employment settings, rather than current science and educational preparation.

Nursing education ranges from technical training to post graduate education, and recent outreach by ICN and WHO has increased nurses' interest, awareness and use of evidence-based practices. Efforts at prevention and mental health promotion are differentiated by level of education and specialty practice as well, but all nurses, direct practitioners, policy developers, or nurse educators, should develop knowledge and skills on substance use disorders. Prevention strategies are most closely linked to social initiatives, are public health oriented, or may involve health teaching, and the provider may not consider the action an "intervention." For example, the inclusion of a drug and alcohol history in the basic individual/family assessment introduces a teachable moment, which can be health education or a targeted intervention such as anticipatory guidance or health teaching in anticipation of conception, pregnancy, and childbearing. All nurses should counsel pregnant women on the implications of smoking, with evidence supporting effective use by nurses of office-based assessment and individualized client counseling (Albrecht *et al.*, 2006).

Counseling on the use of all drugs, including alcohol, should occur for all clients from childhood to older age. As advocates for clients/patients and health, nurses can challenge beliefs and attitudes that addiction and illicit drug use are social choices versus medical disorders, the mechanisms of which are now well documented. When addiction or severe substance use disorders are understood as chronic, relapsing conditions treatable by interpersonal and pharmacotherapeutic interventions, the notion of recovery can be more readily accepted (White, Boyle, & Loveland, 2002). When nurses role model advocacy and engagement with persons suffering from these disorders, they can influence consumer attitudes and reduce stigma. This has implications for both prevention and harm reduction.

Primary prevention using education and information sharing in social contexts

Primary prevention is undertaken in the absence of symptoms and based on the expectation that risk or exposure to illness is likely. Since substance use disorders are multi-determined it is hard to target prevention to factors (Durlak & Wells, 1997). Primary prevention for substance use disorders is more often: 1) targeted at populations known to be vulnerable to developing substance use disorders and/or; 2) focused on limiting exposure to substances. When a strong evidence base exists, such as the relationship between tobacco use and cancer and cardiovascular disease, universal screening is a form of primary prevention. Similarly, screening and advising pregnant women on potential negative fetal effects of alcohol and the risk of fetal alcohol spectrum disorder are supported by strong evidence.

Additional forms of primary prevention at societal levels include legislation in regions, nations and internationally. In the US, using sobriety checkpoints has been demonstrated to decrease alcohol-related vehicular mortality (Elder *et al.*, 2002). National and international policies are often separate and discrete by substance and by illicit or licit status of a drug. One challenge is to arrive at standard definitions of substance use problems and culturally appropriate interventions, which are universally recognized because accessibility of drugs, culture and traditions are highly variable around the world. These variations influence the choice of drugs used for psychotropic effects, accessibility of medical treatment, and the policies of local and national governments. Inasmuch as there is consensus that interventions should occur with SUDS, WHO endorses best clinical practices related to health promotion, education on substance use and screening and brief intervention.

Regulatory and legislative changes within societies, as well as federal and state initiatives to contain substance use and limit access to minors, have created a broad social context of constraint of substance use and provided new information for health teaching by nurses. Major initiatives include response to the 1964 Surgeon's General Report in the United States and the 2008 WHO Global Report on the Tobacco Epidemic. Since that time the "denormalizaton" of tobacco use has made steady progress in both legislative and health care arenas. In the United States, for example, establishing variable forms of anti-smoking legislation in the workplace, restaurants and other gathering places has created barriers for smokers. These can become an impetus for change for the smoker aspiring to be a non-smoker, and have resulted in the reduction of exposure to second-hand smoke. Public education about the harms of smoking (Kim & Shanahan, 2003), anti-smoking media messages (Bala, Strzeszynski, & Cahill, 2008), and increasing cigarette taxes (Wakefield *et al.*, 2008) are all associated with a decrease in smoking prevalence (Kim & Shanahan, 2014; Ritchie, Amos, & Martin, 2010). In the years following such legislative initiatives, nurses in the United States have dropped personal smoking prevalence from 16 percent to 10.73 percent (Sarna, Bialous, Sinha, Yang, & Wewers, 2009). Since research findings suggest that health providers who smoke are less inclined than non-smoking peers to intervene with patient smokers (Tong, Strouse, Hall, Kovac, Schroeder, 2010), this change could increase education and early intervention with smokers. The 2008 WHO Global Report on the Tobacco Epidemic evolved into the WHO Framework Convention on Tobacco Control (WHO FCTC). Its guidelines are foundational for countries to implement and manage tobacco control and include the MPOWER measures. These are intended to assist in the country-level implementation of effective interventions to reduce the demand for tobacco, contained in the WHO FCTC (WHO, 2013b). Many countries now restrict tobacco advertising and place limits on smoking in public areas. When nurse–patient teaching can be informed by current regulatory and legislative guidelines based on evidence, nurses are empowered to inform and educate patients factually and without judgment.

Primary prevention interventions include counseling children, adults, and older adults on health risks associated with substance use. Since substance use exists on a continuum from occasional to excessive daily, to severe substance use disorders and early mortality, prevention of negative health outcomes secondary to substance use can be undertaken at each life stage. Education of children, adolescents, young adults and families may have some effect in decreasing demand through promoting conscious choices by individuals and families to delay the initiation of alcohol use to the post-adolescent years, and/or to establish norms within families that discourage smoking and the use of mind-altering drugs. Research demonstrates that in the adolescent years the brain is still maturing and is more vulnerable to the neurologically damaging effects of alcohol and other drugs even in healthy adolescents (Tapert, Caldwell, & Burke, 2014). Similarly, changes in metabolism, which make older adults more vulnerable to the psychological and physiologic effects of any drug use, are not routinely part of patient education, although this information could significantly reduce vulnerability to harmful use of any drug.

A parallel process has taken place worldwide on alcohol policies at the global, regional, national, and multinational levels. Deterrents that "limit supply" of a drug are generally legal and for alcohol, include prohibitions of sale of alcohol to minors, defined hours for pubs or bars, and limits on the alcohol content in beverages (beers, wines, and liquors). Countries reporting having written national alcohol policies including imposing stricter blood alcohol concentration limits both in beverages sold and in guidelines for driving while intoxicated (driving under the influence) rose in 2012 from those in 2008 (WHO, 2012).

Early/secondary interventions in direct patient care

Nursing organizations and specialty nursing organizations recognize and support important roles for nurses in the identification of substance use disorders (SUDs) and early intervention to change patterns that increase risk for their development. WHO recommends that nurses and midwives be educated on the extent of drug-, tobacco- and alcohol-related problems and acknowledge the importance of screening and brief interventions for hazardous and harmful use of alcohol and other psychoactive substances (Watson, 2010). Further, nurses and midwives are urged to ensure that, where available, standards for screening and brief interventions are implemented. All new patients should be screened and returning patients, screened periodically to identify any emerging or increasing problems.

When used universally, screening is a form of primary prevention, but can also serve as an early intervention. Nurses in both generalist and specialist roles use screening in both ways and these can be considered forms of "primary mental health" care (Haber & Billings, 1995). Screening methods can be very brief such as the NIAAA questions for alcohol use (Table 16.3) or longer (Table 16.4) and are increasingly available for self/consumer administration online (Bickel, Christensen, & Masch, 2011).

A score on a screening instrument opens the door to provider/patient dialogues about substance use and its health implications. For some substance use, screening is undertaken as a universal precaution, for example, screening all primary care patients for risky drinking and tobacco use (US PTF, 2014). When an individual screens negative for tobacco use, for example, the nurse re-enforces health behavior and links it to decreased health risks. Unfortunately, there is little

Table 16.3 NIAAA three question screener

How many days per week do you drink alcohol?
On a typical day when your drink, how many drinks do you have?
What is the maximum number of drinks you had on any given day in the past month?
To avoid the development of health problems related to alcohol use, including a substance use disorder, maximum drinking limits are recommended as:
    For healthy men up to age 65: no more than 5 drinks a day and no more than 15 drinks a week
    For healthy women (and healthy men over age 65): no more than 4 drinks a day and no more than 8 drinks a week

Table 16.4 5As for smoking cessation

Ask: Is the patient a smoker? How many cigarettes/packs per day?

Assess: Describe the smoking pattern. Use a screening test such as the Fagerstrom Questionnaire.

Advise: Tailor the discussion on health implications of smoking to his/her health or diagnosis.

Assist: Use motivational interviewing steps to help the patient evaluate interest, willingness to quit.
   Discuss non-pharmacologic options and over-the-counter (nicotine patches) and prescription aides
   (medications such as Varenicline, Buproprion).

Arrange: For follow-up with a return visit or a visit with a nurse practitioner or physician.

Source: Modified from SAMHSA, 2011a.

evidence to support the timing of an early intervention as a deterrent to the onset of an SUD. Among drugs that are commonly used, alcohol and tobacco are the only drugs for which Screening Brief Intervention (SBI) or Screening Brief Intervention Referral to Treatment (SBIRT) demonstrate some efficacy (SAMHSA, 2011).

The 5As for Smoking Intervention, a brief intervention model (BI), is widely used for smoking cessation and is recommended for nurses' use in generalist and specialist settings (Albrecht *et al.*, 2006; Scanlon 2006). The steps for nurse implementation adapted from SAMHSA (2011) are in Table 16.4.

Motivational interviewing studies have provided evidence that a client-oriented, empathic approach can help to reduce an individual's ambivalence about changing health behaviors and that techniques like "change talk" can shift one's views about the likelihood of behavior change. Motivational Interviewing builds on readiness to change by advising that quitting smoking or reducing alcohol intake based on screening identified data, are possible and desirable. Research provides strong evidence that screening and brief interventions with smoking and excess alcohol use can reduce the frequency of both behaviors. Strong evidence for intervening with marijuana use and heroin with the same model has not yet emerged.

Cross national and multi-site trials of behavioral interventions (BIs) were conducted by WHO in Kenya, Australia, Bulgaria, Costa Rica, United Kingdom, Norway, Mexico, Russia, Wales, Zimbabwe and the United States (WHO Brief Intervention Study Group, 1996). The incorporated motivational interviewing techniques demonstrated significantly reduced alcohol consumption when used by nurses, nurse practitioners, therapists, and research staff in diverse populations and both genders with similarly effective results (Donofrio & Degutis, 2002; Kaner, Lock, Heather, McNamee, & Bond, 2003; Reiff-Hekking, Okene, Hurley & Reed, 2005). Screening using standardized instruments, and the SBI and SBIRT approaches are used with increasing frequency in Canada, the United Kingdom, and Australia. The following describes screening tools validated in several countries and promoted for use by CDC, WHO, NIAAA, and NIDA.

1   The *AUDIT*, an internationally validated screening tool for alcohol use disorders was developed by WHO and used in several languages and cultural settings. The 10-item form can be administered by a provider, or can be self-administered. Research supports its usefulness for screening women and minorities (Reinert & Allen, 2002). This screening tool also has shown promising results with adolescents and young adults; it is less accurate in older patients, though further population specific research is needed (Reinert & Allen, 2002; Chung, Colby, & Barnett, 2000). The AUDIT's first three questions are also used as the AUD-C, found to be equally effective in primary care populations, but not validated for efficacy with special populations such as psychiatric patients.

2   The *ASSIST* is a more comprehensive screening instrument developed by WHO to address the breadth and consequences of worldwide drug abuse. Designed in 1997 for use in primary care settings, the ASSIST is 8 items covering 10 substances: tobacco, alcohol, cannabis, cocaine, amphetamine type stimulants, inhalants, sedatives, hallucinogens, opioids, and other specified drugs (WHO, 2014c). A risk score (low, moderate or high) is provided for each substance and linked to levels of intervention (treatment as usual, BI or specialized treatment referral).

In choosing a screening tool, the nurse should consider the substance use patterns of the population served and choose an appropriate tool. Persons with moderate to severe alcohol disorders may be screened with the CAGE (cut back on drinking, annoyed by others' critcism about drinking, ever feel guilty about drinking, have an "eye opener" to avoid the effects of a sudden drop in BAC the morning after) (Ewing, 1984), adolescents with the CRAFFT (car,

Table 16.5 Recommended screening tools by drug and population

Tool	Screening	Population	Psychometrics
AUDIT Source: WHO 10 questions	Alcohol use disorders (AUD)	Adults in primary and specialty care Accounts for male/female variation	Cronbach's Alpha 0.77 CI 95% 0.75–0.80 Cronbach's Alpha 0.55 CI 95% 0.51–0.59[1]
AUDIT-C Modified from AUDIT First 3 questions of the AUDIT	Alcohol use disorder (AUD)	Older Adults; patients with hazardous/risky drinking Patients with AUD	Sens. 0.66/spec. 0.94(W) Sens.0.95/spec. 0.68(M) Sens. 0.90 spec. 0.45 (M) Sens. 0.79 spec. 0.56 (W)[2]
ASSIST (WHO)	Risky use of alcohol and cannabis, cocaine, amphetamine type stimulants, sedatives, hallucinogenics, inhalants, opioids, other drugs	Adults	Sens. 0.61–1.00 Spec. 0.61–1.00 Internal consistency 0.65–0.86 High test–retest reliability[3]
CRAFFT (Knight, *et al.*, 2002)	Alcohol use disorders Substance use disorders	Adolescents	Reliability is good to excellent range (0.90–0.58). Adjust for diverse groups[4]
Fagerstrom tolerance questionnaire	Degree of nicotine dependence	Adolescents Adults	A valid measure of the heaviness of smoking as measured by biochemical indices[5]
Short Mast-Geriatric (SMAST–G) Short Michigan alcoholism screen	Alcohol use disorders	Older adults	Sensitivity 93.9 Specificity 78.1 Positive Predictive value 87.2 Negative predictive value 88.9[6]

Sources: 1. Kallmen, Wenbery, Ramstedt, & Hallgzen (2014); 2. Bush, Kivlahar, McDonnell, Fihn, & Bradley (1998); 3. Bradley, Bush, Epler (2003); 4. Knight, Sherritt, Shrier, Harrris, & Chang (2002); 5. Heatherton, *et al.* (1991); 6. Blow, Gillespie, Barry, Mudd, & Hill (1998).

Madeline A. Naegle

Table 16.6 Steps for screening, brief intervention, and referral to treatment

Screening: generalist or specialist nurse assesses a patient for risky substance use behaviors using standardized screening tools. A positive score indicates the need for:

A brief intervention: the nurse engages a patient reporting risky substance use behaviors in a short conversation (5–8 minutes), providing feedback and advice. An early intervention will follow screening for approximately 25% of the American population who consume alcohol at levels, that research findings predict will result in health problems, including substance use disorders (CDC, 2014).

For patients who screen positive: the generalist nurse provides a referral to a mental health professional, including a clinical nurse specialist or psychiatric nurse practitioner for brief therapy. For patients who screen positive for a mild, moderate or severe SUD, a referral is made to a provider or facility for the appropriate level of intervention (adapted from SAMHSA, 2011b).

relax, alone, forget, friends, trouble) and older adults with the SMAST-G. Table 16.5 provides additional information about these tools.

Nationally and internationally, SBIRT is now being advocated by SAMHSA and CDC as the optimal model for integrating substance abuse screening into primary and specialty care. Table 16.6 includes a further description of SBIRT.

Psychiatric nurses have many roles in which the use of SBIRT can be incorporated. Patients receiving specialty treatment are often not screened for ATOD. Psychiatric mental health and addictions nursing competencies include skilled screening, motivational interviewing and individual, family and couples counseling (ANA, 2014).

Secondary and tertiary prevention: managing illness, preventing relapse and reducing harm

Nursing roles in the care of persons diagnosed with a substance use disorder are shaped by national policies and resources, standards, and expectations for nursing education and practice (certifications, specialty practice, or advanced practice), capacity and placement of the workforce and population needs (ANA & INTNSA, 2013). In Western countries with current and accessible addiction research, national planning provides for a range of services on a care continuum leveled to use, mild, moderate or severe. In Australia, Canada, and the US, for example, the main components of care consist of identification and intervention, assessment and referral; detoxification, ambulatory treatment programs, residential treatment, hospital and dual diagnoses services, drug and interpersonal strategies, and mutual help (el-Guebaly, 2014). These services are available proportionate to funding and single payer systems, such as those that exist in Canada and Australia. Well-resourced countries can link continuing care more effectively.

Canada and the US have recently initiated campaigns to support the integration of addiction and psychiatric services into primary/general care, and have expanded use of case management models. China, faced with widespread use of heroin and increasing rates of alcohol use disorders, as well as the largest world population of cigarette smokers, has implemented widespread anti-drug programs (Lu & Wang, 2008). Inasmuch as they focus on detoxification, and acute intervention, the nursing workforce will certainly be delivering secondary prevention. Comparing advances in education in China with those of Russia provides a typical picture of how the nursing role changes across countries. Russia is faced with 600,000 deaths from alcohol annually, as well as many individuals with co-occurring illnesses secondary to intravenous drug injection (Mitchell, Nase, & Rar, 2009). Nurses clearly have roles in acute care of these populations for

252

the primary diagnoses as well as co-occurring illness like Hepatitis C and HIV-AIDS. Nursing education, however, does not provide for advanced practice education and certification, which could maximize care outcomes.

The *concepts of harm reduction* and recovery are the umbrella for health promotion strategies for those diagnosed with a SUD and seeking a return to health. Harm reduction refers to the aim to reduce the harms associated with the use of psychoactive drugs in people unable or unwilling to stop (Harm Reduction International, 2014). An example of harm reduction now adopted by the US, and already practiced in other countries is decreasing harm by making Narcan available to health personnel and peers working in needle exchanges to reverse CNS depression from accidental opiate overdose. At the global policy level, the United Nations Office on Drugs and Crime (UNODC), is collaborating with the World Health Organization (WHO), to collect and circulate available best practices on the prevention and treatment of opioid overdose. These will include the use and availability of opioid receptor antagonists such as naloxone and other measures based on scientific evidence (UNODC, 2012). This position exemplifies a balance between tolerance for continued use by addicts and action against addiction and the accessibility of drugs, which produce it.

Similarly, with illness management and support for recovery, nurses can minimize health risks and promote quality of life and maximum health at the tertiary level of intervention. Many nurses participate in drug dependence treatment (basic nursing care of detoxification and withdrawal) and maintenance of abstinence through administration of opioid substitution therapy (methadone maintenance and Buprenorphine/suboxone). The wide variation in the implementation of these practices by nurses is highlighted in Russia and China. Detoxification remains the primary intervention in both countries despite high relapse levels related to underdeveloped ambulatory care services and relapse prevention strategies. China is working hard to make the baccalaureate degree in nursing available, better preparing nurses to work in prevention, treatment, and maintenance of recovery, whereas nursing education in Russia is advancing less quickly.

Conclusion

Substance use and substance use disorders continue to compromise the health of populations worldwide with high costs to the global economy, country-based health care systems, individual health, and quality of family and community life. Long-standing traditions of psychoactive drug use and cultural beliefs that stigmatize those with severe substance use disorders limit access to treatment options and resources, and increase the barriers to help seeking for the largest group of users (men) and for the most vulnerable populations (older adults, adolescents, and pregnant women). Workforce shortages of psychiatric-mental health/addictions professionals constrain capacity at all levels of prevention. Psychiatric-mental health nurses, not all of whom are educated in substance use disorders, fill a variety of roles, primarily in institutions, to meet the needs of patients and families suffering from these disorders. Nursing competencies, defined for both psychiatric nursing and the specialty of addictions nursing in Australia, United Kingdom and the US and several other Western industrialized countries, provide frameworks for the development of primary, secondary, and tertiary prevention interventions. Nurses at all levels, using skills of advocacy and social change, should be practicing at the full scope of their education and experience. This can be within specialist health care delivery systems and community networks, including those with integrated care systems to bring quality nursing care to individuals, families, and communities suffering the stigma, acute and chronic symptoms, and associated consequences of substance use disorders.

Madeline A. Naegle

References

Albrecht, S.A., Maloni, J.A., Thomas, K.K. Jones, R., Halleran, J., & Osborne, J. (2006). Smoking cessation counseling for pregnant women who smoke: Scientific basis for pregnant women who smoke: Scientific basis for practice for AWHONN's SUCCESS project. *Journal of Obstetric, Gynecologic & Neonatal Nursing, 33*(3), 298–305.

Al-Sahab, B. Saqib, M., Hauser, G., & Tamim, H. (2010). Prevalence of smoking during pregnancy and associated risk factors among Canadian women: A national Survey. *BMC Pregnancy and Childbirth, 10,* 24, 1–9.

American Nurses Association. (2014). *Psychiatric-mental health nursing scope and standards of practice, 2nd edition.* Silver Springs, MA: American Nurses Association.

American Nurses Association & International Nurses Society on Addictions. (2013). *Addictions nursing: Scope and standards of practice.* Silver Springs, MA: American Nurses Association.

American Psychiatric Association. (2013). *Diagnostic and statistical manual of mental disorders* (5th ed.). Arlington, VA: American Psychiatric Association.

Bala, M.M., Strzeszynski, L., & Cahill, K. (2008). Mass media interventions for smoking cessation in adults (review). *Cochrane Database of Systematic Reviews 2012,* 4. Doi: 10.1002/14651858.CD004704. pub2.

Bickel, W.K., Christensen, D.R., & Masch, L.A. (2011). A review of computer-based interventions used in assessment, treatment and research of drug addiction. *Substance Use and Misuse, 40*(1), 4–9.

Blow, F.C., Gillespie, B.W., Barry, K.L., Mudd, S.A., & Hill, E.M. (1998). Brief screening for alcohol problems in elderly populations using the Short Michigan Alcoholism Screening Test-Geriatric Version (SMAST-G). *Alcoholism: Clinical and Experimental Research, 22*(Suppl), 131A.

Boborova, N., Rhodes, T., Power, R., Alcorn, R., Neifeld, E., Krasiukov, N., Latyshevskaia, N., & Maksimova, S. (2006). Barriers to accessing treatment in Russia: A qualitative study among injecting drug users in two cities. *Drug and Alcohol Dependence, 82,* Suppl. 1, S57–S63.

Bradley, K.A., Bush, K.R., Epler, A.J., Dorcas, D.J., Davis, T.M, Sporleder, J.J., Maynard, C., & Kivlahan, D.R. (2003). Two brief alcohol-screening tests from the Alcohol Use Disorders identification test (AUDIT): Validation in a female Veterans Affairs patient population. *Archives of Internal Medicine, 163*(7), 821–829.

Bush, K., Kivlahan, D.R., McDonell, M.B., Fihn, S.D., & Bradley, K.A. (1998). The AUDIT alcohol consumption questions (AUDIT-C): An effective brief screening test for problem drinking. *Archives of Internal Medicine, 158*(16), 1789–1795.

Camí, J. & Farré, M. (2003). Drug Addiction. *New England Journal of Medicine, 349,* 975–986.

Center for Disease Control and Prevention (CDC) PRAMS. (2011). Tobacco use and pregnancy. Retrieved May 30, 2015 from www.cdc.gov/reproductivehealth/TobaccoUsePregnancy/.

Center for Disease Control and Prevention (CDC). (2013). About one in five US adult cigarettes smokers have tried an electronic cigarette. *Press Release,* February 28, 2013. Retrieved September 10, 2014 from www.cdc.gov/media.

Center for Disease Control and Prevention (CDC). (2014). Notes from the field: Electronic cigarette us among middle and high school student-United States, 2011–2012. *Morbidity and Mortality Weekly Report.* Retrieved September 10, 2014 from www.cdc.gov/mmwr/preview/mmwrhtml/mm623a6.htm.

Chung, T., Colby, S.M., Barnett, N.P., Rohsenow, D.J., Spirito, A., & Monti, P.M. (2000). Screening adolescents for problem drinking: performance of brief screens against DSM-IV alcohol diagnoses. *Jnl of Studies on Alcohol, 61*(4), 579–587.

Donofrio, G. & Degutis, L.C. (2002). Preventive care in the Emergency Department: Screening and brief intervention for alcohol problems in the emergency department: A systematic review. *Academy of Emergency Medicine, 9,* 627–638.

Dube, S.R., Felitti, V.J., Dong, M., Chapman, D.P., Giles, W.H., & Anda. R.F. (2003). Childhood, abuse, neglect, and household dysfunction and the risk of illicit drug use: The adverse childhood experiences study. *Pediatrics, 1119*(3), 564–572.

Durlak, J.A. & Wells, A.M. (1997). Primary prevention mental health programs for children and adolescents. *American Journal of Community Psychology, 25*(2), 115–152.

Eckholm, E. (2008). A grim tradition, and a long struggle to end it. *New York Times,* April 2, 2008. Retrieved May 30, 2016 from www.nytimes.com/2008/04/02/us/02overdose.html?pagewanted=print.

Elder R.W., Shults R.A., & Sleet, D.A., Nichols, J.L., Zaza, S., & Thompson, R.S. (2002). Effectiveness of sobriety checkpoint for reducing alcohol-involved crashes. *Traffic Injury Prevention, 3,* 266–274.

El-Guebaly, N. (2014). A Canadian perspective on addiction treatment. *Substance Abuse, 35,* 298–303.

Ewing, J.A. (1984). Detecting alcoholism: The CAGE questionnaire. *JAMA: Journal of the American Medical Association,* 252(14), 1905–1907.

Fiore, M.C. (2008). *Clinical practice guidelines for treating tobacco use and dependence: 2008 Update. A US public health service report.* Retrieved August 1, 2014 from: www.ncbi.nlm.nih.gov/pubmed/18617085.

Grant, J.E & Potenza, M.N. (2004). *Pathological gambling: A clinical guide to treatment.* Washington, DC: American Psychiatric Publishing.

Grucza, R.A. & Bierut, J.L. (2006). Co-occurring risk factors for alcohol dependence and habitual smoking. Update on findings from the Collaborative Study on the Genetics of Alcoholism. *Alcohol, Health and Research World, 29*(3), 172–178.

Haber, J. & Billings, C.V. (1995). Primary mental health care: A model for psychiatric mental-health nursing. *Journal of the American Psychiatric Nurses Association,* 1(5), 154–163.

Harm Reduction International (2014). *The global state of harm reduction 2014.* Retrieved 31 May, 2016 from www.ihra.net/contents/1524.

Heatherton, T.F., Kozlowski, L.T., Frecker, R.C., & Fagerström, K.O. (1991). The Fagerström test for nicotine dependence: A revision of the Fagerström Tolerance Questionnaire. *British Journal of Addiction,* 86, 1119–1127.

Jackson, S. & Aveyard, P. (2008). Waterpipe smoking in students: Prevalence, risk factors, symptoms of addiction, and smoke intake. *BMC Public Health,* 8, 174–179.

Johnson, C.A., Palmer, P.H., Chou, C., Zengchang, P., Dunin, Z., Lijun, D., Anderson, J.C., & Unger, J.B. (2006). Tobacco use among youth and adulsts in Mainland China: The China Seven Cities Study. *Public Health, 120*(12), 1156–1169.

Kallmen, H., Wennberg, P., Ramstedt, M., & Hallgren, M. (2014). The psychometric properties of the AUDIT: A survey from a random sample of elderly Swedish adults. *BMC Public Health,* 14, 672.

Kaner, E. Lock, C., Heather, N., McNamee, P., & Bond, S. (2003). Promoting brief alcohol intervention by nurses in primary care: A cluster of randomized controlled trials. *The Cochrane Collaboratione,* 51(3), 277–284.

Keyes, C.L.M. (2007). Promoting and protecting mental helath as flourishing. *American Psychologist, 60*(2), 95–108.

Keyes, K.M., Hatzenbuehler, M.L., Grant, B.F., & Hasin, D.S. (2012). Stress and alcohol: Epidemiologic evidence. *Alcohol research: Current Reviews, 34*(4), 391–400.

Kim, S. & Shanahan, J. (2014). Stigmatizing smokers: Public sentiment toward cigarette smoking and its relationship to smoking behaviors. *Journal of Health Communication, 8*(4), 343–367.

Klingemann, H. & Bergmark, A. (2006). The legitimacy of addiction treatment in a world of smart people. *Addiction, 101*(9), 1230–1237.

Knight, J.R., Sherritt, L., Shrier, L.A., Harris, S.K., & Chang, G. (2002). Validity of the CRAFFT substance abuse screening test among adolescent clinic patients. *Archives of Pediatrics & Adolescent Medicine, 156,* 607–614.

Liu, Z.M., Lu, X.X., Mu, Y., Lian, Z., & Zhou, W.H. (2002). Epidemiologic features of drug users in China. *Chinese Journal of Drug Abuse and Prevention and Treatment,* 8, 27–30.

Lu, L. & Wang, X. (2008) Drug addiction in China. *Annals of the New York Academy of Sciences, 1141,* 304–317.

McCue, M., Slutske, W.,Taylor, J., & Iacono, W. (1997). Personality and substance use disorders: 1. Effects of gender and alcoholism subtype. *Alcoholism Clinical and Experimental Research, 21*(3), 513–520.

Marmot, M. (2005). Social determinants of health inequalities. *The Lancet, 365,* 1099–1104.

Merikangas, K.R. & McClair, V.L. (2012). Epidemiology of substance use disorders. *Human Genetics, 131,* 779–789.

Mitchell, A.J. Vaze, A., & Rao, S. (2009). Clinical diagnosis of depression in primary care: A meta-analysis. *Lancet, 374,* 609–619.

Mulder, R.T. (2005). Alcoholism and personality. *Australian New Zealand Journal of psychiatry, 36,* 44–52.

National Institutes of Alcoholism and Alcohol Abuse (NIAAA) (n.d.). Screening for alcohol use and alcohol related problems. Retrieved May 30, 2016 from http://pubs.niaaa.nih.gov/publications/aa65.h.

NIDA. (2014). Prescription opioids and heroin. Retrieved July 26, 2016 from www.drugabuse.gov/sites/default/files/rx_and_heroin_rrs_layout_final.pdf.

NIDA. (2016). *What is the scope of marijuana use in the United States? Research report.* Retrieved August 1, 2014 from www.drugabuse.gov/publications/research-reports/marijuana/.

O'Brien, C.P. & Jaffe, J. (1992). *Addictive States: Association for research in nervous and mental diseases. meeting proceedings.* New York: Raven Press.

Pearson, G.P. (2010). Editorial: Keeping mental health promotion alive. *Perspectives in Psychiatric Care, 46,* 1–2.

Reiff-Hekking, S., O'Keene, J.K., Hurley, T.G., & Reed, G.W. (2005). Brief physician and nurse practitioner delivered counseling for high-risk drinking: Results at 12-month follow-up. *Journal of General Internal Medicine: Official Journal of the Society for Research and Education in Primary Care Internal Medicine, 21*(1), 7–13.

Reinert, D.F. & Allen, J.P. (2002). Alcohol use disorders identification test (AUDIT): A review of recent research. *Alcoholism: Clinical and Experimental Research 26*(2), 272–279.

Ritchie, D. Amos, A., & Martin, C. (2010). "But it just has that sort of feel about it, a leper": Stigma, smoke free legislation and public health. *Nicotine and Tobacco Research, 12*(6), 622–629.

Sarna, L., Bialous, S.A., Rice, V.A., & Wewers, M.E. (2009). Promoting tobacco dependence treatment in nursing education. *Drug and Alcohol Review, 28,* 507–551.

Scanlon, A. (2006). Nursing and the 5As guideline to smoking cessation interventions. *Australian Nursing Journal, 15*(5), 25–28.

Schuckit, M.A. (1998). Biological, psychological and environmental predictors of alcoholism risk: A longitudinal study. *Journal of Studies on Alcohol, 59,* 486–494.

Shihadeh, A. (2003). Investigation of mainstream smoke aerosol of the argileh water pipe. *Food and Chemical Toxicology, 41,* 143–152.

Stead, L.F., & Lancaster, T. (2012). Behavioral interventions as adjuncts to pharmacotherapy for smoking cessation. *Cochrane Database of Systematic Reviews, 12.* Doi: 10.1002/14651858.CD009670.pub2.

Substance Abuse Mental Health Services Adminstration (SAMHSA). (2011a). Tobacco use cessation policies in substance abuse treatment: Administrative issues. *SAMHSA Advisory, 10*(3), 1–4.

Substance Abuse and Mental Health Services Administration (SAMHSA). (2011b). Screening, brief intervention and referral to treatment (SBIRT) in behavioral health care, 1–30. Retrieved May 30, 2016 from www.samhsa.gov.

Substance Abuse Mental Health Services Administration (SAMHSA). (2015). SBIRT. Retrieved May 30, 2016 from www.http://integration.SAMHSA.gov/clinical practice.

Substance Abuse and Mental Health Services Administration (SAMHSA). (2016). Retrieved May 30, 2016 from www.samhsa.gov/atod/tobacco.

Tang, Y. & Wao, W. (2007). Improving drug addiction treatment in China. *Addiction, 102,* 1057–1063.

Tapert, S.A. Caldwell, L., & Burke, C. (2014). Alcohol and the adolescent brain. National Institute of Alcohol Abuse and Alcoholism. Retrieved May 30, 2016 from http://pubs.niaaa.nih.gov/publications/arh284/205-212.htm.

Tong, E.K., Strouse, R., Hall, J., Kovac, M., & Schroeder, S. (2010). National survey of US health professionals' smoking prevalence, cessation practices, and beliefs. *Nicotine and Tobacco Research, 12*(7), 724–733.

Torre, L.A., Siegel. R.L., Ward, E.M., & Jemal, A. (2014). International variation in lung cancer mortality rates in women. *Cancer Epidemiology, Biomarkers and Prevention.* Doi: 10.1158/1055–9965.EPI-13–1220.

Trull, T.J., Waudby, C.J., & Sher, K.J. (2004). Alcohol, tobacco and drug use disorders and personality disorder symptoms. *Experimental and Clinical Psychopharmacology, 12*(1), 67–75.

United Nations Office on Drugs and Crime (UNODC) World Drug Report. (2012). *Recent statistics and trend analysis.* Retrieved May 30, 2016 from www.unodc.org/document/data-and-analysis.

United Nations Office on Drugs and Crime (UNODC). (2015). *World Drug report finds drug use stable, access to drug and HIV treatment still low: 2015 World Drug Report.* Retrieved May 30, 2016 from www.unodc.org/en/frontpage/2015-world-drug-report/html.

USDHHS. (2014). *Fetal alcohol spectrum disorders among Native Americans.* Retrieved May 30, 2016 from www.samhsa.gov.

U.S. Food and Drug Administration. (n.d.). Vaporizers, E-Cigarettes, and Other Electronic Nicotine Delivery Systems (ENDS). Retrieved July 26, 2016 from www.fda.gov/TobaccoProducts/Labeling/ProductsIngredientsComponents/ucm456610.htm.

U.S. Preventive Services Task Force (USPSTF). (2014). *The Guide to Clinical Preventive Services 2014.* Rockville, MD: USPSTF.

Wakefield, M., Durkin, S., Spittal, M.J., Siahpush, M., Scollo, M., Simpson, J.A., & Hill, D. (2008). Impact of tobacco control policies and mass media campaigns on monthly adult smoking prevalence. *American Journal of Public Health, 98*(8), 1443–1449.

Watson, H. (2010). The involvement of nursing and midwives in screening and brief interventions for hazardous and harmful use of alcohol and other psychoactive substances. WHO publication number

WHO/HRH/HPN/10–6. Retrieved May 30, 2016 from www. whqlibdoc.who.int/hq/2010/WHO_HRH_HPN_10.6_eng.pdf.

Wilsnack, R.W., Wilsnack, S.C., Kristjanson, A.F., Vogeltanz-Holm, N.D., & Gmel, G. (2009). Gender and alcohol consumption: Patterns from the multinational GENACIS project. *Addiction, 104*(9), 1487–1500.

White, W.L., Boyle, M., & Loveland, D. (2002). Alcoholism/addiction as a chronic disease: from rhetoric to clinical reality. *Alcoholism Treatment Quarterly, 20*(3/4), 107–130.

World Health Organization (WHO). (2000). *Surveys of drinking patterns and problems in seven developing countries* WHO/MSD/MSB/01.8 Retrieved August 1, 2014 from www.unicri.it/mih.san.bolletino/dati/alcbrochur.pdf.

WHO. (2012). *World health report (1).* Retrieved from www.who.int/gho/publications/world_health_/en/.

WHO. (2013a). *Comprehensive mental health action plan 2013–2020.* Sixty- Sixth World Assembly Agenda item 13.3. Retrieved August 1, 2014 from www.who.int/whosis/indicators/compendium/2008/2ptu/en.

WHO. (2013b). *MPOWER in action: Defeating the global tobacco epidemic. MPOWER progress. 2007–2012.* Geneva: WHO.

WHO. (2014a). *Alcohol and health global status report.* Retrieved August 1, 2014 from www.who.int/substance_abuse/publications/global_alcohol_report/en/.

WHO. (2014b). *The global information system on alcohol and health (GISAH) management of substance abuse.* Retrieved August 1, 2014 from www.who.int/substance_abuse/activities/gisal.

WHO. (2014c). *Validation of the alcohol, smoking and substance involvement screening test (ASSIST) and pilot brief intervention.* Geneva. Retrieved August 1, 2014 from www.who.int/substance_abuse/activities/assist/en.

WHO. (2016). *International classification of diseases (ICD).* Retrieved August 1, 2014 from WHO Classification of Diseases (ICD) www.who.int/classfications/icd/en.

WHO Brief Intervention Study Group. (1996). A Cross-national trial of brief intervention with heavy drinkers. *American Journal of Public Health, 86*(7), 948–953.

17

MENTAL HEALTH AND AGING

Needs and care of older adults

Karen M. Robinson, Mary L. Corbett
and Teresa McEnroe Clare

Global statistics on aging

There is a change occurring worldwide with an aging demographic. In the past 60 years, the global population of adults 60 years and older has seen a slight increase in growth. During this time, the percent of older adults has risen from 8 percent to 10 percent. Over the next 40 years, the population of adults 60 years and older is projected to increase to approximately 22 percent of the world's population (Bloom *et al.*, 2015) and 80 percent of this group will reside in low-income and middle-income countries (Chatterji, Byles, Cutler, Seeman, & Verdes, 2015). This means that in 40 years, adults 60 years and older will grow from approximately 800 million to 2 billion people worldwide, an unparalleled increase. (Bloom *et al.*, 2015).

When looking at individual countries the numbers continue to be staggering. In 2011, China had approximately 110 million adults 65 years and older. By 2050, it is projected that number will increase to 330 million older adults. In India in 2011, the population of older adults was approximately 60 million. It is estimated that by 2050, the older adult population will expand to 227 million. That change is a 280 percent increase (World Health Organization (WHO), 2011). In 2011 in Australia, adults 65 years and older accounted for approximately 13 percent of the population. In 2031, it is estimated that older adults will rise to 19 to 21 percent of the overall population and in 2051 this group will grow to approximately 26 percent of the population (WHO, 2011).

Historically, developed or high-income countries have had the largest population of older adults. However, this trend is changing with less developed countries seeing a rapid increase in their older adult population. Between 2010 and 2050, the older adult population of developed countries will increase about 71 percent. In comparison, the aging population in less developed countries will rise to more than 250 percent (WHO, 2011). This rate of increase in less developed countries is extraordinary. When looking at France's older adult population growth, it took over 100 years for their older population to rise from 7 percent to 14 percent of the total population. In comparison, Brazil and China will experience that same growth in only 25 years (WHO, 2014a). By 2050, Africa is projected to have 215 million people 60 years and older, which is about 13 times the number of older adults when compared to 2013 (Global Age Watch Index, 2013). As the population ages, many opportunities and challenges arise globally. This chapter will explore global aging, quality of life for older adults, health promotion strategies for depression, dementia and evidence-based care of older adults presenting with dementia. The older adult is defined as an individual 65 years of age and older.

Why is there a change in the aging statistics?

During the twentieth and early twenty-first century, there have been changes that have contributed to an increase in the global aging statistics. One change has been a decline in fertility. Globally, adults over 60 years will exceed the number of children under the age of 15 years by 2050 (Global Age Watch Index, 2013). Since 2000, young children under the age of 5 years of age no longer comprise a greater percentage of the global population when compared to older adults (Global Age Watch Index, 2013). Another change has been an increase in life expectancy at birth and in the older adult population. At the beginning of the twentieth century, infectious and parasitic diseases took the lives of many infants and children. Most children born in 1900, who survived childhood illnesses, did not live past the age of 50 years (WHO, 2011). Public health soon became a focus in many low-, middle-, and high-income countries. The development of vaccinations and antibiotics, as well as proper sanitation, cleaner water, and more nutritious foods helped to prevent deaths among infants and children. The leading cause of death began to shift from communicable diseases to non-communicable diseases. Currently worldwide, the leading causes of death among the older adult population are non-communicable diseases (Beard & Bloom, 2015; WHO, 2011) such as depression, suicide, cancer, diabetes, and cardiovascular diseases.

In 2013, the life expectancy at birth for developed countries was 78 years and for developing regions was 68 years (Global Age Watch Index, 2013). Japan leads the world in life expectancy, with women averaging 87 years and men averaging 80 years (WHO, 2014a). It is projected that by 2050 the life expectancy for developed countries will be 83 years and for developing regions it will be 75 years (Chatterji *et al.*, 2015; Global Age Watch Index 2013). Less developed regions have seen a continuous increase in life expectancy since World War II. As an example, in East Asia, life expectancy in 1950 was 45 years, now life expectancy is approximately 74 years (WHO, 2011). Globally, there has been a steady rise in the population of adults, age 80 years and over. This group is growing more rapidly than the older adult population as a whole. In addition, worldwide the number of centenarians, aged 100 years and over, is expected to grow from approximately 316,600 in 2011 to 3.2 million in 2050 (Global Age Watch Index, 2013). Again, this increase of older adults 80 years and over is unprecedented.

Gaps in life expectancy and quality of life

Even though there is a global rise in life expectancy, there are still gaps associated with health, life expectancy, and quality of life for older adults across low-, middle-, and high-income countries (Chatterji *et al.*, 2015). Unfortunately, some countries in Africa have not seen a great increase in life expectancy due to deaths from the epidemic of HIV/AIDS (WHO, 2011). The country with the worst health and life expectancy in the world is Sierra Leone (Bloom *et al.*, 2015). Often resources to support a healthy life are not available to older adults in developing countries. This necessitates a closer look at the capacity of the particular government and their policies. Poverty is a risk factor for many issues, including mental illness (Yasmay, Dua, Harper, & Saxena, 2013). The United Nations in its September 2015 meeting will discuss the progress of the eight Millennium Development Goals, which focused on eradicating poverty and improving life for all. They will also set new goals, known as the Sustainable Development Goals that will extend to 2030 (United Nations Development Programme, 2015).

As life expectancy increases, quality of life for the added years must be addressed. The Global Age Watch Index of 2013 reported on the quality of life for older adults from 91 nations by ranking the countries from number 1, the best quality of life, to number 91, the worst quality of life. South Africa, a higher-income country, ranked 65 out of 91 on quality of life for older adults. In comparison, Bolivia, a lower-income country, ranked 46, considerably better than South Africa. This suggests that a higher income of a country does not always correlate with a better quality of life for older adults. Bolivia, a lower-income country, has a national plan on aging and provides free health care for older adults. This has resulted in a positive impact on the quality of life for older adult citizens. With the continued global increase in aging, all countries should be encouraged to evaluate the successful aging plans that are working and adopt some of these strategies (Global Health Aging, 2014). More research on aging is needed however from low- and middle-income countries. This research should include studies about mental health, chronic diseases, morbidity, and quality of life (Chatterji *et al.*, 2015). Global standards to evaluate outcomes should be set to support accurate comparisons of research results from all countries.

Healthy aging: signs and symptoms

When studying aging, it is important to be able to distinguish what is healthy aging from pathological changes associated with advanced age. When discussing global mental health, understanding how age affects the brain, the neurological system, and cognition is imperative. Aging is an inevitable process that begins from birth. There are many factors that contribute to one's aging process, such as current state of health, genetics, nutritional status, educational background, social support, cultural and personal beliefs (NIA, 2015; Saxon, Etten, & Perkins, 2015). The concept of age is often subjective and relative to the person experiencing it. Many may not feel their chronological age, even those within the older adult population. However, some may feel older than their chronological age. Regardless of how one feels about their age, there are internal and external signs that indicate the body is aging. Just like other organs of the body, the brain and the central nervous system experience degenerative changes over time. These changes may manifest themselves in a mild or modest decline.

There are many different views of how the brain ages, but there is an understanding that there are some basic age-related changes. The volume of the brain in certain areas, such as the prefrontal cortex and the hippocampus, decreases with age. These areas contribute to learning, organizing, remembering, and other intricate mental tasks (Eliopoulos, 2014; NIA, 2015). There are a reduced number of cerebral and peripheral neurons, as well as a decrease in the level of neurotransmitters, especially dopamine, which can affect communication between neurons (Mattson, 2009; NIA, 2015). Myelin covered axons are degraded or lost, resulting in the decreased communication between neurons. In addition, blood flow in the brain may be diminished because of arterial stenosis and a decrease in new capillary growth (NIA, 2015; Eliopoulos, 2014).

With these age-related neurological changes, there are some clinical signs in the older adult that may appear with changes in functioning and cognition. Some functional changes include: less brisk responses with deep tendon reflexes, decreased sensation of touch, pain and vibrations, and less coordinated movements (Boltz, Capezuti, Fulmer, & Zwicker, 2012). Additionally, because there are changes in the sensory and motor systems, the gait is often modified. The gait may be slower, with a shorter stride and a wider stance (Salzman, 2010). There is a slower response time associated with performing tasks and there is a decrease in physiologic reserve, thus more time is needed to recover from physical exertion (Saxon *et al.*, 2015).

With healthy aging in the older adult, there are some cognitive changes that may be seen. These changes are individualized and may not develop uniformly or at the same rate (NIA, 2015; Saxon *et al.*, 2015). Knowledge and skills gained from experience largely stay intact. This is known as crystallized intelligence. The decline is often seen in fluid intelligence, which involves creative reasoning and problem solving. There may also be a mild decline in executive functioning (Boltz *et al.*, 2015). Older adults may not be able to carry out complex tasks involving attention, learning, and memory as well as younger people, but if given more time to complete the tasks many healthy older adults in their 70s and 80s perform similarly to young adults (NIA, 2015). Researchers think that the older brain can be adaptive by activating alternate brain networks to compensate for a decline in regions. Scientists think that the brain may have a cognitive reserve, which is the brain's ability to produce effective cognition even when there is a disruption. When the cognitive reserve threshold is reached, clinical changes in cognition will become evident after a damaging event. Cognitive reserve varies among individuals depending on many factors such as genetics and lifestyle (NIA, 2015)

Health promotion in gero-psychiatry

Scientists have embraced the concept of health promotion for the brain and have studied the benefits of promoting cognitive training with older adults. One such study was the Advanced Cognitive Training for Independent and Vital Elderly (ACTIVE) in 2006, which included 2,802 adults 65 years and older, who were healthy and living independently. The study involved randomizing the older adults into four groups with three groups receiving computer-based cognitive training and the fourth group receiving no cognitive training. After the initial training and booster sessions, the participants were tested and then tested again once a year for 5 consecutive years. The ACTIVE study found that after the initial training, the processing speed group improved 87 percent. The reasoning group improved 74 percent and the memory group improved 26 percent. After 5 years, the groups who received the training had an easier time with food preparation, money management, and performing housework, than the control group. The ACTIVE study suggests that the saying, "use it or lose it" can be applied to the brain and provides hope that cognitive exercises may be beneficial to a broader population of older adults (NIA, 2015).

Another area of health promotion includes risk modification of non-communicable diseases. Non-communicable diseases remain the major cause of morbidity and mortality in the older adult population regardless of the country's income (Beard & Bloom, 2015). Evidence supports the need for risk modification to prevent or delay non-communicable diseases in the older population. Health promotion and disease prevention may still provide beneficial results with this population (Beard & Bloom, 2015; Yasamy *et al.*, 2013). Researchers are actively studying the possibility that cognitive reserve may be improved by modifying risk factors of diseases and lifestyle choices. This could be beneficial for mental health issues, such as dementia (NIA, 2015).

Studies from Denmark and the USA support health promotion and suggest that risk factor modification and early detection of chronic illnesses can help 30 percent to 40 percent of older people live with less disability and more independently (Chatterji *et al.*, 2015). Education about the benefits of exercise, healthy eating, socialization, and smoking cessation is needed. By promoting healthy lifestyles in the older adults, their mental health can be improved (Yasamy *et al.*, 2013.). The results of a 2-year clinical trial of older adults at risk for cognitive impairment were presented at the 2014 Alzheimer Association International Conference. The study concluded that cognitive decline is slowed by the combination of controlled cardiac risk factors, physical activity, proper nutrition, socialization, and cognitive activities (Alzheimer's Association, 2015).

There are many factors that contribute to the mental health of older adults. These factors include physical health, psychological health, social factors, and genetics. Other more specific issues that may contribute to the mental health of older adults are life stressors, such as the death of significant others and friends, the loss of independence, moving homes, chronic pain, disability, and a decrease in income. These factors may contribute to feelings of isolation, loneliness, and depression. In addition, a change is occurring with the demographic of where the older adult population resides. Historically, many older adults have simulated into their children's homes and lived in multigenerational households. Now many older adults live alone. Approximately 50 percent of women 65 years and older live on their own in some European countries. In sub-Saharan Africa, one million older adults are losing the multigenerational support due to the HIV/AIDS epidemic (Beard & Bloom, 2015). When living alone, the support and resources are often diminished, which may put the older adult population at risk for depression and suicide (Beard & Bloom, 2015).

Health promotion strategies and depression

Depression and dementia are the most common neuropsychiatric disorders that affect adults 60 years and older globally (WHO, 2013). A correlation exists between physical health and mental health. Research has shown there is an increase in depressed mood and impaired well-being in older adults who have coronary heart disease, arthritis and chronic lung disease (Steptoe et, al.2015). Older adults who have cardiac disease have a greater rate of depression, than older adults who do not have cardiac disease. It is understood that untreated depression in cardiac patients can cause their heart disease to worsen (WHO, 2013).

Depression is not part of healthy aging, it is a medical condition. In the older adult population, depression is often under-diagnosed and under-treated (Yasamy *et al.*, 2013). It is known that approximately 80 percent of older adults have a chronic illness and about 50 percent have at least two or more chronic illnesses. A chronic illness can be a contributing factor to depression. The more chronic illnesses an older adult has, the more at-risk they are for co-morbid depression. Signs and symptoms of depression include: a change in appetite, a loss of interest in socializing or hobbies, feelings of hopelessness, worthlessness, irritability, insomnia, changes in cognition, increased physical ailments, and thoughts of or attempted suicide. Too often, these signs and symptoms are missed and attributed as a normal reaction to an illness or life stressor (CDC, 2015). Depression in the older adult can be debilitating and challenging for the patient, the caregiver, the families, and health care systems.

Statistics show that depression is a global issue for older adults and that the diagnosis is challenging especially when coexisting with physical illnesses (Yasamy *et al.*, 2013). Another issue, as seen in the US, is a concern that there are not enough professionals trained in geropsychiatry to care for the growing older adult population with mental health needs (Hoge, Karel, Zeiss, Alegria, & Moye, 2015). Diagnosing early, providing psychological and pharmacological treatments, when appropriate, should be part of the standard of care (Yasamy *et al.*, 2013). The universal goal should be to optimize the well-being of all older adults presenting with symptoms of depression (WHO, 2013; Yasamy *et al.*, 2013).

Health promotion should involve educating patients and communities about depression. Depression is sometimes misunderstood within the older adult population and thought to be a normal part of aging. It is not always understood that with the appropriate treatment, depression can improve (CDC, 2015). Another issue is the negative stigma that is often associated with mental health issues, which can inhibit the desire to seek treatment. Health promotion activities with the older adult population should include comprehensive education about depression, including the signs and symptoms and available treatment options. Education about how to manage and modify risks for chronic diseases is another way to improve the mental health of this population. As previously stated, older adults with chronic diseases such as asthma, arthritis, diabetes, and heart disease, have a higher incidence of depression than older adults without those diseases. By promoting overall healthy aging, the mental health of older adults can be positively impacted (Yasamy *et al.*, 2013).

Health promotion should focus on creating living situations that foster integrated healthy lifestyles. In addition, basic needs of safety, independence, social support, and accessible and affordable health care must also be provided (WHO, 2013). Health promotion strategies can also occur at the government level, by identifying and implementing effective public health plans with a mental health focus (Beard & Bloom, 2015). Australia's approach to mental health provides evidence-based research supporting a health system plan specifically for the older population. In 1992, Australia changed the care of mental health patients from institutional care to community care. Since that time, the policy has expanded its plan and strategies. In 2008, WHO reported on the Australian model of keeping patients in their community and integrating mental health care into primary care (WHO & World Organization of Family Doctors, 2008). The model was studied in the St Vincent District of the inner city, with more than 13,000 adults 65 years and older from various backgrounds. It follows the bio-psycho-social model of care, which focuses on collaborative care, with general practitioners (GPs) being the main care provider. Under this plan, GPs are the first to see the geriatric patients seeking mental health treatment. The GPs receive extensive training in geriatrics and mental health. A team approach is used and is coordinated by the GPs, who are assisted by community geropsychiatric nurses and psychologists. Geriatric psychiatrists are consulted only when needed. The goal is to keep the patient in his or her community, to have the GPs coordinate the care, and to limit the time with specialists (WHO & World Organization of Family Doctors, 2008).

Results of the model studied in the St Vincent District showed that there are many advantages to this bio-psycho-social model. It facilitated communication between all involved and provided continuity of care. There was a level of trust attained by the patients, because the GPs were the main care providers for their mental health needs. The geropsychiatric nurses contributed to the continuity of care by attending appointments with the patient and relaying information from the home visits to the GP. Evidence from this model showed that holistic care initiated and managed by primary care was best. The results of the study showed that the GPs became more effective mental health care providers, which led to a substantial decrease in patients needing to see geriatric psychiatrists. The older patient was more likely to seek care for mental health issues because of the accessibility of primary care and the support provided by the GPs and the geropsychiatric nurses. This primary care model was successful in improving access, quality of care, and decreasing the stigma of having to see a specialist, such as a psychiatrist (WHO & World Organization of Family Doctors, 2008).

A similar effective mental health care approach can be seen in the Ehlazani District of the South African province of Mpumalanga. Practitioners who treat physical ailments have been trained to treat mental health issues. Nurses assist with evaluating both mental and physical ailments. This has been an efficient approach to follow, especially when resources are limited (Chen, 2013). However, it has been noted that in South Africa the older adult population is around 4 million and there are only eight registered geriatricians (Global Health Aging, 2014). This suggests that they have an effective model, but not enough health care providers to facilitate its success. Some developing countries, such as Vietnam, are also using the integration of mental health care into primary care model, but find limitations with lack of resources, such as funding, health care expertise, and treatment facilities (Ng, Than, La, Van Than, & Van Dieu, 2011).

Another health promotion strategy for the older adult population would be implementing a public health plan that focuses on the functional well-being of the older adult, rather than diseases and their treatments (Beard & Bloom, 2015). A functional framework would work to maximize the well-being and functional capacities of all older adults: from the healthy older adult to the frail older adult. In this framework, health systems would provide coordinated geriatric services with a continuum plan of care favoring the older adult population to age in their homes and communities, unless their needs become too great. The plan would have a range of services, such as health promotion, disease prevention/management, acute and chronic care, rehabilitative care, and palliative care. Realizing the limitations of low- and middle-income countries, the current health systems of these countries could start by increasing geriatric training to all health care providers and by adapting their current level of care to the needs of the older adult, as seen with the other models. However, the functional model would also encourage more collaboration between health care and social care to meet the physical and social needs of all older adults (Beard & Bloom, 2015).

One collaborative initiative that promotes the physical and social needs of older adults is the WHO Global Network of Age-Friendly Cities and Communities (2014b), which has more than 200 members and services approximately 100 million older people. This initiative assesses ways to create accessible urban environments for aging populations. Information gained is shared among the global members, with the goal of learning how to improve diverse communities and cities for all older adults. With this model, steps are taken in cities and communities to support socialization of older adults, which is an important factor in combatting isolation and depression. One such step is addressing the basic need for toilets and sitting areas in public places to encourage socialization of older adults outside of their homes. Functional frameworks are an effective way to improve day-to-day life and to address the health and mental needs of the global aging population (Beard & Bloom, 2015; WHO, 2014b).

Screening tools for the older adult

Other effective methods of assisting the older adult population would be the global use of screening tools to evaluate functionality and depression. Three such tools are: the Fulmer SPICES: an overall assessment tool for older adults; the Katz Index of Independence in Activities of Daily Living; and the Geriatric Depression Scale found in Table 17.1. All of these instruments are recommended by The Hartford Institute for Geriatric Nursing (2015). These nursing tools are an inexpensive and effective way of identifying needs within the older adult population and provide a way to standardize care. They allow the nurse to implement a plan of care to prevent further decline and improve the well-being of older adult patients. Through the use of these screening tools, it can be determined if further evaluation of the older patient is needed (Hartford Institute for Geriatric Nursing, 2015).

Dementia care and implications for nursing

Care for persons with dementia (PWD) and their caregivers will be the leading global public health challenge faced by mental health professionals in the next century (Talley & Crews, 2007). The inevitable slow decline apparent in this disease process is why interest for improving quality of care for PWD and their caregivers is a grave concern across the world. The forward, ongoing journey for PWD is characterized by increased dependence and need for support as the disease progresses (Prince, Prina, & Guerchet, 2013a).

Table 17.1 Screening tools

Fulmer SPICES (Fulmer & Wallace, 2012; Hartford Institute for Geriatric Nursing, 2015)
http://consultgerirn.org/uploads/File/trythis/try_this_1.pdf

Katz Independence of ADL's (Shelkey & Wallace, 2012; Hartford Institute for Geriatric Nursing, 2015).
http://consultgerirn.org/uploads/File/trythis/try_this_2.pdf

Geriatric Depression Scale (Greenberg, 2012; Hartford Institute for Geriatric Nursing, 2015)
http://consultgerirn.org/uploads/File/trythis/try_this_4.pdf

Source: Hartford Institute of Geriatric Nursing (2015).

This section of the chapter will describe the clinical picture of dementia and present a global overview of best practices in care for PWD and their caregivers. Exemplars of five national strategies formulated to meet this challenge are also reviewed. Best practices identified from current international literature expected to be useful in implementing dementia strategies are also identified. National strategies formulated in five countries (Australia, England, France, Japan, and the USA) based on the best practices are summarized. Finally, suggestions for implementation of the strategies in low- and middle-income countries are also included.

Clinical picture of dementia

According to Prince *et al.* (2013c) dementia is a clinical syndrome caused by neurodegeneration with Alzheimer's disease, vascular dementia, Lewy body, and frontotemporal dementia being the most common underlying pathology. Aging of the population is the highest risk factor and is having a profound impact on the emerging dementia epidemic. Etiology of dementia is still not known and no identified cure exists. Dementia is characterized by progressive deterioration in cognitive ability as well as in capacity for independent living and is a health and social care priority around the globe. Globally, the majority of care is provided by family members/caregivers referred to as "informal" caregivers. Three clinically distinct stages of Alzheimer's disease (AD) are based on functional and cognitive ability: Stages 1 = mild, 2 = moderate and 3 = advanced. PWD in moderate and advanced stages needs dementia care that is constant, round-the-clock care with supervision included to assure safety. Assistance is needed to carry out activities of daily living such as in help with eating, bathing, and dressing. PWD develop challenging behavioral symptoms due to frustration and difficulty coping with specific situations and limitations. Understanding how to prevent or modify these situations can minimize the challenging behavior and improve quality of life (Prince *et al.*, 2013c).

Prevalence rates

Dementia, including Alzheimer's disease, which produces the most cases of dementia, most likely plays a much larger role in the deaths of older persons around the globe than is usually reported. Improved prevalence rates have resulted from stricter inclusion and exclusion criteria, which have improved previous consensus estimates and resulted in a higher level of evidence from well-conducted studies. New prevalence rate findings thus indicate a near exponential prevalence increase in dementia by gender and age, with a higher prevalence in women than in men, especially in older age groups. The higher prevalence of dementia found in older women might be explained by the increased number of women surviving to older age as well as the differential survival with dementia whereby women seem to live longer with dementia than men (Prince *et al.*, 2013c).

Global prevalence of dementia has significant implications for social, health and public policy. Prevalence for PWD at age 60 and over ranged from 5–8 percent in most world regions. The highest prevalence rate was found in North Africa and the Middle East (8.7 percent) and lowest was in Central Europe (4.6 percent). An estimated 46.8 million people lived with dementia worldwide in 2015. The largest region of people living with dementia was in Asia (22.9 million), followed by Europe with 10.5 million, The Americas with 9.4 million, and Africa with 4 million. Prevalence rates are expected to double every 20 years to produce an estimated 74.7 million persons living with dementia in 2030 and 131.5 million persons in 2050 (Prince *et al.*, 2015). Newer estimates consistently identify increased prevalence rates for 2020 (48.1 million) and 2040 (90.3 million) and can be directly compared to earlier rates of 42.7 million for 2020 and 82 million for 2040 (Sousa *et al.*, 2009). Newest estimates are approximately 12–13 percent higher and represent analysis from systematic reviews including data from a large number of journals published in foreign languages in China and Africa (Prince *et al.*, 2015). Increased life expectancy around the world and improved assessment data may be factors in producing improved prevalence rates. One example of a recent study reported that AD may be the third leading cause of death in the United States (James *et al.*, 2014). The current system of relying on death certificates for causes of death underestimates the impact of AD because the complexity of most dementia deaths occur from secondary causes such as pneumonia or infections. Instead of listing the original disease, the most recent infection is instead recorded on the death certificate.

Economic impact

Dementia is universally found to be a very expensive disease, both for families and governments. The cost of care for PWD is taking an economic toll on the world economy. A recent estimate in the United States of the annual cost of care for all PWD over the age of 70 was $157–215 billion in 2010 (Hurd, Martorell, Delavande, Mullen, & Langa, 2013). Direct care costs for PWD were estimated to be $109 billion, which was notably higher than costs for heart disease ($102 billion) or cancer ($77 billion). When the costs of informal caregivers are included, costs of care for PWD are much higher than those for any other chronic condition (Hurd *et al.*, 2013). Yet, in the case of AD there is no way to prevent the disease or modify the ongoing progression (CDC, 2013). Worldwide the esimated cost of dementia in 2015 is $818 billion and by 2018 dementia will become a trillion dollar disease (Prince *et al.*, 2015).

The largest component of current world spending for care of PWD is related to long-term services and support. As the world population ages, traditional unpaid, informal care by family and friends will become increasingly difficult. Due to decreased availability of caregivers per each PWD much greater support will be needed in the future. PWD have special dementia care needs compared with other persons with long-term care needs. Dementia care needs include more personal care, more hours of care, and increased supervision compared with dependent elders who have a physical illness. Prince *et al.* (2013b) in the World Alzheimer's report about the journey of caring commissioned by Alzheimer's Disease International included an analysis of long-term care for PWD and their caregivers. The report identified that long-term care is primarily focused on dementia care as approximately half of all older people who need personal care have dementia and 80 percent of people in nursing homes are living with dementia. Prince *et al.* (2013b) identified that needs for dementia care start early in the disease and evolve constantly as the disease progresses, requiring advanced planning, monitoring, and care coordination. Additional dementia care needs place increased strain on family caregivers plus dementia care has greater costs. Dementia care needs escalate during the progression of the disease including often to the point of impacting the health of the caregivers. Unpaid contributions of family caregivers must be valued and a reward paid for their work. Policies that build quality into the care system while at the same time containing costs plus achieving equity of access to all will be the greatest challenge in the future health care system (Prince *et al.*, 2013b). The next section reviews best practices in dementia care and includes articles focusing on National Dementia Strategies. Five exemplars of national strategies were chosen because the countries represent industrialized countries capable of implementing the best practice strategies. Implementation of the strategies in low- and middle-income nations will also be discussed.

Best practices in care of PWD

A systematic review by Gallagher-Thompson *et al.* (2012) of 159 articles identifies best practice models that need to be used extensively around the world. National dementia policies identify strategies based on these best care practices and hopefully will be implemented around the world. Gallagher-Thompson *et al.* (2012) advocate for the following best practice recommendations: special emphasis is placed on known effective non-pharmacological interventions being more widely disseminated; best practice recommendations include individual and family counseling programs that are individualized and provide relatively long-term support (1–2 years); psychoeducational programs that use a structured format to teach specific coping skills such as "Coping with Caregiving"; and multi-component programs that include education, respite and support such as the REACH II program (Gallagher-Thompson *et al.*, 2012).

Interventions found to be effective in research settings need to be translated to real-life practice. Barriers that prevent services from being accessible to large segments of the population must be identified and reduced. Significant investment by governments and philanthropic organizations needs to be increased and sustained to support research efforts to improve evidence for effectiveness of interventions for PWD and caregivers. Lack of knowledge is cited as the main reason the recommended best practices do not get implemented more extensively. Workforce practitioners not only need to be better educated regarding early diagnosis, they also need to be educated about the psychosocial and multicomponent interventions that can prove helpful for PWD and caregivers (Gallagher-Thompson *et al.*, 2012). If the best practice interventions were included in dementia guidelines, physicians and other workforce providers might be guided to recommend psychosocial interventions over pharmacological treatment (Vasse *et al.*, 2012).

Comparison of five national dementia strategies (Australia, England, France, Japan, and USA)

International concern for improving care for PWD and their caregivers has led to a number of national strategies, formulated by various stakeholder groups including government officials, policy experts, providers, and family caregivers (WHO, 2012). Initiation of these plans differ; whereas government agencies or officials have developed some, others have been created by advocacy organizations such as the country's national Alzheimer's Association. Many national plans are partnerships between government and advocacy organizations. Rosow *et al.* (2011) defined "national plan" as societal recognition either by the government or by a national advocacy community that policy changes are needed to care for PWD, prevent future cases of disease, and provide support to PWD and caregiver families. Because of the given global epidemic of increased prevalence and costs due to care for PWD, it is hoped these national plans will control the future projections. Several recurring themes were found throughout the national plans. The common themes plus goals of society found in the national plans were identified by Rosow *et al.* (2011) as: increased dementia awareness, early diagnosis, improved access to care, improved support services, patient-centered care, and improved care for caregivers. In the World Alzheimers Report, Prince *et al.* (2013a) recommended six strategies to cope with this coming epidemic. Authors recommended the following themes be used as "principles" in national plans. The themes considered to be principles related to national strategies were: systems must monitor the quality of PWD care; more autonomy and choice must be provided according to preferences of PWD and caregivers; and improved integration and coordination between health and social care systems must occur. Both professional and family caregivers must be trained and compensated as part of the health care system in order to ensure continuity of the workforce. Improved financial and other rewards will enable sustained recruitment and retention of the workforce. Finally, quality of care in institutions should be monitored by objective measures on quality of life (QOL), such as surveys of satisfaction by residents, and routine inspections (Prince *et al.*, 2013a).

National strategies in five countries

This section of the paper will report on national plans in five countries: Australia, England, France, Japan and the United States. The five countries were chosen as exemplars for having national dementia strategies which met the following criteria: they were presented in a Report of the Special Committee on Aging in the United States Senate on December 19, 2012 (United States Senate, 2012); each national strategy was published on the Alzheimer's Disease International (ADI) website (www.alz.co.uk/alzheimer-plans); and each of these five national plans included objectives, action plans, and were published in English. Additionally, the five countries were similar in economies and structure with ability to implement best practices. All national strategies can be found at the ADI website listed above. Other national plans do exist but are still in development and are not as well articulated with several components omitted.

Australia

The initial timeline for implementation of Australia's national plan covered 2005–2010. The Dementia Initiative: Making Dementia a National Health Priority, was implemented in the Federal Budget in 2005 in the amount of AUD 320 million. The Ministerial Dementia Advisory Group for the National Framework for Action on Dementia was established in 2008. The purpose of the Advisory Group was to provide the Minister and Department with expert advice on implementation, monitoring, and evaluation of the Dementia Initiative. The Group also advised on broader issues such as prevention, care and treatments, and issues relevant to health reform. Evaluation of the Dementia Initiative found it made substantial contributions to support of PWD and their caregivers and also was cost effective. Evaluation identified weaknesses in that it did not address primary care and did not include a communication strategy or risk reduction. In 2011 the Initiative was terminated and no longer included in the Federal Budget but it is possible that several of the programs may continue to receive funding even after contracts expire. Brodaty and Cumming (2010) commented about the Australian health system being a combination of public and private service with the goal to provide universal access to health care as well as choice through private health insurance. The government has expanded access to dementia community care packages, improved quality of residential care, and begun initiatives to address behavioral and psychological symptoms of dementia. Gaps found upon evaluation related to the need to promote earlier diagnosis through increased awareness, and initiatives to remove stigma. Education and support also needed to focus on special population groups, such as indigenous, non-English speaking rural communities. Alzheimer's Australia, the powerful advocate for improved services, has initiated a prevention program attempting to delay onset of dementia (Skladzien, Bowditch, & Rees, 2011).

England

Banerjee (2010) provided a historical background on policies that existed before the development of the national dementia strategy for England. Before the national strategy started, only one-third of people with dementia actually received a diagnosis of dementia. Those that did receive a diagnosis received it late in the disease process, often diagnosis occurred during a crisis and too late to prevent harm to PWD and the caregiver family. The first national strategy, Living Well with Dementia: A National Dementia Strategy, (Department of Health, 2009) passed in 2009 with no end date provided. Initial funding occurred in the amount of 150 million pounds. The focus of the strategy was wide ranging including increased awareness, earlier diagnosis, information about quality care, training, community support, end of life (EOL) care and research. The national plan was developed in consultation with key stakeholders. A consultations phase occurred with over 3,000 people initially. A second example of consultation consisted of 50 events held throughout the country with 4,000 in attendance. An implementation plan was developed for the national strategy in 2010. Four priority areas for implementation were: early diagnosis/intervention, improved quality of hospital care, living well in dementia care homes, and reduced use of antipsychotic medication. According to Skladzien *et al.* (2011), the emphasis found on hospital care and antipsychotic medication use came about because of the release of National Reports at this time with reviews on each concern. The delivery of the strategy was carried out through the National Health Service, its local authorities, and other key organizations. Finally in 2011, the evaluation phase released the Good Practice Compendium with examples of successful programs linked to the corresponding strategy objective. See the following website for the Compendium of Best Practices: www.gov.uk/government/publications/living-well-with-dementia-a-national-dementia-strategy-good-practice-compendium.

France

The French National Plan was initiated in 2008 with a projected timeline for implementation through 2013. Funding in the amount of 1.6 billion euros was allocated from the health insurance system and the National Fund for the Autonomy of Elderly Disabled People. Defined measures and outcomes have been chosen to guide the plan evaluation (Skladzien *et al.*, 2011). A pilot committee oversees plan implementation by meeting monthly to check on the progress related to each measure. Thus a summary implementation report has been published every 6 months. The June 2011 implementation report summarized that France successfully grew the nation's research capacity, added new memory clinics/diagnostic centers and reduced the use of antipsychotic drugs. One unmet aim was to increase the number of respite care centers, but this has not been accomplished to date. Pimouguet *et al.* (2013) commented that the plan's main goal was to implement an integrated network of partners involved in elderly care, assistance and support. Specifically, case management was used in complex situations. A coordinated approach proved successful to enhance interaction across the health, medical, social, and research sectors. This model has a flexible system aiming to improve linkages between providers without gatekeeping or specific budget control per case.

Japan

Beginning in 2000, dementia care was funded through a national long-term care (LTC) insurance system. Japan has the fastest aging society in the world. By 2020, nearly one-quarter of the population will be over 65 years of age (Ministry of Health, Labor and Welfare Care, 2013). The philosophy of this system was that society as a whole should support disabled older people in need of assistance (including PWD) but access into the system is dependent upon a score on the Government Certified Disability Index. This measure was sensitive to difficulty with ADL but did not accurately assess the impact of behavioral symptoms of dementia (Skladzien et al., 2011). A specific national dementia plan does not exist at this time. Arai, Arai, and Mizuno (2010) reported some concerns that the care provided through this LTC insurance was not meeting the needs of PWD and their caregivers. Cases with earlier onset dementia did not have access to services through the LTC insurance system. Additionally those with severe behavioral and psychological symptoms of dementia were admitted to psychiatric beds because of unavailable community support (Nakanishi & Nakashima, 2014). These complaints led to development of further strategies beyond the LTC insurance system. An international comparative study was funded (2010–2012) to seek suggestions for future Japanese national policy. Recommendations were that the national government should examine revisions in services as well as support advocacy in joint initiatives with Alzheimer's Association Japan (Nakanishi & Nakashima, 2014). Arai et al. (2010) reported on what these further strategies are. Strategies included: improved understanding of incidence and prevalence of dementia, increased research/development focused on dementia, measures implemented for early diagnosis of dementia with provision of appropriate medical treatment, dissemination of accurate information on appropriate care for dementia, plus support for PWD/caregivers. The focus of additional policy was that support measures be developed specifically for persons with early onset dementia. Implementation of these approaches was expected to result in better coordination between health care and social-care services.

Arai and Zarit (2011) discussed the philosophy of Japanese society in sharing the burden of care for the disabled as a unique perspective. The shared burden philosophy has been implemented in Japanese society by sharing the burden of caregiving through compulsory payment of a LTC insurance premium beginning at age 40. This act of everyone paying into the LTC system may result in a society accustomed to the idea of sharing the burden of caregiving before an individual actually needs assistance. This LTC scheme may also be a means of education to the whole society about disabilities in elders and may actually encourage people to take on care responsibilities without feeling so overwhelmed by having to do all the caregiving themselves. Very few national examples were found of a society sharing the caregiving burden as a whole.

United States

On January 4, 2011, President Barack Obama signed into law the National Alzheimer's Project Act (NAPA) (Public Law 111–375), requiring the Secretary of the US Department of Health and Human Services (HHS) to establish the National Alzheimer's Project to coordinate AD research and services across all federal agencies, accelerate development of treatments to prevent, halt, or reverse AD, improve early diagnosis, coordination of care and treatment of AD, decrease ethnic and racial minority disparities in populations at higher risk for AD, and work with international bodies to fight AD globally.

NAPA established the Advisory Council on AD Research, Care, and Services (Advisory Council) and required the Secretary of HHS, with collaboration from the Advisory Council, to create and maintain a National Plan to overcome AD. The first National Plan to Address AD was released on May 15, 2012 after the Obama Administration's investment in funding it in February 2012. The 2013 update to the plan was released on June 14, 2013. The release of the National Plan to Address AD occurs each spring. This 2014 update reflected national progress made toward meeting the goals set a year ago as well as including new and revised action steps. Five goals of the 2014 plan are to: prevent and effectively treat AD by 2024; optimize care quality and efficiency; expand support for PWD and their caregiving families; enhance public awareness and engagement; and track progress and drive improvement.

Because of advocacy about the ambitious goal to prevent and effectively treat AD by 2024, the US Senate Committee on Appropriations voted to include an additional $104 million in the fiscal year 2014 funding bill for AD research, education, outreach, and care of caregivers. The first goal to prevent and effectively treat AD by 2024 was viewed as an ambitious but critical goal to achieve in order to prevent a great amount of heartbreak and cost in the future (Department of Health and Human Services, 2014).

An overall review of these National Plans led to the following conclusions: a) considerable consensus exists for goals related to diagnosis, treatment, and research; and b) most nations give priority to making a more accurate and early diagnosis, identifying biomarkers and genetic advances, committing resources to reduce the associated stigma of the disease, improving continuity of care, and in developing a trained workforce. A common, shared policy goal among the countries was to craft policies enabling PWD to live at home as long as possible. Countries seem united in efforts to expand the provision of long-term services and support in home and community-based services within their existing health and social services delivery systems. Countries also identified the goal of providing coordinated, integrated care across their health and social services systems for PWD and their caregivers. Plans targeted person-centered care and care coordination as ways to achieve the goals for an integrated care system.

Implementation of strategies in low- and middle-income nations

Dementia strategies from industrialized countries were chosen because of strength in being able to implement policy recommendations. On the other hand, how might these strategies be implemented in developing countries where little is known about PWD? Prince and the Dementia Research Group (2004) report findings from the first systematic, comprehensive assessment of care arrangements of PWD in developing countries and described the status of caregiving in the developing countries of India, China, South East Asia, Latin America, The Caribbean, and Africa. Most caregivers were women who lived in extended three-generation households with the PWD. A quarter to half of all caregiving households included a child. When the caregiver was co-resident, larger households were associated with lower caregiver strain. Levels of caregiver strain were as high as in developed countries. Many caregivers had cut back on hours of employment to provide care and faced additional expenses of paid formal care and health services. Families from the poorest countries were likely to have used expensive private medical services with more than 10 percent of their per capita GNP spending used on PWD health care. High levels of family strain fed into an ongoing cycle of disadvantage because compensatory financial support was negligible (Prince & Dementia Research Group, 2004).

Dias *et al.* (2008) described a home care program for supporting caregivers in India. The program "Helping Carers to Care" train-the-trainer intervention was developed with help from a group of international experts, the Dementia Research Group. The target of the home care intervention was the primary caregiver but also included the extended family. The aim was to provide the caregiver with basic education about dementia and specific training on managing problematic symptoms of dementia. Randomized controlled trials in Argentina, Chile, China, Dominican Republic, India, Mexico, Peru, Russia, and Venezuela have been used to test the intervention. Results identified positive effects on caregiver mental health with greater effects than typically are seen in interventions in high-income countries. Local Community Health Workers (CHW) were used to implement the intervention. CHWs were trained in a two-day training event with content that covered information on dementia and developed skills for management of PWD problematic symptoms. The aim of the Dementia Research group was to use existing, locally available health care resources to provide outreach, needs assessment, and continuing care (Dias *et al.*, 2008).

The key public health challenge in developing countries is poor awareness of dementia. Economic barriers result in fewer health care resources being available to mobilize assessment and outreach for case finding and continuing care (Dias *et al.*, 2008). Consequences resulting from this problem are that PWD and their family caregivers do not seek help, or if they do, services tend not to meet their needs (Prince & Dementia Research Group, 2004). Another major problem in developing countries was the stigma of dementia; as a result PWD were excluded from residential care and denied admission to hospital. For example, in India, raising awareness of the progression of dementia is needed as physicians lack knowledge about how to assess and treat PWD at various stages of the disease. Recommendations included a need for dementia education not only for family caregivers but also especially for physicians. The sad consequence of this lack of awareness was that PWD and families tended to have less support or understanding with resultant increased burden (Gupta, 2009).

Implications for future public health policy

In most nations, dementia historically has not been given as much attention as other physical diseases. This lack of understanding may contribute to a severe lack of funding across the world. Often people think of AD as just a memory problem where you forget where you left your keys. The fact is that AD is universally a fatal brain disease with no identified cure. Primary prevention should target modifiable factors known by current evidence, such as decreasing risk factors related to vascular disease, including diabetes, midlife hypertension, midlife obesity, smoking, and physical inactivity. Cardiovascular risk profiles need to be targeted earlier before midlife. Successful risk reduction of these cardiovascular risk factors could reduce the prevalence of AD by up to 1.1 million cases worldwide (Barnes & Yaffe, 2011). Possible outcomes are that targeted risk reduction initiatives might have an important impact on reduction of the future prevalence and incidence of worldwide dementia. An example of such a risk reduction study, was found in the Right Time Place Care prospective study protocol by Verbeek *et al.* (2012). Home health care policies were examined in eight European countries (Estonia, Finland, France, Germany, Netherlands, Sweden, Spain, United Kingdom). Health policies were chosen that enabled PWD to live at home as long as possible versus be admitted to institutional care. Additional studies are needed to generate primary data to develop best practices on transition from home to institutional care and back home for PWD and their primary caregivers. Outcomes from these national plans and strategies may be very helpful in generating needed future knowledge to improve policy.

Implications for nursing practice

Around the globe programs are being developed that target increased support for PWD and their caregivers. Pressing needs of family caregivers for services to reduce their burden and improve quality of life far outstrip available services even in more developed countries like the United States. Successful models from low-income countries may even help in high-income countries. Gallagher-Thompson *et al.* (2012) suggests that policy makers need to assure increased awareness that effective models of care do exist and must be put into practice. Dissemination is needed for existing nonpharmacological treatments with demonstrated effectiveness. Providing health education and counseling about dementia is also needed to reduce stigma and improve knowledge of the disease as well as available services. Creating awareness at the societal level using radio, television, and social network sites will improve the quality of life for PWD and their caregivers. Barriers that prevent services from being accessible need to be identified and reduced. Excellent programs may exist but may be accessible only to a small percentage of the population. Barriers are similar in both high- and low-income countries and can include cost, low-health literacy, low education and awareness of what these programs can do to help the caregiver and family in improved quality of life. Stigma needs to be reduced regarding diagnosis and treatment of dementia.

The mental health nurse is uniquely qualified to meet the needs of PWD and their caregivers. The mental health nursing workforce has capabilities for providing coordinated, integrated care in the community. Principles underlying interventions in low-income countries can be used to enhance support for mental health nurses across the globe. Not only mental health nurses working in low-income countries experience limited resource, but the global mental health nursing workforce even in high-income countries experience lack of resources in certain parts of all countries. Sustainable interventions have to rely mostly on existing resources or low cost additional resources. Dias *et al.* (2008) discussed that the front-line intervention in a low-income country such as India was a locally recruited individual who had no prior experience with dementia care and was not a health professional. Training was implemented using materials and lay workers supervised by health professionals. Community health workers helped sustain the ongoing program. Mental health nurses have unique knowledge of psychobiology and a holistic approach to care of PWD. Mental health nursing education provides clinical experience in coordination and integration of holistic care and includes preparation for supervision and administration of programs providing support and care to PWD and their caregivers.

References

Alzheimer's Association. (2015). *Brain health*. Retrieved June 9, 2015 from www.alz.org/we_can_help_brain_health_maintain_your_brain.asp.

Arai, Y., & Zarit, S.H. (2011). Exploring strategies to alleviate caregiver burden: Effects of the national long-term care insurance scheme in Japan. *Psychogeriatrics*, *11*(3), 183–189.

Arai, Y., Arai, A., & Mizuno, Y. (2010). The national dementia strategy in Japan. *International Journal Geriatric Psychiatry*, *25*(9), 896–899.

Banerjee, S. (2010). Living well with dementia: Development of the national dementia strategy for England. *International Journal of Geriatric Psychiatry*, *25*(9), 917–922.

Barnes, D.E., & Yaffe, K. (2011). The projected effect of risk factor reduction on Alzheimer's disease prevalence. *The Lancet Neurology*, *10*(9), 819–828.

Beard, J., & Bloom, D. (2015). Towards a comprehensive public health response to population ageing. *The Lancet*, *385*, 658–661.

Bloom, D., Chatterji, S., Kowal, P., Llyod-Sherlock, P., McKee, M., Rechel, B., Rosenberg, L., & Smith, J. (2015). Macroeconomic implications of population ageing and selected policy responses. *The Lancet*, *385*, 649–757.

Boltz, M., Capezuti, E., Fulmer, T., & Zwicker, D. (2012). *Age-related changes in health: Evidence-based geriatric nursing protocols for best practice* (4th ed.). New York: Springer.

Brodaty, H., & Cumming, A. (2010). Dementia services in Australia. *International Journal of Geriatric Psychiatry*, *25*(9), 887–995.

Karen M. Robinson et al.

Centers for Disease Control and Prevention. (2013). Leading causes of death. Retrieved February 25, 2014, from www.cdc.gov/aging/aginginfo/alzheimers.htm.

Centre for Disease Control and Prevention. (2015). Depression is not a normal part of growing older. 2015 update. Retrieved June 8, 2015 from www.cdc.gov/aging/mentalhealth/depression.htm.

Chatterji, S., Byles, J., Cutler, D., Seeman, T., & Verdes, E. (2015). Health, functioning, and disability in older adults-present status and future implications. *The Lancet, 385,* 563–575.

Chen, E. (2013). The integration of mental health into primary care. Retrieved June 6, 2015 from www.hcs.harvard.edu/hghr/online/the-integration-of-mental-health-into-primary-care/.

Department of Health. (2009). *Living well with dementia: A national dementia strategy.* London: Department of Health. Retrieved March 26, 2014 from www.gov.uk/government/uploads/system/uploads/attachment_data/file/168220/dh_094051.pdf.

Department of Health and Human Services (DHHS). (2014). National plan to address Alzheimer's disease: 2014 update. Retrieved July 24, 2016 from http://aspe.hhs.gov/daltcp/napa/NatlPlan2014.shtml.

Dias, A., Dewey, M.E., D'Souza, J., Dhume, R., Motghare, D.D., Shaji, K.S., Menon, R., Prince, M., & Patel, V. (2008). The effectiveness of a home care program for supporting caregivers of persons with dementia in developing countries: A randomised controlled trial from Goa, India. *PLoS One, 3*(6), e2333.

Eliopoulos, C. (2014). *Neurologic function: Gerontological nursing* (8th ed.). Philadelphia, PA: Wolters Kluwer Health | Lippincott Williams & Wilkins.

Fulmer, T. & Wallace, M. (2012). Fulmer SPICES: An overall assessment tool for older adults. *Try This: Best Practices in Nursing Care to Older Adults, 1,* 1–2.

Gallagher-Thompson, D., Tzuang, Y.M., Au, A., Brodaty, H., Charlesworth, G., Gupta, R., Lee, S.E., Losada, A., & Shyu, Y.-I. (2012). International perspectives on nonpharmacological best practices for dementia family caregivers: A review. *Clinical Gerontologist, 35*(4), 316–355.

Global Age Watch Index. (2013). Retrieved May 25, 2016 from www.helpage.org/global-agewatch/reports/global-agewatch-index-2013-insight-report-summary-and-methodology/.

Global Health Aging. (2014). Quality of life for elders: Lessons from South Africa and Bolivia. Retrieved June 6, 2015 from http://globalhealthaging.org/2014/07/05/quality-of-life-for-elders-lessons-from-south-africa-and-bolivia-2/.

Greenberg, S. (2012). The geriatric depression scale (GDS). *Try This: Best Practices in Nursing Care to Older Adults, 4,* 1–2.

Gupta, R. (2009). Systems perspective: Understanding caregiving of the elderly in India. *Health Care for Women International, 30*(12), 1040–1054.

The Hartford Institute for Geriatric Nursing. (2015). New York University, College of Nursing. Retrieved June 9, 2015 from www.hartfordign.org/practice/try_this/.

Hoge, M., Karel, M., Ziess, A., Algeria, M., & Moye, J. Strengthening psychology's workforce for older adults. *American Psychologist, 70*(3), 265–278.

Hurd, M.D., Martorell, P., Delavande, A., Mullen, K J., & Langa, K.M. (2013). Monetary costs of dementia in the United States. *New England Journal of Medicine, 368*(14), 1326–1334.

James, B.D., Leurgans, S.E., Hebert, L.E., Scherr, P.A., Yaffe, K., & Bennett, D. A. (2014). Contribution of Alzheimer disease to mortality in the United States. *Neurology, 82*(12), 1045–1050.

Mattsson, N., Zetterberg, H., Hansson, O., Andreasen, N., Parnetti, L., Jonsson, M., Herukka, S.K., & Blennow, K. (2009). CSF biomarkers and incipient Alzheimer disease in patients with mild cognitive impairment. *JAMA, 302*(4), 385–393.

Ministry of Health, Labor and Welfare. (2013). Health and welfare bureau for the elderly: In anticipation of the arrival of a super aging population. Retrieved March 26, 2014 from www.mhlw.go.jp/english/policy/care-welfare/care-welfare-elderly/dl/health_and_welfare_bureau.pdf.

Nakanishi, M., & Nakashima, T. (2014). Features of the Japanese national dementia strategy in comparison with international dementia policies: How should a national dementia policy interact with the public health-and social-care systems? *Alzheimer's Dementia, 10*(4), 468–476, e463.

National Institute on Aging. (NIA). (2015). *Alzheimer's disease: Unraveling the mystery. The changing brain in healthy aging.* Retrieved June 3, 2015 from www.nia.nih.gov/alzheimers/publications/part-1- basics-healthy-brain/changing-brain-healthy-aging.

Ng, C.H., Than, P.T., La, C.D., Van Than, Q., & Van Dieu, C. (2011). The national community mental health care project in Vietnam: A review for future guidance. *Australasian Psychiatry, 19*(2), 143–150.

Pimouguet, C., Bassi, V., Somme, D., Lavallart, B., Helmer, C., & Dartigues, J.F. (2013). The 2008–2012 French Alzheimer plan: A unique opportunity for improving integrated care for dementia. *Journal of Alzheimer's Disease, 34*(1), 307–314.

Prince, M., & Dementia Research Group. (2004). Care arrangements for people with dementia in developing countries. *International Journal of Geriatric Psychiatry, 19*(2), 170–177.

Prince, M., Guerchet, M., & Prina, M. (2013a). *Policy brief for heads of Government: The global impact of dementia 2013–2050*. King's College London: Alzheimer's Disease International. Retrieved March 26, 2014 from www.alz.co.uk/G8policybrief.

Prince, M., Prina, M., & Guerchet, M. (2013b). *World Alzheimer report 2013: Journey of caring—An analysis of long-term care for dementia*. London: Alzheimer's Disease International. Retrieved March 26, 2014 from www.alz.co.uk/research/worldalzheimerreport2013.pdf.

Prince, M., Bryce, R., Albanese, E., Wimo, A., Ribeiro, W., & Ferri, C.P. (2013c). The global prevalence of dementia: A systematic review and metaanalysis. *Alzheimer's & Dementia, 9*(1), 63–75, e62.

Prince, M., Wimo, A., Guerchet, M., Ali, G., Wu, Y., & Prina, M. (2015). *World Alzheimer report 2015: The global impact of dementia. Analysis of prevalence, incidence, cost and trends*. London: Alzheimer's Disease International.

Rosow, K., Holzapfel, A., Karlawish, J.H., Baumgart, M., Bain, L.J., & Khachaturian, A.S. (2011). Countrywide strategic plans on Alzheimer's disease: developing the framework for the international battle against Alzheimer's disease. *Alzheimer's & Dementia, 7*(6), 615–621.

Salzman, B. (2010). Gait and balance disorders in older adults. *American Family Physician, 82*(1), 61–68.

Saxon, S.V., Etten, M.J., & Perkins, E.A. (2015). *Physical change & aging: A guide for the helping professions* (6th ed.). New York: Springer Publishing.

Shelkey, M., & Wallace, M. (2012). Katz index of independence in activities of daily living. The Hartford Institute for Geriatric Nursing. *Try This: Best Practices in Nursing Care to Older Adults, 2*, 1–2.

Skladzien, E., Bowditch, K., & Rees, G. (2011). National strategies to address dementia: A report by alzheimer's australia. Paper 25. Retrieved March 26, 2014 from www.fightdementia.org.au/common/files/NAT/20111410_Paper_25_low_v2.pdf.

Sousa, R.M., Ferri, C.P., Acosta, D., Albanese, E., Guerra, M., Huang, Y., Jacob, K.S., Jotheeswaran, AT., Rodriguez, J.J.L., Pichardo, G.R., Rodriguez, M.C., Salas, A., Sosa, A.L., Williams, J., Zuniga, T., & Prince, M. (2009). Contribution of chronic diseases to disability in elderly people in countries with low and middle incomes: A 10/66 Dementia Research Group population-based survey. *The Lancet, 374*(9704), 1821–1830.

Steptoe, A., Deaton, A., Stone, A. (2015). Subjective well-being, health, and ageing. *The Lancet, 385*, 640–648.

Talley, R.C., & Crews, J.E. (2007). Framing the public health of caregiving. *American Journal of Public Health, 97*(2), 224–228.

United Nations Development Programme. (2015). Retrieved June 16, 2015 from www.undp.org/content/undp/en/home/mdgoverview/post-2015-development-agenda.html.

United States Senate Special Committee on Aging. (2012). *Alzheimer's disease and dementia: A comparison of international approaches*. (S. Rept. 112–254). Washington, DC: US Government Printing Office. Retrieved March 26, 2014 from www.gpo.gov/fdsys/pkg/CRPT-112srpt254/pdf/CRPT-112srpt254.pdf.

Vasse, E., Vernooij-Dassen, M., Cantegreil, I., Franco, M., Dorenlot, P., Woods, B., & Moniz-Cook, E. (2012). Guidelines for psychosocial interventions in dementia care: A European survey and comparison. *International Journal of Geriatric Psychiatry, 27*(1), 40–48.

Verbeek, H., Meyer, G., Leino-Kilpi, H., Zabalegui, A., Hallberg, I.R., Saks, K., Soto, M.E., Challis, D., Sauerland, D., & Hamers, J.PH. (2012). A European study investigating patterns of transition from home care towards institutional dementia care: The protocol of a RightTimePlaceCare study. *BMC Public Health, 12*(68), 1–10.

World Health Organization and World Organization of Family Doctors. (2008). *Integrating mental health into primary care: A global perspective*. Geneva: WHO.

World Health Organization (WHO). (2011). *Global health and aging*. Retrieved May 30, 2015 from www.who.int/ageing/publications/global_health.pdf.

World Health Organization. (2012). *Dementia: A public health priority*. London: World Health Organization. Retrieved March 26, 2014 from www.who.int/mental_health/publications/dementia_report_2012/en/.

World Health Organization (WHO). (2013). Mental health and older adults. Retrieved June 6, 2015 from www.who.int/mediacentre/factsheets/fs381/en/.

World Health Organization (WHO). (2014a). *Facts about ageing*. Retrieved June 11, 2015 from www.who.int/ageing/about/facts/en/.

World Health Organization (WHO). (2014b). *Global network for age friendly cities and communities*. Retrieved June 11, 2015 from www.who.int/ageing/projects/age_friendly_cities_network/en/.

Yasamy, M., Dua, T., Harper, M., & Saxena, S. (2013). *Mental health of older adults, addressing a growing concern*. Geneva: WHO, Department of Mental Health & Substance Abuse.

18

STRATEGIES FOR MENTAL HEALTH PROMOTION IN CHILDREN AND ADOLESCENTS

Irene Eunhee Kim, Andrew Cashin and Edilma L. Yearwood

Introduction

Childhood mental health is defined by the World Health Organization (WHO) as "having a positive sense of identity, the ability to manage thoughts and emotions, as well as to build social relationships, and the aptitude to learn and to acquire an education, ultimately enabling full active participation in society" (WHO, 2013, p. 6). WHO (2012) also stated that

> young people with a good sense of mental well-being possess problem-solving skills, social competence and a sense of purpose, which helps them rebound from any setbacks that they encounter, thrive in the face of poor circumstances, avoid risk-taking behavior and continue a productive life.
>
> *(WHO, 2012, p. 6)*

Children and adolescents are challenged with serious obstacles to their mental health regardless of whether they live in developing or developed countries (Achenbach & Rescorla, 2007; Belfer, 2008). These obstacles include abandonment, neglect, child abuse, family instability, parent psychopathology, poverty, dislocation, exposure to traumatic events such as violence, disaster, and, in some parts of the world, child prostitution and child soldiering (Masten, 2014). Additionally, children constitute up to half of the population in many developing countries with basic needs for nutrition, water and sanitation taking precedence over child mental health concerns (Belfer & Nurcombe, 2007; Patel, Flisher, Nikapota, & Malhotra, 2008).

Epidemiological data consistently report the global prevalence of child and adolescent mental disorders to be approximately 20 percent (Kieling *et al.*, 2011; Klasen & Crombag, 2013; WHO, 2012) and suicide to be the second leading cause of death in the 15–19 years age category worldwide (Patton *et al.*, 2009; WHO, 2012). Mental health challenges and disorders can result when children's vulnerabilities and risk factors outweigh their resilience and protective factors. Child mental disorders can manifest themselves in many domains and in many different ways. It is now understood that mental disturbances at a young age can lead to ongoing impairment in adult life (Belfer, 2008; Flament *et al.*, 2007; Kessler *et al.*, 2005; Merikangas, Nakamura, & Kessler, 2009) and up to 50 percent of adult mental disorders have their origin in childhood (Belfer, 2008). Thus, the lack of attention to the mental health of children and adolescents not only leads to mental disorders with lifelong consequences to the quality of life for individuals, but to a reduced capacity of societies to be safe and productive.

In 1989, the Convention on the Rights of the Child (CRC) was adopted by the United Nations General Assembly (United Nations Children's Fund (UNICEF), 2009; WHO, 2005a). CRC, the most universally endorsed and comprehensive human rights treaty of all time (WHO, 2005a), was a major and historic milestone in the effort to promote mental health and well-being in children around the world. It advocated for children having the right to survive and develop, and to be protected from violence, abuse and exploitation. The treaty also called for the views of children to be respected, and actions concerning them to be taken in their best interests (UNICEF, 2009). However, despite this effort to identify characteristics and environments that support healthy growth and development of children, the magnitude and impact of mental health problems were not properly recognized by many governments and policy makers in the world and continue to be unrecognized to this day, as many countries have chosen not to endorse the CRC.

Recently, the WHO has started playing a major role in raising public awareness of child mental health and facilitating the establishment of appropriate services (Belfer, 2008; Kieling *et al.*, 2011). In 2002, it convened an expert panel to deliberate the status of children with mental disorders, especially in developing countries, and issued its report, *Caring for Children and Adolescents with Mental Disorders: Setting WHO directions* (WHO, 2003) to establish a framework for understanding the overall scope of the problems associated with launching a system of care for the treatment of child mental disorders. In 2005, WHO also published *The Child and Adolescent Mental Health Atlas* (WHO, 2005a), which is one of the first systematic efforts to collect data on treatment resources available for children and adolescents with mental disorders worldwide. The WHO ATLAS project was complemented by another publication, *Child and Adolescent Mental Health Policies and Plans* (WHO, 2005b), in order to provide practical information and guidelines for developing mental health policies and strategies. These efforts demonstrated the WHO's recognition of the fundamental worldwide absence of mental health policy for children and its negative impact on healthy development. In these documents, nurses, as the largest group of health care providers, were being asked to serve as frontline providers in delivering services to children with mental disorders (WHO, 2011). While these documents provide us with epidemiological data on child disorders and policy recommendations, there is also a need for robust guidelines for child mental health promotion especially in low- and middle-income environments.

This chapter will describe risks, protective factors, and global issues impacting children's mental health. It will further explore common mental health challenges and disorders, mental health promotion strategies, prevention programs for this population and opportunities for nurses, as the largest health care providers globally, to meet the mental health needs of children, adolescents and their families.

(Throughout this chapter, the term "children" will include adolescents unless otherwise specified.)

Etiology of childhood psychiatric and behavioral syndromes

Before embarking upon a discussion of variance from "normal" development of behavior and cognition in the form of syndromes and disorders, and in the case of illness acute variance, it is always worthwhile to briefly review what we consider to be normal.

Although the unified theories of cognitive development (Piaget), identity (Erickson), and moral reasoning (Kohlberg) have been critiqued, they remain valuable in that they provide a base from which to articulate variance. It must be noted that heterogeneity of people is the rule rather than the exception within age groups, but also within countries and cultures (Smetana, Campione-Barr and Metzger, 2006). Varied ways of thinking about development have been presented through consideration of information processing (largely development of attention, memory, and use of images) and the socially mediated aspects represented in ecology, among others. Table 18.1 provides a quick overview of development as represented in the staged approach used by Piaget, Erickson, and Kohlberg. Piaget's work focused on the development of mental schemata and the assimilation of these into daily life (Piaget, 1952). Erickson focused on the development of identity (1952/1998) and Kohlberg on moral development in the context of shifting views from those traditionally held that moral education was the province of the family and church alone, which left little space to consider the role of school professionals and others in this endeavor (Kohlberg and Hersh, 1977).

Summary of developmental theorists

It is of note that adolescence is a time of upheaval and crisis that is in and of itself developmentally normal. Preceding the theorists featured in Table 18.1, Mitchell (1924) provided an apt description of the depth of normal teenage upheaval in the context of rapid physiological change and cognitive development:

> The adolescent youth is an unbalanced and lumbering creature. He finds it difficult to make his way around in a world littered with obstacles. He is constantly running into furniture. He is awkward in making delicate distinctions and in observing the nice decisions of society. His hands and feet are large. He finds the world an uncharted sea in which he is constantly making mistakes. Our customary attitude toward him is one of reproof and condemnation. We urge him to conform to set standards but the very nature of his mechanism at this time makes conformity impossible ... The adolescent girl in her development parallels that of the youth. Her awkwardness may be not so marked and she seems to recover from it more quickly.
>
> *(Mitchell, 1924, pp. 51–53)*

The causes of most psychiatric disorders and behavioral challenges involve some combination of biological and psychosocial factors. Furthermore, child psychiatric symptoms are mitigated by the child's cognitive, social, emotional, and developmental stages and socio-cultural context. The extent and nature of the influence of the child's surroundings, such as family, peers, school, community, and cultural group, depend on the developmental stage and age of the child (Patel, Flisher, & Cohen, 2006; Paula, Duarte, & Bordin, 2007). Also, culture can create specific sources of distress and impairment in children, and influence how symptoms are interpreted (Kieling *et al.*, 2011).

The concept of risk and protective factors

Researchers explain the etiology of mental disorders in children in association with risk and protective factors. A risk factor is a variable associated with an increased risk of psychopathology whereas a protective factor is a variable that moderates the effects of risk exposure. Furthermore, risks can be either modifiable (can be influenced or altered) or non-modifiable (cannot be

Table 18.1 Comparison of child developmental theories

Piaget *4 stages of cognitive development*	Erickson *8 stages of identity formation*	Kohlberg *6 stages of moral development*
Sensorimotor 0–2 years Thinking with the bodily sensorimotor equipment	Trust vs. mistrust The first social achievement is letting mother out of sight Trust is developed in oneself and the capacity of the body An inner population of memories and anticipated sensations is developed that has correspondence with outer people and things	The punishment and obedience orientation Responds to rules and norms of good and bad, but based on consequences of punishment or reward at the individual level
Preoperational 2–7 years Schemata developed that are no longer attached to activity alone There is an increase in representational (symbolic) thinking	Autonomy vs. shame A stage of development of autonomy of free will be characterized by holding in and letting	The instrumental- relativist orientation Action is largely that which satisfies one's own needs Social relations are seen through a market type place lens of profiting from action
Concrete operational 7–11 years Thought is organized in a more logical fashion Thinking becomes more agil	Initiative vs. guilt Corresponds with ambulating and infantile genitality a time when a sense of making is added to the social armory Insight is gained into the role and functions of people and institutions How to participate is grasped	The interpersonal concordance of "good boy—nice girl" orientation Approval is sought through doing what is considered "nice"
Formal operational 11+ years The capacity is developed for abstraction applied in systematic and scientific thinking Hypothetico-deductive reasoning develops	Industry vs. inferiority Child learns to win praise and acceptance by sustained production of things The value of sustained attention and diligence is learnt	The law and order orientation A stage of doing duty informed by authority figures, rules and a principle of social order maintenance
	Identity vs. role diffusion This marks the end of childhood and the beginning of being a youth (adolescence) Marked by rapid physiological changes and a questioning of all the learning acquired from the earlier stages Concerned with how they appear to others and how to apply industry fruitfully	The social-contract legalistic orientation, generally with utilitarian overtones Focus is dominated by a legal point of view, but peppered with awareness that society may need to change this view based on utility and rational discussion
	Intimacy vs. isolation The ability to relate fully, both emotionally and sexually in relationships is developed A balance is negotiated between work, love, and recreation	The universal-ethical-principle orientation Right is seen as an individual judgment based on self-selected ethical principles This represents a shift from internalization of concrete rules
	Generativity v stagnation Interest in assisting and promoting the next generation is cultivated	
	Ego integrity vs. despair Acceptance is developed of the meaning of one's life	

Source: Erikson, 1952/1998; Kohlberg & Hersh, 1977; Piaget, 1952.

influenced or altered). Children are more vulnerable to developing psychiatric and behavioral symptoms when risk factors surpass protective factors. In the meantime, protective factors can act by promoting alternative, compensatory processes that enhance self-esteem and a sense of personal effectiveness (Nurcombe, 2007). The more opportunities children have to experience the positive effects of protective factors, the more likely they are to be able to sustain mental health later in life (WHO, 2012). In general, both risk factors and protective factors can be understood in the context of three domains—biological, psychological, and social. Table 18.2 provides a description of risk and protective factors for children's mental health.

Global risk factors

In addition to the aforementioned risk factors within low, middle-, and high-income communities, there are worldwide crises that can also impact child mental health. Many children may show resilience in response to these global phenomena especially with the appropriate scaffolding from adults and community resources. However, severe traumas will place vulnerable children at a significantly higher risk of experiencing mental health problems.

Displacement

According to the *UNHCR Statistical Yearbook 2012* (United Nations High Commissioner for Refugees (UNHCR), 2013), 45.2 million people were forcibly displaced worldwide as a result of war, political violence, and/or related threats as of the end of 2012. Disaggregated information on age showed that children under the age of 18 represented an average of 49 percent of the total population affected by these traumas (UNHCR, 2013). Displaced children may experience enormous trauma in the form of violence, crime, or other humiliations, disruption of family and loss of parents and relatives, physical and psychological injury, and economic dispossession, (Patel *et al.*, 2006; Reed, Fazel, Jones, Panter-Brick, & Stein, 2012). These occurrences may be characterized by multiple events happening in multiple contexts that persist over time. Refugee families often encounter resettlement stressors such as poverty and poor housing, as well as acculturative stressors and discrimination, which can pose increased risks for emotional and behavioral health in refugee children (Betancourt *et al.*, 2015; Reed *et al.*, 2012; Ziaian, de Anstiss, Antoniou, Baghurst, & Sawyer, 2013). The results of most studies show high prevalence estimates of psychological problems in refugee children, particularly with respect to anxiety, depression, and posttraumatic stress disorder (Belfer, 2008; Porter & Haslam, 2005; Reed *et al.*, 2012).

Disasters

Children are one of the most vulnerable groups for post-disaster psychological morbidity (Kar, 2009; Norris *et al.*, 2002). Disasters can be classified as either natural disasters or man-made disasters (Masten & Osofsky, 2010). Natural disasters refer to phenomena such as earthquakes, floods, hurricanes, tornados, or tsunamis that can kill thousands of people and destroy entire communities. Man-made disasters include fires, acts of mass violence such as war, genocide, terrorism, and mass shootings, as well as industrial accidents, transportation accidents, and disease outbreaks.

Following catastrophic disasters, post-traumatic reactions in directly affected children may reach epidemic proportions, remain high for a lengthy period, and ultimately endanger the well-being of all children residing in the affected region. A child's psychological reaction to a disaster

Table 18.2 Description of risk and protective factors for children's mental health

Domain	Risk factors	Protective factors
Biological factors	Genetic susceptibility for mental disorders Chromosomal abnormality Exposure to intrauterine toxins such as alcohol, illegal drugs, and tobacco Premature birth Perinatal trauma and low birth weight Environmental exposure to lead Malnutrition Traumatic brain injury HIV infection and other physical illnesses	Good intellectual functioning Age-appropriate physical development Good physical health
Psychological	Difficult temperament or behavioral inhibition Maladaptive personality traits Consequences associated with emotional, sexual, physical abuse or neglect Learning difficulties	Easy temperament style Good self-esteem Age-appropriate social skills High level of problem-solving ability Ability to learn from experience
Social *Family factors*	Disrupted attachment Poor parenting Marital discord Parent's psychopathology such as parental depression, substance abuse, and antisocial personality Single parent or blended families Poverty Death of family member	Secure attachments to parents Good support from at least one parent Cohesive family environment Opportunities for positive involvement in familial activities
School factors	Peer rejection, bullying and negative peer group influence Academic failure Inadequate educational provision or training opportunities	The quality of schools Peer networking Positive relationships with teachers Opportunities for involvement in school life with accompanying sense of belonging Positive academic achievement
Community factors	Poor access to or lack of resources Discrimination, marginalization, and stigma Exposure to violence Overcrowding	Adequate community resources for sports and skill building Positive cultural experiences Positive role modeling Rewards for community involvement A connection with community organizations including religious organizations

Source: Kieling *et al.*, 2011; Manikam, 2002. Adapted from Patel, Flisher, Hetrick, & McGorry, 2007.

depends upon degree of exposure, extent of loss of family members, trauma-related parental distress, previous exposure to stressful events, and proximity to traumatic events (Kar, 2009; Ying, Wu, Lin, & Chen, 2013). Common psychiatric manifestations among children include acute stress reaction, adjustment disorder, depression, panic disorder, post-traumatic stress disorder (PTSD) and other anxiety disorders (Belfer & Nurcombe, 2007; Kar, 2009; Weems *et al.*, 2007; Yule & Smith, 2008). The prevalence of PTSD varied from around 5 percent to over 43 percent (Kar, 2009) and man-made disasters tend to have a higher prevalence of PTSD than natural disasters (Kar, 2009; Kumar & Fonagy, 2013; Norris *et al.*, 2002).

Child trafficking: soldiering and sexual exploitation

Child trafficking fundamentally violates the right and dignity of all children and is one of the most alarming global issues threatening children today. The International Labor Organization (ILO) estimated that 5.5 million children aged 17 and below were victims of forced labor globally at any point in time during the period 2002–2011 (ILO, 2012). This estimate reflects most forms of human trafficking that children are subject to, including sexual exploitation and forced labor (ILO, 2012). The children, who are trafficked within their home countries or transported away from their homes, are treated as commodities to be bought, sold, and resold. These children are trapped in jobs into which they are coerced or deceived and which they cannot leave even though they have a right to be protected under the UN Convention on the Rights of the Child and their governments are obliged to safeguard them. Instead, these children are made to serve as domestic slaves, field or factory workers, unwitting organ donors, prostitutes, or even child soldiers (Conradi, 2013; Rafferty, 2013). Here, we will further explore two of the worst forms of forced child labor, child soldiering and child sexual exploitation.

Child soldiering

The brutal outcomes of war in some parts of world may be the creation of child soldiers at an age better suited for school. The United Nation's Children's Fund (UNICEF) (2007) has defined the child soldier as, "a child associated with an armed force or armed group" as

> any person below 18 years of age who is or who has been recruited or used by an armed force or armed group in any capacity, including but not limited to children, boys, and girls used as fighters, cooks, porters, messengers, spies, or for sexual purposes.
>
> *(UNICEF, 2007, p. 7)*

Children are introduced into armed organizations in a variety of ways such as kidnapping, force, and manipulation (Betancourt *et al.*, 2013a; Conradi, 2013; McMullen *et al.*, 2013), but no matter what inducements are offered, it is generally accepted that children cannot give voluntary consent to join such groups (Conradi, 2013).

It is estimated that about 300,000 children may be involved in armed forces activities in more than 87 countries at any given moment (Coalition to Stop the Use of Child Soldiers, 2008). These children, who are the victims of child trafficking, become perpetrators of violence once they are absorbed into the armed groups. They are forced to commit violent acts, and participate in mass atrocities (Coalition to Stop the Use of Child Soldiers, 2008). The very environment of violence and abuse results in serious health and mental health risks as well as social stigma upon return (McMullen *et al.*, 2013).

Findings of the systemic review for all articles related to former child soldiers by Betancourt *et al.* (2013b) concluded that abduction, age of conscription, exposure to violence, gender, and community stigma are associated with increased internalizing and externalizing mental health problems. On the other hand, family acceptance, social support, and educational/economic opportunities are associated with improved psychosocial adjustment in these child soldiers. Although there are variations in prevalence rates of mental health problems, most of the researchers have agreed that former child soldiers have a higher prevalence of PTSD, depression and suicidal ideation, (Belfer & Nurcombe, 2007; Ertl, Pfeiffer, Schauer-Kaiser, Elbert, & Neuner, 2014). Betancourt *et al.* (2013b) also reported a greater prevalence of anxiety disorder and conduct disorder among former child soldiers compared to a control group.

Child sexual exploitation

Child sexual exploitation is one of the most destructive forms of abuse, but is pervasive throughout the world in developing countries as well as industrialized nations such as North America and Europe. ILO (2012) estimated that about one million children are the victims of forced sexual exploitation worldwide at any point in time during the period 2002–2011; children therefore constituted 21 percent of 4.5 million total victims, both child and adult. Not surprisingly, girls and women represent 98 percent of those 4.5 million total victims (ILO, 2012). In addition, girls who are trafficked are especially likely to be forced into the sex trades such as prostitution and pornography (Rafferty, 2013). Barnitz (2001) points out that the average age of children brought into commercial sexual exploitation is estimated to be 13 or 14.

Children are entrapped in sexual exploitation in a variety of ways and remain vulnerable (ILO, 2009; Rafferty, 2013; Willis & Levy, 2002); homeless, runaway, or abandoned children are frequently pushed into prostitution and actively recruited by pimps and traffickers; girls are sometimes enticed or kidnapped and then forced into prostitution; poverty-stricken families sell their children in a desperate attempt to purchase food. Sexual exploitation disrupts normal life experiences and has a cascading effect on children's well-being, development, and health. The short- and long-term effects on children victimized by this traumatic experience are profound; the immediate risks include emotional, sexual, and physical abuses and even torture and murder (Barnitz, 2001; ILO, 2009; Rafferty, 2013; Willis & Levy, 2002); it will also put these children at greater risk of mental health issues such as post-traumatic stress disorder, depression and suicidal ideation, anxiety, aggressive behavior and substance abuse (Rafferty, 2013; Willis & Levy, 2002; Wondie, Zemene, Reschke, & Schroder, 2011); they are also vulnerable to sexually transmitted diseases, HIV infection, unwanted pregnancy, and reproductive illnesses (ILO, 2009; Mitchell, Finkelhor, & Wolak, 2010; Willis & Levy, 2002).

Impact of human immunodeficiency virus/acquired immunodeficiency syndrome (HIV/AIDS)

Millions of children worldwide live in communities heavily burdened with HIV/AIDS; children who are facing such disruption confront a number of serious risks, both direct and indirect, which threaten their overall development and health. They may acquire HIV infection transmission from their mothers during pregnancy or more commonly during delivery; they may become infected in adolescence or later by means of sexual transmission (Betancourt *et al.*, 2013a). In addition, children may suffer from the loss of family and friends who form the basis of their supportive environment.

In 2012, 2.1 million adolescents were living with HIV globally and approximately two-thirds of new HIV infections in adolescents aged 15–19 years were among girls (UNICEF, 2013). Betancourt *et al.* (2013a) expressed their concern that young women are at greater risk of contracting the virus through sexual activity as well as through sexual exploitation and abuse in many parts of the globe. Furthermore, about 230,000 children, 90 percent of whom live in 21 countries in sub-Saharan Africa and India, were newly infected with HIV in 2012 (UNICEF, 2013). Also, an estimated 17.8 million children throughout the world have lost one or both parents to HIV/AIDS in the same year (UNICEF, 2013).

The effects of living with HIV/AIDS, of having an affected parent or being orphaned by AIDS can increase the risk for mental illnesses in children. Children and adolescents with HIV/AIDS need not only to cope with fears of dying, but also to face unique illness-related stressors including stigma and discrimination, isolation, and complex disclosure issues (Murphy, Moscicki, Vermund & Muenz, 2000; Orban *et al.*, 2010), while trying to adjust to declining physical functioning. For young people in the HIV/AIDS affected families—either living with infected parents or having lost one or both parents—risks are numerous and include poverty, the pressure to drop out of school to care for sick parents or get a job to support the family, and the psychological burden associated with witnessing illness and coping with death (Belfer, 2008; Betancourt *et al.*, 2013a; Cluver, Orkin, Gardner, & Boyes, 2012; Hong 2010; Sturgeon & Orley, 2005). Many of these stressors are chronic and adversely impact children's lives on multiple levels. Children affected by HIV/AIDS are highly vulnerable to mental disorders and have shown a high prevalence for depression (Cluver *et al.*, 2012; Zhao *et al.*, 2009; Zhao, Zhao, Zhao, & Stanton, 2014), anxiety, and post-traumatic stress disorder (PTSD) (Cluver *et al.*, 2012). In conclusion, it is clear that the presence of HIV/AIDS in the family has far-reaching consequences that can seriously affect the mental health and well-being of children.

Resilience

Globally, tens of millions of children each year are exposed to terrifying phenomena such as disasters, political violence, displacement, child trafficking, pandemics, malnutrition, neglect, and abuse that threaten child development and well-being (Masten, 2014). In spite of such significant adversities or risks, there are some children who adapt successfully. These children are often called "resilient"(Garmezy, 1991; Rutter, 1987), "invulnerable" (Caffo & Belaise, 2007) and "stress-resistant" (Luthar & Zigler, 1991; Rutter, 1987). Rutter (2012) has defined "resilience" as "reduced vulnerability to environmental risk experiences, the overcoming of a stress or adversity, or a relatively good outcome despite risk experiences" (p. 336). In understanding the concept of "resilience," two pivotal conditions are necessary: exposure to significant threat or severe adversity and the achievement of positive adaptation despite major assaults on the developmental process (Luthar, Cicchetti, & Becker, 2000).

According to Kieling and colleagues (2011), resilience is related to the concept of protective factors, but it focuses more on a child's ability to regulate his/her own behavior and emotions to endure chronic stress or overcome trauma. Although early studies were mostly focused on personal qualities of "resilient children," such as self-esteem (Masten & Garmezy, 1985), and social competence (Luthar & Zigler, 1991), there has been a change of paradigm in resilience as research has progressed. It has been acknowledged that resilience may often stem from factors external to the child (Luthar *et al.*, 2000). Garmezy (1991) has emphasized that resilience is best understood in three domains: the child, the family, and the community. He has suggested that the presence of some caring adults such as grandparents, kindly concerned teachers, or the presence of an institutional structure, such as a caring agency or a church, could foster resilience in children in the absence of responsive parents or in the presence of marked marital discord (Garmezy, 1991). Walsh (2003; 2007) has conceptualized the new notion of "family resilience," which has shifted attention from family as a protective factor for the child to family as the functional unit of resilience. The concept of "community resilience" has also been formulated by Landau (2007; 2010) based on her global experience in disaster recovery. She defined "community resilience" as "the community's inherent capacity, hope, and faith to withstand major trauma, overcome adversity, and to prevail, with increased resources, competence, and connectedness" (Landau, 2007, p. 352).

Many scholars who are concerned with the impact of extreme adversity on children have found that children can actually grow stronger through such adversity with the support of family and community (Masten, 2014; Masten & Narayan, 2012; Landau, 2010; Walsh, 2007). Rutter (2012) has also supported this finding with the introduction of two new concepts: the notion of "steeling effects," where engagement with stress serves to prepare the individual for better subsequent adaptation, and the notion of "turning point effects," where negative life experience or adversity eventually serve to give more opportunities to individuals in life.

Assessing children and adolescents

Childhood impairment can be defined as a deficiency in adaptive functioning for the child's developmental stage within his/her specific cultural context (Paula *et al.*, 2007). There has traditionally been a focus on disorders when discussing child and adolescent mental health. However, maintaining this focus only serves to foster stigma and a pathologizing approach rather than supporting a mental health promotion perspective. Thus, culture-specific tools are important to properly assess both resilience and impairment in children. Unfortunately, nomenclatures that describe mental disorders in this section are based on the two most frequently used diagnostic classifications of mental illnesses, the American Psychiatric Association's *Diagnostic and Statistical Manual of Mental Disorders* (DSM) and the World Health Organization's *International Classification of Diseases* (ICD). These classifications are grounded in Western conceptualizations (Schwab-Stone, Ruchkin, Vermeiren, & Leckman, 2001), which may fail to integrate meaningful cultural perspectives and context in classifying mental and behavioral disorders of children from other parts of the world and limit the understanding of mental disorders and challenges in these children (Belfer, 2008).

The following neuropsychiatric symptoms are identified as the most significant challenges in children across the world based on frequency of occurrence and degree of associated impairment. Merikangas, Nakamura, and Kessler (2009) have reported that about one-third of children experience a mental disorder over their lifetime. The most prevalent conditions in children are anxiety, followed by behavioral, mood, and substance use (Belfer, 2008; Merikangas *et al.*, 2009). In particular, adolescents with mental health problems demonstrate high rates of suicidal behaviors and of tobacco, alcohol, and other drug use (Centers for Disease Control and Prevention, 2013; Flament *et al.*, 2007). Nurses need to be knowledgeable about the diagnoses and clinical features associated with major childhood behavioral and mental disorders, as a necessary prerequisite for both needs assessment and the provision of good child mental health care.

Developmental challenges

Consistent with all the syndromes considered by child and adolescent psychiatric nurses, neurodevelopmental disorders have onset in a period characterized by intense development. However this particular subset of disorders affect the youngest of our population, and are frequently recognized in early childhood (American Psychiatric Association, 2013). The context of social impairment is often seen in early play and relationships with family and peers and occupational function is seen in pre-school or early school performance. Developmental deficits can involve limitations of learning, of executive functioning, of intelligence or impairment of social skills (American Psychiatric Association, 2013) as well as limitations in physical functioning.

Diagnosis of behavioral disorders is a probabilistic statement (Szatmari, Archer, Fisman, Streiner, & Wilson, 1995). That is, a behavioral diagnosis as a professional construct is a descriptor of behaviors that fit most closely with those exhibited by the young person. Validated tools are often used to record observations and aid in answering how the intensity and frequency of observed behaviors, or performance, compares to population means. This is important information in terms of distinguishing when to make the determination that behavior is outside the range of that typically expected within the developmental and cultural context, and within the bounds of a diagnostic category. Clinician judgment is also required as many of the neurodevelopmental disorders impact an individual's ability to actively participate in the assessment process (American Psychiatric Association, 2013). Social impairment, impairments of attention, and physical impairment can all impact on testability. Further, the thinking and information style in some groups, such as impaired abstraction in autism (Cashin & Barker, 2009; Cashin, Gallagher, Newman, & Hughes, 2012) and other forms of intellectual disability (American Psychiatric Association, 2013) may impact on the person's ability to understand questions designed for a neurotypical population. Disorders that involve perception, such as some communication disorders may interfere with decoding messages or responding. In the subset of neurodevelopmental disorders there is a propensity for co-morbidity of physical or behavioral disorders (American Psychiatric Association, 2013).

As the neurodevelopmental disorders are diagnosed in early childhood there is also frequently a change of diagnosis as further development in the child allows for the emergence of a fuller understanding of the profile of psychiatric disability. One common example is when a child in preschool is observed to have problems with attention and focus and is diagnosed with attention deficit hyperactivity disorder (ADHD) and a trial of stimulant medications may be started. The child then enters school, and is observed to be defiant and to not follow directions, and a diagnosis of oppositional defiance disorder (ODD) is added. As part of refusing to follow directions it is observed that the child has high preference routines and activities, and later obsessive-compulsive disorder (OCD) may be added. Soon after a more complete picture emerges when difficulty interacting with peers is observed and a diagnosis of an autism spectrum disorder (ASD) is made. As a more thorough probabilistic statement is made and diagnosis refined, it is important to consider whether true comorbidity exists, or whether the new diagnosis better explains earlier understandings and requires removal of the earlier diagnoses.

Stretching the above example into adolescence further demonstrates the need to understand diagnosis as being within the context of a particular time and available data. Many of the disorders in the category of neurodevelopmental disorders, although often diagnosed in childhood are pervasive and lifelong (American Psychiatric Association, 2013). Nomenclature in the DSM refers to *disability* as opposed to *delay* to reflect this feature. Delay has the unfortunate implication that catch-up will occur. We are in many countries used to delayed public transport and familiar with the expectation that, although perhaps late, we will arrive at the destination. For some neurodevelopmental disorders, such as those of speech and communication this analogy may apply.

Many of the disorders in this category are characterized by deficits or excess in behaviors, and delay or failure to reach milestones of development (American Psychiatric Association, 2013).

The behavior, while the focus of intervention, often does not adequately inform the therapeutic approach. It is essential to understand the thinking and information processing style of those who are participating in treatment (Cashin, 2005, 2008; Cashin & Barker, 2009; Cashin, Browne, Bradbury, & Mulder, 2013). Autism, for example, is characterized by a specific cognitive processing style that makes modification of treatment essential (Rotheram-Fuller & MacMullen, 2011). Intellectual disability impacts upon volume of information that can be processed and speed of processing, and this must be taken into consideration when assessing or treating a child with a developmental delay.

Behavioral disorders

Table 18.3 provides a description of common behavioral disorders and their associates symptoms including attention-deficit/hyperactivity disorder (ADHD); oppositional defiant disorder (ODD); conduct disorder (CD); and substance use disorders (SUD).

Psychiatric disorders

Table 18.4 contains a description of common psychiatric disorders seen in children and adolescents with associated symptoms, etiology, global prevalence rates and recommended treatment.

Self-harm: non-suicidal self-injury and suicide in children and adolescents

Self-harm is one of the most serious global health problems for adolescents and young adults (de Kloet *et al.*, 2011; Muehlenkamp, Claes, Havertape, & Plener, 2012; Nock, 2012). WHO (2010b) defines self-harm as "a broader term referring to intentional self-inflicted poisoning or injury which may or may not have a fatal intention or outcome"(p. 73). Self-harm is generally divided into suicidal self-injury (SSI) and non-suicidal self-injury (NSSI) (Nock, 2012). SSI refers to suicide ideation, suicide plans, suicide attempts, and suicide death (Nock, 2012) while NSSI refers to the direct, deliberate destruction of one's own body tissue in the absence of any intent to die (Cloutier, Martin, Kennedy, Nixon, & Muehlenkamp, 2010; Favazza, 1998; Jacobson, Muehlenkamp, Miller, & Turner, 2008; Nock, 2012). Both NSSI and suicidal behavior disorder are included as conditions for further study in the DSM-5 (APA, 2013). Muehlenkamp and colleagues (2012) conducted a systematic review of current (2005–2011) empirical studies reporting on the prevalence of NSSI and self-harm in adolescent samples across the globe and found a mean lifetime prevalence of 18.0 percent for NSSI behavior and 16.1 percent for self-harm.

NSSI is also called self-mutilation, self-injurious behaviors, or para-suicidal behaviors. The term NSSI has been formulated to distinguish self-injurious behavior from suicidal attempts because they present as separate entities with differentiable motivations (see Table 18.5) (Cloutier *et al.*, 2010; Jacobson *et al.*, 2008; Muehlenkamp, 2005; Nock & Kessler, 2006). Nock and Kessler (2006) reported that the US prevalence of suicide attempts decreased from 4.6 percent to 2.7 percent after a reanalysis of data from the National Comorbidity Study when intent to die was required as prerequisite for a suicidal attempt. However, it is important to note that there are youngsters who engage in both SSI and NSSI behaviors (Andover, Morris, Wren, & Bruzzese, 2012; Cloutier *et al.*, 2010; Jacobson *et al.*, 2008; Nock, Joiner, Gordon, Lloyd-Richardson, & Prinstein, 2006). Moreover, NSSI is a risk factor for suicide attempts (Andover *et al.*, 2012; Nock, *et al.*, 2006; Plener, Libal, Keller, Fegert, & Muehlenkamp, 2009) and 70 percent of adolescents who self-injure have at least one suicide attempt (Nock *et al.*, 2006). Global suicide and self-harm behaviors in youth are addressed further in Chapter 12.

Table 18.3 Behavioral disorders

Disorder	Characteristics	Etiology	Treatment	Global factors
Attention deficit hyperactivity disorder (ADHD)	Inattention, impulsivity, hyperactivity, failure to pay close attention to details, difficulty organizing tasks and activities, excessive talking, fidgeting or inability to remain seated in appropriate situations (APA, 2013; WHO, 2010a) Symptoms present before age 12 and affect performance in social, academic and work settings (APA, 2013)	Genetics Neurobiological (Pliszka & AACAP Work Group on Quality Issues, 2007a) Environmental (APA, 2013, p. 62)	Pharmaco-therapy Adjunctive psychosocial intervention including parent training, classroom behavioral intervention and social skills training (Pliszka et al., 2007a; Young & Amarasinghe, 2010)	For children aged 5–19 years, the global pooled prevalence of ADHD in 2010 was 2.2% and 0.7% for males and females, respectively (Erskine et al., 2013)
Oppositional defiant disorder (ODD)	Negativistic, disobedient, hostile behavior toward authority figures; angry/irritable mood; argumentative/defiant; vindictiveness (APA, 2013; WHO, 2010a); onset between age 8–adolescent (Steiner, Remsing & AACAP Work Group on Quality Issues, 2007) Poor school performance despite normal intelligence; risk for low self-esteem and mood dysregulation (Steiner, Remsing, & AACP Work Group on Quality Issues, 2007; Gale, 2011) Disorder associated with substantial risk of secondary mood, anxiety, impulse-control, and substance use disorders (Nock, Kazdin, Hiripi, & Kessler, 2007)	Biological Psychological Social (Steiner et al., 2007)	Individual problem-solving skills training Parent management training Adjunctive pharmaco-therapy (Steiner et al., 2007)	The pooled prevalence of ODD was estimated as 3.3%, which was associated with significant heterogeneity (Canino, Polanczyk, Bauermeister, Rohde, & Frick, 2010)
Conduct disorder (CD)	The most severe type of behavioral disorder (Buitelaar et al., 2013) Repetitive violation of the rights of others and violation of age-appropriate norms; bullying, threatening/intimidation of others; cruelty to animals, people; destruction of property; deliberate fire-setting; truancy; theft and violation of rules (APA, 2013)	Temperamental Environmental Genetic Physiological (APA, 2013)	Individual skill-building approaches Parent management training Adjunctive pharmaco-therapy (Buitelaar et al., 2013; National Institute for Health and Care Excellence (NICE), 2013)	The pooled global prevalence of CD in 2010 for children aged 5–19 years was 3.6% (3.3–4.0) and 1.5% (1.4–1.7) for males and females, respectively (Erskine et al., 2013)

Substance use disorder (SUD)	A maladaptive pattern of psychoactive substance use with clinically significant levels of impairment or distress Impairment including family conflict or dysfunction, interpersonal conflict, and academic failure, risk-taking behavior An increase in the likelihood of legal problems due to possession, and exposure to hazardous situations Substances are defined for alcohol, amphetamine (or amphetamine-like), caffeine, cannabis, cocaine, hallucinogens, inhalants, nicotine, opioids, phencyclidine and sedative, hypnotic, or anxiolytic agents (APA, 2013)	Genetic (Dick & Agrawal, 2008) Neurobiological (Clark, Chung, Thatcher, Pajtek, & Long, 2012) Environmental such as family and peer factors (Thatcher & Clark, 2008)	Family therapy CBT with motivational enhancement Non–substance using peer support Comprehensive services such as housing, academic assistance, and recreation (Bukstein & AACAP Work Group on Quality Issues, 2005)	The median estimate of alcohol or drug abuse or dependence in community surveys of adolescents is 5% with a range from 1% to 24% (Merikangas et al., 2009)

Table 18.4 Psychiatric/mental disorders

Disorders	Characteristics	Etiology	Treatment	Global factors
Anxiety disorders Generalized anxiety disorder and social anxiety disorder are the two most prevalent types of anxiety disorders (Merikangas et al., 2009)	**Generalized anxiety disorder** Excessive and irrational worries about competence, approval, appropriateness of past behavior, and the future The dominant symptoms—restlessness or feeling keyed up, being easily fatigued, trouble concentrating, irritability, muscle tension, and sleep disturbance (APA, 2013; WHO, 2010a)	Temperamental Environmental Genetics (APA, 2013) Neurobiological (Strawn, Wehry, DelBello, Rynn, & Strakowski, 2012).	Pharmaco-therapy, *CBT (Connolly, Bernstein & AACAP Work Group on Quality Issues, 2007; Khalid-Khan, Santibanez, McMicken & Rynn, 2007; Silverman, Pina, & Viswesvaran 2008; Strawn et al., 2012)	The median prevalence rate of all anxiety disorders of children and adolescents was 8% (Merikangas et al., 2009)
	Social anxiety disorder A persistent fear of being embarrassed in social situations, in performance situations, or in one or more social settings (APA, 2013; WHO, 2010a)			
Mood disorders	**Depressive disorders** Depressed or irritable mood, loss of interest and pleasure, increased or decreased appetite or sleep, decreased activity, poor concentration, lack of energy, and exaggerated guilt May have self-injurious or suicidal ideation (APA, 2013; Birmaher, Brent, & AACAP Work Group on Quality Issues, 2007)	Temperamental (APA, 2013) Genetic Environmental factor (APA, 2013; Birmaher et al., 2007)	CBT or IPT Pharmaco-therapy Supportive management Family involvement School involvement Psychoeducation (Birmaher et al., 2007)	A worldwide prevalence rate of major depressive disorder in youth range from 0.6% to 3% (Merikangas et al., 2009)

Disorder	Description	Etiology	Treatment	Prevalence
Bipolar disorder	Characterized by extreme episodic mood dysregulation accompanied by symptoms (e.g.,decreased need for sleep, hypersexuality, impulsivity) that significantly impair multiple domains of functioning Differentiated from adult-onset bipolar disorder by increased rates of rapid cycling, mixed mood states, psychiatric comorbidity, and developmentally-specific psychosocial impairment Higher chance of neurocognitive deficits, poor academic performance and disruptive school behavior (West et al., 2014)	Genetic Environmental (APA, 2013; Birmaher et al., 2007)	Pharmaco-therapy Psychotherapy Psychoeducation (AACAP, 2007; WHO, 2010b) Child- and family-focused cognitive-behavioral therapy (West et al., 2014)	A meta-analysis of the existing international studies of pediatric bipolar disorders for young people ages 7 to 21 years reported an overall rate of 1.8% (Van Meter, Moreira, & Youngstrom, 2011)
Early-onset schizophrenia	Onset before 18 years of age Two or more psychotic symptoms such as hallucinations, delusions, disorganized speech, disorganized or catatonic behavior, and/or negative symptoms (APA, 2013; McClellan, Stock, & AACAP Committee on Quality Issues, 2013) Onset before 13 years of age appears to be quite rare. The rate of onset then increases during adolescence, with the peak ages of onset for the disorder ranging from 15 to 30 years (McClellan et al., 2013)	Genetic Environmental (APA, 2013) Neuroanatomical abnormalities (McClellan et al., 2013)	Antipsychotic medications combined with psychoeducational, psychotherapeutic, and educational interventions (McClellan et al., 2013)	The worldwide prevalence of schizophrenia is generally held to be approximately 1%, but the prevalence of early-onset schizophrenia has not been adequately studied (McClellan et al., 2013)

The incidence of suicide is rare before puberty, but becomes increasingly frequent through adolescence (Dervic, Brent, & Oquendo, 2008). In the 15–19- year-old age category, the second leading cause of death is suicide (Patton *et al.*, 2009; WHO, 2013). Mental disorders or behavioral challenges have been identified as a root cause in 90 percent of youth death by suicide (Bridge, Goldstein, & Brent, 2006; WHO, 2006), and the most common links with suicide attempts are major depressive disorder (MDD) (Jacobson *et al.*, 2008), anxiety disorder, PTSD, disruptive behavior disorders and substance use disorder (Chartrand, Sareen, Toews, & Bolton, 2012). Teens engaged in NSSI also show similar patterns of psychiatric disorders, including high rates of MDD, PTSD, oppositional defiant disorder, and substance use disorder (Nock *et al.*, 2006; Nock & Kessler, 2006). Additionally, NSSI is one of the hallmark symptoms of borderline personality disorder (BPD) in the DSM-5 (APA, 2013). However, NSSI and BPD can also occur independently (In-Albon, Ruf, & Schmid, 2013). Nock and colleagues (2006) confirmed that only about 50 percent of those who engage in NSSI suffer from BPD. Table 18.5 contains a comparison between non-suicidal self-injurious behaviors and suicidal self-injurious behaviors.

Taliaferro and Muehlenkamp (2014) analyzed the data from the 2010 Minnesota Student Survey to identify risk factors associated with suicidal ideation and suicide attempts among adolescents. The risk factors included childhood physical and sexual abuse, parental substance abuse, cultural taboo about same-sex sexual attraction or experience, weight dissatisfaction and maladaptive dieting behavior, alcohol and other drug use, depression, anxiety disorders, hopelessness, involvement in bullying, running away from home, dating violence, physical fighting, self-injury, physical or mental health problems, and chronic family dysfunction or violence (Taliaferro & Muehlenkamp, 2014). They also identified protective factors against suicidal ideation or behavior among youth: parent connectedness, school engagement, involvement in certain extracurricular activities particularly sports, academic achievement, close supportive friendships, and connections to non-parental adults (Taliaferro & Muehlenkamp, 2014).

Mental health promotion strategies and evidence-based prevention programs

Mental health promotion refers to actions undertaken to improve conditions and environments as a means of supporting individual competence, mental health and well-being. The focus is on identifying and fostering strengths and supporting community assets that can then serve as resources to further promote overall health (Kobau *et al.*, 2011), with less focus on illness and pathology. Mental health promotion strategies must address and work to correct the social determinant of health factors that impede mental health and overall well-being. Positive psychology focuses on empowerment strategies, positive attributes and ways in which individuals and communities can thrive. The WHO Global School Health Initiative developed in 1995 supports school environments that strengthen their capacity to develop healthy settings for living, learning and working. These schools focus on caring for self and others, healthy decision-making, strive to shape health related behaviors, develop and adhere to policies supporting equity, peace, social justice, and stability.

Mental Health: A Report of the Surgeon General (US Department of Health and Human Services, 1999) highlighted the importance of preventive intervention as a central activity for the improvement of children's mental health. Childhood is a critical time for preventing mental disorders since there is a high degree of continuity between child disorders and those in adulthood (Klasen & Crombag, 2013; McDougall, 2010). Thus, it is pivotal to intervene early in a child's life in order to prevent or reduce the likelihood of long-term impairment (McDougall, 2010; SAMHSA, 2007).

Table 18.5 Comparison between non-suicidal self-injury (NSSI) and suicidal self-injury (SSI)

Feature	NSSI	SSI
Intent	Affect regulation, self-punishment, interpersonal influence, sensation seeking, interpersonal boundaries, anti-dissociation, anti-suicide	To cease existence, eliminate life, to escape a painful situation
Lethality	Low, rarely requires medical attention	High, requires medical attention
Chronicity	Repetitive in nature, chronic (10–15 years)	Infrequent
Methods	Tendency to use multiple methods: skin cutting, severe scratching, self-biting, skin-picking, burning, head-banging, hitting, preventing wound healing, some forms of body piercing, branding or carving words or symbols into skin, object insertion	Often one chosen method: ingestion, vehicular exhaust, hanging/strangulation, gun use, running into traffic, cutting
Reactions	Elicits fear, disgust, hostility, revulsion	Elicits care, compassion, concern
Aftermath	Sense of relief, calm, satisfaction	No relief of distress
Demographics	Adolescents and young adults, equally males and females	Usually older men complete
Global prevalence	The mean lifetime prevalence of 18.0% (SD = 7.3) for NSSI	The mean proportion of adolescents reporting a lifetime suicidal attempt is 9.7% and suicidal ideation is 29.9%

Source: Bridge *et al.*, 2006; Cloutier *et al.*, 2010; Evans, Hawton, Rodham, & Deeks, 2005; Klonsky & Muehlenkamp, 2007; Muehlenkamp *et al.*, 2012; Wilkinson & Goodyer, 2011; Yearwood & Bosnic, 2012; Young, Sproeber, Groschwitz, Preiss, & Plener, 2014. Adapted from Muehlenkamp, 2005.

Mental health promotion strategies

As discussed in the previous section, exposure to risk factors and lack of protective factors will increase prevalence of mental health challenges. Preventive intervention in child mental health must be multifaceted, targeting both individual and community dynamics and structures that influence healthy psychological development in children. The goal would be to develop and support appropriate resources that would then promote capacity, foster resilience, and increase overall effectiveness of protective factors (Manikam, 2002; Nurcombe, 2007; Shea & Shern, 2011). Timely and effective interventions will reduce the burden of mental health disorders on children and their family, and also reduce the costs to health systems and communities (Catalano *et al.*, 2012; Hahlweg, Heinrichs, Kuschel, Bertram, & Naumann, 2010; SAMHSA, 2007).

Preventive health care interventions are generally classified as primary, secondary, and tertiary as proposed by the Commission on Chronic Illnesses (CCI) (1957). Primary prevention refers to interventions targeting the general population to prevent future health problems and involves education, while secondary prevention involves screening and prompt intervention for those who are beginning to show signs of difficulty by early identification and effective treatment (CCI, 1957). Tertiary prevention aims to reduce the severity of the impairment associated with an existing disorder, support rehabilitation success, prevent relapse, and achieve the highest level of functioning (CCI, 1957).

The Institute of Medicine (IOM) (1994) has recognized issues in applying this traditional classification to mental health and has redefined intervention phases into prevention, treatment, and maintenance. In order to describe the different service needs in the prevention phase, IOM has adapted the framework of Gordon (Gordon, 1987), which divides preventive intervention strategies as universal, selective, and indicated, based on the population groups to whom interventions are directed. Universal prevention targets the entire population of a particular area, whereas selective intervention targets specific groups or individuals whose risk of developing a mental disorder is significantly higher than average due to exposure to some risk factors (IOM, 1994). Indicated prevention involves targeting those individuals who exhibit subclinical symptoms of a disorder (IOM, 1994).

The IOM commissioned development of the framework is summarized in Figure 18.1.

Prevention phase (primary intervention)

Prevention strategies in this phase involve either universal prevention or selective prevention; both strategies target those individuals who are currently functioning normally in order to prevent future problems. Durlak, Weissberg, Dymnicki, Taylor, and Schellinger (2011) reviewed 213 school-based universal prevention programs and confirmed significant improvement in social and emotional skills, attitudes, behavior, and academic performance in children. Sometimes specific intervention strategies might be necessary to address children's needs depending on the nature of targeted mental health issues. The prevention interventions that focus on helping children build coping skills and social competence, and also reinforcing proper parenting skills might be most effective in children regardless of the circumstances (El Din, 2004; Masten & Monn, 2015).

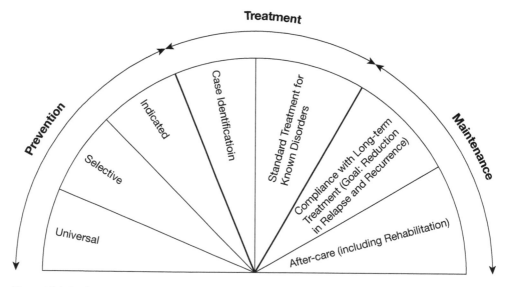

Figure 18.1 Reducing risks for mental disorders: frontiers for preventive intervention research, 1994

Source: Reprinted with permission by the National Academy of Sciences, Courtesy of the National Academies Press, Washington, DC.

Parenting skills

Parenting plays a crucial role in a wide variety of child social, emotional, behavioral, and intellectual outcomes (Landry, Smith, & Swank, 2006; Shapiro, Printz & Sanders, 2008). Researchers have reported that parental attachment contributes positively to self-esteem and life satisfaction and negatively to measures of depression, anxiety, and feelings of alienation (Grant *et al.*, 2006; Manikam, 2002). Dysfunctional parent–child interactions increase the risk of mental disorders, particularly when they are prolonged and accompanied by other adverse factors (Dodge, Coie, & Lynam, 2006). Conversely, enhanced parenting can even mitigate or buffer the adverse effects of environmental adversities on early childhood development (Domian, Baggett, Carta, Mitchell, & Larson, 2010; Leidy, Guerra, & Toro, 2010).

Therefore, it is crucial to teach parents optimal parenting skills in order to help build positive relationships with their children. Studies have shown that interventions targeted towards parenting have been efficacious in improving parental perceptions, children's social skills and school adjustment, and also produced reductions in behavioral problems (Barlow & Stewart-Brown, 2000; Cartwright-Hatton, McNicol, & Doubleday, 2006). Parenting training is also known to promote family coping, consistency, cohesion, and use of family support networks, each of which support the development of family resilience (Masten & Monn, 2015; Webster-Stratton, 2009).

Coping and social skills

Psychosocial stress is a significant and pervasive risk factor for psychopathology in childhood. But, in reality, children need to handle a wide range of challenging social situations every day. The ways in which children cope with stress are potentially important mediators and moderators of the impact of stress on current and future adjustment and psychopathology (Compas *et al.*, 2001). Also, a child's ability in social interaction with his/her environment may be the best way to predict the child's mental health (Compas, Connor-Smith, Saltzman, Thomsen, & Wadsworth, 2001; Grossman & Liang, 2008; Gumpel, 2007). Thus, preventive mental health interventions for children may be desirable to promote the coping and social skills of children (Durlak & Wells, 1997; Greenberg, Domitrovich & Bumbarger, 2001; Spence, 2003).

Treatment phase (secondary prevention)

This phase can be summarized as early identification and intervention. It involves *indicated* prevention, that is, prompt intervention for those who are just beginning to show signs of difficulty. First of all, target problems need to be identified for intervention. When children are screened and identified in a primary care or school setting, those with early disturbances should be referred to proper treatment (Durlak *et al.*, 2011). Then, the most effective evidence-based treatment modalities have to be selected in order to build resources and capacities in children and their families (Verhulst, 2004; WHO, 2005b). It is critical to evaluate outcomes of mental health services and effectiveness of the treatment by comparing the baseline measures at the time of assessment with measures upon completion of intervention (Verhulst, 2004).

Maintenance phase (tertiary prevention)

This phase focuses on relapse prevention. Children with mental disorders need proper support from family and school in order to prevent relapse or deterioration and also maintain optimal functioning (El Din, 2004). It is important for teachers and other school personnel to understand the nature of a child's problems and work together with mental health providers and family.

Global evidence-based preventive programs

"Evidence-based prevention" can be defined as

> the conscientious, explicit and judicious use of current best evidence to make decisions about interventions for individuals, communities and populations that facilitate the currently best possible outcomes in reducing the incidence of diseases and in enabling people to increase control over and to improve their health.
>
> *(Hosman & Jané-Llopis, 2005, as cited in WHO, 2004, p. 18)*

Additionally, Nation and colleagues (2003) have identified nine characteristics that are consistently associated with effective prevention programs: being comprehensive, using varied teaching methods, providing sufficient dosage, including theory-driven strategies, providing opportunities for positive relationships, being appropriately timed, incorporating relevant socio-cultural values and practices, integrating outcome evaluations, and involving well-trained and sensitive staff.

Most of the evidence-based mental health preventive interventions have been developed in high-income countries, such as the USA, Canada, Australia, and northern European countries (Klasen & Crombag, 2013; WHO, 2004). WHO (2004) has published *Prevention of Mental Disorders: Effective interventions and Policy Options* to facilitate the use of evidence-based interventions worldwide, especially for low-income countries where there is a lack of prevention knowledge in spite of enormous public mental health problems. WHO (2004) has also advised that service providers need to take into consideration cultural adaptation when they implement evidence-based programs from other countries or cultures in communities and target populations that differ from the ones that were originally developed and tested.

Klasen and Crombag (2013) have performed a systematic review of all randomized controlled trials in child and adolescent mental health in low- and middle-income countries, and have indicated that affordable and feasible interventions can be developed to improve the functioning of affected children, their families and their communities worldwide. In addition, they have found that parent training is a highly effective intervention in lessening conduct symptoms in behavioral disorders. Also, children who are exposed to war, disaster, and other traumatic experiences can be well treated in low resource settings even in unstable environments with proper interventions (Klasen & Crombag, 2013).

Fayyad and colleagues (2010) adopted the parenting skills intervention that was developed by the Integrated Services Taskforce of "the World Psychiatric Association Child Mental Health Presidential Programme" in order to check the feasibility of dissemination of the evidence-based intervention in a developing country. The program was delivered to 87 mothers of children with behavior problems in Lebanon by social and health workers with little or no mental health background who were trained for this program over four half-day sessions. This pilot project revealed that the intervention was effective in decreasing both the abnormal range of the children's behaviors from 54.4 percent to 19.7 percent, and mothers' use of severe corporal punishment from 40.2 percent to 6.1 percent.

Patel and colleagues (2007) have proposed "a population-based, youth focused model" to improve the range of affordable and feasible interventions to youth in both developing and developed countries. The model recommends integrating youth mental health programs into all existing youth programs, including general health, education, and welfare programs, since those programs are less stigmatized and more accessible to young people and can provide youth-friendly services under the same location (Patel *et al.*, 2007).

The following four preventive mental health programs are cited by WHO (2004) as global exemplary evidence-based prevention interventions. These are mostly a universal prevention or a selective prevention, which mental health nurses who work in community and school settings can utilize.

Incredible Years

The Incredible Years (IY) is one of the best-validated and well-established intervention programs for parents, teachers, and children that aims at treating and preventing conduct problems in children aged 0 to 12 years old (Presnall, Webster-Stratton, & Constantino, 2014; Webster-Stratton, & Herman, 2010; Webster-Stratton, Rinaldi, & Reid, 2011). Carolyn Webster-Stratton, a nurse practitioner, researcher and psychologist developed the intervention. The intervention is based on research conducted at the University of Washington Parenting Clinic in the United States in 1984 (Trotter & Rafferty, 2014; Webster-Stratton *et al.*, 2011). The program interventions have been implemented with positive results in over 24 countries including Germany, Ireland, Netherlands, New Zealand, Norway, Portugal, Republic of Korea, Russian Federation, Turkey, United States, and Wales (United Kingdom) (United Nations Office on Drugs and Crime, (UNODC), 2010). IY has been published in 10 languages, Chinese, Danish, Dutch, French, Norwegian, Portuguese, Russian, Spanish, Swedish, and Turkish (UNODC, 2010).

IY Training Series is a set of three separate, complementary, multifaceted, and developmentally based curricula for children, parents, and teachers, which can be used independently or together (Webster-Stratton, & Herman, 2010). IY is underpinned by social learning theory and comprises behaviorally based group training programs in order to promote positive interactions and reduce coercive interaction cycles between the child and the parent, and to improve the child's problem-solving behavior, social competence and emotional regulation (Webster-Stratton *et al.*, 2011; WHO, 2004). There are treatment versions of the parent and child programs as well as prevention versions for high-risk populations. The child and teacher programs span the age range of 3–8 years. The parenting programs span the age range of 0–12 years. IY uses videotape-modeling methods and includes modules for parents, school teachers, and children.

IY Series programs have been the subject of extensive empirical evaluation over the past three decades. All three programs have been widely endorsed by various review groups (Reinke, Stormont, Webster-Stratton, Newcomer, & Herman, 2012). IY parent and child interventions have proven efficacious in multiple randomized control studies for young children with primary diagnoses of ODD or CD, 40 to 50 percent of whom also had high levels of inattentive and hyperactive symptoms (Webster-Stratton, Reid, & Beauchaine, 2013). Also, in classrooms where teachers received the IY Classroom Management Training, children were observed to have higher school readiness scores, including engagement and on-task behavior and increased prosocial behaviors, as well as significantly reduced peer aggression in classrooms (Reinke *et al.*, 2012). IY has been selected as an exemplary best practice program for violence prevention by the US Office of Juvenile Justice and Delinquency Prevention (Center for the Study and Prevention of Violence, 2004; Webster-Stratton & Herman, 2010) and is also considered a "model program" by the World Health Organization (WHO, 2004).

Promoting alternative thinking strategies

The promoting alternative thinking strategies (PATHS) is a multi-year, universal and selective primary prevention program that was developed by Mark Greenberg and Carol Kusche in the United States in early 1990s (Kusche & Greenberg, 1994). Teachers, while simultaneously enhancing the educational process in the classroom, use this comprehensive program for kindergarten through sixth grade. It is based on the ABCD (Affective–Behavioral–Cognitive–Dynamic) model, which places primary importance on the developmental integration of affect, behavior, and cognitive understanding (Kusche & Greenberg, 1994). The PATHS has been selected as an exemplary Blueprint model program by the US Office of Juvenile Justice and Delinquency Prevention (Center for the Study and Prevention of Violence, 2004) and is also considered a "model program" by the World Health Organization (2004). The PATHS program has been implemented in many countries such as the United States, Belgium, United Kingdom, Norway, Canada, Australia, and Israel (Flament *et al.*, 2007).

The PATHS curriculum provides teachers with systematic, developmentally based lessons, materials, and instructions to enhance children's social competence and reduce aggression and acting-out behavior in the classroom (Kusche & Greenberg, 1994). The PATHS materials consist of a manual and six volumes of lessons, which are divided into three major units, each containing developmentally sequenced lessons to integrate and build on previous learning. There is also a supplementary unit that contains 30 lessons, which reviews and extends concepts covered. Each unit contains aspects of five themes: self-control, emotional understanding, interpersonal problem-solving skills, positive self-esteem, and improved peer communication/relationships. Each volume includes teacher scripts, pictures, photographs, activity sheets, posters, home activities, and parent letters and information. It is recommended to initiate the program at the entrance to schooling and continue through Grade 5 and be taught three times per week for a minimum of 20–30 minutes per day. Although primarily focused on school and classroom settings, information and activities are also included for home use by parents.

The PATHS program has demonstrated efficacy in developing greater emotional knowledge and social competence and less social withdrawal among children receiving the program than children who did not participate (Crean & Johnson, 2013; Domitrovich, Cortes, & Greenberg, 2007; Greenberg, Kusche, Cook, & Quamma, 1995). The PATHS program has shown a 32 percent reduction in teachers' reports of students exhibiting aggressive behavior; a 36 percent increase in teachers' reports of students exhibiting self-control; and a 20 percent increase in students' scores on cognitive skills tests in various studies that used a control group (SAMHSA 2007). A recent study evaluated PATHS embedded within the Fast Track prevention model using a sample of almost 3,000 children who were randomly selected to begin the program in first grade and were followed for 3 years. The authors found positive effects for reduced aggression, increased prosocial behavior, and increased academic engagement for those children who received the program. Program effects were particularly robust for children in disadvantaged schools and for those who initially showed higher rates of aggression (Conduct Problems Prevention Research Group, 2010). Similar results were found using the PATHS curriculum with a sample of elementary students in the United Kingdom and Turkey, in which participant children were rated as showing improvement in emotional vocabulary, recognizing feelings in self and others, cooperation, empathy, and self-control (Arda & Ocak, 2011; Curtis & Norgate, 2007; Kelly, Longbottom, Potts, & Williamson, 2004).

Triple P-positive parenting program

Triple P (TP), which designates a "positive parenting program," is a comprehensive multilevel system of parenting intervention that was designed to prevent behavioral, emotional and developmental problems in children from birth to age 16 (Hahlweg *et al.*, 2010; UNODC, 2010; Sanders, Kirby, Tellegen, & Day, 2014). The program was developed by Sanders and colleagues at the Parenting and Family Support Center of the School of Psychology at the

University of Queensland, Australia (Sanders, 2008; Sanders, Markie-Dadds, & Turner, 2003). The program began on a small scale as a home-based, individually administered training program for parents of disruptive preschool children (Sanders & Glynn, 1981), but, over the past 30 years, has evolved into a comprehensive evidence-based public health model of intervention (Sanders, 2008). The ultimate goal of TP is to enhance the knowledge, skills, and confidence of parents at a whole-of-population level and, in turn, to reduce the prevalence rates of behavioral and emotional problems in children and adolescents (Sanders, 2008).

TP emphasizes the centrality of parent–child interactions to promote family protective factors and reduce risk factors by using social learning models (de Graaf, Speetjens, Smit, de Wolff, & Tavecchio, 2008). It gives parents simple and practical strategies to confidently manage their children's behavior, develop effective, non-violent strategies, provide a safe, nurturing environment, and build positive, caring family relationships, which enhance children's healthy development and prevent problems from developing.

The program involves five levels of intervention on a tiered continuum in order to meet the differing needs of parents within a comprehensive system of parenting support (de Graaf et al., 2008; Sanders et al., 2014). The five levels of intervention incorporate programs that vary according to intensity, contact with practitioners, and delivery format: Level 1 is a form of universal prevention that delivers psychoeducational information on parenting skills to interested parents and is a media and communication strategy, including television, radio, online, and print, on positive parenting; Level 2 is a brief intervention consisting of 1 or 3 sessions for parents of children with mild behavioral problems using telephone or face-to-face contacts or group seminars; Level 3 consists of narrow-focused interventions including 3 to 4 individual face-to-face or telephone sessions, or a series of 2-hour group discussion sessions that target children with mild to moderate behavioral difficulties and includes active skills training for parents; Level 4 includes 8–10 sessions delivered through individual, group or self-directed (online or workbook) formats that target individual parents of children at risk; and Level 5 includes enhanced interventions using adjunct individual or group sessions for families where parenting difficulties are complicated by other sources of family distress (de Graaf et al., 2008; Sanders et al., 2014).

TP has been recognized as an effective example of the parenting program by WHO (2004), and is number one on the United Nations' ranking of parenting programs, based on ample research-based evidence indicating the effectiveness based on 4 meta-analyses of Triple-P studies, 10 independent randomized control trials, 47 randomized control trials, 28 quasi-experimental studies and 11 studies containing pre- and post-intervention evaluation (UNODC, 2010). In addition, TP has been implemented successfully in 25 countries including Australia, Belgium, Canada, China, the Netherlands Antilles (Curaçao), Germany, Iran (Islamic Republic of), Ireland, Japan, New Zealand, Netherlands, Singapore, Sweden, Switzerland, United Kingdom, and United States (UNODC, 2010). The program is also published in 10 languages: Chinese (Mandarin/-Cantonese), Dutch, English, Flemish, French, German, Japanese, Papiamento (the Netherlands Antilles), and Spanish (UNODC, 2010).

The Olweus bullying prevention program

One of the most well-known and widely implemented anti-bullying programs is "the Olweus Bullying Prevention Program (OBPP)" that was developed by Dan Olweus in Norway (El Din, 2004; Limber, 2011; Stephens, 2011; Ttofi & Farrington, 2009). The OBPP is a multilevel, multicomponent school-based program designed to prevent or reduce bullying and related victimization, and achieve better peer relations among elementary, middle, and junior high school students aged 6 to 15 (Olweus & Limber, 2010; Limber, 2011). It was started as a nationwide campaign in Norway after three adolescent boys in northern Norway committed suicide as the result of severe bullying and victimization in 1983 (Olweus & Limber, 2010; Limber, 2011).

The OBPP has been implemented in six large-scale evaluations involving more than 40,000 students in Norway, which have yielded average reductions by 20 percent to 70 percent in students' report of bullying and victimization, as well as reductions in antisocial behaviors such as vandalism and truancy (Olweus & Limber, 2010; Limber, 2011). Ttofi & Farrington (2009) have performed a most comprehensive systemic review and meta-analysis of the effectiveness of anti-bullying programs and have concluded that the programs inspired by the work of Dan Olweus worked best and the OBPP should be the basis of future anti-bullying initiatives. It has been replicated internationally with positive results in the United States, Canada, Japan, Australia, and many European countries, including United Kingdom, Germany, and Belgium (Limber, 2011; Olweus & Limber, 2010; Stephens, 2011; Ttofi & Farrington, 2009). This program is considered a "model program" by the World Health Organization (2004).

The OBPP attempts to restructure the existing school environment to minimize opportunities and rewards for bullying and to increase awareness and knowledge of teachers, parents, and students about bullying (Olweus & Limber, 2010). The intervention consists of workshops for teachers and parents, and booklets, videos, and social skills and problem-solving training for students (Olweus & Limber, 2010). School staff members are primarily responsible for introducing four key principles: (a) show warmth and positive interest in their students; (b) set firm limits to unacceptable behavior; (c) use consistent nonphysical, non-hostile negative consequences when rules are broken; and (d) function as authorities and positive role models (Olweus & Limber, 2010). These principles have been incorporated into specific interventions at four levels: the school, the classroom, the individual, and, in some contexts, the community

Table 18.6 Components of the OBPP

School-level	• Establish a bullying prevention coordinating committee (BPCC) • Conduct trainings for the BPCC and all staff • Administer the Olweus Bullying Questionnaire (Grades 3–12) • Hold staff discussion group meetings • Introduce the school rules against bullying • Review and refine the school's supervisory system • Hold a school-wide kick-off event to launch the program • Involve parents
Classroom-level	• Post and enforce school-wide rules against bullying • Hold regular (weekly) class meetings to discuss bullying and related topics • Hold class-level meetings with students' parents
Individual-level	• Supervise students' activities • Ensure that all staff intervene on-the-spot when bullying is observed • Meet with students involved in bullying (separately for those who are bullied and who bully) • Meet with parents of involved students • Develop individual intervention plans for involved students, as needed
Community-level	• Involve community members on the BPCC • Develop school–community partnerships to support the school's program • Help to spread anti-bullying messages and principles of best practice in the community

Source: Reprinted from Olweus & Limber (2010).

(Olweus & Limber, 2010; Limber, 2011). Table 18.6 provides a summary of the components of the OBPP at each of these four levels.

Low educational attainment and evidence-based interventions

Low educational attainment is a worldwide problem, especially in developing countries. *The Millennium Developmental Goals Report 2013* (United Nations (UN), 2013) has set one of its major global goals as achieving universal primary education in order to enhance proper education and prevent poor academic performance in children. This report indicates that 57 million children globally are still denied their right to primary education and more than half of these children live in sub-Saharan Africa. It further reports that 123 million youths aged 15 to 24 lack basic reading and writing skills and 61 percent of them are young women (UN, 2013). Moreover, in lower-income countries, only 37 percent of adolescents complete lower secondary education and the rate is as low as 14 percent for the poorest (UNESCO, 2014). Even high-income countries that provide free or mandatory secondary education still have problems. In Europe, about 14 percent of all 18- to 24-year-olds either complete a low level of education or end their education without a certificate, which are of little use in the labor market (Theunissen, Griensven, van Verdonk, Feron, & Bosma, 2012). A 2009 survey showed that 8 percent of 16- to 24-year-olds in the US did not have a high school degree and were not enrolled in school (Aud *et al.*, 2011).

Low educational attainment is described as children who do not enroll, do not progress, or drop out (Petrosino, Morgan, Fronius, Tanner-Smith, & Boruch, 2015), and poverty is known to be a key factor of this phenomena (UN, 2013). Children from the poorest households are at least three times more likely to be out of school than children from the richest households in developing countries (UN, 2013). It is common for children to work to earn money to support their family or to stay home to take care of younger siblings. In some cultures, girls are not encouraged to pursue education and are expected to help out at home. Additionally, the cost of schooling, poor school infrastructure, teacher shortages, and safety and sanitation problems are some other factors that impede children's education in developing countries (Birdsall, Levine & Ibrahim, 2005). Meanwhile, variables associated with low educational attainment in developed countries include poor or single-parent households, minority status, poor academic performance, school disengagement, dissatisfaction with teachers, peer rejection, chaotic school environment, alcohol and substance abuse, adolescent pregnancy, mental illnesses, low parental expectation, and family disruption (El Din, 2004; Fan & Wolters, 2014; Graeff-Martins *et al.*, 2007; Nurcombe, 2007).

Low educational attainment has long-lasting negative consequences for individuals, families, and communities, as indicated by low earnings, more dependence on public assistance, poor health outcomes, life-dissatisfaction, social alienation, depression, alcohol and drug abuse, criminal activities, and higher chance of an intergenerational cycle (Fall & Roberts, 2012; Flisher, Townsend, Chikobvu, Lombard, & King, 2010; Henry, Knight, & Thornberry, 2012). On the other hand, education can help individuals escape poverty, improve health outcomes, and stop poverty from being passed down through the generations (Petrosino *et al.*, 2015; UNESCO, 2014).

Due to the disparate and varied reasons for low educational attainment, there may not be one common solution to this problem. However, regardless of the cause of low educational attainment, early intervention may be crucial. Increased access to schooling is a necessary first step towards universal primary education in developing countries (UN, 2013). According to Petrosino and colleagues (2015), who have done a systematic review of impact studies on school enrollment interventions in developing countries, the interventions with the largest average effects are the ones that focus on improving school or community infrastructures, such as building new schools, repairing schools, and improving roads/access to schools. These developments increase student enrollment, student attendance and academic progress, as well as decrease school dropout (Petrosino *et al.*, 2015). Graeff-Martins and colleagues (2006) have assessed the feasibility and initial efficacy of a package of universal preventive intervention designed to reduce school dropout in developing countries. This intervention was implemented in a city public school in Brazil and yielded significant effects in dropout and absenteeism (Graeff-Martins *et al.*, 2006). The package consisted of two workshops with teachers, five letters to parents, three meetings with parents and school, a telephone helpline, 1-day cognitive intervention and a mental health assessment with possible referral to resources available in the community for students absent more than 10 days (Graeff-Martins *et al.*, 2006). In Honduras, a number of middle-school alternative programs have been implemented to expand post-primary school coverage for at-risk youngsters who live in rural and urban areas. These programs have been successful in reaching a vulnerable population in the country, although dropout rates are generally high (Marshall *et al.*, 2014).

In developed countries, most of the intervention programs are school-based programs, which aim to prevent school dropout and absenteeism. It is reported that the role of teachers as tutor-counselors is the most crucial and has a significant impact on school success, engagement, and educational achievement of youngsters (Graeff-Martins *et al.*, 2007). Also, students and families, who feel marginalized in their relations with teachers and peers, need further support to connect at school and engage with students' learning (Christenson & Thurlow, 2004; Graeff-Martins *et al.*, 2007). Tanner-Smith and Wilson (2013) report that dropout programs have generally been shown to be effective at reducing school dropout, and the relationship between absenteeism and later school dropout is well-established based on their findings from a systematic review and meta-analysis of literature on school dropout prevention and intervention programs. The most frequently used dropout intervention modalities can be classified as school/class restructuring, supplemental academic training, mentoring counseling, alternative school, cognitive behavioral/skills training, attendance monitoring/financial rewards, vocational/employment oriented, and multi-service packages (Tanner-Smith & Wilson, 2013).

The US Department of Health and Human Services Substance Abuse and Mental Health Services Administration (SAMHSA, 2007) have introduced "Reconnecting Youth (RY)" as an effective evidence-based dropout prevention program. RY is a selective school-based program for youth in ninth through twelfth grade (ages 14 to 18), who are at risk for school dropout. The central program goals are to decrease drug involvement, increase school performance and decrease emotional distress. It uses a partnership model involving peers, school personnel, and parents and caregivers. Since RY was developed in 1985 by Leona Eggert, child/adolescent psychosocial nurse specialist, and Liela Nichola in the United States, it has been implemented in all 50 states as well as internationally (e.g., in Canada, Germany, Malaysia, Russia, and Spain) to reach hundreds of thousands of youth (SAMHSA, 2007).

Role for nurses

Mental Health Atlas 2011(WHO, 2011) reports that nurses represent the largest professional group working in the mental health field worldwide, with the median rate of nurses in this sector at 5.8 per 100,000 population. This is greater than the rate of all other mental health workers combined. In particular, nurses have been primary providers in delivering necessary care to children with mental health challenges in most low- and middle-income countries where mental health professionals are scarce (WHO, 2007). In some developed countries, psychiatric/mental health nurses have expanded their roles, with adequate educational preparation, to advanced functioning, which includes diagnosing, prescribing medication, and providing various types of supportive therapies including brief, trauma-focused, group, and individual to children in need. This model needs to be applied to and scaled up for use in low- and middle-income environments that are resource poor.

Therefore, it will be greatly beneficial to develop and offer educational opportunities to nurses and expand their roles accordingly in order to provide timely and effective services to children with mental and behavioral disorders and their families. Above all, nurses need to be recognized as essential and untapped human resources, capable of providing these crucial services.

Conclusion

About 20 percent of children suffer from mental disorders worldwide, accounting for a significant portion of the global burden of disease (Belfer & Nurcombe, 2007; Kieling *et al.*, 2011). Burden involves higher rates of health care utilization, necessary educational accommodation, and potential burden to both the criminal justice and social service systems (Belfer, 2008; Merikangas *et al.*, 2009). In addition, mental health challenges and behavioral symptoms cause enormous burden to children and their families. In low-income communities resources are insufficient, inequitably distributed and poorly used, contributing to a 90 percent treatment gap (Malhotra & Padhy, 2015). If untreated, childhood difficulties persist into adulthood resulting in poor quality of life, erosion of self-esteem and lost productivity.

Engaging in mental health promotion and prevention efforts is a necessary component when addressing barriers to human flourishing associated with the social determinants of health. Supportive resources for children include parents, teachers, nurses, and primary care providers, but ideally must be extended to many other groups involved in nurturing young people where they work, play, and learn. The specialist child and adolescent mental health nurse clinician has a strong role to play in education, policy development, and promotion of mental health literacy within communities. In addition nurses can use their expertise when conducting comprehensive assessments and providing evidence-based treatment within a culturally aware, respectful, and inclusive framework.

References

Achenbach, T.M., & Rescorla, L.A. (2007). *Multicultural understanding of child and adolescent psychopathology: Implications for mental health assessment*. New York: Guilford.

American Academy of Child and Adolescent Psychiatry (AACAP) Committee on Quality Issues (CQI). (2007). Retrieved July 24, 2016 from www.jaacap.com/content/pracparam.

American Psychiatric Association. (2013). *Diagnostic and statistical manual of mental disorders* (5th ed.), Washington, DC: Author.

Andover, M.S., Morris, B.W., Wren, A., & Bruzzese, M.E. (2012). The co-occurrence of non-suicidal self-injury and attempted suicide among adolescents: Distinguishing risk factors and psychosocial correlates. *Child and Adolescent Psychiatry and Mental Health*, 6, 11.

Arda, T.B., & Ocak, Ş. (2011). Social competence and promoting alternative thinking strategies: PATHS preschool curriculum. *Educational Sciences: Theory & Practice*, 12(4), 2691–2698.

Aud, S., Hussar, W., Kena, G., Bianco, K., Frohlich, L., Kemp, J., & Tahan, K. (2011). *The condition of eduj309 cation 2011 (NCES 2011–2033)*. US Department of Education, National Center for Education Statistics. Washington, DC: US Government Printing Office.

Barlow, J., & Stewart-Brown, S. (2000). Behavior problems and group based parent education programs. *Journal of Development & Behavioral Pediatrics*, 21, 356–370.

Barnitz, L. (2001). Effectively responding to the commercial sexual exploitation of children: A comprehensive approach to prevention, protection, and reintegration services. *Child Welfare*, 80(5), 597–610.

Belfer, M.L. (2008). Child and adolescent mental disorders: The magnitude of the problem across the globe. *Journal of Child Psychology and Psychiatry*, 49(3), 226–236.

Belfer M.L., & Nurcombe, B. (2007). The epidemiology and burden of child and adolescent mental disorder. In H. Remschemidt, B. Nurcombe, M.L. Belfer, N. Sartorius & A. Okasha (Eds.), *The mental health of children and adolescents: An area of global neglect* (pp. 27–42). West Sussex, UK: John Wiley & Sons.

Betancourt, T.S., Meyers-Ohki, S.E., Charrow, A., & Hansen, N. (2013a). Annual research review: Mental health and resilience in HIV/AIDS-affected children—a review of the literature and recommendations for future research. *Journal of Child Psychology & Psychiatry*, 54(4), 423–444.

Betancourt, T.S., Borisova, I., Williams, T.P., Meyers-Ohki, S.E., Rubin-Smith, J.E., Annan, J., & Kohrt, B.A. (2013b). Research review: Psychosocial adjustment and mental health in former child soldiers—A systematic review of the literature and recommendations for future research. *Journal of Child Psychology & Psychiatry*, 54(1), 17–36.

Betancourt, T.S., Abdi, S., Ito, B.S., Lilienthal, G.M., Agalab, N., & Ellis, H. (2015). We left one war and came to another: Resource loss, acculturative stress, and caregiver-child relationships in Somali refugee families. *Cultural Diversity & Ethnic Minority Psychology*, 21(1), 114–125.

Birdsall, N., Levine, R., & Ibrahim, A. (2005). *Toward universal primary education: Investments, incentives, and institutions*. London: United Nations Development Programme.

Birmaher, B., Brent, D., & AACAP Work Group on Quality Issues. (2007). Practice parameter for the assessment and treatment of children and adolescents with depressive disorders. *Journal of the American Academy of Child Adolescent Psychiatry*, 46(11), 1503–1526.

Bridge, J.A., Goldstein, T.R., & Brent D.A. (2006). Adolescent suicide and suicidal behavior. *Journal of Child Psychology and Psychiatry* 47(3/4), 372–394.

Buitelaar, J.K., Smeets, K.C., Herpers, P., Scheepers, F., Glennon, J., & Rommelse, N.N. (2013). Conduct disorders. *European Child & Adolescent Psychiatry*, 22(Suppl 1), S49–S54.

Bukstein, O.G., & AACAP Work Group on Quality Issues. (2005). Practice parameter for the assessment and treatment of children and adolescents with substance use disorders. *Journal of the American Academy of Child Adolescent Psychiatry*, 44(6), 609–621.

Caffo, E., & Belaise, C. (2007). Violence and trauma: Evidence-based assessment and intervention in children and adolescents: A systemic review. In H. Remschemidt, B. Nurcombe, M.L. Belfer, N. Sartorius, & A. Okasha (Eds.), *The mental health of children and adolescents: An area of global neglect* (pp. 137–164). West Sussex, UK: John Wiley & Sons.

Canino, G., Polanczyk, G., Bauermeister, J.J., Rohde, L.A., & Frick, P. (2010). Does the prevalence of CD and ODD vary across cultures? *Social Psychiatry & Psychiatric Epidemiology*, 45(7), 695–704.

Cartwright-Hatton, S., McNicol, K., & Doubleday, E. (2006). Anxiety in a neglected population: Prevalence of anxiety disorders in pre-adolescent children. *Clinical Psychology Review*, 26(7), 817–833.

Cashin, A. (2005). Autism: Understanding conceptual processing deficits. *Journal of Psychosocial Nursing and Mental Health Services*, 43(4), 22–30.

Cashin, A. (2008). Narrative therapy: A psychotherapeutic approach in the treatment of adolescents with Asperger's Disorder. *Journal of Child and Adolescent Psychiatric Nursing*, 21(1), 48–56.

Cashin, A, & Barker, P. (2009). The triad of impairment in autism revisited. *Journal of Child and Adolescent Psychiatric Nursing*, 22(4), 189–193.

Cashin, A., Gallagher, H., Newman., C., & Hughes, M. (2012). Autism and the cognitive processing triad: A case for revising the criteria. *The Diagnostic and Statistical Manual. Journal of Child and Adolescent Psychiatric Nursing*, 25, 141–148.

Cashin, A., Browne, G., Bradbury, J., & Mulder, A. (2013). The effectiveness of Narrative Therapy with young people with autism. *Journal of Child and Adolescent Psychiatric Nursing*, 26(1), 32–41.

Catalano, R.F., Fagan, A.A., Gavin, L.E., Greenberg, M.T., Irwin Jr, C.E., Ross, D.A., & Shek, D.T. (2012). Worldwide application of prevention science in adolescent health. *The Lancet*, 379 (9826), 1653–1664.

Center for the Study and Prevention of Violence. (2004). Blue prints for violence prevention. Retrieved May 14, 2014 from www.ncjrs.gov/pdffiles1/ojjdp/204274.pdf.

Centers for Disease Control and Prevention. (2013). Mental health surveillance among children United States, 2005–2011. *Morbidity and Mortality Weekly Report*, 62(Suppl 2), 1–35. Retrieved January 3, 2014 from CDC website: www.cdc.gov/mmwr/preview/mmwrhtml/su6202a1.htm.

Chartrand, H. Sareen, J., Toews, M., & Bolton, J. M. (2012). Suicide attempts versus non-suicidal self-injury among individuals with anxiety disorders in a nationally representative sample. *Depression & Anxiety*, 29(3), 172–179.

Christenson, S.L., & Thurlow, M.L. (2004). School dropouts: Prevention considerations, interventions, and challenges. *Current Directions in Psychological Science*, 13(1), 136–39.

Clark, D.B., Chung, T., Thatcher, D.L., Pajtek, S., & Long, E.C. (2012). Psychological dysregulation, white matter disorganization and substance use disorders in adolescence. *Addiction*, 107(1), 206–214.

Cloutier, P., Martin, J., Kennedy, A., Nixon, M.K., & Muehlenkamp, J.J. (2010). Characteristics and co-occurrence of adolescent non-suicidal self-injury and suicidal behaviours in pediatric emergency crisis services. *Journal of Youth & Adolescence*, 39(3), 259–269.

Cluver, L.D., Orkin, M., Gardner, F., & Boyes, M.E. (2012). Persisting mental health problems among AIDS-orphaned children in South Africa. *Journal of Child Psychology & Psychiatry*, 53(4), 363–370.

Coalition to Stop the Use of Child Soldiers. (2008). *Child soldiers: Global report 2008*. London: Coalition to Stop the Use of Child Soldiers.

Commission on Chronic Illness. (1957). *Chronic illness in the United States (Vol. 1)*. Cambridge, MA: Harvard University Press.

Compas, B.E., Connor-Smith, J.K., Saltzman, H., Thomsen, A.H., & Wadsworth, M.E. (2001). Coping with stress during childhood and adolescence: Problems, progress, and potential in theory and research. *Psychological Bulletin*, 127(1), 87–127.

Conduct Problems Prevention Research Group. (2010). The effects of a multi-year randomized clinical trial of a universal social-emotional learning program: The role of student and school characteristics. *Journal of Consulting and Clinical Psychology*, 78(2), 156–168.

Connolly, S.D., Bernstein, G.A., & AACAP Work Group on Quality Issues. (2007). Practice parameter for the assessment andtreatment of children and adolescents with anxiety disorders. *Journal of the American Academy of Child Adolescent Psychiatry*, 46(2), 267–283.

Conradi, C. (2013). Child trafficking, child soldiering: Exploring the relationship between two "worst forms" of child labor. *Third World Quarterly*, 34(7), 1209–1226.

Crean, H.F., & Johnson, D.B. (2013). Promoting Alternative Thinking Strategies (PATHS) and elementary school aged children's aggression: Results from a cluster randomized trial. *American Journal of Community Psychology*, 52(1/2), 2691–2698.

Curtis, C., & Norgate, R. (2007). An evaluation of the Promoting Alternative Thinking Strategies curriculum at Key Stage 1. *Educational Psychology in Practice*, 23(1), 33–44.

de Graaf, I., Speetjens, P., Smit, F., de Wolff, M., & Tavecchio, L. (2008). Effectiveness of the Triple P-Positive Parenting Program on Parenting: A meta-analysis. *Family Relations*, 57(5), 553–566.

de Kloet, L., Starling, J., Hainsworth, C., Berntsen, E., Chapman, L., & Hancock, K. (2011). Risk factors for self-harm in children and adolescents admitted to a mental health inpatient unit. *Australian and New Zealand Journal of Psychiatry*, 45, 749–755.

Dervic, K., Brent, D.A., & Oquendo, M.K. (2008). Completed suicide in childhood. *Psychiatric Clinics of North America*, 31(2), 271–291.

Dick, D.M., & Agrawal, A. (2008). The genetics of alcohol and other drug dependence. *Alcohol Research & Health*, 31(2), 111–118.

Dodge, K.A., Coie, J.D., & Lynam, D. (2006). Aggression and antisocial behavior in youth. In W. Damon, R.M. Lerner, & N. Eisenberg (Eds.), *Handbook of child psychology: Social, emotional, and personality development* (6th ed.) (Vol. 3, pp. 719–788). New York: Wiley.

Domian, E.W., Baggett, K.M., Carta, J.J., Mitchell, S., & Larson, E. (2010). Factors influencing mothers' abilities to engage in a comprehensive parenting intervention program. *Public Health Nursing*, 27(5), 399–407.

Domitrovich, C.E., Cortes, R C., & Greenberg, M.T. (2007). Improving young children's social and emotional competence: A randomized trial of the Preschool PATHS® Curriculum. *Journal of Primary Prevention*, 28(2), 67–91.

Durlak, J.A., & Wells, A.M. (1997). Primary prevention mental health programs for children and adolescents: A meta-analytic review. *American Journal of Community Psychology*, 25(2), 115–152.

Durlak, J.A., Weissberg, R.P., Dymnicki, A.B., Taylor, R.D., & Schellinger, K.B. (2011). The impact of enhancing students' social and emotional learning: A meta-analysis of school-based universal interventions. *Child Development*, 82(1), 405–432.

El Din, A.S. (2004). Prevention and intervention in school setting. In H. Remschemidt, M.L. Belfer, & I. Goodyer (Eds.), *Facilitating pathways: Care, treatment, and prevention in child and adolescent mental health* (pp. 326–334). Berlin, Germany: Springer.

Erickson, E. (1952/1998). Eight stages of man. In C. Cooper, and L. Pervin (Eds.). *Personality: Critical concepts in psychology* (pp. 67–77). London: Routledge.

Erskine, H.E., Ferrari, A.J., Nelson, P., Polanczyk, G.V., Flaxman, A.D., Vos, T., & Scott, J.G. (2013). Research review: Epidemiological modelling of attention-deficit/hyperactivity disorder and conduct disorder for the Global Burden of Disease Study 2010. *Journal of Child Psychology & Psychiatry*, 54(12), 1263–1274.

Ertl V., Pfeiffer A., Schauer-Kaiser E., Elbert T., & Neuner F. (2014). The challenge of living on: Psychopathology and its mediating influence on the readjustment of former child soldiers. *Plos One*, 9 (7), e102786.

Evans, E., Hawton, K., Rodham, K., & Deeks, J. (2005). The prevalence of suicidal phenomena in adolescents: A systematic review of population-based studies. *Suicide and Life-Threatening Behavior*, 35(3), 239–250.

Fall, A., & Roberts, G. (2012). High school dropouts: Interactions between social context, self-perceptions, school engagement, and student dropout. *Journal of Adolescence*, 35(4), 787–798.

Fan, W., & Wolters, C.A. (2014). School motivation and high school dropout: The mediating role of educational expectation. *British Journal of Educational Psychology*, 84(1), 22–39.

Favazza, A. (1998). The coming of age of self-mutilation. *The Journal of Nervous and Mental Disease*, 186(5), 259–268.

Fayyad, J.A., Farah, L., Cassir, Y., Salamoun, M.M. & Karam, E.G. (2010). Dissemination of an evidence-based intervention to parents of children with behavioral problems in developing country. *European Child & Adolescent Psychiatry*, 19, 629–636.

Flament, M.F., Nguyen, H., Furino, C., Schacher, H., MacLean, C., Wasserman, D., & Remschmidt, H. (2007). Evidence-based primary prevention programmes for the promotion of mental health in children and adolescents: A systemic worldwide review. In H. Remschmidt, B. Nurcombe, M.L. Belfer, N. Sartorius, & A. Okasha (Eds.), *The mental health of children and adolescents: An area of global neglect* (pp. 65–135). West Sussex, UK: John Wiley & Sons.

Flisher, A.J., Townsend, L., Chikobvu, P., Lombard, C.F., & King, G. (2010). Substance use and psychosocial predictors of high school dropout in Cape Town, South Africa. *Journal of Research on Adolescence*, 20(1), 237–255.

Gale, B.M. (2011). Oppositional defiant disorder. In C. Draper & W.T. O'Donohue (Eds.), *Stepped care and e-health* (pp. 181–202). New York: Springer.

Garmezy, N. (1991). Resiliency and vulnerability to adverse developmental outcomes associated with poverty. *American Behavioral Scientist*, 34(4), 416–430.

Gordon, R. (1987). An operational classification of disease prevention. In J. Steinberg & M. Silverman (Eds.), *Preventing mental disorders: A research perspective* (pp. 20–26). Rockville, MA: US Department of Health and Human Services: National Institute of Mental Health.

Graeff-Martins, A.S., Oswald, S., Comassetto, J.O., Kieling, C., Goncalves, R.R., & Rohde, L.A. (2006) A package of interventions to reduce school dropout in public schools in a developing country. A feasibility study. *European Child & Adolescent Psychiatry*, 15(8), 442–449.

Graeff-Martins, A.S., Dmitrieva, T., El Din, A.S., Caffo, E., Flament, M.F., Nurcombe, B., Rydelius, P.-A., Remschmidt, H., Rohde, L.A. (2007). School dropout: A systemic worldwide review concerning risk factors and preventive interventions. In H. Remschmidt, B. Nurcombe, M.L. Belfer, N. Sartorius, & A. Okasha (Eds.), *The mental health of children and adolescents: An area of global neglect* (pp. 165–177). West Sussex, UK: John Wiley & Sons.

Grant, K.E., Compas, B.E., Thurm, A.E., McMahon, S.D., Gipson, P.Y., Campbell, A.J., & Westerholm, R.I. (2006). Stressors and child and adolescent psychopathology: Evidence of moderating and mediating effects. *Clinical Psychology Review*, 26(3), 257–283

Greenberg, M.T., Domitrovich, C., & Bumbarger, B. (2001). The prevention of mental disorders on school-aged children: Current state of the field. *Prevention and Treatment*, 4(1), 1–62.

Greenberg, M.T., Kusche, C.A., Cook E.T., & Quamma, J.P. (1995). Promoting emotional competence in school-aged children: The effects of the PATHS Curriculum. *Development and Psychopathology*, 7, 117–136.

Grossman, J.M., & Liang, B. (2008). Discrimination distress among Chinese American adolescents. *Journal of Youth & Adolescence*, 37, 1–11.

Gumpel, T.P. (2007). Are social competence difficulties caused by performance or acquisition deficits? The importance of self-regulatory mechanisms. *Psychology in the Schools*, 4(4), 351–372.

Hahlweg, K., Heinrichs, N., Kuschel, A., Bertram, H., & Naumann, S. (2010). Long-term outcome of a randomized controlled universal prevention trial through a positive parenting program: Is it worth the effort? *Child and Adolescent Psychiatry and Mental Health*, 4, 14.

Henry, K., Knight, K., & Thornberry, T. (2012). School disengagement as a predictor of dropout, delinquency, and problem substance use during adolescence and early adulthood. *Journal of Youth & Adolescence*, 41(2), 156–166.

Hong, Y., Li, X., Fang, X., Zhao, G., Lin, X., Zhang, J., Zhao, J., Zhang, L. (2010). Perceived social support and psychosocial distress among children affected by AIDS in China. *Community Mental Health Journal*, 46(1), 33–43.

Hosman, C., Jané-Llopis, E. (2005). Effectiveness and evidence: Levels and perspectives. In C. Hosman, E. Jané-Llopis, & S. Saxena (Eds.), *Prevention of mental disorders: Effective interventions and policy options.* Oxford: Oxford University Press.

In-Albon, T., Ruf, C., & Schmid, M. (2013). Proposed diagnostic criteria for the DSM-5 of nonsuicidal self-injury in female adolescents: Diagnostic and clinical correlates. *Psychiatry Journal*, 2013, Article ID 159208. Retrieved October 22, 2014 from http://dx.doi.org/10.1155/2013/159208.

Institute of Medicine. (1994). *Reducing risks for mental disorders: Frontiers for preventive intervention research.* Washington, DC: National Academies Press.

International Labour Organization (ILO). (2009). *Training manual to fight trafficking in children for labour, sexual, and other forms of exploitation: Understanding child trafficking.* Turin, Italy: International Training Centre of the ILO.

International Labour Organization (ILO). (2012). *ILO global estimate of forced labour 2012: Results and methodology.* Geneva: Author.

Jacobson, C.M., Muehlenkamp, J.J., Miller, A.L., & Turner, J.B. (2008). Psychiatric impairment among adolescents engaging in different types of deliberate self-harm. *Journal of Clinical Child & Adolescent Psychology*, 37(2), 363–375.

Kar, N. (2009). Psychological impact of disasters on children: Review of assessment and interventions. *World Journal of Pediatrics*, 5(1), 5–11.

Kelly, B., Longbottom, J., Potts, F., & Williamson, J. (2004). Applying emotional intelligence: Exploring the Promoting Alternative Thinking Strategies curriculum. *Educational Psychology in Practice*, 20(3), 221–240.

Kessler, R.C., Berglund, P., Demler, O., Jin, R., Merikangas, K.R., & Walters, E.E. (2005). Lifetime prevalence and age-of-onset distributions of DSM-IV disorders in the National Comorbidity Survey Replication, *Archives of General Psychiatry*, 62(6), 593–602.

Khalid-Khan, S., Santibanez, M., McMicken, C., & Rynn, M.A. (2007). Social anxiety disorder in children and adolescents: Epidemiology, diagnosis, and treatment. *Pediatric Drugs*, 9(4), 227–237.

Kieling, C., Baker-Henningham, H., Belfer, M., Conti, G., Ertem, I., Omigbodun, O., Rohde, L.A., Srinath, S., Ulkuer, N., & Rahman, A. (2011). Child and adolescent mental health worldwide: Evidence for action. *The Lancet*, 378(9801), 1515–1525.

Klasen, H., & Crombag, A. (2013). What works where? A systematic review of child and adolescent mental health interventions for low- and middle-income countries. *Social Psychiatry & Psychiatric Epidemiology*, 48(4), 595–611.

Klonsky, E.D., & Muehlenkamp, J.J. (2007). Self-injury: A research review for the practitioner. *Journal of Clinical Psychology*, 63(11), 1045–1056.

Kobau, R., Seligman, M.E., Peterson, C., Diener, E., Zack, M.M., Chapman, D., & Thompson, W. (2011). Mental health promotion in public health: Perspectives and strategies from positive psychology. *American Journal of Public Health*, 101(8), e 1–9.

Kohlberg, L., & Hersh, R. (1977). Moral development: A review of theory. *Theory Into Practice*, 12(2), 53–59.

Kumar, M., & Fonagy, P. (2013). Differential effects of exposure to social violence and natural disaster on children's mental health. *Journal of Traumatic Stress*, 26(6), 695–702.

Kusche, C.A., & Greenberg, M.T. (1994). *The PATHS curriculum.* South Deerfield, MA: Channing-Bete.

Landau, J. (2007). Enhancing resilience: Families and communities as agents for change. *Family Process*, 46(3), 351–365.

Landau, J. (2010). Communities that care for families: The LINC Model for enhancing individual, family, and community resilience. *American Journal of Orthopsychiatry*, 80(4), 516–524.

Landry, S.H., Smith, K.E., & Swank, P.R. (2006). Responsive parenting: Establishing early foundations for social, communication, and independent problem-solving skills. *Developmental Psychology*, 42(4), 627–642.

Leidy, M.S., Guerra, N.G., & Toro, R.I. (2010). Positive parenting, family cohesion, and child social competence among immigrant Latino families. *Journal of Family Psychology*, 24(3), 252–260.

Limber, S.P. (2011). Development, evaluation, and future directions of the Olweus Bullying Prevention Program. *Journal of School Violence*, 10(1), 71–87.

Luthar, S.S., & Zigler, E. (1991). Vulnerability and competence: A review of research on resilience in childhood. *American Journal of Orthopsychiatry*, 61, 6–22.

Luthar, S.S., Cicchetti, D., & Becker B. (2000). The construct of resilience: A critical evaluation and guidelines for future work. *Child Development*, 71(3), 543–562.

McClellan, J., Stock, S., & AACAP Committee on Quality Issues. (2013). Practice parameter for the assessment and treatment of children and adolescents with schizophrenia. *Journal of American Academy of Child and Adolescent Psychiatry*, 52(9), 976–990.

McDougall, Tim. (2010). Early intervention with children can prevent problems in later life. *Mental Health Practice*, 13(10), 30–32.

McMullen, J., O'Callaghan, P., Shannon, C., Black, A., & Eakin, J. (2013). Group trauma focused cognitive-behavioural therapy with former child soldiers and other war-affected boys in the DR Congo: A randomised controlled trial. *Journal of Child Psychology and Psychiatry*, 54(11), 1231–1241.

Malhotra, S., & Padhy, S. (2015). Challenges in providing child and adolescent psychiatric services in low resource countries. *Child Adolescent Psychiatric Clinics of North America*, 24, 777–797.

Manikam, R. (2002). Mental health of children and adolescents. In N.N. Singh, H.O. Thomas, & A.N. Singh (Eds.), *International perspectives on child and adolescent mental health* (Vol. 2, pp. 1–36). Oxford, UK: Elsevier Science.

Marshall, J.H., Aguilar, C.R., Alas, M., Castellanos, R.R., Castro, L., Enamorado, R., & Fonseca, E. (2014). Alternative education programmes and middle school dropout in Honduras. *International Review of Education*, 60(1), 51–77.

Masten, A.S. (2014). Global perspectives on resilience in children and youth. *Child Development*, 85(10), 6–20.

Masten, A.S., & Garmezy, N. (1985). Risk, vulnerability, and protective factors in developmental psychopathology. In B. Lahey, & A. Kazdin (Eds.), *Advances in clinical child psychology* (Vol. 8, pp. 1–52). New York: Plenum Press.

Masten, A.S., & Osofsky, J.D. (2010). Disasters and their impact on child development: introduction to the special section. *Child Development*, 81(4), 1029–1039.

Masten, A.S., & Monn, A.R. (2015). Child and family resilience: A call for integrated science, practice, and professional training. *Family Relations*, 64(1), 5–21.

Masten, A.S., & Narayan, A. J. (2012). Child development in the context of disaster, war and terrorism: Pathways of risk and resilience. *Annual Review of Psychology*, 63, 227–257.

Merikangas, K.R., Nakamura, E.F., & Kessler, R.C. (2009). Epidemiology of mental disorders in children and adolescents. *Dialogues in Clinical Neuroscience*, 11(1), 7–20.

Mitchell, D. (1924). *Psychology of the child*. New York: Robert K. Hass.

Mitchell, K., Finkelhor, D., & Wolak, J. (2010). Conceptualizing juvenile prostitution as child maltreatment: Findings from the national juvenile prostitution study. *Child Maltreatment*, 15(1), 18–36.

Muehlenkamp, J.J. (2005). Self-injurious behavior as a separate clinical syndrome. *American Journal of Orthopsychiatry*, 75(2), 324–333.

Muehlenkamp, J.J., Claes, L., Havertape, L., & Plener, P.L. (2012). International prevalence of adolescent non-suicidal self-injury and deliberate self-harm. *Child Adolescent Psychiatry Mental Health*, 6, 1–9.

Murphy, D.A., Moscicki, A.B., Vermund, S.H., & Muenz, L.R. (2000). Psychological distress among HIV(+) adolescents in the REACH study: Effects of life stress, social support, and coping. The Adolescent Medicine HIV/AIDS Research Network. *Journal of Adolescent Health*, 27(6), 391–398.

Nation, M., Crusto, C., Wandersman, A., Kumpfer, K.L., Seybolt, D., Morrisey-Kane, E., & Davino, K. (2003). What works in prevention. *American Psychologist*, 58(6/7), 449–457.

National Institute for Health and Care Excellence (NICE). (2103). *Antisocial behaviour and conduct disorders in children and young people: Recognition, intervention and management*. Manchester, UK: Author.

Nock, M.K. (2012). Future directions for the study of suicide and self-injury. *Journal of Clinical Child & Adolescent Psychology*, 41(2), 255–259.

Nock, M.K., & Kessler, R.C. (2006). Prevalence of and risk factors for suicide attempts versus suicide gestures: Analysis of the National Comorbidity Survey. *Journal of Abnormal Psychology*, 115(3), 616–623.

Nock, M.K., Kazdin, A.E., Hiripi, E., & Kessler, R.C. (2007). Lifetime prevalence, correlates, and persistence of oppositional defiant disorder: Results from the National Comorbidity Survey Replication. *Journal of Child Psychology & Psychiatry*, 48(7), 703–713.

Nock, M.K., Joiner T.E. Jr., Gordon K.H., Lloyd-Richardson E., & Prinstein M.J. (2006). Non-suicidal self-injury among adolescents: Diagnostic correlates and relation to suicide attempts. *Psychiatry Research*, 144(1), 65–72.

Norris, F.H., Friedman, M.J., Watson, P.J., Byrne, C.M., Diaz, E., & Kaniasty, K. (2002). 60,000 disaster victims speak: Part I. An empirical review of the empirical literature, 1981–2001. *Psychiatry: Interpersonal and Biological Processes*, 65(3), 207–239.

Nurcombe, B. (2007). The principles of prevention in child and adolescent mental health. In H. Remschemidt, B. Nurcombe, M.L. Belfer, N. Sartorius, & A. Okasha (Eds.), *The mental health of children and adolescents: An area of global neglect* (pp. 53–64). West Sussex, UK: John Wiley & Sons.

Olweus, D., & Limber, S. P. (2010). Bullying in school: Evaluation and dissemination of the Olweus bullying prevention program. *American Journal of Orthopsychiatry*, 80(1), 124–134.

Orban, L.A., Stein, R., Koenig, L.J., Conner, L.C., Rexhouse, E.L., Lewis, J.V., & LaGrange, R. (2010). Coping strategies of adolescents living with HIV: Disease-specific stressors and responses. *AIDS Care*, 22(4), 420–430.

Patel, V., Flisher, A., & Cohen, A. (2006). Mental Health. In M.H. Merson, R.E. Black, & A.J. Mills (Eds.), *International public health: Diseases, programs, systems, and policies* (2nd ed.) (pp. 355–391). Sudbury, MA: Jones & Bartlett.

Patel, V., Flisher, A.J., Hetrick, S., & McGorry, P. (2007). Mental health of young people: A global public-health challenge. *The Lancet*, 369, 1302–1313.

Patel, V., Flisher, A.J., Nikapota, & A., Malhotra, S. (2008). Promoting child and adolescent mental health in low- and middle-income countries. *Journal of Child Psychology and Psychiatry*, 49(3), 313–334.

Patton, G.C., Coffey, C., Sawyer, S.M., Viner. R.M., Haller, D.M., Bose, K., & Mathers, C.D. (2009). Global patterns of mortality in young people: a systematic analysis of population health data. *The Lancet*, 374, 881–892.

Paula, C.S., Duarte, C.S., & Bordin, I.A.S. (2007). Prevalence of mental health problems in children and adolescents from the outskirts of Sao Paulo City: Treatment needs and service evaluation. *Revista Brasileira de Psiquiatria*, 29(1), 11–17.

Petrosino, A., Morgan, C., Fronius, T., Tanner-Smith, E.E., & Boruch, R.F. (2015). What works in developing nations to get children into school or keep them there? A systematic review of rigorous impact studies. *Research on Social Work Practice*, 25(1), 44–60.

Piaget, J. (1952). *The origins of intelligence in children*. New York: International Universities Press.

Plener, P.L., Libal, G., Keller, F., Fegert, J.M., & Muehlenkamp, J.J. (2009). An international comparison of adolescent non-suicidal self-injury (NSSI) and suicide attempts: Germany and the USA. *Psychological Medicine*, 39(9), 1549–1558.

Pliszka, S.R., & AACAP Work Group on Quality Issues (2007). Practice parameter for the assessment and treatment of children and adolescents with attention-deficit/hyperactivity disorder. *Journal of the American Academy of Child Adolescent Psychiatry*, 46(7), 894–921.

Porter, M., & Haslam, N. (2005). Pre-displacement and post-displacement factors associated with mental health of refugees and internally displaced persons: A meta-analysis. *JAMA*, 294(5), 602–612.

Presnall, N., Webster-Stratton, C.H., & Constantino, J.N. (2014). Parent training: Equivalent improvement in externalizing behavior for children with and without familial risk. *Journal of the American Academy of Child & Adolescent Psychiatry*, 53(8), 879–887.

Rafferty, Y. (2013). Child trafficking and commercial sexual exploitation: A review of promising prevention policies and programs. *American Journal of Orthopsychiatry*, 83(4), 559–575.

Reed, R.V., Fazel, M., Jones, L., Panter-Brick, C., & Stein, A. (2012). Mental health of displaced and refugee children resettled in low-income and middle-income countries: Risk and protective factors. *The Lancet*, 379(9812), 250–265.

Reinke, W.M., Stormont, M., Webster-Stratton, C., Newcomer, L.L., & Herman, K.C. (2012). The Incredible Years Teacher Classroom Management Program: Using coaching to support generalization to real-world classroom settings. *Psychology in the Schools*, 49(5), 416–428.

Rotheram-Fuller, E., & MacMullen, L. (2011). Cognitive behavioral therapy for children with autism spectrum disorders. *Psychology in the Schools*, 48(3), 263–271.

Rutter, M. (1987). Psychosocial resilience and protective mechanisms. *American Journal of Orthopsychiatry*, 57, 316–331.

Rutter, M. (2012). Resilience as a dynamic concept. *Development and Psychopathology*, 24(2), 335–344.

Sanders, M.R. (2008). Triple P-Positive Parenting Program as a public health approach to strengthening parenting. *Journal of Family Psychology*, 22(3), 506–517.

Sanders, M.R., & Glynn, E.L. (1981). Training parents in behavioral self-management: An analysis of generalization and maintenance effects. *Journal of Applied Behavior Analysis*, 14(3), 223–237.

Sanders, M.R., Markie-Dadds, C., & Turner, K.M.T. (2003). Theoretical, scientific and clinical foundations of the Triple P-Positive Parenting Program: A population approach to the promotion of parenting competence. *Parenting Research and Practice Monograph* (1), 1–21.

Sanders, M.R., Kirby, J.N., Tellegen, C.L., & Day, J.J. (2014). The Triple P-Positive Parenting Program: A systematic review and meta-analysis of a multi-level system of parenting support. *Clinical Psychology Review*, 34(4), 337–357.

Schwab-Stone, M., Ruchkin, V., Vermeiren, R., & Leckman, P. (2001) Cultural considerations in the treatment of children and adolescents: Operationalizing the importance of culture in treatment. *Child and Adolescent Psychiatric Clinics of North America*, 10(4), 729–743.

Shapiro, C.J., Prinz, R.J., & Sanders, M.R. (2008). Population-wide parenting intervention training: Initial feasibility. *Journal of Child and Family Studies*, 17, 457–466.

Shea, P., & Shern, D. (2011). *Primary prevention in behavioral health: Investing in our nation's future*. Alexandria, VA: National Association of State Mental Health Program Directors (NASMHPD).

Silverman, W.K., Pina, A.A., & Viswesvaran, C. (2008). Evidence-based psychosocial treatments for phobic and anxiety disorders in children and adolescents. *Journal of Clinical Child & Adolescent Psychology*, 37, 105–130.

Smetana, J., Campione-Barr, N., & Metzger, A. (2006). Adolescent development in interpersonal and societal contexts. *Annual Reviews Psychology*, 57, 255–84.

Spence, S.H. (2003). Social skills training with children and young people: Theory, evidence and practice. *Child and Adolescent Mental Health*, 8(2), 84–96.

Steiner, H., Remsing, L., & AACAP Work Group on Quality Issues. (2007). Practice parameter for the assessment and treatment of children and adolescents with oppositional defiant disorder. *Journal of the American Academy of Child Adolescent Psychiatry*, 46(1), 126–141.

Stephens, P. (2011). Preventing and confronting school bullying: A comparative study of two national programmes in Norway. British *Educational Research Journal*, 37(3), 381–404.

Strawn, J.R., Wehry, A.M., Del Bello, M.P., Rynn, M.A., & Strakowski, S. (2012). Establishing the neurobiologic basis of treatment in children and adolescent with generalized anxiety disorder. *Depression & Anxiety*, 29(4), 328–339.

Sturgeon, S., & Orley, J. (2005). Concepts of mental health across the world. In H. Herrman, S. Saxena, & R. Moodie (Eds.), *Promoting mental health: Concepts, emerging evidence, practice* (pp. 59–69). Geneva: World Health Organization.

Substance Abuse and Mental Health Services Administration, Center for Mental Health Services (2007). *Promotion and prevention in mental health: Strengthening parenting and enhancing child resilience*. DHHS Publication No. CMHS-SVP-0175. Rockville, MD: Author.

Szatmari, P., Archer, L., Fisman, S., Streiner, D., & Wilson, F. (1995). Asperger's syndrome and autism: Differences in behavior, cognition, and adaptive functioning. *Journal of the American Academy of Child and Adolescent Psychiatry*, 34(12), 1662–1671.

Taliaferro, L.A., & Muehlenkamp, J.J. (2014) Risk and protective factors that distinguish adolescents who attempt suicide from those who only consider suicide in the past year. *Suicide & Life-Threatening Behavior*, 44(1), 6–22.

Tanner-Smith, E.E., & Wilson, S.J. (2013). A meta-analysis of the effects of dropout prevention programs on school absenteeism. *Prevention Science*, 14(5), 468–478.

Thatcher, D.L., & Clark, D.B. (2008). Adolescents at risk for substance use disorders. *Alcohol Research & Health*, 31(2), 168–176.

Theunissen, M., Griensven van, I., Verdonk, P., Feron, F., & Bosma, H. (2012). The early identification of risk factors on the pathway to school dropout in the SIODO study: A sequential mixed-methods study. *BMC Public Health*, 12(1), 1033–1040.

Trotter, H., & Rafferty, H. (2014). A follow-up to the Incredible Years Parenting Programme: The reflections of mothers one to two years later. *Educational & Child Psychology*, 31(4), 40–57.

Ttofi, M.M., & Farrington, D.P. (2009). What works in preventing bullying: Effective elements of anti-bullying programmes. *Journal of Aggression, Conflict and Peace Research*, 1(1), 13–24.

United Nations. (2013). *The millennium development goals report 2013*. New York: Author.

United Nations Children's Fund. (2007). *The Paris principles: Principles and guidelines on children associated with armed forces or armed groups*. Retrieved August 7, 2014 from UNICEF website: www.unicef.org/emerg/files/ParisPrinciples310107English.pdf.

United Nations Children's Fund. (2009). *The state of the world's children, special edition: Celebrating 20 Years of the Convention on the Rights of the Child*. New York: Author.

United Nations Children's Fund. (2013). *Towards an AIDS-free generation: Children and AIDS: Sixth stocktaking report, 2013*. New York: Author.

United Nations Educational, Scientific and Cultural Organization. (2014). *EFA global monitoring report 2013/4: Teaching and learning—achieving quality for all*. Paris: UNESCO.

United Nations High Commissioner for Refugees. (2013). *UNHCR statistical yearbook 2012*. Geneva: Author.

United Nations Office on Drugs and Crime. (2010). *Compilation of evidence-based family skills programmes*. Retrieved June 17, 2014 from www.unodc.org/documents/prevention/family-compilation.pdf.

US Department of Health and Human Services. (1999). *Mental health: A report of the Surgeon General*. Rockville, MD: US Department of Health and Human Services, Substance Abuse and Mental Health Services Administration, Center for Mental Health Services, National Institutes of Health, National Institute of Mental Health.

Van Meter A.R., Moreira, A.L., & Youngstrom, E.A. (2011). Meta-analysis of epidemiologic studies of pediatric bipolar disorder. *Journal of Clinical Psychiatry*, 72(9), 1250–1256.

Verhulst, F.C. (2004). Epidemiology as a basis for the conception and planning of services. In H. Remschmidt, M.L. Belfer, & I. Goodyer (Eds.), *Facilitating pathways: Care, treatment, and prevention in child and adolescent mental health* (pp. 3–15). Berlin, Germany: Springer.

Walsh, F. (2003). Family resilience: A framework for clinical practice. *Family Process*, 42(1), 1–18.

Walsh, F. (2007). Traumatic loss and major disasters: Strengthening family and community resilience. *Family Process*, 46(2), 207–227.

Webster-Stratton, C. (2009). Affirming diversity: Multi-cultural collaboration to deliver the Incredible Years Parent Programs. *The International Journal of Child Health and Human Development*, 2(1), 17–32.

Webster-Stratton, C., & Herman, K.C. (2010). Disseminating Incredible Years Series early intervention programs: Integrating and sustaining services between school and home. *Psychology in the Schools*, 47(1), 36–54.

Webster-Stratton, C., Rinaldi, J., & Reid, J.M. (2011). Long-term outcomes of Incredible Years Parenting Program: Predictors of adolescent adjustment. *Child & Adolescent Mental Health*, 16(1), 38–46.

Webster-Stratton, C., Reid, M.J., & Beauchaine, T.P. (2013). One-year follow-up of combined parent and child intervention for young children with ADHD. *Journal of Clinical Child & Adolescent Psychology*, 42(2), 251–261.

Weems, C.F., Pina, A.A., Costa, N.M., Watts, S.E., Taylor, L.K., & Cannon, M. F. (2007). Predisaster trait anxiety and negative affect predict posttraumatic stress in youths after Hurricane Katrina. *Journal of Consulting and Clinical Psychology*, 75(1), 154–159.

West, A.E., Weinstein, S.M., Peters, A.T., Katz, A.C., Henry, D.B., Cruz, R.A., & Pavuluri, M.N. (2014). Child- and family-focused cognitive-behavioral therapy for pediatric bipolar disorder: A randomized clinical trial. *Journal of the American Academy of Child & Adolescent Psychiatry*, 53(11), 1168–1178.

Wilkinson, P., & Goodyer, I. (2011) Non-suicidal self-injury. *European Child & Adolescent Psychiatry*, 20(2), 103–108.

Willis, B.M., & Levy, B.S. (2002). Child prostitution: Global health burden, research needs, and interventions. *The Lancet*, 359, 1417–1422.

Wondie, Y., Zemene, W., Reschke, K., & Schroder, H. (2011). Early marriage, rape, child prostitution, and related factors determining the psychosocial effects severity of child sexual abuse in Ethiopia. *Journal of Child Sexual Abuse*, 20(3), 305–321.

World Health Organization. (2003). *Caring for children and adolescents with mental disorders: Setting WHO Directions*. Geneva: Department of Mental Health and Substance Abuse.

World Health Organization. (2004). *Prevention of mental disorders: Effective interventions and policy options*. Geneva: Author.

World Health Organization. (2005a). *Atlas: Child and adolescent mental health resources—global concerns, implications for the future*. Geneva: Author.

World Health Organization. (2005b). *Mental health policy and service guidance package: Child and adolescent mental health policies and plans*. Geneva: Author.

World Health Organization. (2006). *Preventing suicide: A resource for counselors*. Geneva: Department of Mental Health and Substance Abuse.

World Health Organization. (2007). *Atlas: Nurses in mental health 2007*. Geneva: Author.

World Health Organization. (2010a). *International statistical classification of diseases and related health problems, 10th revision*. Geneva, Author.

World Health Organization. (2010b). *mhGAP intervention guide for mental, neurological and substance use disorders in non-specialized health settings: Mental Health Gap Action Programme (mhGAP)*. Geneva: Author.

World Health Organization. (2011*). Mental health atlas 2011*. Geneva: Author.

World Health Organization. (2012). *Adolescent mental health: Mapping actions of nongovernmental organizations and other international development organizations*. Geneva: Author.

World Health Organization. (2013). *Mental health action plan 2013–2020*. Geneva: Author.

Yearwood, E.L., & Bosnick, E. (2012). Deliberate self-harm: Nonsuicidal self-injury and suicide in children and adolescents. In E.L. Yearwood, G.S. Pearson, & J.A. Newland (Eds.), *Child and adolescent behavioral health* (pp. 187–204). West Sussex, UK: John Wiley & Sons.

Ying, L., Wu, X., Lin, C., & Chen, C. (2013). Prevalence and predictors of posttraumatic stress disorder and depressive symptoms among child survivors 1 year following the Wenchuan earthquake in China. *European Child & Adolescent Psychiatry*, 22(9), 567–575.

Young, R., Sproeber, N., Groschwitz, R.C., Preiss, M., & Plener, P.L. (2014). Why alternative teenagers self-harm: Exploring the link between non-suicidal self-injury, attempted suicide and adolescent identity. *BMC Psychiatry*, 14(1), 1–25.

Young, S., & Amarasinghe, J.M. (2010). Practitioner review: Non-pharmacological treatments for ADHD—a lifespan approach. *Journal of Child Psychology and Psychiatry*, 51(2), 116–133.

Yule, W., & Smith, P. (2008) Post-traumatic stress disorder. In M. Rutter, D.V.M. Bishop, D.S. Pine, S. Scott, J. Stevenson, E. Taylor, & A. Thapar (Eds.), *Rutter's child and adolescent psychiatry*, (5th ed) (pp. 686–697). Oxford: Blackwell.

Zhang, J., Zhao, G., Lib, X., Hong, Y., Fang, X., Barnett, D., & Zhang, L. (2009). Positive future orientation as a mediator between traumatic events and mental health among children affected by HIV/AIDS in rural China. *AIDS Care*, 21(12), 1508–1516.

Zhao, Q., Li, X., Zhao, J., Zhao, G., & Stanton, B. (2014). Predictors of depressive symptoms among children affected by HIV in rural China: A 3-year longitudinal study. *Journal of Child and Family Studies*, 23, 1193–1200.

Ziaian, T., de Anstiss, H., Antoniou, G., Baghurst, P., & Sawyer, M. (2013). Emotional and behavioural problems among refugee children and adolescents living in South Australia. *Australian Psychologist*, 489(2), 139–148.

19

STRATEGIES FOR HEALTH PROMOTION AFTER VIOLENCE EXPOSURE

Leilani Marie Ayala, Michael Hazelton,
and Vicki P. Hines-Martin

Introduction

Pinker (2011) has argued that we are living through one of the most peaceful times in the history of humankind. While this may be the case in historical comparative terms, the recent shooting down of Malaysian Airlines Flight 17 (MH17) serves as a tragic reminder of the globalization of risk (Beck, 1992) and we might add violence. For many of us, the violence associated with war, terrorism, civil disturbance or crime is something we watch on television or read about online – from our location in McLuhan's (1964) 'global village'; we might be aware of and concerned about distant wars and local crime rates, but these are often vague and remote apprehensions. Nonetheless, as 9/11, the downing of MH17 and the attack on Atatürk Airport indicate, the potential for exposure to violence now extends well beyond concerns over crime in our local community. For some, exposure to violence will be as primary victims – those directly affected by violence. For others, exposure will be as secondary victims – the family, friends and work colleagues of the primary victim. The notion of secondary victimhood may also be extended to include those who attend the crime scene, support the victims or investigate the crime.

In this chapter we consider the mental health impacts of exposure to violence and how these might be addressed using health promotion strategies. While the approach adopted is heavily influenced by the service contexts of our own countries – the United States and Australia – the discussion will be contextualized within broader international concerns and responses: we will thus explore violence and its health implications both locally and globally; in the home, classroom and workplace; interpersonally and collectively; and in relation to both the primary and secondary victims of violence.

The range of topics that could be addressed under the rubric of violence and mental health is enormous and we have had to make choices regarding particular areas of focus in this chapter. What follows reflects our own concerns and expertise but also addresses topics likely to be of interest to clinical practitioners and researchers worldwide. Claims regarding contemporary human peacefulness (Pinker, 2011) would not sit easily with the day-to-day work experience of many health professionals. Indeed, the health impacts of violence, whether these are approached broadly as social determinants of health, or more specifically in relation to the impact of violence on health care providers, is currently a hot topic internationally. Homicide and overall crime rates have been declining in recent years in many countries, including Australia and Britain. While such trends are encouraging, we should nonetheless note that approximately half a million homicides are officially recorded each year with homicide rates increasing in many parts of the world such as the Caribbean and South America (Morrall, Hazelton & Shackleton, 2013). Beyond consideration of homicide rates, many more people are regularly exposed to violence through war, civil disturbance and terrorism; or as part of their role in the workplace; or in relation to family life and wider social and occupational connections. While relationships between social determinants and health are notoriously difficult to disentangle, levels of hostility and homicides, as well as levels of mental health and well-being have been shown to vary according to the degree of social inequality (Pickett & Wilkinson, 2009). Indeed, as Wilkinson and Pickett (2009) have argued, violence and many other social problems (e.g. bullying, poor educational achievement, rates of imprisonment) are likely to be more prevalent in unequal societies.

The link between violence and social and economic development has come to be a major focus internationally with supranational organizations such as the United Nations (UN) and the World Health Organization (WHO) undertaking major initiatives in the last two decades to better understand and respond to the problem of violence. The WHO Global Campaign for Violence Prevention seeks to implement the recommendations of the *World Report on Violence and Health 2002* (Krug, Dalhberg, Mercy, Zwi & Lozano, 2002) and the *Global Status Report on Violence Prevention 2014* (WHO, 2014b). The broad intention is to draw attention to the health and social development impacts of violence and to facilitate violence prevention

Table 19.1 UN sustainable development goal 16 and targets

Goal 16	*Promote peaceful and inclusive societies for sustainable development, provide access to justice for all and build effective, accountable and inclusive institutions at all levels*		
16. 1	Significantly reduce all forms of violence and related death rates everywhere	16. 7	Ensure responsive, inclusive, participatory and representative decision-making at all levels
16. 2	End abuse, exploitation, trafficking and all forms of violence against and torture of children.	16. 8	Broaden and strengthen the participation of developing countries in the institutions of global governance
16. 3	Promote the rule of law at the national and international levels and ensure equal access to justice for all.	16. 9	By 2030, provide legal identity for all including birth registration
16. 4	By 2030, significantly reduce illicit financial and arms flows, strengthen the recovery and return of stolen assets and combat all forms of organized crimes	16. 10	Ensure public access to information and protect fundamental freedoms, in accordance with national legislation and international agreements
16. 5	Substantially reduce bribery and corruption in all their forms	16. a	Strengthen relevant national institutions, in particular in developing countries, to prevent violence and combat terrorism and crime
16. 6	Develop effective, accountable and transparent institutions at all levels	16. b	Promote and enforce non-discriminatory laws and policies for sustainable development

Source: Source: From Open Working Group Proposal for Sustainable Development Goals by Open Working Group of the General Assembly on Sustainable Development Goals © 2014 United Nations. Reprinted with the permission of the United Nations.

through evidence-based public health strategies (who.int/violence_injury_prevention/violence/global_campaign/en). Other important violence and health related initiatives include the Institute of Medicine's (IOM) Forum on Global Violence Prevention and the Geneva Declaration on Armed Violence and Development. The IOM Forum is intended to bring together experts on many aspects of violence prevention to consider the evidence on and make recommendations for improving violence prevention policies and practices, both domestically and internationally (www.iom.edu). Adopted in 2006, the Geneva Declaration is a diplomatic initiative designed to enhance sustainable development internationally through strategies to reduce armed violence in conflict and non-conflict settings by 2015 (genevadeclaration.org). Table 19.1 outlines Sustainable Development Goal 16 from the UN sustainable development goals (sustainabledevelopment.un.org).

In the next section we discuss issues surrounding the definition of violence used in this chapter and outline various types of violence – self-directed violence, interpersonal violence and collective violence. We then consider health outcomes of the victims of violence, addressing these in two categories: the *primary victims of violence* (i.e. those who are directly exposed to violence) and *secondary victims of violence* (i.e. those who are close relatives, associates, or close work colleagues of victims; those who have witnessed a violent crime; or those who must intervene to offer help to victims and/or investigate violent incidents). Throughout the chapter we refer to various strategies for health promotion following exposure to violence.

Definition and types of violence

There are various ways of defining violence. In this chapter we have used the definition developed by the World Health Organization as outlined in the *World Report on Violence and Health* (Krug *et al.*, 2002), which approaches violence as:

> The intentional use of physical force or power, threatened or actual, against oneself, another person, or against a group or community, that either results in or has a high likelihood of resulting in injury, death, psychological harm, maldevelopment or deprivation.
>
> *(Krug et al., 2002, p. 5)*

This definition has been purposefully developed to take into account acts of omission such as neglect, as well as the more obvious violent acts of commission such as homicide. The definition also stresses intentionality, so as to differentiate between, for example, purposeful violence resulting in injury and unintentional incidents such as road traffic injuries.

The *World Report on Violence and Health* (Krug *et al.*, 2002) also proposes a useful typology of violence, based on the characteristics of those who commit the violence:

- *Self-directed violence* includes the sub-categories of suicidal behaviour (e.g. suicidal thoughts, attempted suicides and completed suicides), self-abuse (e.g. self-mutilation) and high-risk behaviors with potential for injury. Self-directed violence will not be addressed in this chapter but is found in Chapter 12.
- *Interpersonal violence* is differentiated into family and intimate partner violence (e.g. violence occurring between family members and intimate partners, inside or outside the home) and community violence (e.g. violence between individuals who may or may not know each other, largely occurring outside of the home). Much of what is covered in this chapter fits within the broad rubric of interpersonal violence.

- *Collective violence* addresses violence committed for social, political and economic purposes. Included are crimes of hate perpetrated by organized groups, acts of terrorism, mob violence, war and other forms of state violence, and violence directed towards disrupting economic activity. Some coverage of collective violence will be provided in this chapter.

Primary victims of violence

Bullying

Bullying as a significant example of interpersonal violence is a public health concern associated with serious (mental) health problems whether the one involved is the bully, the victim or the bystander. Importantly, bullying can be approached as a significant modifiable risk factor for mental illness, highlighting the need for effective prevention strategies targeting (Scott, Moore, Sly & Norman, 2013) the attitudes and behaviours that sustain bullying victimization.

The prevalence of bullying has increased dramatically in countries such as the United States and Australia, with large numbers of students missing school to avoid being bullied and up to 35 per cent of students being exposed to bullying daily in the form of teasing, rumors, intimidation and physical confrontation (Mayers-Adams, 2008; Scott *et al.*, 2013). Traditionally, bullying has been perceived as a normal part of growing up; a kind of 'rite of passage'. More recently, media and public attention has focused on bullying-associated suicide, with at least 250 cases being reported worldwide in the English language press in the last half century and many of these occurring in the last decade. Moreover, there are indications that a high proportion of perpetrators in school shootings had been bullied or harmed by their peers prior to the shooting incidents (Schroeder *et al.*, 2012).

Exposure to bullying significantly increases the risk of developing physical, psychosocial and psychiatric problems, including higher risk of suicide (Borrowsky, Taliaferro & McMorris, 2013; Feekes, Pijpers, & Verloove-Vanhorick, 2004; Fung & Rain, 2012; Gini, 2007). The growth in bullying in the United States has prompted legislators to enact laws prohibiting bullying in a majority of states, with many of these including electronic harassment or 'cyberbullying'. The problem has not as yet been addressed specifically in Australian legislation, although harassment or threats are included under national crimes legislation (Kozlowska & Durheim, 2013).

What is bullying?

In what is perhaps the most widely used definition of bullying, Olweus (1993) has proposed that a person is bullied when they are exposed, repeatedly and over time, to negative actions from one or more people with an associated imbalance of power. Bullying has also been described as a 'systematic abuse of power'. The power exercised by the bully may occur in many forms, including direct physical contact as well as indirect methods, such as verbal abuse, the spreading of rumours, intentional exclusion from a group, indecent gestures and cyberbullying (Olweus, 1993; 1994; Smith *et al.*, 2008).

Bullies, victims, bystanders

The bully has a strong need to dominate and subdue others and to get his or her own way. They are typically impulsive, easily angered, often defiant and aggressive towards adults, including parents and teachers. They lack empathy towards victims and often celebrate violence. Children exposed to intimate partner violence are more likely to display physically aggressive forms of bullying such as pushing, shoving others and fighting (Bauer *et al.*, 2006). If the bullies are boys, they are often physically stronger than other boys and are perceived to be more popular by their peers. Individuals with a history of exposure to bullying are more likely to bully others, to have negative attitudes to school and to engage in unhealthy behaviours such as tobacco and alcohol use (Nansel *et al.*, 2001).

Bullies are also more likely to have authoritarian parents whose use of power-assertive techniques of discipline and physical punishment, model bullying-like behaviour (Barboza *et al.*, 2009), or lack involvement and warmth towards their children (Olweus, 1993; 1994). It has also been suggested that adolescents with inadequate social support systems, either at school or in the family, may engage in bullying behaviours as a means of empowering themselves (Barboza *et al.*, 2009). At the same time, victims of bullying may not have developed self-confidence and independence due to having overprotective parents who are critical or permissive and distant. Boys who are victims of bullying may be physically weaker and may react to aggression by withdrawing from the situation; they may relate better to adults than other children and are often rejected and isolated by their peers (Cook, Williams, Geuvarra, Kim & Sadek, 2010). There may be passive victims who do not retaliate and those who do and become bullies themselves. So-called bully-victims have experienced being both bully and victim. Such an individual will likely have negative attitudes and beliefs about themselves and poor social problem-solving skills. Bully-victims will often struggle academically; will be rejected and isolated by their peers; but at the same time will be negatively influenced by those with whom he or she interacts (Cook *et al.*, 2010).

The actions (or inactions) of bystanders may facilitate or mitigate bullying victimization. Bystanders may witness bullying but they are neither the bully nor the victim (Twemlow, Fonagy & Sacco, 2004). At least four bystander roles have been identified in the bullying process: *assistants* join the ringleader; *reinforcers* provide encouragement to the bully; *outsiders* withdraw from bullying situations; and *defenders* support and comfort the victim (Salmivalli & Pokisparta, 2012). Although bystanders may not have direct involvement in bullying activity they are nonetheless at risk of developing similar psychological symptoms as those who are. These symptoms can include increased anxiety, depression and absenteeism, substance abuse and self-harming behaviours, including suicide (Rivers & Noret, 2013).

Violence in the health workplace

Workplace violence can be understood as 'any incident where staff are abused, threatened or assaulted in circumstances relating to their work, involving explicit or implicit challenge to their safety, wellbeing or health' (Lynch, Appleboam & McQuillan, 2003). Workplace aggression and violent behaviour is a common phenomenon. Large numbers of people, in a range of occupations, have been shown to regularly experience aggression from multiple sources while at work. Such exposure may arise from customers, clients, or patients; from the members of the general public; or from co-workers. In general, aggression and violent behaviour from external sources is more prevalent than from work colleagues (Hills & Joyce, 2013). In response to increases in violence in the health workplace, many countries have augmented occupational health and safety legislation along with industry standards and codes of practice to ensure staff are sufficiently trained to deal with instances of violence and aggressive situations in the work place (ASIS Health care Security Council, 2011; International Council of Nurses, 2009; International Labour Office, 2002; Victorian Department of Human Services, 2003).

Nurses are especially likely to be subjected to physical or verbal abuse in the workplace (Ogundipe *et al.*, 2010; Stone, McMillan & Hazelton, 2015), with some studies indicating that nurses are at greater risk than police officers (McKinnon & Cross, 2008). The risk of exposure to workplace violence (and resultant injury) has been reported to be high; among nursing staff as high as 77–87 per cent (Lynch *et al.*, 2003; Wand & Coulson, 2006). A study from Britain found unqualified and junior staff to be more at risk than senior trained staff; that there was a higher incidence of violence associated with patients with co-morbid mental illness and substance use disorders; and that environmental factors such as ward layout, boredom and staff attitudes can increase violence (McKinnon & Cross, 2008). In Australia, registered nurses have been reported to be the second largest employee group to claim worker's compensation as a result of exposure to violence (Kennedy, 2005). A consistent finding of research undertaken in Australia (Crilly, Chaboyer & Creedy, 2004; Lam, 2002) and internationally (Pich & Kable, 2014) is that a majority of nurses experience workplace violence on a regular basis.

Patient initiated aggression and violence towards staff has been increasingly reported in a range of health service locations including acute inpatient mental health units, emergency departments and general practice surgeries (Hills & Joyce, 2013; Lynch *et al.*, 2003; Magin, Adams, Sibbritt, Joy & Ireland, 2005; 2005; O'Connell, Young, Brooks, Hutchings & Lofthouse, 2000). There is a high prevalence of workplace violence in mental health services, with mental health nurses being the occupational group most likely to be affected. The most common psychiatric diagnoses likely to be associated with risk of aggression and violence are severe or acute psychotic episodes and co-morbid personality disorders and substance use disorders. Substance intoxication has been reported as the major risk factor for aggression and violence in emergency departments (Crilly *et al.*, 2004; Lynch *et al.*, 2003). In some emergency departments violence is considered to be an almost daily occurrence and the timing tends to follow social patterns of substance use with incidents more likely to occur during the evenings and on the weekends (Crilly *et al.*, 2004; Kennedy, 2005). It is also important to note that violent incidents are almost certainly under-reported (Lynch *et al.*, 2003) with some commentators suggesting that perhaps as few as 1 in 5 violent episodes are brought to the attention of management (Farrell & Cubit, 2005). It has sometimes been suggested that under-reporting of violent incidents in health workplaces reflects a perception that the problem is 'part of the job' and unlikely to be addressed by managers (Lyneham, 1999; Pich, Hazelton, Sundin & Kable, 2010).

Medical practitioners have also faced a growing problem with workplace violence. In general practice occupational violence is common, with one Australian study reporting a 64 per cent 12-month incidence (Magin *et al.*, 2005). Documentation of the types of violence encountered indicates that 'low-level' violence, especially verbal abuse, is the most prevalent form of violence. While 'high-level' violence, such as physical assault, sexual abuse and stalking, occurs less often, the level of occurrence is nonetheless worrying. No matter what level of violence the individual has been exposed to, the psychological sequelae of violence occur frequently in general practitioners and can have a significant impact on the provision of services to patients (Coles, Koritsas, Boyle & Stanley, 2007; Harris, 1989; Magin *et al.*, 2006; Magin *et al.*, 2008;) and negatively affect the recruitment and retention of doctors (Alexander & Fraser, 2004; Coles *et al.*, 2007; Hobbs, 1991), and we would add, other health care practitioners including nurses.

One of the strategies that has been widely implemented in response to concerns over health workplace violence in countries such as the United States, Australia, New Zealand and Britain is 'zero tolerance' (Elston, Gabe, Denney, Lee & O'Beirne, 2002; Lynch *et al.*, 2003; Wand & Coulson, 2006). While zero tolerance policies may be appropriate in workplaces other than health care, they may not be consistent with current therapeutic approaches to the management of aggressive and violent behaviour in patients. Adherence to zero tolerance may undermine therapeutic decision-making on the part of practitioners and the capacity of patients to respond to such approaches may be compromised due to their current health crisis. Critics of the use of zero tolerance in general practice in the United Kingdom have argued that such polices are difficult to implement, ineffective and largely a political tool (Elston *et al.*, 2002; Magin, Adams & Joy, 2007).

It has been suggested that zero tolerance risks exacerbating aggression and violence (Lynch, Appleboam & McQuillan, 2003) and that aggression minimization and de-escalation strategies offer better prospects for effectively managing such episodes (Farrell & Cubit, 2005; Lynch *et al.*, 2003; Royal College of Nursing, 2005). Although violence in the workplace is a well-recognized problem the psychological impact on staff and associated costs remains under-researched. Farrell and Cubit (2005) evaluated 28 aggression management programs, with approximately half of these being drawn from organizations and services within the health sector. While most of the programs reviewed covered personal safety issues for staff and patients and legal issues, many failed to adequately address psychological and organizational costs associated with aggression and violence in the workplace, such as: rates of absenteeism and sick leave, property damage, security costs, reduced job satisfaction and issues associated with workforce recruitment and retention.

Intimate partner violence

So far in this chapter much of the discussion has addressed interpersonal violence involving children and adolescents at school and at home, and violence in the health workplace, where this may be perpetrated by health service users. A feature of these forms of violence exposure is that they largely take place within the public domain. We now consider violence involving intimate partners, which to a considerable extent occurs in the private domain.

Intimate partner violence (IPV) is a global health concern that affects both men and women of all ages from diverse ethnic and socioeconomic backgrounds. This form of violence involves the intentional inflicting of physical, psychological or sexual harm by a current or former spouse or intimate partner who is or has been in a heterosexual or same-sex relationship (Black, Basile, Breiding, Smith, Walters, Merick, Chen & Stevens, 2010). There are four main categories of IPV (Breiding, Basile, Smith & Mahendra, 2015) *physical violence*, which involves the use of force with the potential to causing injury or harm; 2) *sexual violence*, where another individual is forced against their will to engage in sexual acts – this is further categorized into rape or penetration of victim, victim was made to penetrate someone else, non-physically pressured unwanted penetration, unwanted sexual contact, non-contact unwanted sexual experiences; 3) *Stalking*, which involves repeated and unwanted attention and contact that causes fear or concerns for one's own safety or the safety of someone else; *psychological aggression* – the use of verbal and non-verbal means to control another person or to cause harm.

The 2010 National Institute of Intimate Partner and Sexual Violence Survey in the United States reported that more than 1 in 3 women (35.6 per cent) and more than 1 in 4 men (28.5 per cent) have experienced rape, physical violence and/or stalking by an intimate partner in their lifetime and that for up to 69 per cent of these the first instance occurred before the age of 25. Physical violence is experienced by 1 in 4 women (24.3 per cent) and 1 in 7 (13.8 per cent) men at some point in their lives and about 9.4 per cent of high school students have reported being victims of physical aggression (i.e. being hit, slapped, or physically hurt on purpose) by their girlfriend or boyfriend (Black *et al.*, 2011).

Although women have been found to use physical aggression more than men, male perpetrators cause more fatal injury (Karakut & Silver, 2013). Psychological (emotional) abuse has been found to be the most common form of IPV with almost half of all men (48.4 per cent) and women (48.8 per cent) having experienced it in their lifetime. It is also the most common form of IPV reported by females across population groups, followed by physical and then sexual abuse (Williams, Ghandour & Kub, 2008). Young women are more susceptible to psychological abuse possibly through isolation associated with the importance they place in being in a romantic relationship (Karakut & Silver, 2013). Although IPV affects both genders, female victimization (4.9 per 1,000) is far greater than that for males (1.1 per 1,000) (Lauritsen & Rezey, 2013). The World Health Organization (2016) has recently reported that worldwide about 35 per cent of women have experienced physical and/or sexual violence from an intimate partner and as much as 38 per cent of all female homicides were committed by their partners.

Three broad categories of risk for IPV have been identified (World Health Organization, 2012):

- *individual factors* (e.g. young age, low educational attainment, witnessing or experiencing violence as a child, harmful use of alcohol and drugs);
- *relationship factors* (e.g. conflict or dissatisfaction in relationship, male dominance in family, economic stress, man having multiple partners); and
- *community and societal factors* (e.g. gender-inequitable social norms, poverty, low social and economic status of women, weak legal sanctions against IPV within marriage, lack of women's civil rights).

The victims of IPV may suffer from chronic physical illnesses, mental health problems and economic difficulties. Women exposed to IVP have been shown to be at greater risk of developing adverse health outcomes (Bonomi, Anderson, Rivara & Thompson, 2007; Ulloa & Hammett, 2016), including stress-related problems such as fibromyalgia, eating disorders, fertility problems, irritable bowel and other gastrointestinal disorders and cardiovascular diseases (Jannone, 2011; Knapp, 2011; Stene, Jacobsoson, Dyb, Tverdal & Schei, 2013). A high prevalence of problems associated with reproductive coercion has also been reported, including unwanted pregnancies and termination of pregnancies and sexually transmitted infections and HIV among female victims (Hess *et al.*, 2012; Miller *et al.*, 2014). Victims may also suffer from a range of serious psychological and mental health problems including low self-esteem, low self-worth, post-traumatic stress disorder, depression, alcohol and substance abuse, suicidal ideation and suicide attempts (Devries *et al.*, 2013; Sabri *et al.*, 2013). Severe mental health problems may disrupt decision-making thus contributing to delayed help-seeking and prolonged exposure to violence. Similarly, a person's psychological and physical state may affect job performance and stability and thus threaten financial and domestic welfare.

Mental health prevention and promotion strategies for intimate partner violence

It has been recommended that both men and women be screened for intimate partner violence as part of preventative health visits. However, medical practitioners and nurses often fail to ask about IPV due to time pressures, lack of training, differences in personal and cultural beliefs and practices and such institutional barriers as lack of privacy and space (Beynon, Gutmanis, Tutty, Wathen & MacMillian, 2012; Guruge, 2012). This gap in practice can be addressed by providing a training curriculum on IPV screening for medical residents and nurse educators (Papadakaki, Petriduo, Kogevinas & Lionis, 2013; Tufts, Clements, Karlowicz, 2009). Adolescents and higher education students should be evaluated for recent or previous dating violence involvement. First-time mothers and women with disabilities, who are dependent on their partners for physical and medical needs, should also be routinely screened. It is critical that victims of IPV are supported to access community resources and referred to appropriate health and community support agencies.

The following are some examples of community support programs:

- *The nurse-family partnership*: an intensive evidence-based home visitation program for first time mothers from a low-income background in which nurses conduct home visits prenatally until the child reaches two years of age, has been shown to decrease exposure to IPV.
- *Mothers Advocates in the Community (MOSAIC)*: a nonprofessional mentor support program, which aims to reduce IPV among pregnant women and recent mothers, accepts referrals from primary care practitioners.
- *Kid's Club*: a 10-week community based program designed for mothers and children exposed to IPV.
- *Project Support*: assists mothers in managing children displaying conduct problems.

Evidence-based therapies for IPV include psychological interventions such as:

- *Cognitive behaviour therapy for battered women* (CBT-BW): combines CBT techniques with psychoeducation, stress management, exposure, assertiveness training, safety planning and self-advocacy to increase self-esteem and decrease depression in women who have left abusive relationships and are not abusing alcohol and other substances (Iverson *et al.*, 2011).
- *HOPE Program* (Helping to Overcome PTSD through Empowerment): involves short-term cognitive-behavioural intervention focusing on stabilization, safety and empowerment, for residents of women's shelters with current safety concerns; aims to reduce PTSD symptoms by teaching relaxation techniques and coping skills (Johnson, Zlotnick & Perez, 2011).
- *Trauma-Focused Cognitive Behaviour Therapy* (TF-CBT): brief CBT intervention designed to reduce PTSD symptoms and anxiety in IPV victims (Ramirez *et al.*, 2014).

In addition to the more formal psychological interventions outlined above, a range of other measures can be used in IPV prevention, including classes addressing dating and healthy relationships, academic achievement programs, peer mediation, family therapy, recreational programs, services for adults who were abused as children and after-school programs.

As a professional group, nurses can play a pivotal role in preventing and addressing issues of IPV. Nurses and nurse practitioners should be trained to screen patients who are at risk for IPV and to make effective recommendations for referral and follow-up. More broadly, nurses can exercise leadership in public education initiatives addressing violence prevention and reduction, and in the development of outreach programs that are culturally sensitive and address the needs of both victims and perpetrators of abuse.

Female genital mutilation/cutting (FGM/C)

Definition and prevalence

As has been identified throughout this chapter, some populations are at higher risk for being a victim of violence. Violence toward women as a group includes *Female genital mutilation/cutting* (FGM/C). The World Health Organization and other human rights organizations (UNAIDS, UNDP, UNECA, UNESCO, UNFPA, UNHCHR, UNHCR, UNICEF, UNIFEM & WHO, 2008) identify that FGM/C includes all procedures in which there is removal of all or part of the external female genitals, or other injury to the female genitals for non-medical reasons (WHO, 2014a). Although the exact number of girls/women who have had FGM/C is unknown, the WHO (WHO, 2014a) estimates that more than 125 million are living at this time. The literature identifies that this procedure occurs most commonly between the ages of 0 and 15 years although the procedure has been done in adulthood. The practice is primarily done in African countries but has been identified in almost every nation worldwide as a result of population migration (Brigham and Women's Hospital, 2014; Dorkenoo, 2012). More than 18 per cent of all FGM is performed by health care providers, and the trend towards medicalization is increasing (WHO, 2015b).

FGM/C and global policy

FGM is recognized internationally as a violation of the human rights (health, security, physical integrity, dignity and life) of girls and women. Many countries have specific legislation against the practice, including the US (US Congress, 1996). In 2008, the Eliminating Female Genital Mutilation: An Interagency Statement – UNAIDS, UNDP, UNECA, UNESCO, UNFPA, UNHCHR, UNHCR, UNICEF, UNIFEM and WHO was published to jointly identify the practice as *mutilation* and to note the gravity and detrimental nature of this practice. They also identify that FGM/C is a culture-bound practice without religious sanction is paternalistic and reinforces male power over female choice and reproductive self-direction within their cultural group. There continues to be significant cultural pressure on, and stigma against, those who do not adhere to the practice where it is valued, which can be exerted even when families have migrated to settings in which this practice is not accepted and is illegal.

FGM/C and mental health

The negative physical outcomes from FGM/C are well documented and are related to reproductive, sexual and urinary functioning (WHO, 2015b). Research about the mental health outcomes for women who have had this procedure is still developing. Current literature identifies that girls and women who have had FGM/C experienced significantly higher prevalence of PTSD, depression, anxiety disorder and somatic disturbance. Research has also identified coping mechanisms among these girls and women that ranged from adaptive to traumatized and these mechanisms greatly affected interactions with providers and therapeutic interventions (Kizilhan, 2011; Vloeberghs *et al.*, 2011; Mulango, McAndrew & Martin, 2014).

FGM/C and the importance of nursing

Mulango *et al.* (2014) provided a comprehensive synthesis of current research on the psychological aspects of girls and women with FGM/C and the following recommendations were made for nurses (and other health care providers). Foundational to any care is knowledge about the practice of FGM/C, and cultural sensitivity, which includes an understanding of the cultural norms and pressures that support the practice. Women who experience this procedure may identify that having this done, was traumatic, but may also see the outcome as a demonstration of their cultural identity and themselves as 'good ' women of that society. Nurses must understand that is difficult for families to abandon the practice without support from the wider community. Even as the harm to girls is known, the perceived social benefits of the practice are viewed as higher than its disadvantages (UNICEF, 2005). Therefore, any negative judgement from providers targeted toward these women may serve as significant barriers to care. Mental health nurses are essential in helping women and communities better view this practice through a focus on empowerment, and helping women through identifying and addressing life-long negative outcomes. Prevention of FGM/C also requires a culturally appropriate approach focused on harm prevention, health promotion and empowerment of mothers to protect at-risk girls. An integration of mental and physical health care is recommended. Prevention should also be directed toward education of health care providers regarding the ethical and legal standards against medical FGM/C; 'Do no harm' must be a guiding principle.

Finally, WHO (2015b) identifies that it is committed to supporting research and research dissemination in the following areas:

> the dynamics of social and cultural change that lead to the abandonment of the practice, the prevalence of immediate health complications, girls' experiences of the practice, psychological consequences of FGM, care procedures for girls and women and birth care procedures that might reduce the risks from FGM for mothers and their babies, the impact of legal measures to prevent the practice, and its medicalization.
>
> *(WHO, 2015b, p. 1)*

Nurses and other health care professionals are in key roles in a variety of community settings to conduct research and share research findings in these important priority areas toward the betterment of women's health.

Child maltreatment and elder abuse

Two groups that have been identified as being especially vulnerable to abuse and violence are the very young and older people. Indeed, child maltreatment and elder abuse have emerged as serious public health concerns and were addressed in specific chapters in the *World Report on Violence and Health* (Krug *et al.*, 2002: 57–86; 123–146).

Child maltreatment

A widely accepted definition of child maltreatment (sometimes referred to as child abuse) is abuse and neglect that occurs to children under 18 years of age. Included in the definition are all types of physical and/or emotional ill-treatment, sexual abuse, neglect, negligence and commercial or other forms of exploitation, which may compromise the child's health, survival, development or dignity, in the context of a relationship of responsibility, trust or power. Being exposed to intimate partner violence is sometimes considered a form of child maltreatment (WHO, 2014a). Child maltreatment is considered to be a global problem with serious long-term consequences; detection and response strategies are often hampered by a lack of data – especially in low- to middle-income countries, and the very complexity of the issues being addressed. Nonetheless, studies indicate up to a quarter of all adults having been physically abused as children, with 1 in 5 women and 1 in 13 men reporting abuse of a sexual nature as a child. It is estimated that annually more than 41,000 homicide deaths occur worldwide in children, with the overall extent of emotional abuse and neglect being substantial but difficult to estimate accurately. The consequences of maltreatment include depression, obesity, engaging in high-risk sexual behaviours, unintended pregnancy and alcohol and drug misuse. The recommended intervention approach is based on public health practices and principles and involves multi-sectoral collaboration in programmes designed to support parents and teach parenting skills. An important principle is that in child maltreatment, children are the victims and are never to blame for what has occurred. A closely associated issue, child soldiers, is dealt with further on in this chapter.

Elder abuse

As defined by the World Health Organization (2015a) elder abuse involves single or repeated acts, or failure to take action, occurring within any relationship where there is an expectation of trust, which causes harm or distress to an older person. Elder abuse constitutes a violation of human rights and may include physical, sexual, psychological, emotional abuse; financial and materials abuse; abandonment; neglect; and serious loss of dignity and respect. Between 4 and 6 per cent of older people report recent exposure to abuse and the health consequences range from serious physical injuries to long-term psychological damage. The prevalence of elder abuse is predicted to increase in the coming decades as many countries experience rapidly ageing populations; by 2025 it is predicted that the global population of people aged 60 years and above will reach 1.2 billion, more than double the 542 million reached in 1995. In response to concerns surrounding elder abuse, health services in many countries are developing and implementing prevention and response guidelines such as those recently disseminated by the Health Department of the State of Victoria in Australia (Victorian Health Department, 2012). The basic approach as set out in the Victorian guideline involves public health strategies to raise community awareness of elder abuse; empower older people to understand and exercise their legal, financial and social rights; engage professionals to identify and respond to elder abuse; and facilitate multi-agency support for people experiencing elder abuse.

Human trafficking

According to a report from the International Labor Organization (Besler, 2005) an estimated 2.5 million persons are being trafficked at any given time within countries or across national borders. More than half (1.4 million) are estimated to be victims of sexual exploitation and 1.1 million as victims of economic exploitation. Human trafficking is now considered to be the second largest criminal industry in the world, second to drug dealing and tied with illegal arms dealing, where profits are estimated to be as high as $31.6 billion (Besler, 2005). The UN Protocol to Prevent, Suppress and Punish Trafficking in Persons Especially Women and Children defines human trafficking as:

> the recruitment, transportation, transfer, harboring or receipt of persons, by means of threat or use of force or other forms of coercion, of abduction, of fraud, of deception, of the abuse of power or of a position of vulnerability or of the giving or receiving of payments or benefits to achieve the consent of a person having control over another person, for the purpose of exploitation.
>
> *(United Nations, 2000)*

Human trafficking or modern-day slavery can be categorized into seven different types (US Department of State, 2014a; 2014b):

a) *Sex trafficking* is when a person is coerced, forced and threatened to engage in commercial sex acts. Use of alcohol and drugs are usually involved as a means of controlling the victim or is used by the trafficked victim as a coping method.

b) *Child sex trafficking* is when a child (under the age of 18) is recruited, lured, transported, obtained or maintained to perform a commercial sex act regardless of whether force, coercion and fraud is used.

c) *Forced labour* also called 'labour trafficking' is when an individual has been recruited, transported, transferred and harbored and is forced to work by means of physical threats, deception, psychological coercion and abuse of the legal system. Migrant workers are vulnerable to this type of trafficking.

d) *Bonded labour or debt bondage* in some countries individuals, for example, in South Asia, are forced to work in servitude to pay off their ancestor's debts. Migrant workers who leave their country of origin by obtaining financial support from a labour agency may also contribute to debt bondage. Those who work under employment-based programs may have their legal status tied to their employer and may fear asking for rightful compensation for fear of being deported.

e) *Involuntary domestic servitude* is a form of human trafficking where an individual working for and living in a private residence is underpaid and basic benefits given to others are withheld such as having a day off.

f) *Forced child labour* is when a child is compelled to work for someone else's financial gains and the child is prevented from leaving.

g) *Unlawful recruitment and use of child soldiers* is the unlawful recruitment of children through force, coercion and deception by armed forces to be combatants or other forms of employment. Some children are abducted to become combatants while others are used for other purposes such as spies, cooks, messengers and servants. Young girls may be forced to marry or engage in sexual acts with male combatants.

Human trafficking laws

The Protocol to Prevent, Suppress and Punish Trafficking in Persons, was adopted by General Assembly Resolution 55/25. This protocol helped establish a legally binding global definition of human trafficking. In the United States the Trafficking Victims Protection Act of 2000 (TVPA) authorized the establishment of Trafficking In Persons (TIP) reporting. The TIP is used as a tool to engage foreign governments in discussion of anti-human trafficking reforms and determination of where resources are most needed. The ultimate goal of this US Government anti-trafficking policy is to free victims, prevent trafficking and bring traffickers to justice.

Health consequences of human trafficking

Although limited studies have addressed the physical, mental and sexual health consequences of trafficking, the available evidence shows that sexual exploitation is associated with violence and a range of serious health issues. Physical and sexual abuse has been reported before or during exploitation of female victims. Headache, back pain, fatigue, dizziness, stomach pain, pelvic pain and skin problems are the most commonly reported problems. According to Sabella (2011), victims of sex trafficking might also present with bald patches where their hair was pulled out, bruises, lacerations, scars, burns and bite marks. Sexually transmitted infections (STI) have also been reported but HIV infection data is only available from studies conducted in Nepal and India.

Trafficked victims who are forced to work under unfavorable environmental conditions may suffer from malnutrition, dehydration, exhaustion, heatstroke or stress, hypothermia, frostbite and respiratory and skin problems. Common psychological sequela found in trafficking victims, include post-traumatic stress disorder, suicidal ideation, depression, anxiety and addiction. Figure 19.1 depicts the health consequences of trafficking. Figure 19.1 depicts the health consequences of trafficking.

Nursing implications

Nurses in various clinical settings are in a vital position to help promote and fight against human trafficking by learning how to identify victims, make proper referrals, appropriately intervene

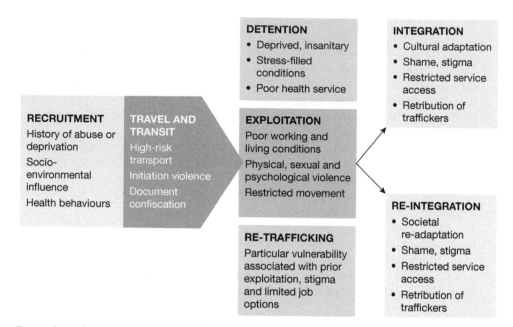

Figure 19.1 Influences on health and well-being at various stages of trafficking

Source: Reprinted from *Human trafficking and health: A conceptual model to inform policy, intervention and research*, 73, Cathy Zimmerman, Mazeda Hossain and Charlotte Watts, pp. 327–335, Copyright 2011, with permission from Elsevier.

and advocate for and provide care and support to post-trafficked victims. Nurse educators can help increase awareness about human trafficking by including the topic in the academic curriculum, which includes discussion about laws governing human trafficking, victim identification, referral process, how to respond safely if victims are identified and in-depth provision of care post-trafficking. *Caring for Trafficked Persons: Guidance for Health Providers* (Zimmerman & Borland, 2009) was developed to provide guidance in identifying, diagnosing and intervening to help trafficking victims.

Armed conflict

Armed conflict, which includes the popular notion of 'war', can be approached as a form of collective violence. While medicine, through its longstanding association with the military and the state, has often been involved in responding to the health effects of warfare, public health responses to collective violence are a relatively recent development (Krug *et al.*, 2002). In countries such as the US and Australia, exposure to collective violence in the form of warfare is typically limited to members of the armed forces their families, friends and close colleagues. We might send our army, navy and airforce personnel off to war, but only a small proportion of the population of our countries face the consequences of direct exposure to armed conflict. The experience is very different for people living in war zones.

The application of public health perspectives to collective violence led to the identification of risk factors for violent conflicts, including increasing inequality, rapidly changing demographic composition, lack of democratic processes, political instability and severe economic decline (Krug *et al.*, 2002, p. 220). The health consequences of living in war-affected communities include; increased mortality (e.g. increased infant mortality); morbidity and disability resulting from the combination of weapons-related deaths; communicable (e.g. decline in immunization coverage; increased environmental hazards such as water and air pollution) and non-communicable diseases (e.g. reduced access to health services) as social and health infrastructure degrades (Krug *et al.*, 2002, p. 222). If armed conflict can have negative consequences for military personnel, civilian populations in war-torn areas are especially vulnerable, often facing lack of food and water, malnutrition, increased risk of communicable diseases, precarious environmental conditions, severe psychosocial distress and little or no access to health care (Krug *et al.*, 2002, pp. 222–228). For many civilians caught up in armed conflict, the initial experience of living in a war zone can be followed – often for years, by that of being a refugee or internally displaced person. Displaced populations have been shown to have greatly increased morbidity and mortality rates (Krug *et al.*, 2002, 225).

One important group to be considered in relation to the health implications of armed conflict is child soldiers. Child soldiers are usually defined as children under 18 years of age who are recruited formally or informally as combatants, non-combatant military personnel, suicide bombers, human shields, messengers, spies or for sexual purposes. The number of child soldiers has been estimated to be at least 300,000. In addition to the risks of direct involvement in combat (i.e. death, loss of hearing, sight and limbs), the longer term health consequences for child combatants often relate to the frailty of their bodies and the types of duties undertaken, including injuries from carrying heavy loads, malnutrition, infectious diseases and for girls especially, sexually transmitted diseases. Following demobilization, child soldiers are likely to need medical-psychiatric and psychological treatment for ongoing psychosocial problems, including symptoms of post-traumatic stress syndrome and other forms of chronic anxiety, regressed behaviour, poor impulse control and increased substance abuse (Krug *et al.*, 2002).

Secondary victims of violence

An often overlooked group in current debates surrounding victimization and mental health includes the secondary victims of violence. While the numbers of people involved in primary and secondary victimization globally are significant, the emotional impact on secondary victims – the families, friends and colleagues of primary victims is poorly understood (Morrall, Hazelton & Shackleton, 2011; Morrall *et al.*, 2013). In addition, secondary victimhood can be extended to take account of the professionals who attend – in the case of homicide and other violent crimes – the crime scenes, investigate the crimes and provide support to the families, often over lengthy periods of time.

The secondary victims of violence may comprise 'a substantial part of the population' (Armour, 2002). Writing in relation to the United States, Hertz, Prothrow-Stith and Chery (2005) calculated that in excess of 16 million people were affected by homicide alone. This figure is comprised of 5 million adults who had experienced the murder of an immediate family member, 6.6 million people who had experienced the murder of a relative other than an immediate family member and 4.8 million who had experienced the murder of a close friend. If the family and friends of the perpetrator and the professionals who investigate the crime and provide support to the victim's family are also included, the scope of secondary victimhood extends much further.

While the victims of crime are nowadays more directly incorporated into the criminal justice systems of countries such as the United States, Australia and Britain (Karmen, 2009), the specific needs of secondary victims are often overlooked or treated insensitively, which can contribute to ongoing re-traumatization (Morrall *et al.*, 2013). In Australia, the Victims of Crime Assistance League (New South Wales) have captured the dilemma often faced by primary and secondary victims of crime: 'They say that responses from supposed professional workers in the field, the police, courts and comments and reactions from friends, family and others, often just astound and re-victimize them in their grief' (Victims of Crime Assistance League, 2013).

The health impact of secondary victims have often been understood and treated using a framework analogous to (sudden) bereavement (Morrall *et al.*, 2011). However, it has been argued that the intensity of bereavement experienced by the loss of a loved one through homicide or some other form of violent crime, can be distinguished from other types of grieving, such as those associated with the loss of human life from illness and accidents (Malone, 2007). Moreover, the suffering experienced by the secondary victims may be compounded if the violent crime has been sadistic and/or sexualized in nature and by the often prolonged procedures by which a perpetrator is (or is not) apprehended and brought to trial, and the often lengthy processes of trial, appeal and re-trial. Under such circumstances feelings of 'unfinished business' or 'lack of closure' may remain for years; the grieving process may also be further complicated by the intrusiveness of the media (Morrall *et al.*, 2013).

Hertz, Prothrow and Chery (2005) have suggested that the usual therapeutic approach to bereavement is inadequate for secondary victimhood in that it may not capture the intensity of the homicide survivor's experience, some aspects of which present as similar to the symptoms of post-traumatic stress disorder. In Britain, the National Institute for Health and Clinical Excellence (2005) guidelines for the management of post-traumatic stress disorder includes case studies of people who have experienced PTSD after the unnatural or sudden deaths of close relatives. The emotional intensity of the bereavement experience in such circumstances would likely approximate the unrelenting emotional agony described by many people who have lost a loved one to a violent crime (Morrall *et al.*, 2011; 2013).

While much of the literature on secondary victimization addresses the experiences and needs of the immediate family and close associates of primary victims, there is growing awareness that the emotional anguish experienced by individuals can also extend to neighborhoods, communities and even countries (in the case of the latter this might be conceptualized as tertiary victimhood), especially in the aftermath of atrocities such as 9/11, MH17 and attack on Atatürk Airport.

Mental health and exposure to violence

Recognition of the health impacts of violence have led to violence being declared a leading worldwide public health problem (Krug *et al.*, 2002). Turning to mental health it has been suggested that the mistreatment of humans by other humans may be the most important illness-causing factor (Middleton *et al.*, 2014). Much of what has been covered in this chapter falls within the category of interpersonal violence and it is perhaps not surprising that to date, mental health promotion and prevention strategies targeting violence have concentrated on this level of engagement.

If violence is pathogenic for mental illness, it has also been suggested that various types of violence are in principle modifiable and that significant reductions in these could result in reduced rates of mental illness (Scott *et al.*, 2013). For example, it has been suggested that bullying is a significant modifiable risk factor for mental illness (Kozlowska & Durheim, 2013; Scott, *et al.*, 2013) and as outlined above, a range of effective prevention initiatives have been developed in response to this form of interpersonal violence. At the same time, it is important to note how changing patterns of violence may imply varying etiological factors for mental illness. With the rapid emergence of cyberbullying, the main platform of intervention is shifting from the school environment to multiple sites within which electronic communication devices can be used, both within and beyond the school (Scott *et al.*, 2013).

While violence prevention can be considered an emerging public health field, a range of evidence-based practice innovations have been developed in the last two decades. Kress, Noonan, Freire, Marr and Olsen (2012) outline a list of what they consider to be the top 20 violence and injury practice innovations since the establishment of the National Center for Injury Prevention and Control (NCIPC) in the United States in 1992. Included in the list are initiatives designed to connect and train practitioners using online resources for violence education and training (e.g. the VetoViolence program); youth violence prevention strategies (e.g. Urban Networks to Increase Thriving Youth – UNITY); intimate partner violence primary prevention programs (e.g. Domestic Violence Prevention Enhancement and Leaderships Through Alliances program – DELTA); approaches to directly engage boys and men in the prevention of violence against women (e.g. Men of Strength Clubs; Men Stopping Violence); and strategies for preventing child maltreatment (e.g. Positive Parenting Program – Triple P).

Kress *et al.* (2012), also outline a modified version of Cohen and Swift's (1999) Spectrum of Prevention, suggesting its applicability as a comprehensive framework for building vertically and horizontally integrated violence prevention interventions.

Following this approach, effective violence prevention initiatives would seek to:

1   strengthen individual knowledge and skills in preventing violence and promoting safety;
2   promote community education using health promotion and safety information;
3   educate providers to transmit health and safety skills and knowledge to others;
4   foster coalitions and networks addressing health and safety concerns and actions;
5   change organizational practices by adopting regulations and shaping norms to improve health and safety;
6   influence policy and legislation through strategies to shape process and outcomes; and
7   develop infrastructure to build data systems, organizational capacity and resources to support interventions.

It is clear that in the last few decades a much greater emphasis has been placed on understanding and responding to the relationship between exposure to violence and mental health problems. However, following Kress *et al.* (2012) our efforts so far ought to be considered as a firm beginning from which future innovations will be developed. In terms of responses to interpersonal violence much remains to be done in developed countries such as the United States, Australia and Britain. In many parts of the developing world violence remains endemic and is likely intensifying. Moreover, as the MH17 tragedy reminds us, violence can no longer be regionally contained. Given the recent upsurge in violence in the Eastern Ukraine, Iraq, Syria, Yemen, Somalia and many other regions globally, the need for effective interventions for responding to the mental health implications of exposure to violence has never been greater and will likely continue to increase in the coming years.

Summary

In this chapter we have considered the consequences for mental health of being exposed to various forms of violence and how these might be addressed using health promotion and illness prevention strategies. While much of the discussion has involved circumstances in our own countries, we have sought to contextualize these globally. In considering the health and mental health impacts of violence, the chapter has sought to address that which occurs in the home, the classroom, the workplace – in peaceful communities and those affected by armed conflict; to think about violence and its consequences for both individuals and collections of people;

and in relation to those who are the primary and secondary victims of violence. It is clear that we are never far from violent acts – whether these are being watched on television or experienced first-hand. Public health responses to the health and mental health consequences of violence are a relatively recent development that will likely grow in importance in the coming decades. Such developments will both challenge and provide many leadership opportunities for mental health nurses.

References

Alexander, C. & Fraser, J. (2004). Occupational violence in an Australian health care setting: Implications for managers. *Journal of Healthcare Management, 49* (6), 377–390.

Armour, M. (2002). Experiences of covictims of homicide. *Trauma, Violence & Abuse, 3* (2), 109–124.

ASIS Healthcare Security Council (2011). *Managing disruptive behavior and workplace violence in health care.* Alexandria, VA: ASIS International.

Barboza, G., Schiamberg, L., Oehmke, J., Korzeniewski, S., Post, L. & Heraux, C. (2009). Individual characteristics and multiple contexts of adolescent bullying: Ecological perspective. *Journal of Youth and Adolescence, 38* (1), 101–121.

Bauer, N., Herrenkohl, T., Lozano, P., Rivara, F., Hill, K. & Hawkins, J. (2006). Childhood bullying and exposure to intimate partner violence. *Pediatrics, 118* (2), 235–242.

Beck, U. (1992). *Risk Society: Towards a new modernity.* London: Sage.

Besler, P. (2005). *Forced labour and human trafficking: Estimating the profits.* Geneva: International Labour Organization.

Beynon, C., Gutmanis, I., Tutty, L., Wathen, C. & MacMillian, H. (2012). Why physicians and nurses ask (or don't) about partner violence: A qualitative analysis, *BMC Public Health 12*, 473.

Black, M., Basile, K., Breiding, M., Smith, S., Walters, M., Merrick, M., Chen, J. & Stevens, M. (2011). *The National intimate partner and sexual violence survey (NISVS): 2010 summary report.* Atlanta, GA: National Center for Injury Prevention and Control, Centers for Disease Control and Prevention.

Bonomi, A., Anderson, M., Rivara, F. & Thompson, R. (2007). Health outcomes in women with physical and sexual intimate partner violence exposure. *Journal of Women's Health, 16*, 987–997.

Borrowsky, I., Taliaferro, L. & McMorris, B. (2013). Suicidal thinking and behavior among youth involved in verbal and social bullying: Risk and protective factors. *Journal of Adolescent Health 53*, S4–S12.

Breiding, M.J., Basile, K.C., Smith, S.G., Black, M.C. & Mahendra, R.R. (2015). *Intimate partner violence surveillance: Uniform definitions and recommended data elements, version 2.0.* Atlanta (GA): National Center for Injury Prevention and Control, Centers for Disease Control and Prevention.

Brigham and Women's Hospital. (2014). Female genital cutting: statistics. Retrieved 25 May 2016 from www.brighamandwomens.org/Departments_and_Services/obgyn/services/africanwomenscenter/research.aspx.

Cohen, L. & Swift, S. (1999). The spectrum of prevention: Developing a comprehensive approach to injury prevention, *Injury Prevention, 5*, 203–207.

Coles, J., Koritsas, S., Boyle, M. & Stanley, J. (2007). GPs, violence and work performance: 'Just part of the job?' *Australian Family Physician, 36* (3), 189–191.

Cook, C., Williams, K., Geuvarra, N., Kim, T., Sadek, S. (2010). Predictors of bullying and victimization in childhood and adolescence: A meta-analytic investigation, *School of Psychology Quarterly, 25* (2), 65–83.

Crilly, J., Chaboyer, W. & Creedy, D. (2004). Violence towards emergency department nurses by patients. *Accident & Emergency Nursing, 12* (2), 67–73.

Devries, K., Mak, J., Bacchus, L., Child, J., Falder, G., Petzold, M., Astbury, J. & Watts, C. (2013). Intimate partner violence and incident depressive symptoms and suicide attempts: A systematic review of longitudinal studies, *PLoS Med, 10* (5), e10011439.

Dorkenoo, E. (2012). Female genital mutilation: Report of a research methodological workshop on estimating the prevalence of FGM in England and Wales Workshop. London: Equality Now. Retrieved 25 May 2016 from www.equalitynow.org/sites/default/files/UK_FGM_Workshop_Report.pdf.

Elston, M.A., Gabe, J., Denney, D., Lee, R. & O'Beirne, M. (2002). Violence against doctors: A medical(ised) problem? The case of the National Health Service general practitioners. *Sociology of Health & Illness, 24* (5), 575–598.

Farrell, G. & Cubit, K. (2005). Nurses under threat: A comparison of 28 aggression management programs. *International Journal of Mental Health Nursing, 14* (1), 44–53.

Feekes, M., Pijpers, F. & Verloove-Vanhorick, P. (2004). Bullying behavior and associations with psychosomatic complaints and depression in victims. *The Journal of Pediatrics*, *144* (1), 17–22.

Fung, A.L. & Rain, A. (2012). Peer victimization as a risk factor for schizotypal personality in childhood and adolescence. *Journal of Personality Disorders*, *26* (3), 428–434.

Gini, G. (2007). Association between bullying behaviors, psychosomatic complaints, emotional and behavioural problems. *Journal of Pediatrics and Child Health*, *44* (9), 492–497.

Guruge, S. (2012). Nurse's role in caring for women experiencing intimate partner violence in the Sri Lankan context. *International Scholarly Research Network*, 1–9. Doi: 10.5402/2012/486273.

Harris, A. (1989). Violence in general practice. *British Medical Journal*, *298* (6666), 63–64.

Hertz, M., Prothrow-Stith, D. & Chery, C. (2005). Homicide survivors: Research and practice implications. *American Journal of Preventative Medicine*, *29* (5S2), 288–295.

Hess, K., Javanbakht, M., Brown, J., Weiss, R., Hsu, P. & Gorbach, P. (2012). Intimate partner violence and sexually transmitted infections among young adult women, *Sexual Transmitted Diseases*, *39* (5), 1–12.

Hills, D. & Joyce, C. (2013). A review of research on the prevalence, antecedents, consequences and prevention of workplace aggression in clinical medical practice. *Aggression and Violent Behaviour*, *18*, 554–569.

Hobbs, F.D. (1991). Violence in general practice: A survey of general practitioners' views. *British Medical Journal*, *302* (6772), 329–332.

International Council of Nurses. (2009). Violence: A worldwide epidemic. *Nursing Matters*. Retrieved 5 August 2015 from: www.icn.ch/images/stories/documents/publications/fact-sheets/19k-FS-Violence.pdf.

International Labour Office. (2002). *Framework guidelines for addressing workplace violence in the health sector*. Geneva: ILO.

Iverson, K., Gradus, J., Resick, P., Suvak, M., Smith, K. & Monson, C. (2011). Cognitive-behavior therapy for PTSD and depression symptoms reduces risk for future intimate partner violence among interpersonal trauma survivors. *Journal of Consulting and Clinical Psychology*, *79* (2), 193–202.

Jannone, L. (2011). Community services for victims of interpersonal violence. *Nursing Clinics of Northern America*, *46* (4), 471–476.

Johnson, D., Zlotnick, C. & Perez, S. (2011). Cognitive-behavioral treatment for PTSD in residents of battered women's shelters: Results of a randomized clinical trial. *Journal of Consulting and Clinical Psychology*, *79* (4), 542–551.

Karakut, G. & Silver, K. (2013). Emotional abuse in intimate partner relationships: The role of gender and age. *Violence Victimization*, *28* (5), 804–821.

Karmen, A. (2009). *Crime victims: An introduction to victimology* (7th edn). London: Wadsworth.

Kennedy, M.P. (2005). Violence in emergency departments: Under-reported, unconstrained, and unconscionable. *Medical Journal of Australia*, *183*, 362–365.

Kizilhan, J.I. (2011). Impact of psychological disorders after female genital mutilation among Kurdish girls in Northern Iraq. *European Journal of Psychiatry*, *25* (2), 92–100.

Knapp, R. (2011). Impact of interpersonal violence on health care. *The Nursing Clinics of Northern America*, *46* (4), 465–70.

Kozlowska, K. & Durheim, E. (2013). Is bullying in children and adolescents a modifiable risk factor for mental illness? *Australian and New Zealand Journal of Psychiatry*, *48* (3), 288–289.

Kress, H., Noonan, R., Freire, K., Marr, A. & Olson, A. (2012). Top 20 violence and injury practice innovations since 1992. *Journal of Safety Research*, *43*, 257–263.

Krug, E.G., Dalhberg, L.L., Mercy, J.A., Zwi, A.B. & Lozan, R. (2002). (eds). *World report on violence and health*. Geneva: World Health Organization.

Lam, L.T. (2002). Aggression exposure and mental health among nurses. *Australian e-Journal for the Advancement of Mental Health*, *1* (2), 1–12.

Lauritsen, J. & Rezey, M. (2013). Bureau of Justice Statistics technical report: *Measuring the prevalence of crime with the national crime victimization* survey (Rep. No. NCJ 241656). Retrieved 25 May 2016 from www.bjs.gov/content/pub/pdf/mpcncvs.pdf.

Lynch, J., Appleboam, R. & McQuillan, P. (2003). Survey of abuse and violence by patients and relatives towards intensive care staff. *Anaesthesia*, *59* (9), 838–839.

Lyneham, J. (1999). Violence in NSW emergency departments. *Australian Nursing Journal*, *2* (2), 22–25.

McKinnon, B. & Cross, W. (2008). Occupational violence and assault in mental health nursing: A scoping project for a Victorian Mental Health Service. *International Journal of Mental Health Nursing*, *17* (1), 9–17.

McLuhan, M. (1964). *Understanding the media: The extensions of man.* New York: McGraw-Hill.

Magin, P.J., Adams, J. & Joy, E. (2007). Occupational violence in general practice: Internatitonal and Australian perspectives. *Australian Family Physician, 36* (11), 955–957.

Magin, P.J., Adams, J., Sibbritt, D., Joy, E. & Ireland, M. (2005). *Experiences of occupational violence in Australian urban general practice: A cross-sectional study of GPs. Medical Journal of Australia, 183* (7), 352–356

Magin, P.J., Adams, J., Ireland, M., Joy, E., Heaney, S. & Darab, S. (2006). The response of general practitioners to the threat of violence in their practices: Results from a qualitative study. *Family Practice, 23* (3), 273–278.

Magin, P.J., Adams, J., Sibbritt, D., Joy, E. & Ireland, M. (2008). Effects of occupational violence on Australian general practitioners' provision of home visits and after-hours care: A cross-sectional study. *Journal of Evaluation in Clinical Practice, 14* (2), 336–342.

Malone, L. (2007). In the aftermath: Listening to people bereaved by homicide. *Journal of Community and criminal Justice, 54* (4), 383–393.

Mayers-Adams, N. (2008). School violence: Bullying behaviors and the psychosocial school environment in middle schools. *Children and Schools, 30*, 211–221.

Middleton, W., Stavropoulos, P., Dorahy, M., Kruger, C., Lewis-Fernandez, R., Martinez-Taboas, A., Sar, V. & Brand, B. (2014). Institutional abuse and social silence: An emerging global problem. *Australian and New Zealand Journal of Psychiatry, 48* (1), 22–25.

Miller, E., McCauley, H., Tancredi, D., Decker, M., Anderson, H. & Silverman, J. (2014). Recent reproductive coercion and unintended pregnancy among female family planning clients, *Contraception, 89* (2), 122–128.

Morrall, P., Hazelton, M. & Shackleton, W. (2011). Homicide and health: The suffering of secondary victims and the role of the mental health nurse. *Mental Health Practice, 15* (3), 14–19.

Morrall, P., Hazelton, M. & Shackleton, W. (2013). Psychotherapy and social responsibility: The challenging case of homicide. *Psychotherapy and Politics International, 11* (2), 102–113.

Mulango, P., McAndrew, S. & Martin, C.H. (2014). Crossing borders: Discussing the evidence relating to the mental health needs of women exposed to female genital mutilation. *International Journal of Mental Health Nursing, 23*(4), 296–305.

Nansel, T., Overpeck, M., Ruan, W., Scheidt, P., Simmons-Morton, B. & Pilla, R. (2001). Bullying behaviors among US Youth: Prevalence and association with psychosocial adjustment. *Journal of the American Medical Association, 258*, 2094–2100.

National Institute for Health and Clinical Excellence. (2005). *Post-traumatic stress disorder: The management of PTSD in adults and children in primary and secondary care.* London: NICE.

O'Connell, B., Young, J., Brooks, J., Hutchings, J. & Lofthouse, J. (2000). Nurses' perceptions of the nature and frequency of aggression in general ward settings and high dependency areas. *Journal of Clinical Nursing, 9* (4), 602–610.

Ogundipe, O.K., Aladesanmi, T., Adigun, A.I., Taiwo, O., Etonyeaku, A.C., Ojo, O.E. & Obimakinde, S.O. (2010). Violence in the emergency department: A multicentre survey of nurses' perceptions. *Injury Prevention, 16* (supp 1), A26.

Olweus, D. (1993). *Bullying at school: What we know and what we can do.* Cambridge, MA: Blackwell.

Olweus, D. (1994). Bullying at school: Basic facts and effects of a school-based intervention program. *Journal of Child Psychology and Psychiatry and Allied Disciplines, 35*, 1171–1190.

Papadakaki, M., Petriduo, E., Kogevinas, M. & Lionis, C. (2013). Measuring the effectiveness of an intensive IPV training program offered to Greek general practitioners and residents of general practice, *BMC Medical Education, 13*, 46.

Pich, J. & Kable, A. (2014). Patient-related violence against nursing staff working in emergency departments: A systematic review. *JBI Database of Systematic Reviews and Implementation Reports, 12* (9), 398–453.

Pich, J., Hazelton, M., Sundin, D. & Kable, A. (2010). Patient related violence against emergency department nurses. *Nursing and Health Sciences, 12*, 268–274.

Pickett, K.E. & Wilkinson R.G. (2009). Greater equality and better health. *BMJ 339*, b4320.

Pinker, S. (2011). *The better angels of our nature: Why violence has declined.* London: Viking.

Ramirez, M., Lyman, R., Jobe-Shields, L., Preethy, G., Dougherty, R., Daniels, A., Ghose, S., Huang, L. & Delpin-Rittman, M. (2014). Trauma-focussed cognitive behavioural therapy: Assessing the evidence. *Psychiatric Services, 65* (5), 591–602.

Rivers, I. & Noret, N. (2013). Potential suicide ideation and its association with observing bullying at school. *Journal of Adolescent Health, 53* (1), S32–S36.

Royal College of Nursing. (2005). *Violence: The short-term management of disturbed/violent behaviour in in-patient psychiatric settings and emergency departments.* Clinical Practice Guidelines commissioned by the National Institute for Health and Clinical Excellence (NICE). London: NICE.

Sabella, D. (2011). The role of the nurse in combating human trafficking. *American Journal of Nursing, 111* (2), 28–37.

Sabri, B., Bolyard, R., McFadgion, A., Stokman, J., Lucea, M., Callwood, G., Coverston, C. & Campbell, J. (2013). Intimate partner violence, depression, PTSD and use of mental health resources among ethnically diverse black women, *Social Work in Health Care, 52* (4), 351–369.

Salmivalli, C. & Pokisparta, E. (2012). Making bullying prevention a priority in Finnish schools: the KiVa antibullying program. *New Directions for Youth Development, 133*, 41–53.

Schroeder, B., Messina, A., Schroeder, D., Good, K., Barto, S., Saylor, J. & Masiello, M. (2012) The implementation of a statewide bullying prevention program: preliminary findings from the field and the importance of coalitions. *Health Promotion Practice, 13* (4), 489–495.

Scott, J., Moore, S., Sly, P. & Norman, R. (2013). Bullying in children and adolescents: A modifiable risk factor for mental illness. *Australian and New Zealand Journal of Psychiatry, 48* (3), 209–212.

Smith, P.K., Mahdavi, J., Carvalho, M., Fisher, S., Russell, S. & Tippet, N. (2008). Cyberbullying: Its nature and impact in secondary school pupils. *Journal of Child Psychology and Psychiatry and Allied Disciplines, 49*, 376–385.

Stene, L., Jacobsen, G., Dyb, G., Tverdal, A. & Schei, B. (2013). Intimate partner violence and cardio-vascular rick in women: A population-based cohort study in women. *Journal of Women's Health, 22* (3), 250–258.

Stone, T., McMillan, M. & Hazelton, M. (2015). Back to swear one: A review of English language literature on swearing and cursing in Western Health settings. *Aggression and Violent Behavior, 25* (Part A), 65–74.

Tufts, K.A., Clements, P.T. & Karlowicz, K.A. (2009). Integrating intimate partner violence content across curricula: Developing a new generation of nurse educators, *Nurse Education Today, 29* (1), 40–47.

Twemlow, S., Fonagy, P. & Sacco, F. (2004). The role of the bystander in the social architecture of bullying and violence in schools and communities. *Annals of the New York Academy of Sciences, 1036* (1), 215–232.

Ulloa, E. & Hammett, J. (2016). The effect of gender and perpetrator-victim role on mental health outcomes and risk behaviors associated with intimate partner violence. *Journal of Interpersonal Violence*, 31 (7), 1184–1207.

UNAIDS, UNDP, UNECA, UNESCO, UNFPA, UNHCHR, UNHCR, UNICEF, UNIFEM & WHO. (2008). *Eliminating female genital mutilation: An interagency statement.* Geneva: WHO.

UNICEF. (2005). *Female genital mutilation/female genital cutting: A statistical report.* New York: UNICEF.

United Nations. (2000). Protocol to prevent, suppress and punish trafficking in persons especially women and children, supplementing the United Nations convention against transnational organized crime. Ratified by UN General Assembly Resolution 55/25 (15 November 2000). Retrieved 24 May 2016 from www.ohchr.org/EN/ProfessionalInterest/Pages/Protocol TraffickingInPersons.aspx.

United Nations General Assembly on Sustainable Development Goals. (2014). Goal 16. Retrieved 7 July 2016 from https://sustainabledevelopment.un.org/content/documents/1579SDG%20Proposal.pdf.

US Congress. (1996). US Title 118, Part 1, Paragraph 116: Female genital mutilation. Retrieved 25 May 2016 from www.law.cornell.edu/uscode/pdf/uscode18/lii_usc_TI_18_PA_I_CH_7_SE_116.pdf.

US Department of State. (2014a). *Diplomacy in Action, Trafficking in Persons Report 2014.* Washington, DC: US Department of State. Retrieved July 24, 2016 from www.state.gov/j/tip/rls/tiprpt/index.htm.

US Department of State. (2014b). *Diplomacy in Action. US Laws in Trafficking in Persons 2014.* Washington, DC: US Department of State. Retrieved July 24, 2016 from www.state.gov/j/tip/laws.

Victims of Crime Assistance League. (2013). Responses to murder and suspicious death. Retrieved 15 March, 2013, from http://vocal.org.au/crime-types-3/murder-suspicious-death/criminal-suspicious-death/.

Victorian Department of Human Services. (2003). *Industry standard for the prevention and management of occupational violence and aggression in Victoria's mental health services.* Melbourne: Department of Human Services.

Victorian Health Department. (2012). *Elder abuse prevention and response guidelines for action 2012–14. Health Priorities Framework, 2012–2022.* Melbourne: Victorian Health Department.

Vloeberghs, E., Knipscheer, J., van der Kwaak, A., Naleie, Z. & van den Muijsenbergh, M. (2011). *Veiled pain: A study in the Netherlands on the psychological, social and relational consequences of female genital mutilation.* Uthrech: Pharos.

Wand, T. & Coulson, K. (2006). Zero Tolerance: A policy in conflict with current opinion on aggression and violence management in health care. *Australasian Emergency Nursing Journal, 9* (4), 163–170.

Wilkinson. R. & Pickett, K. (2009). *The spirit level: Why more equal societies almost always do better.* London: Allen Lane.

Williams, J., Ghandour, R. & Kub, J. (2008). Female perpetration of violence in heterosexual intimate relationship: Adolescence through adulthood. *Trauma Violence Abuse, 9* (4), 227–249.

World Health Organization. (2012) *Understanding and addressing violence against women: Human Trafficking.* Retrieved 6 August 2015 from http://apps.who.int/iris/bitstream/10665/77394/1/WHO_RHR_12.42_eng.pdf?ua=1.

World Health Organization. (2014a). *Child maltreatment.* Fact sheet No. 150. Retrieved 6 August 2015 from www.who.int/mediacentre/factsheet/fs150/en/.

World Health Organization. (2014b). *Global status report on violence prevention.* Geneva: WHO.

World Health Organization. (2015a). *Elder abuse.* Fact sheet No. 357. Retrieved 6 August 2015 from www.who.int/mediacentre/factsheet/fs357/en/#.

World Health Organization. (2015b). *Sexual and reproductive health: Female genital mutilation and other harmful practices.* Retrieved 25 May 2016 from www.who.int/reproductivehealth/topics/fgm/overview_fgm_research/en/.

World Health Organization. (2016). *Violence against women.* Fact sheet No. 239. Retrieved 24 May 2016 from www.who.int/mediacentre/factsheets/fs239/en/.

Zimmerman, C. & Borland, R. (2009). (eds). *Caring for trafficked persons: Guidance for health providers.* Geneva: International Organization for Migration.

20

EVIDENCE-BASED MENTAL HEALTH PRACTICE IN A GLOBAL CONTEXT

Steven Pryjmachuk

Introduction

Evidence-based practice (EBP) is one of the six cross-cutting themes of the World Health Organization's *Comprehensive Mental Health Action Plan* (World Health Organization (WHO), 2013). This fact should not be surprising to those of us in the developed world who are involved in mental health research, education and practice since it has been a principle guiding the way in which we work for several decades. When thinking globally, however, it is important for us in the developed world to remember that our perspectives on EBP are framed by certain advantages – well-funded health, research and education facilities in particular – that persons in the developing world do not necessarily enjoy. Consequently, while the principal aim of this chapter is to examine the role that EBP can play in identifying and delivering effective, patient-centred mental health care, taking a *global* rather than Western or developed-world perspective also necessitates some discussion of the difficulties that our colleagues in less-developed countries might face when trying to implement EBP.

This chapter is not intended to be a manual on 'how to do EBP'. Instead, it focuses on a conceptual exploration of EBP (the theory) and a critical discussion of the processes and methods involved in carrying it out (the practice) so that those familiar and unfamiliar with EBP can make a judgement about its value to mental health care. Some economic, political, cultural and philosophical challenges that emerge when EBP's global applicability is considered are highlighted. Any reader eager to learn more about EBP is encouraged to follow up on the primary sources (articles, websites and other resources) cited within the text.

What is evidence-based practice?

EBP in health care has its roots in evidence-based medicine, a field pioneered in the 1960s and 1970s by the British epidemiologist Archie Cochrane (who the Cochrane Collaboration is named after) and later by Canadian physician David Sackett. The most widely known definition of evidence-based medicine is from Sackett and his colleagues: 'the conscientious, explicit and judicious use of current best evidence in making decisions about the care of individual patients' (Sackett, Rosenberg, Gray, Haynes & Richardson, 1996, p. 71). They add: 'it requires a bottom up approach that integrates the best external evidence with individual clinical expertise and patients' choice' (Sackett *et al.*, p. 72).

While originating in medicine, the definition by Sackett *et al.* (1996) is applicable to most practice-based disciplines, which explains why it has been embraced by all health care disciplines. Evidence-based mental health practice, for example, could easily be defined as the 'conscientious, explicit, and judicious use of current best evidence in making decisions about the *mental health* care of individuals'.

The definition by Sackett *et al.* (1996) makes it clear that EBP is intrinsically connected to the notion of *clinical decision-making*; indeed, one simple way of conceptualizing EBP is to see it as a framework for effective clinical decision-making. To understand EBP – and thus clinical decision-making – key elements require deconstruction.

First, the evidence is expected to be *current* and *best*. On the surface *current* simply implies that it is the most recent evidence that should be considered, but the most recent evidence may not be available or accessible both for benign and for more malevolent reasons. That *best* evidence is required opens questions about what is 'best' and according to whose standards? Moreover, the use of this best evidence needs to be *conscientious*, *explicit* and *judicious*, which implies that there is a moral ('conscientious') element to EBP, that the process should be transparent and open to scrutiny ('explicit'), and that higher-order cognitive skills ('judicious') are required. Second, EBP is about the care of *individual* patients, which implies that what is best in terms of evidence for one patient or service user may not necessarily be best for another. Finally, and perhaps most importantly, practitioners should not be restricted to any particular source of evidence; indeed, EBP works best when the evidence is triangulated from a variety of sources.

Sources of evidence

From the perspective of Sackett *et al.* (1996), there are three principal evidence sources: (1) external evidence; (2) the expertise of practitioners; and (3) the patient/service user perspective.

External evidence essentially means the scientific or *research* evidence. Research is especially important in practice-based disciplines like nursing because it is the means by which theory and practice are reconciled and it is the medium through which knowledge develops (Pryjmachuk, 1996). However, while important, research evidence alone is insufficient to drive EBP because it has to be interpreted by the person using it (the nurse or health care practitioner) so that its contextual relevance to a particular clinical situation or patient/service user can be determined.

From a nursing perspective, clinical expertise can be seen as the internalised, intuitive application of integrated theoretical and practical knowledge (Benner, 1984). An understanding of research is a necessary component of clinical expertise because it is difficult to become expert without the ability to reconcile or integrate theory and practice. Moreover, while clinical experience is an aspect of clinical expertise, it is important to note that the two are not synonymous in that a practitioner can be experienced yet not expert (McHugh & Lake, 2010).

Regarding the patient/service-user perspective, the rise of consumerism and increasing access to information sources like the internet has empowered developed-world populations to challenge the paternalism that has traditionally been associated with health care provision. In mental health care, the 'recovery' approach has had a particularly significant impact in shifting the balance of power from professionals to patients/service users to the point that the focus now is on what practitioners do *with* patients/service users rather than what they do *to* them. Recovery is an approach that embraces concepts as varied as hope, choice, independence, diversity, eclecticism and community (Shepherd, Boardman & Slade, 2008). It requires that practitioners put patients/service users and their significant others at the heart of decision-making; indeed, *shared* decision-making is an essential element of recovery (Warren, 2012).

To outline the importance of shared decision-making to EBP, and the need to consider more than just the research evidence when applying EBP, consider the following. When faced with an 'uncertainty' in practice, health care practitioners have a number of ways of responding or making a decision. They can simply guess or apply some random intervention, but in situations that can be life-or-death this is an incredibly risky strategy. They can assume that there is, in fact, no uncertainty and do what has always been done in these circumstances, acting ritualistically and without question. However, while this option may be less risky than merely guessing and while it may work in areas where there is low uncertainty (for example, using *clinical guidelines*), the downside is that acting ritualistically assumes that patients/service users are homogenous and that there are incontrovertible explanations for their behaviour. As a third option, they could make a more informed decision using the principles of EBP.

Consider the case (Burrow, 2011) of an agitated elderly woman with dementia wandering around her neighbourhood and shouting out unintelligible words, a situation her husband finds particularly distressing. An inexpert ('guessing') decision might mean that the nurse does nothing but offer reassurance to the husband because she or he simply sees the person's behaviour as an inevitable consequence of dementia. Medicating the person would be an example of ritualised care; a somewhat ironic situation given the recent evidence suggesting that the use of anti-psychotic medications to control agitation in dementia is more likely to do harm than good (Huybrechts *et al.*, 2012). An EBP approach, however, would consider the nurse's expertise, the research evidence and the patient/service-user's perspective as well as that of her husband such that an *expert* nurse might know that hunger or pain in people with dementia might present in this way and that, as a result, the patient should be assessed appropriately.

Evidence hierarchies

It is at this point that we encounter our first major issue in EBP, one that concerns the value put on the specific types of evidence – i.e., how the 'best' evidence is determined. Tables 20.1 and 20.2 outline two examples of 'hierarchies of evidence'.

In these two examples, certain types of evidence seem to be given more importance than others. Two less obvious, but perhaps more important, observations can be made. Patient/service-user perspectives are lacking from these hierarchies, and expert opinion appears at the bottom in both. This implies that scientific research evidence is deemed to be more important than either expert opinion or the patient perspective. Also, a hierarchy exists within the differing types of scientific research, with studies involving quantitative designs (including reviews and meta-analyses of quantitative studies) appearing near the top whereas studies involving qualitative designs (or reviews of qualitative designs) appear near the bottom. In particular, most hierarchies put studies involving the randomised, controlled trial (often abbreviated to RCT) at the top because there is a perception – particularly in medicine – that it is the 'gold-standard' of research designs.

Not everyone, however, agrees with this view and there are major criticisms of the RCT as gold-standard (see Cartwright, 2007; Grossman & McKenzie, 2005; Kaptchuk, 2001). Most of the criticism centres not on the robustness of the RCT as a research design (most agree it has good *internal* validity) but on its *external* validity, i.e. the extent to which the results are – the evidence is – applicable to real-life situations. Indeed, Kaptchuk (2001) states that the central value of the RCT may be more about 'fairness' than 'truth' (p. 546), and Smith (2003), somewhat

Table 20.1 The Melnyk and Fineout-Overholt (2011) hierarchy of evidence

Level	Details
Level 1	Systematic review/meta-analysis of randomised controlled trials; clinical guidelines based on systematic reviews or meta-analyses
Level 2	One or more randomised controlled trials
Level 3	Controlled trial (no randomisation)
Level 4	Case–control or cohort study (uncontrolled trials)
Level 5	Systematic review of descriptive/qualitative studies
Level 6	Single descriptive or qualitative study
Level 7	Expert opinion

Table 20.2 The SIGN levels of evidence (Scottish Intercollegiate Guidelines Network, 2011)

Grade	Details
1++	High quality meta-analysis, systematic reviews of RCTs, or RCTs with a very low risk of bias
1+	Well conducted meta-analyses, systematic reviews, or RCTs with a low risk of bias
1−	Meta-analyses, systematic reviews, or RCTs with a high risk of bias
2++	High quality systematic reviews of case control or cohort studies
	High quality case control or cohort studies with a very low risk of confounding or bias and a high probability that the relationship is causal
2+	Well conducted case control or cohort studies with a low risk of confounding or bias and a moderate probability that the relationship is causal
2−	Case control or cohort studies with a high risk of confounding or bias and a significant risk that the relationship is not causal
3	Non-analytic studies, e.g. case reports, case series
4	Expert opinion

mockingly, questions medicine's lavish adherence to the RCT by asking why the use of parachutes as an intervention to prevent death and major trauma due to gravitational challenge has not been subjected to the RCT!

The process of EBP

The Sicily consensus statement on EBP (Dawes *et al.*, 2005) argued that there were five steps to EBP. Tilson *et al.* (2011) summarised these steps using five single words:

1   *ask* (translating uncertainty to an answerable question);
2   *search* (systematically retrieving the best evidence available);
3   *appraise* (critically appraising the evidence for validity and clinical relevance);
4   *integrate* (applying the search and appraisal results to practice);
5   *evaluate* (evaluating the application of the evidence to practice).

We will consider each of these steps in turn and, in doing so, the cultural, economic, political and philosophical barriers to EBP that were alluded to earlier will become apparent.

Step 1. Ask: uncertainties in practice

This first step in the EBP process concerns *uncertainty* in clinical practice. In medicine and health care, 'uncertainty' has a large and diverse literature associated with it (Han, Klein & Arora, 2011). For our purposes, however, it is enough to state that uncertainty simply means that the nurse or health care practitioner is faced with something in their day-to-day clinical practices that she or he is unsure about. The uncertainty might arise from a variety of sources: a government drive to cut down on the costs of health care; a consultation with a patient or service user; a discussion with a colleague; or as a result of something completely new or unexpected happening in practice. In capable and reflective practitioners, uncertainty will always generate questions ('What do I do now?' 'How do I deal with this?' 'Who can help me?'), but the skill in EBP is to ensure that the questions generated by uncertainty are ones that are *answerable*. This means that questions need to be targeted and specific.

PICO

A commonly used framework for conceptualising answerable questions in EBP is the 'PICO' framework (Strauss, Richardson, Glasziou & Haynes, 2011):

P = patient or population group of interest
I = potential intervention (or treatment or course of action)
C = any comparisons that might be made
O = any relevant outcomes.

Box 20.1 contains an example of how PICO can be used to conceptualise what might be considered the developed world's 'standard' medical uncertainty – one in which the effectiveness of a specific intervention (medication) for a particular condition (psychosis) is considered in terms of an outcome that focuses on symptom reduction.

This paradigm appears to be straightforward enough. There are problems with it, however, even before its global applicability is considered. For one, the patient group (P) typically centres on a diagnostic category, even to the point of using formal diagnostic systems such as the WHO's *International Statistical Classification of Diseases and Related Health Problems (ICD-10)* (WHO, 2010) or the American Psychiatric Association's *Diagnostic and Statistical Manual of Mental Disorders (DSM-5)* (APA, 2013). While this diagnostic approach might work well in physical medicine where more objective evidence of disease tends to be available and there is often little cultural dispute over diagnoses (e.g., tuberculosis or cerebrovascular accident), the same cannot be said for psychiatry. With psychiatric diagnoses not only do researchers and practitioners have to contend with broad conceptual critiques such as the view that schizophrenia may be nothing more than a 'scientific delusion' (Bentall, 2003; Boyle, 2002), concerns have also been raised about their global validity. As White (2013) points out, psychiatric diagnostic systems tend to erroneously assume that the various diagnostic categories are culturally independent, and membership of the panels that formulate these systems tends to be heavily biased towards the West and the developed world. Watters (2010) even goes so far as to suggest that Western psychiatry is being marketed and globalised (by the US in particular) in much the same way as other bastions of American culture like McDonalds, Hollywood or Nike.

A second issue concerns outcomes (O). While the example in Box 20.1 reflects the commonly held view that a positive outcome should be a reduction in symptoms of some sort, White (2013) adds that there is no global consensus on what a positive outcome might be in

---

Box 20.1: Effective medication for schizophrenia

Uncertainty: a health care funder is unsure which antipsychotic medications they should be buying to treat schizophrenia.

P: people with schizophrenia (as defined by ICD-10 criteria)

I: antipsychotic medications

C: no treatment (placebo) *or* different medications (e.g. 'typical' medications like haloperidol or chlorpromazine vs 'atypical' medications like risperidone or olanzapine)

O: a reduction in negative and positive symptoms

Answerable question: What antipsychotic medications are the most effective treatments in schizophrenia?

---

mental health, and that outcomes are often culturally sensitive. Even locally, the various parties involved might not be able to agree on what defines a positive outcome. In particular, patients/ service users and their significant others may have wildly different expectations regarding outcomes. A service user may want symptoms to be reduced but not at the expense of the excessive weight gain associated with anti-psychotic medications; a husband, wife or partner may see an improved sex life as a more important outcome; and a health care practitioner might see less reliance on health care services and more self-management as a better outcome. Indeed, differing perspectives are not restricted merely to outcomes; they can be reflective of the uncertainty itself.

Whose uncertainty?

In considering uncertainty, it has typically been health care funders (in many cases governments), researchers, and practitioners who have dictated uncertainties. But more recently in the West – in line with a general move towards recovery-focussed care – patient/service-user perspectives have begun to be incorporated into uncertainty. For example, the *James Lind Alliance* in the United Kingdom (www.jla.nihr.ac.uk) identifies and prioritises particular health care uncertainties though collaboration between patients, carers and clinicians. Lloyd and White (2011) report on work by the Alliance involving uncertainties in schizophrenia noting that 'the money rarely goes to the studies that those with mental illness would chose' (p. 277). Indeed, when a collaborative approach to uncertainty is undertaken, the sorts of uncertainties that emerge tend to be less about mental illness and more about mental health and recovery from mental illness: the uncertainties cited by Lloyd and White (2011, p. 277), for instance, include 'What training is needed to recognise the early signs of recurrence?', 'How can sexual dysfunction due to anti-psychotic-drug therapy be managed?' and 'What are the benefits of hospital treatment compared with home care for psychotic episodes?'.

Involving patients/service users in the development of clinical questions does raise practical issues. Petit-Zeman and Locock (2013) note that in the West the danger that decisions end up being influenced by educated, middle-class patients instead of educated, middle-class professionals is real. Globally, the difficulties may be more acute, particularly in countries that are paternalistic, authoritarian, or with no history of citizen-involvement.

PICO's flexibility

Despite these criticisms, PICO is flexible enough to operate outside of a strict medical model. Box 20.2 gives an example of how PICO can be used to deal with an uncertainty in a much more patient-centred way.

Note that Boxes 20.1 and 20.2 use all four PICO elements because they are uncertainties about the *effectiveness* of an intervention, treatment or course of action; i.e., whether it works or not. PICO is flexible enough to be used as a framework when the uncertainty is somewhat broader, as is often the case in primary care or in mental health promotion or prevention. Box 20.3 provides an example where C and O are redundant.

Box 20.2: A young person hearing voices

Uncertainty: a parent asks a nurse what they should do to try and help their 15-year-old son who is distressed by voices he hears. They add that they would prefer that he did not take medication in the first instance because he and they are worried about side effects.

P: young people who hear voices

I: specific intervention(s) or treatment(s) for hearing voices

C: the different interventions for hearing voices (excluding medication because of the family's preference)

O: some indicator of improvement, e.g. a reduction in voice-hearing symptoms or the young person is able to 'live well' with the voices

Answerable question: What is the best non-pharmacological way to help a young person hearing voices?

Box 20.3 Ethnic minorities' access to mental health services

Uncertainty: an audit of a primary care mental health service suggests that disproportionately fewer service users from ethnic minorities access the service, but no one is sure why.

P: ethnic minorities (this could be conceptualised as a whole or broken down into relevant specific minorities, e.g. Black, Latino, South East Asian)

I: access to mental health services

C: (not applicable in this case)

O: (not applicable in this case)

Answerable question: What are the experiences of ethnic minorities when accessing mental health services?

The examples contained in Boxes 20.1–20.3 demonstrate that PICO can help health care practitioners conceptualise answerable questions relatively easily, whether those questions are broad or specific. PICO is also particularly useful in providing the groundwork for step 2 of the EBP process, searching.

Step 2. Search: finding the evidence

Once an uncertainty has been conceptualised as an answerable question, the next step is to look for the evidence that will help practitioners deal with that uncertainty. At this point, a practitioner might also want to restrict their search to a specific type of study and so PICO is sometimes modified to PICOS, with the 'S' standing for *study type*. It is sometimes advisable to include study type as a criterion because questions concerning *effectiveness* ('Does it work?') usually require different evidence from questions focusing on *experiences* or *opinions* ('What was it like?').

While PICO(S) can help determine *what* needs to retrieved, there is also a need to determine *where* to look for the evidence. The practitioner could ask a colleague what they think, look in a textbook, or search the internet using a search engine like *Google*. These are not especially robust approaches, however, and the usual approach in the developed world at least is to make use of subject databases.

Subject databases

Subject databases are regularly updated, are often commercially owned and produced and catalogue all the published material relating to a particular discipline. Databases most relevant to mental health care are the US National Library of Medicine's *MEDLINE* (medicine), EBSCO Publishing's *CINAHL* (nursing and the allied health disciplines) and the American Psychological Association's *PsycINFO* (psychology).

Databases are normally searched for one of two reasons: to identify evidence that can help a practitioner make a clinical decision or, alternatively, to actually *create* evidence, usually in the guise of some sort of evidence synthesis such as a systematic review, meta-analysis, or meta-synthesis. Regardless of the purpose, the principles are the same: search terms need to be identified and relevant material obtained from the various databases. However, searching in order to create, rather than merely identify evidence requires substantially more resources and necessitates a *systematic* approach. A systematic approach results in transparent and repeatable searches, with identified limitations or biases in the search process being made explicit.

If a practitioner searches databases merely to assist in clinical decision-making, using a systematic approach will still be beneficial. Being systematic in terms of the *where* means keeping a record of the databases searched and the date on which they were searched. Being systematic in terms of the *what* requires clear conceptualisations of each of the requisite PICO(S) elements via specific 'inclusion' and 'exclusion' criteria. Table 20.2 gives an illustration of how this might work for the clinical example that was described in Box 20.2.

Using PICO(S) to establish inclusion and exclusion criteria also helps with the search strategy, which is the process of identifying the actual terms that will be used to search the databases. In the example outlined in Box 20.2 and Table 20.2, the nurse will need to determine relevant search terms for P, I and S. At this point, search terms are not necessarily required for C and O because they could restrict the search too much although these elements will certainly come into play when the *relevance* of any particular evidence is considered (step 3 of the EBP process). The search strategy for this example will thus involve searching for papers in relevant databases

Table 20.3 Inclusion and exclusion criteria for the answerable question 'What is the best non-pharmacological way to help a young person distressed by hearing voices?'

	P	I	C	O	S
Inclusion criteria	'Young people hearing voices', defined as those aged 14–25 years who hear voices (evidence of auditory hallucinations)	Psychological or psychosocial approaches to dealing with voice hearing	Any intervention for voice hearing including medication No treatment (e.g. being on a waiting list for treatment) or 'treatment as usual'	Some indicator of improvement, e.g. a reduction in voice-hearing symptoms or the young person is able to live well with the voices	Because it is an effectiveness question, consider only 'trials', defined as at minimum a study with a before and after measure
Exclusion criteria	Those below 14 and above 25 years Young people who do not hear voices (experience auditory hallucinations) Young people who hear voices but who are not distressed by them	Medications as an intervention for hearing voices	No interventions for voice hearing will be excluded as comparators	Outcomes not associated with voice-hearing	Expert opinion; case studies; qualitative studies; correlational studies

that report *trials* (S) of *interventions* (I) for *young people* (P) who *hear voices* (another P dimension). For a robust search, consider also substituting synonyms for the italicised terms, for example, 'adolescent', 'teen' or 'youth' for *young people* and 'psychosis' and 'hallucination' for *hearing voices*. The US National Library of Medicine's *Medical Subject Headings* thesaurus (MeSH®) is an integral part of *MEDLINE* and can be helpful here (www.nlm.nih.gov/mesh).

Accessing search resources

At this point, significant barriers to EBP arise for those in the less-developed world. We in the developed world can access, often via the *internet*, these predominantly *English-language* resources *cost-free* because our employers, who are usually well-resourced health care service providers or educational institutions, tend to cover the costs involved. Each of the italicised terms here can be a barrier in the less-developed world, however. The infrastructure for the internet may be non-existent or prohibitively expensive and materials may be in a non-native language and hence require (expensive) translation services. Perhaps more insidious are the deliberate barriers put into place by the commercial interests of global publishing, health care and pharmaceutical corporations.

Academic publishing is largely controlled by a few major international publishers who have traditionally had a monopoly on the distribution and publication of academic research articles, i.e. the evidence. Even if a practitioner or researcher in a less-developed country has internet access, they might find that they are required to pay as much as $40 to access and download a single research article, which can be prohibitively expensive when, for example, in 2012 the average monthly gross pay of a health care professional in Thailand was approximately $700 and a mere $120 in Ethiopia (International Labour Organisation, 2013).

There have been recent moves to address this particular barrier through 'open access' whereby the costs of publication are borne by the authors and researchers (or, more likely, employers or research funders) in return for few or no restrictions on public access. While this removes one particular barrier for researchers and practitioners in the less-developed world, it ironically adds a barrier that may be insurmountable for those in low-income countries because the upfront costs of open access are often in the region of $1–2,000, which few institutions, let alone individuals, in those countries can afford. The WHO might want to encourage more research in less-developed countries to counter the dominance of more-developed countries (WHO, 2013), but there is little point in encouraging research if the costs associated with dissemination are exorbitant. Moreover, open access is not necessarily as altruistic as it might seem. One of the main reasons it has gained ground in the West is irritation from research funders (usually governments and public bodies) at the public being charged to access findings from research for which they have already paid. This explains to a large degree why the US National Institute of Health, the British National Institute for Health Research and the British Medical Research Council have all recently insisted that any publications arising from research they have funded must be publicly and freely available.

A second major issue in accessing search resources is one that affects all users and not just those with restricted budgets: the fact that the materials available are not necessarily an accurate reflection of the full evidence available because of systemic biases in the publication process. Some of these biases simply reflect the vagaries of human nature; others are more malevolent. Most academics are aware of *publication bias*, a bias in which positive findings are more likely to be published than negative findings because positive findings have a salience that negative findings do not. While this is a rather benign explanation for publication bias, there is a far more disconcerting one: there is evidence (Goldacre, 2013) that major pharmaceutical companies have wilfully suppressed the results of many studies that do not put their products (medicines) in a good light.

Awareness of publication bias is particularly important in EBP because it can have real implications for patient safety. A good mental health example concerns the use of anti-depressant medications in young people. Whittington *et al.* (2004) identified five published and nine unpublished RCTs concerning the use of selective serotonin reuptake inhibitors (SSRIs) in young people. Taking the published trials alone, the risk-benefit profiles in prescribing paroxetine and sertraline to young people were ambivalent or weakly beneficial and thus did not necessarily detract from their use with this client group. However, when the unpublished trials were combined with the published trials, the risks with these two medications appeared to far outweigh their benefits, strengthening the case against their use with young people.

When no evidence is found

If little or no external evidence is available, greater weight is usually given to the other forms of evidence – clinical expertise and the patient/service-user perspective – until adequate external evidence becomes available. In the developed West, a lack of evidence for a particular uncertainty is often seen as an opportunity or a 'gap in the literature' and is often used as a rationale to request research funding. From a global perspective, two further issues emerge: research tends to be conducted in more-developed countries (WHO, 2013) that, contextually, creates significantly greater gaps in the literature in less-developed countries; and research is expensive, so the less-developed and usually low-income countries are further disadvantaged. When extensive research does occur in the developing world, ethical concerns often arise particularly when developed world corporations are seen to be exploiting the ready supply of cheap, naïve participants to further their own goals or profits (Goldacre, 2013; Macklin, 2004).

Step 3. Appraise: the relevance and validity of the evidence

Once any potential evidence is identified, the next step in the EBP process is to appraise it. Appraisal is essentially concerned with identifying the *best* evidence from that available. There are two levels to evidence appraisal: the first is to make a judgement against the PICO inclusion/exclusion criteria to determine its relevance to the uncertainty; the second relates to judgements about the veracity of the evidence. To a large extent, the latter is about guarding against *bias* when making such judgments. The biases can, as we have already seen, operate as a result of political, economic and cultural influences; biases can also be influenced by the philosophical and theoretical preferences (psychodynamic vs cognitive, for example) of the researcher or practitioner. In addition, most research methods will have inherent biases, and biases can also be present in the way in which evidence is reported or not reported.

Internal and external validity

In appraising the veracity of evidence, reference is usually made to the two types of validity we encountered briefly earlier on: internal validity and external validity. External validity refers to the degree to which a finding is generalisable; in other words, it is concerned with the applicability and *clinical* relevance of the evidence. Biases that emerge here may be subtle; for example, the study may have been funded by an organisation with a vested interest in the research such as a commercial enterprise or government. On the other hand, biases may be more blatant. For example, RCTs conducted in a laboratory or artificially controlled setting ('efficacy' studies) often do not produce the same outcomes when applied to real-life clinical scenarios where 'effectiveness' rather than efficacy is the issue.

Internal validity, on the other hand, is concerned with the robustness of the research design; biases here might actually invalidate study results. Research studies with low internal validity (often referred to as 'poor quality' studies) rarely have good external validity because it is hard to draw conclusions from findings when the research design is questionable. However, while well-designed studies usually have good internal validity (and are thus 'high quality' studies), they may not necessarily have good external validity, as noted earlier when critiquing the RCT as a gold-standard design.

Appraisal tools

When appraising the validity or quality of studies, true clinical experts with the requisite knowledge and experience are often able to do this intuitively. For novices and those less confident, and in circumstances in which a greater degree of objectivity is required (a systematic review, for instance), a variety of standard appraisal tools exist that are almost always a product of the developed West and often only available in English, again disadvantaging the less-developed world.

One of the most widely used appraisal tools for RCTs is the *Cochrane Risk of Bias Tool* (Higgins & Green, 2011), a tool that examines the major sources of bias in RCTs such as a lack of true randomisation or the insufficient blinding of participants. The British *Critical Appraisal Skills Programme* (CASP) (www.casp-uk.net) has appraisal tools available for a variety of research designs including RCTs, systematic reviews, and qualitative studies (see Box 20.4 for an adapted version of the qualitative research appraisal tool). The University of Auckland, New Zealand has developed a unique (though somewhat complex for the uninitiated) pictorial approach to critical appraisal (Jackson *et al.*, 2006).

An interesting observation about the CASP tool in Box 20.4 is the 'can't tell' option. Having a 'not sure' or 'unclear' option is a common feature of appraisal tools because a study's quality is determined not only by how well the study has been conducted but also by how well the study has been written up. When reviewing an academic paper, it can sometimes be difficult to tell whether a bias is evident or not, or whether the researchers have carried out the study well because the information is simply not reported in the paper. This might be a result of author carelessness but often it is can be attributed to another vagary of the publication process – word limits imposed by most academic journals.

Critical thinking

Underpinning appraisal is the notion of *critical thinking*. Critical thinking requires personal traits and higher order cognitive abilities like flexibility, creativity, inquisitiveness, information seeking, logical reasoning and analytical skills (Scheffer & Rubenfeld, 2000). Closely allied to critical thinking is the notion of *reflection*, a concept discussed further in step 5 of the EBP process.

It is beyond the scope of this chapter to offer anything more than a cursory examination of critical thinking but it needs mentioning because critical thinking has a strong cultural dimension to it, often being seen as construct of Western thought (Atkinson, 1997). For those living in

---

Box 20.4: The CASP qualitative research appraisal tool

10 questions to help you make sense of qualitative research

1 Was there a clear statement of the aims of the research? ❑ Yes ❑ Can't tell ❑ No

2 Is a qualitative methodology appropriate? ❑ Yes ❑ Can't tell ❑ No

AT THIS POINT IS IT WORTH CONTINUING?

3 Was the research design appropriate to address the aims of the research? ❑ Yes ❑ Can't tell ❑ No

4 Was the recruitment strategy appropriate to the aims of the research? ❑ Yes ❑ Can't tell ❑ No

5 Was the data collected in a way that addressed the research issue? ❑ Yes ❑ Can't tell ❑ No

6 Has the relationship between researcher participants been adequately considered? ❑ Yes ❑ Can't tell ❑ No

7 Have ethical issues been taken into consideration? ❑ Yes ❑ Can't tell ❑ No

8 Was the data analysis sufficiently rigorous? ❑ Yes ❑ Can't tell ❑ No

9 Is there a clear statement of findings? ❑ Yes ❑ Can't tell ❑ No

10 How valuable is the research?

Source: Adapted from the Critical Appraisal Skills Programme Qualitative Research Checklist (21 May 2013 version), under a creative commons licence CC BY-NC-SA 3.0 (see www.casp-uk.net).

---

countries or cultures where obedience, particularly to the state or to authority, is a cultural expectation or where a strict medical hierarchy exists (with nurses usually near the bottom), critical thought can be a difficult concept to grasp. Furthermore, as Ryan and Louie (2007) remark, just because critical thought is seen to be a Western concept does not necessarily mean it should be a desirable one.

Step 4. Integrate: application to practice and clinical decision-making

In order to integrate the evidence into practice, decisions need to be made about the applicability of the evidence. It is at this point that the notion of clinical decision-making really comes into play. The health care practitioner may be armed with the best (research) evidence and may have extensive clinical experience in their specialty; but without reference to the context (which encompasses geographical, cultural, organisational, or patient-specific factors), it will be insufficient and poor clinical decisions might arise as a result. For example, there may be substantial evidence that written self-help materials can help people with anxiety but allocating this form of treatment to someone who cannot read is a poor clinical decision. This example also highlights the importance of *shared* decision-making; there is little point in recommending anxiolytic medication if a patient/service user has explicitly stated that they do not want to take medication.

Different models of service delivery

One contextual factor that is especially important when considering the global applicability of EBP is the different organisational models that health services operate under around the world. Reid (2010) outlined five specific models, which vary according to the degree of universal cover, who pays for the service, and who provides it. This raises questions over whether evidence pertaining to one particular model is applicable outside of that model. A particularly ironic case in point relates to the UK in that, according to Reid, the countries with the closest models to the UK National Health Service are New Zealand and Spain, followed perhaps by the rest of Europe and Japan. Yet a substantial amount of the evidence underpinning British EBP is imported from the US, probably because the UK and US share the same language, and the US dominates in health care research.

Clinical guidelines

In some jurisdictions, practitioners are supported in EBP by the production of clinical guidelines. Organisations producing guidelines include both the National Institute for Health and Care Excellence (NICE) (www.nice.org.uk) and the Scottish Intercollegiate Guidelines Network (SIGN) (www.sign.ac.uk) in the UK, the Joanna Briggs Institute in Australia (www.joannabriggs. org) and the US Preventive Services Taskforce (www.uspreventiveservicestaskforce.org) in the US. Clinical guidelines are 'best practice' recommendations for people with specific diseases or conditions. The recommendations can have varying levels of *strength* from top grade recommendations arising from meta-analysis or systematic review evidence to *good practice points* based on the clinical expertise of the guideline development group. Nonetheless, it is important to note that guidelines are designed to help health professionals in their work and are by no means substitutes for clinical knowledge and skill. Indeed, if clinical knowledge and skill are taken out of the equation, they become nothing more than an aid to ritualised practice.

While organisations that develop clinical guidelines usually provide them as open-access documents, the same issues of global applicability arise. Guidelines tend to be devised in the more-developed countries and in the context of well-funded health, research and education facilities.

Equivocal evidence

Even when armed with the best evidence, making a clinical decision can be extremely difficult when the evidence is equivocal, particularly when political or ethical factors enter the fray. In 2007, a debate in the *British Medical Journal* over whether young people should be given antidepressants pitched two psychiatrists against each other (Cotgrove, 2007; Timini, 2007). Both made reference to the evidence but drew different conclusions. Cotgrove (yes) argued that meta-analysis and systematic review evidence demonstrated the effectiveness of SSRIs while Timini (no) questioned why *any* intervention was necessary given that most childhood distress is self-limiting, further adding that marketing spin seemed to have been given precedence over scientific accuracy. To some extent, this debate highlights the fact that questions exist over the status and credence assigned to different research types and drives home the fact that EBP can be as much an art as it is a science.

Step 5. Evaluate: reflect on performance

At this point, those of us familiar with the nursing process might be able to see some parallels with the EBP process (see Figure 20.1). Like steps 1 and 2 of the EBP process, the assessment phase of the nursing process is all about asking questions and obtaining relevant information. Like step 3, the planning phase of the nursing process requires appraisal of the information obtained. The implementation phase of the nursing process is like step 4 of the EBP process concerned with applying theory to practice, and evaluation is the common later phase in both processes. As with the nursing process, it could be argued that the EBP process should be cyclical because evaluation in both cases requires further action: re-assessment in the case of the nursing process and a re-examination of the uncertainty and/or the evidence in the case of the EBP process.

Reflection

In both processes, the evaluative phase or step is important because it enables individual and discipline-wide expertise to develop systematically rather than arbitrarily. The key to evaluation in both processes is the notion of *reflection*. Reflection is to a large extent a critical self-examination of a practitioner's own practices in order to develop and enhance her or his performance, ultimately to the benefit of the patient/service user. Reflection is thus a necessary component of clinical expertise. Schön (1983) distinguishes between reflection *on* action where the reflection happens *after* an event and reflection *in* action, which happens *during* an event. Reflection in action is a deeper skill that is the hallmark of true clinical expertise.

Because reflection is closely related to critical thinking, similar issues apply when considering it globally. Reflection, like critical thinking, may be a Western socio-cultural construct that does not necessarily translate outside of this context (Finlay, 2008).

Conclusion

In this chapter, we have discussed how those in the less-developed and developed world might struggle in implementing Western-style EBP because of economic, political, cultural and

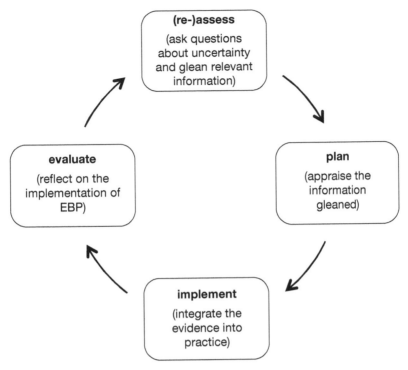

Figure 20.1 Comparing the nursing and EBP processes

philosophical constraints. However, this does not necessarily exclude colleagues in the less-developed and developing world from adopting the principles of EBP because EBP is flexible enough to allow for cultural idiosyncrasies. Indeed, the WHO (2013) argues that cultural considerations are a necessary dimension of EBP. Even in the developed world EBP is being conceptualized with more flexibility. Greenhalgh, Pawson, Walshe and Harvey (2004) argued that EBP should be concerned with 'What works, for whom, how, and in what circumstances?' rather than merely with 'Does this intervention work?'

This conceptualisation of EBP is also particularly good when considering public health, primary care and psychosocial approaches to mental health care, approaches that do not necessarily embrace the rigid medical paradigms that underpin much of the 'evidence' relating to mental *illness*. Public health and primary care interventions are difficult to test in the laboratory because with preventative interventions in particular, there is often no 'illness' to treat and the long-term nature of outcomes means that longitudinal research is needed. Proctor *et al.* (2009) argued that mental health care might benefit if more *implementation* research were conducted or research that focused on the gap between ostensibly effective interventions and what actually happens in clinical practice.

White (2013) suggests that the focus on globalisation in psychiatry should shift from mental illness where it currently appears to be, to *mental health*, arguing that mental health is a more inclusive aspiration and creates greater potential for clinicians, academics, patients/service users and policy makers to work globally together with a shared purpose. This is a particularly salient point because in less austere times the WHO (2004) observed that mental health promotion and mental disorder prevention were the only sustainable ways of reducing the global burden caused by mental ill-health.

By thinking broadly in terms of the 'best' evidence, trying to understand the perspectives of service users and their significant others, and making the most of their knowledge and skills, nurses and health care practitioners around the world can use the principles of EBP to make a real difference in the lives of those affected by mental distress.

References

American Psychiatric Association. (2013). *Diagnostic and statistical manual of mental disorders* (5th edn). Arlington, VA: American Psychiatric Publishing.

Atkinson, D. (1997). A critical approach to critical thinking in TESOL. *TESOL Quarterly, 31*(1), 71–94.

Benner, P. (1984). *From novice to expert: Excellence and power in clinical nursing practice.* Menlo Park, CA: Addison-Wesley.

Bentall, R.P. (2003). *Madness explained: Psychosis and human nature.* Harmondsworth, UK: Penguin.

Boyle, M. (2002). *Schizophrenia: A scientific delusion?* (2nd edn). London: Routledge.

Burrow, S. (2011). Helping older people with mental health problems. In S. Pryjmachuk (ed.), *Mental health nursing: An evidence-based introduction.* London: Sage, pp. 253–290.

Cartwright, N. (2007). Are RCTs the gold standard? *Biosocieties, 2*(1), 11–20.

Cotgrove, A. (2007). Should young people be given antidepressants? Yes. *British Medical Journal, 335*, 750.

Dawes, M., Summerskill, W., Glasziou, P., Cartabellotta, A., Martin, J., Hopayian, K., Porzsolt, F., Burls, A., & Osborne, J.(2005). Sicily statement on evidence-based practice. *BMC Medical Education, 5*(1). Doi: 10.1186/1472–6920–5-1.

Finlay, L. (2008). *Reflecting on reflective practice: Practice-based professional learning centre discussion paper 52.* Milton Keynes, UK: Open University. Available at: www.open.ac.uk/opencetl/files/opencetl/file/ecms/web-content/Finlay-(2008)-Reflecting-on-reflective-practice-PBPL-paper-52.pdf (accessed 18 December 2013).

Goldacre, B. (2013). *Bad pharma: How medicine is broken, and how we can fix it.* London: 4th Estate.

Greenhalgh, T., Pawson. R., Walshe, K. & Harvey. G. (2004). RCT may not be the 'gold standard' (*BMJ* online rapid response article). Available at: www.bmj.com/rapid-response/2011/10/30/rct-may-not-be-gold-standard (accessed 18 December 2013).

Grossman, J. & McKenzie. F.J. (2005). The randomized controlled trial: gold-standard, or merely standard? *Perspectives in Biology and Medicine, 48*(4), 516–553.

Han, P.K.J., Klein, W.M.P. & Arora, N.K. (2011). Varieties of uncertainty in health care: a conceptual taxonomy. *Medical Decision-making, 31*, 828–838.

Higgins, J.P.T. & Green, S. (eds) (2011). *Cochrane handbook for systematic reviews of interventions.* Oxford: The Cochrane Collaboration. Available at: http://handbook.cochrane.org (accessed 18 December 2013).

Huybrechts, K.F., Gerhard, T., Crystal, S., Olfson, M., Avorn, J., Levin, R., Lucas, J.A. & Schneeweiss (2012). Differential risk of death in older residents in nursing homes prescribed specific antipsychotic drugs: population based cohort study. *British Medical Journal, 344*, e977.

International Labour Organisation. (2013). *ILOSTAT database: Mean nominal monthly earnings of employees by sex and occupation (selected ISCO level 2).* Available at: www.ilo.org/ilostat (accessed 18 December 2013).

Jackson, R., Ameratunga, S., Broad, J., Connor, J., Lethaby, A., Robb, G., Wells, S., Glasziou, P. & Heneghan, C. (2006). The GATE frame: critical appraisal with pictures. *Evidence-based Medicine, 11*, 35–38.

Kaptchuk, T.J. (2001). The double-blind, randomized, placebo-controlled trial: gold-standard or golden calf? *Journal of Clinical Epidemiology,* 54, 541–549.

Lloyd, K. & White, J. (2011). Democratizing clinical research. *Nature, 474*, 227–278.

McHugh, M.D. & Lake. E.T. (2010). Understanding clinical expertise: nurse education, experience, and the hospital context. *Research in Nursing and Health, 33*(4), 276–287.

Macklin, R. (2004). *Double standards in medical research in developing countries.* Cambridge: Cambridge University Press.

Melnyk, B.M. & Fineout-Overholt, E. (2011). *Evidence-based practice in nursing and health care: A guide to best practice,* 2nd edn. Philadelphia, PA: Williams & Wilkins.

NICE (National Institute for Health and Care Excellence). (2011). Clinical guidelines (web page). Available at http://guidance.nice.org.uk/CG (accessed 18 December 2013).

Petit-Zeman, S. & Locock, L. (2013). Health care: bring on the evidence. *Nature, 501*, 161–162.

Proctor, E.K., Landsverk, J., Aarons, G., Chambers, D., Glisson, C. & Mittman, B. (2009). Implementation research in mental health services: an emerging science with conceptual, methodological and training challenges. *Administration and Policy in Mental Health and Mental Health Services Research*, *36*(1), 24–34.

Pryjmachuk, S. (1996). A nursing perspective on the interrelationships between theory, research and practice. *Journal of Advanced Nursing*, *23*(4), 679–84.

Reid, T.R. (2010). *The healing of America: A global quest for better, cheaper, and fairer health care*. New York: Penguin Press.

Ryan J. & Louie, K. (2007). False dichotomy? 'Western' and 'Confucian' concepts of scholarship and learning. *Educational Philosophy and Theory*, *39*(4), 404–417.

Sackett D., Rosenberg W.M.C., Gray, J.A.M., Haynes, R.B., & Richardson, W.S. (1996). Evidence-based medicine: what it is and what it isn't. *British Medical Journal*, *312*, 71.

Scheffer, B.K & Rubenfeld, M.G. (2000). A consensus statement on critical thinking in nursing. *Journal of Nursing Education*, *39*(8), 352–60.

Schön, D. (1983). *The reflective practitioner: How professionals think in action*. London: Temple Smith.

Scottish Intercollegiate Guidelines Network. (2011). *SIGN 50: A guideline developer's handbook*. Edinburgh, UK: Scottish Intercollegiate Guidelines Network. Available at: www.sign.ac.uk/pdf/sign50.pdf (accessed 18 December 2013).

Shepherd, G., Boardman, J. & Slade, M. (2008). *Making recovery a reality*. London: Sainsbury Centre for Mental Health.

Smith, G. (2003). Parachute use to prevent death and major trauma related to gravitational challenge: systematic review of randomised controlled trials. *British Medical Journal*, *327*, 1459.

Strauss, S.E., Richardson. W.S., Glasziou, P. & Haynes, R.B. (2011). *Evidence-based medicine: How to practice and teach it*, 4th edn. Edinburgh, UK: Churchill Livingstone.

Tilson, K., Kaplan, S.L., Harris, J.L., Hutchinson, A., Ilic, D., Niederman, R., Potomkova, J. & Zwolsman, S.E. (2011). Sicily statement on classification and development of evidence-based practice learning assessment tools. *BMC Medical Education*, *11*(78). Doi: 10.1186/1472–6920–11–78.

Timini, S. (2007). Should young people be given antidepressants? No. *British Medical Journal*, *335*, 751.

Warren, B.J. (2012). Shared decision-making: a recovery cultural process. *Journal of Psychosocial Nursing and Mental Health Services*, *50*(12), 4–5.

Watters, E. (2011). *Crazy like us: The globalization of the American psyche*. New York: Simon & Schuster.

White, R. (2013). The globalisation of mental illness. *The Psychologist*, *26*(3), 182–185.

Whittington, C.J., Kendall, T., Fonagy, P., Cottrell, D., Cotgrove, A. & Boddington, E. (2004). Selective serotonin reuptake inhibitors in childhood depression: systematic review of published versus unpublished data. *The Lancet*, *363*, 1341–1345.

WHO (World Health Organization). (2004). *Prevention of mental disorders: Effective interventions and policy options: summary report*. Geneva: WHO. Available at: www.who.int/mental_health/evidence/en/prevention_of_mental_disorders_sr.pdf (accessed 2 December 2013).

WHO (World Health Organization). (2010). *International statistical classification of diseases and related health problems, 10th revision*. Geneva: WHO. Available at: http://apps.who.int/classifications/icd10/browse/2010/en (accessed 2 December 2013).

WHO (World Health Organization). (2013). *Comprehensive mental health action plan 2013–2020*. Geneva: WHO. Available at: http://apps.who.int/gb/ebwha/pdf_files/WHA66/A66_R8-en.pdf (accessed 25 October 2013).

PART III

Cultural voices and human rights
Case exemplars

The following exemplars provide a depiction of the issues and contexts in which mental health nursing care is provided and experienced by each of the authors. Each setting has its own unique cultural and professional contexts and may or may not be similar within the setting of the reader. We hope that the unique and common nursing experiences offered in this section provide a rich description and complex picture of mental health nursing in all its forms.

21

DEINSTITUTIONALIZED CARE

Jamaican psychiatric workers' viewpoints

Andrea Pusey-Murray and Hermi Hyacinth Hewitt

Introduction: cultural context

The estimated population of Jamaica at the end of 2009 was 2,698,800 with an estimated growth rate of approximately 0.2 percent (ESSJ, 2009). The ethnic make-up of the Jamaican population is 91.2 percent black, 6.2 percent mixed (Chinese, Indian, Caucasian), and 2.6 percent unknown (Jamaica Demographic Profile, 2013). The majority (36 percent) of the population falls between 25–54 years of age (Jamaica Demographic Profile, 2014). This chapter contextualizes the origin of the Jamaican population and the traditions, cultural and structural influences pertaining to mental health. It provides a historical overview of the care of the mentally ill from institutionalization to deinstitutionalization. Finally it highlights the views of psychiatric workers towards deinstitutionalization.

Historical perspectives

The indigenous peoples of Jamaica, the Tianos, were enslaved by the Spaniards in 1492 and were reportedly brutally treated. In 1655 the British captured Jamaica from the Spaniards, and between them both the Tianos became extinct. Hickling and Gibson (2012) noted that "by the time the British captured the island of Jamaica from the Spanish in 1655, the majority of the indigenous population had been eradicated by genocidal violence or lethal infectious diseases imported by the Spanish colonizers" (p. 431). The British then proceeded to populate Jamaica by enslaving Africans to work on the Jamaican plantations.

It has been reported that the Tianos used "unguents (ointments) and salvent herbs blended with foods which they hung from fruit trees for those they called 'mind-riven' (mentally ill) who were allowed to wander at large" (Hickling & Gibson, 2012, p. 438). The nature of slavery focused attention on the enslaved population as a tool of production rather than as human beings with emotions, feelings, and mental needs. Consequently this vast black population had to resort to their own traditions that they brought with them to attend to any malady they experienced and were also subjected to whatever was given them by the slave owners.

The British having built the Lunatic Asylum at the Kingston Public Hospital shifted the care of mentally ill slaves from their owners to the colonial government as the prelude to abolition and emancipation (Hickling & Gibson, 2012). The authors emphasized that the "state did not take responsibility for the care of ordinary black people until post emancipation and the new mental hospital (1860) was built partly to accommodate the increase in numbers, with the addition of ex-slaves to the patient pool" (Hickling & Gibson, 2012, p. 431). The first formalized services for patients with psychiatric illness started in Jamaica in 1862 at the "Lunatic Asylum," its structure was similar to the General Penitentiary where hardened convicted criminals were confined. The Asylum was renamed "Bellevue Hospital" in 1947. Bellevue Mental Hospital served as the sole long-stay facility and primary source of inpatient mental health care for several decades, until deinstitutionalization was enforced in 1972 (Hickling, Robertson-Hickling, & Paisley, 2011). During a time period that spanned over 300 years, the black population experienced the most horrendous treatment throughout slavery and colonialism (Bowerbank, 1860; Rouse, 1860). The belief system of obeah (an Afro-Creole religion that uses folk magic as a means of protection) and cultural practices passed down from ancestors preserved myths and practices associated with the treatment of mental illness. There was an ingrained belief that mentally ill individuals needed to be protected from self as well as from society in restricted spaces such as a hospital.

Between 1655 and 1939 care of the mentally ill remained custodial and followed the pattern of treatment given to slaves by their owners. During that period when Jamaica was colonized by the Spanish, they "attributed the excellent results achieved by these indigenous treatments as sorcery" (Beaubrun et. al 1976, p. 438).

Custodial care for the mentally ill continued in Jamaica until the early 1950s when Maxwell Jones' (Jones, 1952) concept of the therapeutic community, the establishment of vocational therapy and a thrust towards community and family reintegration of patients from the asylum occurred (Collis & Green, 1976). In the early 1970s some psychiatrists led by Beauburn introduced the community mental health care movement, thus introducing deinstitutionalization to Jamaica (Hickling, 1975). Hickling (1995) indicated that this

> programme saw the integration of psychiatric services with general primary and secondary health care services; the establishment of a cadre of specialist community psychiatric nurses known as mental health officers; the implementation of new mental health legislation in 1974, and reduction of the 3,000 patient mental hospital population to 1,200 persons by 1990.
>
> (as cited in Hickling & Gibson, 2012, p. 439)

It is the opinion of the authors that some of the practices and perceptions held about mental illness and also the shift from hospitalized to deinstitutionalized services had its genesis in slavery, colonialism, and neo-colonialism and persists in the practice of mental health services today.

Description of the issue

Mental health remains one of the priority health issues in Jamaica. It has been suggested by mental health experts that trauma and stress are possible underlying causes for the high levels of homicide and other acts of criminality prevalent in the society (ESSJ, 2009). Hickling indicated that Ottey in 1973 pioneered the first steps towards the integration of mental health and primary care services in a rural parish hospital; and Beaubrun (1977) introduced the first steps towards the integration of mental health and primary care services that took place in the parish of St Thomas at the outpatient clinic at the Princess Margaret Hospital. The pilot project, pioneered by Ottey (1973) and early mental health officers provided the model for island-wide services. The initial implementation of the community mental health service in 1974 precipitated an immediate reduction in admissions to the mental hospital by 52 percent in the first two years (Hickling, 1976). Eventually, primary care mental health services were established in nearly 400 clinics island-wide.

Evidence indicates that society places stigma on institutionalized services. Hickling and colleagues (2011, p. 169) found that

> The Bellevue Mental Hospital and homelessness were identified as major causes of stigma (and that) . . . Attitudes toward the mentally ill have improved and stigma has decreased since the increase of community involvement with the mentally ill. This reduction in stigma seems to be a result of the rigorous deinstitutionalization process and the development of a robust community mental health service in Jamaica.

The authors made a connection between the dismantling of the archaic colonial custodial system of care at the mental hospital, the deinstitutionalization processes and the interrelationship between the colonial victimization of Jamaicans with African belief systems such as the Rastafari, and the creation of mental health systems of incarceration designed to excise these belief systems from the mainstream of colonial society (Hickling *et al.*, 2011). Despite the effort of the British to discredit and discontinue the African traditions and practices of the slaves, the efforts were futile. Instead, the slaves found ways to preserve their traditions, many of which had been passed on to succeeding generations.

Brief analysis/aftermath and update

Although deinstitutionalized care for mentally ill patients started approximately three decades ago, to date there are still some mentally ill patients in the two government facilities in the country who could be treated in their communities. The historical perspective of custodial care is still engrained in the psyche of some health workers who believe that most patients cannot cope or exist in a deinstitutionalized environment.

To garner evidence on opinions of deinstitutionalization the authors, who were also study investigators, sought to understand the views held by psychiatric workers who are currently serving in the health system. Focus groups of psychiatric workers in two state-run hospitals in Jamaica were conducted. One of the hospitals exclusively treats the mentally ill, and the other has a floor within the medical hospital for treating individuals with a mental illness. The group discussions were held with psychiatric workers who were working in these two hospitals between 17 months and 25 years. Participants included registered nurses, assistant nurses, psychiatric nursing aides, and ward assistants. Both males and females participated in the study. Ethical clearance to conduct the study was received from the Ministry of Health Research and Ethics Committee, the South East Regional Health Authority Ethics Committee, and the University of Technology Research Ethics Committee.

Perceptions of psychiatric workers

The cultural beliefs underpinning the care of persons with mental illness were evident in the focus group discussions conducted in 2014. The findings presented are part of a larger study on the perceptions of psychiatric workers towards deinstitutionalized care. The perceived restrictive nature of hospitalized care was evident in the results. For example some psychiatric workers referred to hospitalized care as analogous to imprisonment. In describing institutionalized or hospital care a psychiatric worker indicated: "In terms of bad, as [another speaker] had stated, they feel imprisoned when they are in the hospital; they don't have that amount of freedom as they should, yeah."

Even in situations where psychiatric workers acknowledged that deinstitutionalization was best for the patient there was reticence towards community acceptance, reservation about a person's ability to be rehabilitated and become functional and an independent citizen. There is a preference towards custodial care as illustrated by the following perceptions:

> Yes, they can be treated in their community if they are not chronic. If they are chronic, they pose a danger to themselves or their community at large, so if they are in the hospital that would be better. If they do not have a good family support they are at a disadvantage being treated in the community.
>
> Yes, they can be treated in the community as long as they have family members who understand their illness and also the community at large is aware that such a person has that illness, they will care for them.
>
> Depending on the nature of the diagnosis, they may not require a more established institution for that treatment, so yes they could be treated in the community.
>
> There are advantages in institutionalisation relating to follow up. While in institution they will not do things that they would do outside without supervision by trained personnel. So you would consider institutionalisation as beneficial in that sense.

Psychiatric health workers expressed both positive and negative opinions of deinstitutionalization. Based on their opinions, institutionalized patients cannot be rehabilitated and are relegated to the state of dependency and confinement.

> In terms of these—you're talking about these same patients? It can have positive and negative effects, because there are patients who have been in an institution for 30 years. If these individuals are just taken back into the community without proper guidance, there are a lot of issues that can occur.
>
> You [patients] have lost the idea of what really happens out there; time has passed you. So, a lot of them will be, I would say, would eventually have what you call culture shock, 'cause they would not be able to deal with what is happening now in the community. Some patients would not even know where to find a particular place that they were used to [from] the time that they left the community.
>
> Family members that are not used to having a patient with them for so many years will find it difficult to deal and cope with this individual. There will also be interpersonal relations problems, as well, as many of them will not have adequate placement in terms of housing facilities and facilities that are adequate for them.

Psychiatric health workers perceived that mentally ill patients would relapse or will be neglected and noncompliant with medications. They anticipated that the treatment regime would not be followed once the patients were no longer under institutionalized care. A variety of reasons were expressed:

> Most times the clients go home with medications that they should take to maintain their stability, but they come back into hospital with medications untaken. If they were in institutions, they would have taken their medications and remained stable. Sometimes relatives for various reasons—such as work, etc.—do not keep up with their leg of the race (caring for the patient).

Deinstitutionalisation can be good because some persons do not want to be associated with a psychiatric ward, they would be compliant with medications because they want to stay well and not to come on the ward. If the relatives are aware of the conditions, then I think that is a plus for them as well.

The good part of the community is if they have the family support to continue with their treatment, to get comfort they need. The bad side is that sometimes they get medication from the field workers (community mental health workers) and it ends there so they rotate back to the institution. And the community staff is very limited. For example, this community with 2 or 3 persons, it's very hard to give the effective care to each person.

There seems to be a domineering attitude towards mentally ill patients and almost an expression of ownership. Psychiatric workers perceived that confinement to an institution would make the patient become submissive. It suggests that the workers have become accustomed to a modicum of control over mentally ill patients and do not want to relinquish their roles. These perceptions were present in both the urban and rural hospital, regardless of the length of time that they had been working with patients. Their perceptions are described in the following statements:

Most patients who live outside the institution tend to relapse as they do not have proper guidance. The family cannot offer support, as they cannot cope when the patients refuse to take their medications. They might have problems meeting their nutritional and social needs because the caregiver or family member cannot afford it.

Working with the mentally ill you realize what they came in for. For example, how aggressive they can be when they are ill, whether they hurt people. And now they're in the institution, they're stabilized, and you see this nice, sweet little person, and he's saying "Yes ma'am, no ma'am, yes nurse," you don't know what he can go back to if he just relapse even for a minute, and I think a lot of people don't understand that these are some of the clients we have in our hospitals. They are stable now, but if they go back on the road . . . you're gonna have an increase in violence, rapists, pedophiles, and I think we have to be very careful how we . . . deinstitutionalize them and get them back into society.

I think a vast majority of society does not readily accept mental illness; therefore, their tolerance level towards the behavior that these patients can portray could be very uncomfortable for them, and they in turn could be a threat to the patient rather than the patient threatening them.

Institutionalisation is good if they are being monitored on a 24-hour basis, so the client can cooperate with whatever you want them to do, whether to bathe or to eat or participate in activities and help them to interact with others.

Custodial care is deeply ingrained in the institution towards patients. Workers are both fearful of losing their hold over the patient and also of patient relapse. They perceive that they are more prepared to control the illness than family members, as deinstitutionalization would relinquish their authority over the patient.

The perceptions of mental health workers corroborate Hickling's findings of benefits to institutionalized services.

There are advantages in institutionalization relating to follow up. While in institution they will not do things that they would do outside without supervision by trained personnel. You have persons who for reasons take their relatives for admission and then abandon them and I guess that puts additional strain on the institution. However, if the family members are not involved, I don't think it (deinstitutionalization) would be beneficial to the client, because there would be no supervision and follow up day to day.

The advantages of the patients being in an institution are that they are in a therapeutic environment. They are offered, whether it is psychological, psychiatric care, and they have nursing and medical care if it is also deemed necessary. The opportunity to be around well-caring persons who seem to have their interest at heart, and they're now among persons with the same condition, so they know that they're not alone, so they get a sense of belonging. The aim is to bring them up to an optimal level of well-being where they're now able to go back and function in society.

Unpreparedness of the community to cope and absence of a community support system are two areas of concern identified by the psychiatric workers. A perception of deinstitutionalization is the lack of support available for patients and the consequences.

I am not in 100 percent agreement with it because, after a person [has] been in an institution . . . as a matter of fact, the Bellevue Hospital was designed for the mentally ill, you understand? And we don't want to take that away from our patients, because as we look at these and other hospitals, they are there for that purpose, so I am not in agreement to deinstitutionalize altogether our patients.

But for them now to go back out into the community, for some of them, there is no family support; the stigma that is there; they don't want to go to the health center for the medication because there is a stigma at the health center because psychiatry is housed in a little corner, so everybody knows once you go to the room. So persons don't want to, so when they go back into the community, the fear of the treatment brings them right back to square one so you get them right back here into the institution.

The view of the psychiatric workers is corroborated by the Canadian Alliance on Mental Illness and Mental Health (2007).

If the patients return to their community where society does not understand their illness, or a society who feels that they cannot sit beside somebody who has bipolar disorder, or somebody diagnosed with schizophrenia, that is where the breakdown is going to be and that is where the risk of relapse increases.

Community members are not very keen on helping people with mental illness and this is true because even if you look in our situation here . . . I'm going to go back to a Jamaican tale that we say here. When you are sick in your family, everybody inquire about you and they want to visit you and they want to take a little soup for you if they're allowed. Now if you're mentally ill, the family wants to hide it, they never tell you what's really wrong with the person, they never come to look for them, and if they do, they come and whisper, and as soon as the patient get back home, he is branded as someone who is never ever going to be stable, is never ever going to be able to do things that he use to before. So, the community is not very supportive of these individuals, and again it takes education and the effort of all to make this thing possible.

The negative part of deinstitutionalization is the fact that pushing deinstitu-tionalization when we do not have the support system in place is causing . . . is pushing us to something that we might regret later. There must be systems that are set up, right; halfway houses that are very important . . . Before we do deinstitutionalization, patients must be able to learn skills; they must be able to have good occupational therapy, yes? They must be able to go . . . to be able to be allowed into the community to socialize, even to go to church to see how they integrate with people. So the system must be set up and right now we don't have a system, so that's the negative part for me right now.

We don't have proper initiatives in the community for going on a daily basis, especially for skills training to be able to live off that. Sometimes on the road they are set ablaze or chopped or killed.

If not educated the community will see these individuals as mad and will treat them as such. So they will isolate them and stigmatize them and they will not get their support. Also the family members will be stigmatized also and that person will be shut away in a corner. So unlike here where we are educated and they'll be able to go about and we interact with them, these persons while they're in the community will be locked away in a small room and isolated from the larger community.

Substance use and abuse presented challenges:

So the same man now will look on you and selling you the weed (ganja) and all of that. Nobody is going to say "No, don't sell him any weed because if you sell him the weed him a relapse and go back a Bellevue" and so on.

They [family] should also be concerned with patient safety in the home and ensure that follow-up care is done and that persons are compliant with their medication.

When that is being done, patients would be saying, "Hey, I have the freedom to smoke (ganja) as much as I want because the community don't understand the person, there's still going to be negative influence and feedback.

Caregiver perspectives

Pusey-Murray and Miller (2013) studied caregivers of the mentally ill in their communities and found that some are not able to cope due to a number of factors, including the patient denying that they were mentally ill, inadequate support at home, and threats made to the caregiver by the patient. A caregiver indicated inability to cope with the relative as her health was being affected "It gives me high blood pressure, sometimes he doesn't want to wash his clothes. He often refuses to attend clinic because he says he isn't sick."

It is believed that changing attitudes and fighting stigma require more than just improving the understanding of the signs and symptoms of mental health problems and illnesses. The best way to break down stigma is through "contact-based education"—meeting and talking with people who can share their experiences of mental illness and recovery (Canadian Alliance on Mental Illness and Mental Health, 2007). The psychiatric workers' perceptions range from pessimism, and negative outcomes to recommendations on the support needed for success. The introduction of community mental health in the 1970s created a paradigm shift and demonstrated the rehabilitative possibility of patients with psychiatric illness. There is no doubt that patients and their families have benefited.

Based on the focus group discussions psychiatric workers had grave concerns about the patients being returned to their respective communities without the necessary support systems being in place such as family support, affordability of their medications, and human and material resources.

The absence of systems to support deinstitutionalization was expressed by a psychiatric worker who stated:

> They must be able to go . . . to be able to be allowed into the community to socialize; even to go to church to see how they integrate with people. So the system must be set up and right now we don't have a system, so that's the negative part for me right now.

If the correct support systems and resources are not in place it can place undue burden on the family and indeed the person who is the "care giver."

Pusey-Murray and Miller (2013) also found that the caregivers recognized the importance and value of social interaction with family members and the community, both for themselves and for their sick relative. Caregivers also highlighted problems of cost, accessibility, and availability of medications. Some caregivers were hindered financially, due to their age and/or lack of employment, from purchasing the medications that were prescribed. The psychiatric workers on the other hand voiced similar concerns about the families.

Pusey-Murray, Bourne, Warren, LaGrenade, and Charles (2010), postulated that patients believed in external factors apart from medications that could be used to control their illness such as praying, use of Obeah, fasting, smoking marijuana or cigarettes, and use of sour-sop leaves. There is strong evidence that spiritual rituals, obeah and bushes play an integral part of health practice in Jamaica. In their study, Pusey-Murray and Miller (2013) also indicated that the obeah man was consulted to boost up the medication effects. Respondents indicated that in addition to the prescribed medication for mental illness the caregiver also gave the patient "what the bush doctor ordered"(Pusey-Murray & Miller, 2013).

Implications for nurses practicing within global communities

It is imperative that nurses become familiar with the contextual milieu of mental illness and are sensitive to the historical and cultural perspectives associated with persons for whom care is provided. The historical perspective situates the deep perceptions and beliefs that can impact health and response to health care. Jamaicans have had a strong heritage of external dominance, which influenced all its institutions and functions inclusive of health care and health care beliefs. The African ancestry of the majority of the population imprinted beliefs and cultural practices that are still in existence today. To provide holistic and comprehensive care the nurse must delve into the background of each patient to gain a greater understanding of influences and factors that contribute to the best outcomes and to quality care. This journey will also assist the nurse to be reflective, empathetic towards others and understanding of what drives or restricts patient progress. The approach can stimulate practice-focused research and drive evidence to support and enhance treatment. Jamaicans are a migratory population and can be found in any country of the world. Knowing the context of their ancestry and cultural beliefs and practices can break down barriers and create relationships and partnerships that can focus on promoting mental health.

According to Lefley, (1998) a psycho-educational approach, in which the nurse educates the family about the illness and offers supportive understanding of the family experience, may help in this situation. Caregivers who accompany loved ones to the health centers or hospitals should be included in the teaching sessions being conducted by the health care provider. Culturally, clients with a mental health problem or their caregivers may seek the services of these healers; hence the community mental health officers may need to educate these persons from time to time. Caregivers as well as clients may gravitate to the healers for treatment due to lack of financial resources, and their belief that the illness is caused by demons. This is corroborated by one psychiatric worker who stated:

> Due cognizance must be taken to ingrained cultural beliefs that form an integral part of health care practices in communities. If the support systems and adequate resources are lacking, it will be easier to resort to alternative means that could exacerbate the mental illness.

The nursing process is essential in order to effectively provide care to meet holistic needs of individuals. Implementation should include maintaining a therapeutic nurse–patient relationship, incorporating cultural beliefs in the care provided and understanding the impact of multiple factors on the individual. The influence of prescribed medication and non-prescribed medications can result in serious side effects; therefore the nurse must involve all relevant stakeholders in the planning of care for the mentally ill.

Summary/conclusion

Between the Spaniards and the British the indigenous population of Jamaica, the Tianos, became extinct. Most Jamaicans are of African descent having been enslaved by the British. Based on the heritage and political, social and economic contextual milieu there are cultural practices and beliefs that continue to influence the way of life of the population. Scholars attest to the inclusion of nontraditional alongside traditional practices in health care including mental illness (Hickling & Gibson, 2012; Pusey-Murray & Miller, 2013). History attests that persons of African descent with mental illness had horrific treatment whether on the slavery plantation or within the "lunatic asylums." Custodial care and paternalistic care is deeply inculcated in the culture of mental illness in Jamaica. Even with the paradigm shift towards community care nearly 50 years ago, some mental health workers have reservations about the capability of patients to successfully navigate their communities and the readiness of families and communities to accommodate to deinstitutionalized care. There is no doubt that deinstitutionalization can be successfully implemented; however, there is reservation regarding preparedness of families and communities to sustain deinstitutionalized service.

It is imperative that an aggressive campaign be mounted to sensitize and educate communities to the benefits of deinstitutionalization and to eliminate the associated stigma experienced by the mentally ill patients. The authors believe that the psychiatric workers are expressing the reality that they observe when patients are taken out of their care in the hospital and return in a worse state. A much more concerted effort must be made to involve all categories of psychiatric health care workers in the decision-making process towards deinstitutionalization. Their views will be pertinent to the success of deinstitutionalized mental health services. Simultaneously, the support services within communities must be sharpened and expanded with the introduction of community mental health officers to foster deinstitutionalized mental health care that can be rigorously pursued for a positive outcome for all.

References

Beaubrun, M.H. (1977). *Mosaic of cultures.* World Health. Geneva: WHO.

Beaubrun, M.H., Bannister P., Lewis, L.F., Mahy, G.E., Royes, K.C., Smith, P. (1976). *The history of psychiatry in the West Indies.* In Howells G. (Ed.), *History of world psychiatry.* New York: Brunnel/Mazel.

Bowerbank, L. (1860). *The Case of Ann Pratt, Reviewed and answered in a letter to his Excellency the Governor.* Kingston, Jamaica: George Henderson, Savage.

Canadian Alliance on Mental Illness and Mental Health. (2007). *Mental health literacy: A review of the literature.* Retrieved from: www.camimh.ca/files/literacy/LIT_REVIEW_MAY_6_07.pdf.

Collis, R., & Green, P. (1976). Community psychiatry and the Pan American Health Organization: The Jamaican experience. *Bulletin of the Pan American Health Organization,* 10, 233–240.

Economic and Social Survey Jamaica (ESSJ) (2009). Planning Institute of Jamaica, Kingston, Jamaica. Retrieved from www.scribd.com/doc/47531459/Economic-Social-Suurvey-Jamaica-2009.

Hickling, F.W. (1975). An analysis of the 1873 Mental Hospital Law in Jamaica and its effect on mental treatment facilities. *Jamaica Law Journal,* October, 64–69.

Hickling, F.W. (1976). The effects of a community psychiatric service on mental hospital admissions in Jamaica. *West Indian Medical Journal,* 25, 101–107.

Hickling, F.W. (1995). Community psychiatry and deinstitutionalization in Jamaica. *Hospital Community Psychiatry,* 45, 1122–1126.

Hickling, F.W., & Gibson, R.C. (2012). Decolonization of psychiatric public policy in Jamaica. *West Indian Medical Journal.* 61(4), 437–441.

Hickling, F.W., Robertson-Hickling, H., & Paisley, V. (2011). Deinstitutionalization and attitudes toward mental illness in Jamaica: A qualitative study. *Rev Panam Salud Publica.* 29(3), 169–76.

Jamaica Demographic Profile. (2014). Retrieved from: www.indexmundi.com/jamaica/demographics_profile.html.

Jones, M. (1952). *Social psychiatry: A study of therapeutic communities.* London: Tavistock.

Lefley, H. (1998). The family experience in cultural context: Implications for further research and practice. In Lefley, H. (Ed.), *Families coping with mental illness: The cultural context* (pp. 97–105). San Francisco, CA: Jossey-Bass.

Ottey, F. (1973). *A psychiatric service for eastern Jamaica.* Thesis. Mona, Jamaica: University of the West Indies.

Pusey-Murray, A., & Miller, P. (2013). "I need help": Caregivers' experience caring for their relatives with mental illness in Jamaica. *Mental Health in Family Medicine,* 10(2), 113–121.

Pusey-Murray, A., Bourne, P., Warren, S., LaGrenade, J., & Charles, C. (2010). Medication compliance among mentally ill patients in public clinics in Kingston and St Andrew, Jamaica. *Journal of Biomedical Science and Engineering,* 3, 602–611.

Rouse, R. (1860). New *lights on dark deeds being jottings from the diary of Richard Rouse.* Kingston, Jamaica: Hall & Myers.

22

KOREAN AMERICANS, DEPRESSION AND NURSING CARE

Kunsook S. Bernstein

Introduction and background

Korean Americans are the fourth largest Asian American group in the United States, at 0.4 percent of the population; Chinese Americans make up the largest Asian group at 0.9 percent, followed by Filipino Americans at 0.7 percent, Asian Indians at 0.6 percent, and Japanese Americans at 0.3 percent (Kalibatseva & Leong, 2011). Korean Americans are also one of the fastest growing ethnic minorities in the United States (Hoeffel, Rastogi, Kim, & Shahid, 2012). In addition, a recent analysis by the Pew Research Center found that 78 percent of Korean Americans ages 18 years and older were born outside of the United States (Pew Research Center, 2012). One study of Korean Americans ($N = 304$) found that they had higher depression scores than the general population (Bernstein, Park, Shin, Cho, & Park, 2011), and another found that 23 percent reported having depressive symptoms but only 8.5 percent used mental health services (most did not perceive the need for psychological help, even when they had depressive symptoms) (Park, Cho, Park, Bernstein, & Shin, 2013). Another study of 860 Korean immigrants found that they reported higher levels of depressive symptoms and of psychological distress than other Asian ethnic groups (Noh, Avison, & Kaspar, 1992). Korean Americans who abandoned their Korean identity, traditions, and values scored higher for depression than did those who maintained their traditional values and identity (Oh, Koeske, & Sales, 2002). Depression was often under diagnosed in another study and therefore not treated due to barriers that included limited access to services and lack of culturally appropriate therapies (Lee, Hanner, Cho, Han, & Kim, 2008). A study of 230 older Korean American immigrants reported that the women scored higher on depressive symptoms than the men did and that their cultural background and values deeply influenced, and thus limited, their help-seeking behaviors and attitudes toward mental health services (Jang, Kim, & Chiriboga, 2011). The Korean word for depression, "woo-ul-jeung," translates as "a state of being out-of-balance," reflecting a culture in which health and well-being are seen as a balance between body and mind (Shin, 2002). Korean culture is informed by Confucianism and its emphasis on family integrity, group conformity, and traditional gender roles, influencing how people of Korean descent conceptualize depression, express depressive symptoms, and seek help (Park & Bernstein, 2008). The Korean cultural norm is to suppress personal emotions, avoid confrontation, and emphasize harmony within groups and in relationships (Park & Bernstein, 2008). Furthermore, the ideal Korean woman has been traditionally viewed as self-sacrificing, discreet, soft-spoken, and submissive (Kim, 1998). The "wise mother and good wife" concept has been influential in modern Korean life (Kŭm, 2003; Pak, 2006), and its influence is apparent in Korean American women's mental health-related behaviors and attitudes toward treatment (Bemak & Chung, 2000).

Cultural barriers to mental health services

Studies indicate that Korean Americans' cultural values and their negative experiences with conventional mental health services can often limit their use of mental health services, especially among immigrants (Lee *et al.*, 2008). In particular, Western-style psychotherapy, which often emphasizes self-disclosure and emotional expression, may contrast with Asian Americans' preferences for receiving help, such as assistance from family or friends (Leong & Lau, 2001). Also, there are significant differences between Western and Korean conceptions of emotion. For example, the Korean word "han" describes a syndrome of regret or resentment about the neglect of parents or children that would be labeled "shame" or "guilt" in Western society (Pang, 1998). Korean women with "han" have a tendency to internalize their feelings, and have few emotional outlets and social supports (Cho, Bernstein, Roh, & Chen, 2013), as do women with the Korean culture-bound syndrome "hwa-byung," which translates as "fire illness" or "anger syndrome" (Min, Suh, & Song, 2009). In addition, when given an opportunity to share their life stories, Asian women, including Korean women, tend to focus on relationships and family rather than on themselves (Haight, Nomura, & Nomura, 2000). A lack of culturally tailored therapeutic interventions has been a major barrier for Korean Americans, preventing them from seeking timely mental health services for a range of mental health problems including depression (Bernstein *et al.*, 2011). Furthermore, the consequences of untreated depression can be costly not only for the treatment of depression but also loss of productivity of the individuals suffering from depression: for instance, the National Alliance on Mental Illness (NAMI) estimates the direct and indirect workplace costs of depression to be more than $34 billion per year (NAMI, 2011). However, there are no data available on the direct and indirect costs associated with depression among Korean Americans.

Case example

Clinical presentation

Mrs. K, age 45, has been married for 28 years and lives with her husband in Koreatown, New York. She has an only son who is 27 years old, attending a doctoral program at a prestigious college in Korea. She has been working as a helper in a Korean restaurant and her husband also works in a Korean market as a laborer. She admitted that she has been depressed since her early twenties, often thought of committing suicide but never acted on it and has never been treated for depression. She presented with the following symptoms of depression: feeling trapped and living in a pitch black place (depressed mood); disappointment with life in general; severe insomnia (2–3 hours of sleep per night); no energy with chronic fatigue and feeling completely wasted physically; poor appetite (5 pound weight loss within past month); and difficulty with living a normal life since nothing matters, often leading to preoccupation with suicide. She acknowledged that she has been depressed with no intention to seek treatment due to no health benefit and financial constraints. She was brought to the free mental health clinic serving Korean Americans accompanied by her younger sister seeking help. Mrs. Kim was initially reluctant to engage in the interview, and became tearful and claimed that there was no hope for her and nothing would help so ending her life would be the only option. She expressed feeling ashamed that she could not shake off these feelings and blamed her husband, who she felt was not supportive of her. She claimed that her husband had no idea what she has been going through, and continued to expect her to serve him and fulfill his daily needs. She was angry and disappointed, and could not bear to stay in the relationship with him and planned to leave him as soon as she could once her son graduated from the college. She reported that her life has been in constant turmoil, with feelings of worthlessness, and saw her self image as an "empty rusty can" and expressed seeing no point in continuing. When asked whether she had an imminent plan or intent to end her life, she stated that she promised her son not to take her own life and also could not bear the thought of facing "God" if she took her own life. She also reported that she had been diagnosed with thyroid cancer and had a partial thyroidectomy 10 years ago and was currently in remission.

Brief analysis/aftermath and update

Case analysis of depressive symptoms

Mrs. K meets the *Diagnostic and Statistical manual of Mental Disorders'* (DSM-5) (American Psychiatric Association, 2013) diagnostic criteria of major depressive disorder, which is during the same 2-week period, at least one of the following symptoms: either depressed mood or loss of interest or pleasure, plus four of the following symptoms of disturbed sleep, loss of appetite, psychomotor agitation or retardation, fatigue, feelings of worthlessness, excessive guilt, poor concentration, and recurrent thoughts of death and suicidal ideation. Her depressive symptom manifestation might be somewhat different from the diagnostic criteria of DSM-5, but her symptoms of depression clearly meet the criteria of major depressive disorder with: 1) depressed mood manifested by feeling trapped and living in a pitch dark black place; 2) lack of interest in life manifested by difficulty with living since nothing matters in life; 3) severe insomnia (2–3 hours of sleep per night); 4) fatigue manifested by feeling completely wasted physically; 5) feelings of worthlessness and suicidal ideation for the last several years. Bernstein, Lee, Park, and Jyoung, (2008) reported that the meanings of the culture-specific symptom manifestation and expression of depressive symptom by Koreans could be significant to those inside or knowledgeable about this subculture, but they might differ from the predominant Western understanding of depression as a brain chemical imbalance, which is expressed mainly as a depressed mood (e.g. feeling blue or down). Additionally, linguistic limitation may apply, as it does to all cultures. For example, while Americans often describe their depressive moods by saying "I feel blue," Koreans usually use "black" to express depressed feelings (Kim, 2002). Koreans often describe their general environment as having the same qualities as their moods. For instance, a common phrase that Korean immigrants use to express feelings of depression is "Everything that surrounds me is dark and black" (Kim) as expressed by Mrs. K's statement of "pitch dark black." Also, since Korean culture is significantly influenced by Confucianism, openly expressing one's feelings is seen as a reflection of negative well-being; the family's or society's needs, not the individual's, are the priority, so expressing one's emotions is not socially acceptable (Lee, Moon, & Knight, 2004). Therefore, Koreans tend to express their emotions metaphorically, as expressed by Mrs. K., "I see my life as an empty rusty can."

Traditional Korean culture and values

Confucianism still remains a major force in shaping the social behavior, ethics, and moral principles of Koreans (Kim, 1998) despite the rapid industrialization that has caused Korean society to be exposed to Western culture and to adopt many Western values (Kŭm, 2003). Along with Confucianism, which is characterized by filial piety, the worship of ancestors, respect for authority, and a relatively rigid social hierarchy based on age, sex, and social class (Kim, 2001), Taoism and Buddhism have also influenced Korean culture (Kwon-Ahn, 2001). The guiding principles of Taoism and Buddhism, which have shaped the Korean national character as a way of life are strength on overcoming difficulties, enduring hardships, and maintaining calm in the face of trying circumstances (Kwon-Ahn, 2001).

Since Korean family life and traditional Korean values are based on Confucian philosophy, a person is often judged by how well he or she practices filial piety, which regulates the intergenerational relationship between parents and children throughout the life cycle, and it regulates many other relationships through the principle of seniority (Kŭm, 2003; Kim, 2001). One result of this emphasis on filial piety in Korean society is that the family unit is more important than the individual, and an individual is expected to sacrifice his or her personal desires in favor of the needs and welfare of the family (Kim, 2001) to maintain group solidarity (Lee *et al.*, 2004). Additionally, Confucianism rigidly defines the role of women by stressing the differences between the roles of husbands and wives (Kim, 2001). Traditionally, a Korean woman's life is always constrained by her cultural obligations, making it difficult for her to carve out her own identity (Kim, 2001); divorce is considered shameful and tends to carry a greater stigma than it does in Western culture, in large part because of the disgrace it can bring to the entire family (Park, Murgatroyd, Raynock, & Spillet, 1998). In traditional Korean society, the husband is the main breadwinner and is supposed to make all major decisions affecting the family, while the wife is to serve him and other family members with devotion (Kim, 2001) including working hard alongside her husband for the welfare of the whole family since the wife's hard work is viewed as her required duty to the family, not a virtue or a choice (Pak, 2006).

Mrs. K is no exception to this cultural influential force, which has shaped and influenced her family structure, gender role, and marital relations, even though she has been exposed to Western notions of individualism, gender equality, self-respect, and freedom. She always put herself after her husband and son in the family despite her resentment and anger toward her husband, but never toward her son who has been her only hope and joy in life. As a wife, she prepares her husband's meals every day after working all day long, cleans the house, and does laundry and other household chores. She sees these as her duties and responsibilities. Even though she has expressed the desire to leave her husband, this idea remains as a personal desire and thought for the last 15 years, and she has not acted on it and has no plan to do so in the near future. In other words, she has been influenced by and lives based on Confucian philosophy that she practices filial piety in her daily life by serving her husband as a devoted wife and sacrifices herself to support her son's schooling regardless of her own emotional turmoil compounded with her depression.

Aftermath and update

Following the initial intake, Mrs. K.'s treatment for her depression initiated with the plan of: 1) psychotherapy with journaling; 2) psychotropic medications (antidepressant), which were suggested but Mrs. K. refused; and 3) family therapy with the husband but Mrs. K. refused. Mrs. K. went through 8-weeks of structured logotherapy combined with autobiography, which were designed to specifically treat depressed Korean women. Since expressing emotions is not valued traditionally, a notion that persists in Korean society and among Korean Americans, psychotherapy with journaling was chosen as a therapeutic modality for Mrs. K. The purpose of the therapy was to ultimately find a purpose in her life through searching for meaning in life through guided writing of a self-autobiography. Upon the completion of the 8-week treatment, Mrs. K.'s depression was lifted as evidenced by changes in the CES-D score from 46 pre-treatment to 14 post-treatment. She also reported a significant improvement in her relationship with the husband and has been actively involved in her church and social activities.

Intervention model: enhanced logo-autobiography

Logo autobiography (LA) was designed for depressed Korean American women to write about their experiences of such culture-bound phenomena as han and hwa-byung, which are familiar terms for them, and it was found to have assisted them in lessening depressive symptoms and in finding meaning in their lives (Bernstein, Cho, Cho, & Roh, 2013; Cho, et al., 2013). An enhanced form of LA, the E (enhanced) LA program incorporates coping and psychological growth by expanding the original 6-week program to 8 weeks. ELA as the experimental intervention seeks to capture the benefits of both logotherapy and autobiography: finding meaning in life through guided writing about one's own life story. Logotherapy is based on Frankl's three concepts—the freedom of will, the will to meaning, and the meaning of life—which together guide people to focus on their power to forge meaning rather than focus on the debilitating nature of a crisis (Frankl, 1969). The autobiography as a therapeutic intervention is a written self-narrative that allows the writer to reflect on how she has faced her life's problems, drawing on the human capacity for self-description and self-analysis (Sommer, 2003); the guided autobiography explores an individual's own life through structured, self-reflective journaling (Cho *et al.*, 2013). In blending these two approaches, ELA emphasizes cognitive change: it provides a structured method for unlearning negative thought patterns and learning new, more positive ones. The intended outcome is that the participant will manage her personal obstacles more productively and find meaning through the structured exploration of self-reflection, self-description, and self-analysis (Cho *et al.*, 2013).

Summary/conclusion

Depression is prevalent among Korean Americans who have to deal with stress caused by social and cultural differences from residing in mainstream America. Many people who suffer from depression are inadequately diagnosed and treated, which often leads to serious psychosocial and functional impairments.

Confucianism and its emphasis on family integrity, group conformity, and traditional gender roles influence Korean culture. Culture influences how people of Korean descent conceptualize depression, express depressive symptoms, and seek help. The Korean cultural norm is to suppress personal emotions, avoid confrontation, and emphasize harmony within groups and in relationships. Furthermore, the ideal Korean woman has been traditionally viewed as a self-sacrificing mother, discreet and good wife, and this belief is still influential in modern Korean life, and its influence is apparent in Korean American women's mental health-related behaviors and attitudes toward treatment. However, conventional psychotherapy has been viewed as ineffective, costly, intrusive, and time consuming by many Asian Americans, including Korean Americans, who generally prefer directive, structured, problem-solving approaches that focus on alleviating specific symptoms. Culturally sensitive and appropriate therapeutic modality for depressed Korean American women might be beneficial to guide them to express emotion through a self-reflective life review focusing on family relationships and the moral and social values that dominate their lives.

References

American Psychiatric Association. (2013). *Diagnostic and statistical manual of mental disorders (DSM-5)* (5th ed.). Washington, DC: American Psychiatric Publishing.

Bemak, F., & Chung, R.C. (2000). Psychological intervention with immigrants and refugees. In J.F. Aponte, & J. Wohl (Eds.), *Psychological intervention and cultural diversity* (2nd ed., pp. 200–213). Boston, MA: Allyn & Bacon.

Bernstein, K., Cho, S. H., Cho S. Y., & Roh, S. (2013). Logo-autobiography and its effectiveness on depressed Korean immigrant women: a replication study. *Journal of Nursing Education and Practice, 3*(6), 51–60.

Bernstein, K.S, Lee, J.S., Park, S.Y., & Jyoung, J.P. (2008). Symptom manifestations and expressions among Korean immigrant women suffering with depression. *Journal of Advanced Nursing, 61*(4), 393–402.

Bernstein, K. S., Park, S., Shin, J., Cho, S., & Park, Y. (2011). Acculturation, discrimination, and depressive symptoms among Korean immigrants in New York City. *Community Mental Health Journal, 47*(1), 24–34.

Cho, S., Bernstein, K.S., Roh, S., & Chen, D. (2013). Logo-autobiography and its effectiveness on depressed Korean immigrant women. *Journal of Transcultural Nursing, 24*(1), 33–42.

Frankl, V.E. (1969). *The will to meaning: Foundations and applications of logotherapy.* New York: World Publishing.

Haight, B., Nomura, T., & Nomura, A. (2000). Life review as an Alzheimer's intervention: results of an American-Japanese project. *Dimensions, 7*(4), 4–8.

Hoeffel, E.M., Rastogi, S., Kim, M.O., & Shahid, H. (2012). *The Asian population: 2010 census briefs.* Washington, DC: US Department of Commerce, Economics & Statistics Administration, US Census Bureau; March 2012. Retrieved January 5, 2014 from www.census.gov/prod/cen2010/briefs/c2010br-11.pdf.

Jang, Y., Kim, G., & Chiriboga, D. A. (2011). Gender differences in depressive symptoms among older Korean American immigrants. *Social Work In Public Health, 26*(1), 96–109.

Kalibatseva, Z., & Leong, F.T.L. (2011). Depression among Asian Americans: review and recommendations. *Depression Research & Treatment, 2011*(320902). Doi:10.1155/2011/320902.

Kim, E.J. (1998). The social reality of Korean-American women: toward crashing with the Confucian ideology. In Y.I. Song, & A. Moon (Eds.), *Korean American women: From tradition to modern feminism* (pp. 23–33). Westport, CT: Praeger.

Kim, M.T. (2001). *Yookyojeok Jyontonggya Hyundae Hankook [Confucianism and the Contemporary Korean].* Seoul, Korea: Cheolhakgya Hyunshilsa.

Kim, M.T. (2002). Measuring depression in Korean Americans: development of the Kim Depression Scale for Korean Americans. *Journal of Transcultural Nursing, 13*(2), 109–117.

Kŭm, C. (2003). *Hyŏndae Han'guk Yugyo wa chŏnnt'ong [Adaptation of Confucian organizations to the contemporary Korean society].* Seoul, Korea: Seoul National University Press.

Kwon-Ahn, Y. (2001). Substance abuse among Korean-Americans: a social-cultural perspective and framework for intervention. In S. Straussner (Ed.), *Ethnocultural issues in addiction treatment* (pp. 418–436). New York: Guildford Press.

Lee, H., Moon, A., & Knight, B.G. (2004) Depression among elderly Korean immigrants: exploring socio-cultural factors. *Journal of Ethnic & Cultural Diversity in Social Work 13*(4), 1–26.

Lee, H.B., Hanner, J.A., Cho, S.J., Han, H.R., & Kim, M.T. (2008). Improving access to mental health services for Korean-American immigrants: moving toward a community partnership between religious and mental health services. *Psychiatry Investigation, 5*(1), 14–20.

Leong, F.T.L., & Lau, A.S.L. (2001). Barriers to providing effective mental health services to Asian Americans. *Mental Health Services Research, 3*(4), 201–214.

Min, S.K., Suh, S.Y., & Song, K.J. (2009). Symptoms to use for diagnostic criteria of hwa-byung, an anger syndrome. *Psychiatry Investigation, 6*(1), 7–12.

National Alliance on Mental Illness. (2011). The impact and cost of mental illness: the case of depression. Retrieved January 7, 2014 from www.nami.org/Template.cfm?Section=Policymakers_Toolkit& Template=/ContentManagement/ContentDisplay.cfm&ContentI D=19043.

Noh, S., Avison, W.R., & Kaspar, V. (1992). Depressive symptoms among Korean immigrants: assessment of a translation of the Center for Epidemiologic Studies Depression scale. *Psychological Assessment, 4*(1), 84–91.

Oh, Y., Koeske, G. F., & Sales, E. (2002). Acculturation, stress, and depressive symptoms among Korean immigrants in the United States. *Journal of Social Psychology, 142*(4), 511–526.

Pak, J.H.C. (2006). *Korean American women: Stories of acculturation and changing selves.* New York: Routledge.

Pang, K.Y.C. (1998). Symptoms of depression in elderly Korean immigrants: Narration and the healing process. *Culture, Medicine and Psychiatry, 22,* 93–122.

Park, S.Y., & Bernstein, K.S. (2008). Depression and Korean American immigrants. *Archives of Psychiatric Nursing, 22*(1), 12–19.

Park, H., Murgatroyd, W., Raynock, D.C., & Spillett, M.A. (1998). Relationship between intrinsic-extrinsic religious orientation and depressive symptoms in Korean Americans. *Counseling Psychology Quarterly, 11*(3), 315–324.

Park, S.Y., Cho, S.H., Park, Y., Bernstein, K.S., & Shin, J. (2013). Factors associated with mental health service utilization among Korean American immigrants. *Community Mental Health Journal.* Doi: 10.1007/s10597-013-9604-8.

Pew Research Center (2012). Social and demographic trends: the rise of Asian Americans. Retrieved January 7, 2014 from www.pewsocialtrends.org/2012/06/19/the-rise-of-asian-americans/.

Shin, J.K. (2002). Help-seeking behaviors by Korean immigrants for depression. *Issues in Mental Health Nursing, 23*(5), 461–476.

Sommer, R. (2003). The use of autobiography in psychotherapy. *Psychotherapy in Practice, 59*(2), 197–205.

23

THE PHILIPPINES

Nurses' role in bullying prevention

Leilani Marie Ayala

Introduction

The Center for Disease Control has defined bullying as "any unwanted aggressive behavior(s) by another youth or group of youths who are not siblings or current dating partners that involves an observed or perceived power imbalance and is repeated multiple times or is highly likely to be repeated" (Gladden, Vivolo-Kantor, Hamburger, & Lumpkin, 2013). Two broad types of bullying can be discerned – traditional bullying and cyberbullying (Scott, Moore, Sly, & Norman, 2013). Traditional bullying can be either direct or indirect. The direct variant is more prevalent among males and involves overt displays of physical and/or verbal aggression directed at another person (e.g. pushing, punching, kicking, shoving, throwing things, verbal insults, taunts, name calling). This type of bullying is more commonly reported since it is easily observable (Wang, Ianotti, & Nansel, 2009). The indirect variant can be considered as "relational-aggression"; verbal methods are used to threaten relationships or undermine the social standing of victims. The victims are excluded from important social activities through spreading rumors, ostracizing and backstabbing. This form of bullying is more common among females and being less observable is not as likely to be reported.

Bullying is a global public health concern that has short- and long-term deleterious effects on the person's psychological and physical health. It is prevalent worldwide, which affects 5–57 percent of youths from high-income countries and a wide prevalence range of 12–100 percent in low- and middle-income countries (Fleming & Jacobsen, 2009). The Philippines was one of the countries that participated in the Global School-based Student Health Survey (GSHS) where a total of 7,338 students completed the survey of which 37.1 percent (2,722) reported being bullied. Among those who had been bullied, 63 percent were aged 12 years and younger, which is a higher prevalence rate when compared to the total percentage score of the other countries included in the survey (32.3 percent). In addition, the study showed that children exposed to bullying have a significantly increased risk of developing depressive symptomatology such as sadness or hopelessness, loneliness, insomnia, suicidal ideation, and risky health behaviors such as smoking, drinking, and drug-related involvement (Fleming & Jacobsen, 2009); thus making bullying an important issue to address in this cultural group.

Bullying in the Philippines

The Philippines, located in Southeast Asia, is an archipelago made up of 7,107 islands with an estimated population of about 96 million. The Philippines is a mix of Eastern and Western cultures having been under Spanish (1565–1898) and American (1898–1946) colonization for several years. Religious beliefs and practices, primarily Catholicism, were from the Spanish influence, while the emphasis on the importance of education was from the Americans. In post-colonial times, the Western influence is evident in the Filipino's perception of beauty. Individuals with a high-bridged nose and lighter skin—also known as "mestizas"—are regarded as beautiful and more superior than Filipinos with brown skin and a flat nose (David, 2013, p. 44). The latter are perceived as inferior and not as desirable compared to those with European physical attributes. This post-colonial mentality is evident by the surge of whitening products, such as skin lightening clinics and bleaching among Filipinos. Philippines ranked the highest in consumer rates for bleaching products among its contemporaries in Hong Kong, Taiwan, Malaysia, and Korea (Synovate, 2004). Individuals who have a darker complexion are perceived as unattractive and oftentimes subjected to teasing and bullying, thus skin whitening is considered as a social and economic investment (Mendoza, 2014) among Filipinos.

Religious beliefs of Filipinos may also contribute to their negative perception of the Lesbian, Gay, Bisexual and Transgender (LGBT) community, who like the darker skinned Filipinos, are often the target of bullying. The bullies are believed to get a "free pass" because their behavior conforms to socially acceptable norms (Tan, 2013). Aguiling-Dalisay *et al.*, 2001 (as cited in Manalastas & Del Pilar, 2005) identified that being gay is "sinful" and that gay sex is unnatural and "filthy" (Tan, Ujano-Batangan & Cabado-Espanola, 2001). Furthermore, Mostajo, Saz-Page, & Rasing, stated (as cited in Manalastas & Del Pilar, 2005) that gays and lesbians are perceived as sick or abnormal, oftentimes subjected to anti-gay jokes, forced to be in an intimate relationship with the opposite sex and frequently called "bakla" (gay) instead of their given name. Filipinos were found to have a largely negative attitude toward lesbians and gays, where 1 in every 4 Filipinos expressed not wanting to have a gay or lesbian neighbor (Manalastas & Del Pilar, 2005). Victimization experiences among gay and bisexual Filipino men places them at risk for suicide and even at higher risk for suicidal ideation compared to their heterosexual counterparts (Manalastas, 2013).

Culture of teasing and bullying

The culture of teasing is also present among Filipinos. According to Roces and Roces (2009), children are controlled by the elders through teasing, which is used as a way to keep children in line. Roces further added that teasing is used as a tool to "feel someone out" and it helps reveal the individuals' views and attitudes about sensitive issues without directly disclosing their personal thoughts. Therefore, it is not surprising to find that, in a Philippine study, teasing was the most common form of peer victimization and aggression among sixth graders (Calaguas, 2011) and a high prevalence rate of name-calling, teasing and gossiping were reported among high school students (Ouano, Buot, & Dela Rosa, 2013). In 2008, 2,442 children from 58 public schools were surveyed and results showed that ridicule and teasing by peers were the most common form of bullying experiences (50–65 percent) among students from grade school to high school (Plan Philippines, 2008).

Anti-bullying law in the Philippines

On September 6, 2013, Philippine President Benigno Aquino III signed into law Republic Act 10672, otherwise known as the Anti-Bullying Act of 2013. The law defined bullying as

> any severe, or repeated use by one or more students of a written, verbal, or electronic expression, or a physical act or gesture, or any combination thereof, directed at another student that has the effect of actually causing or placing the latter in a reasonable fear or physical or emotional harm or damage to his property; creating a hostile environment at school for the other student; infringing on the rights of another student at school; or materially and substantially disrupting the education process or the orderly operation of a school.
>
> *(Anti-Bullying Act of 2013, 2013, pp. 1–4)*

The law includes definitions of cyberbullying and gender-based bullying, and mandates for all private and public schools to adapt a bullying prevention program. In December 2013, the Department of Education issued guidelines for the implementation of the anti-bullying law and included procedures in reporting, record-keeping, referral process, and handling and monitoring incidents of bullying. The Department of Education launched the Child Protection Policy (CPC) in May 2012 to promote zero tolerance for any act of child abuse, exploitation, violence, discrimination, and other offenses. A nationwide campaign was conducted and a series of training of trainers was done. The CPC was in charge of facilitating training programs and ensuring that the anti-bullying policy was adopted and implemented by the schools. The CPC has been tasked to handle bullying cases in public and private school and will be composed of the school head/administrator, guidance counselor/teacher, teacher, parent, student, and community representative. The school head or CPC may refer those involved in bullying to trained professionals outside the school such as social workers, guidance counselors, psychologists, or child protection specialists for further evaluation as deemed necessary. If bullying results in death or serious physical injury, the case will be dealt with in accordance with the provisions stipulated in the Juvenile Justice and Welfare Act (Republic Act 9344) (2005) and the school head will notify the Women and Children's Protection Desk (WPCD) of the local Philippine National Police.

Examples of bullying prevention activities in the Philippines

1   The bullying prevention efforts in the Philippines are not limited to the school system. The Philippine Pediatric Society has opened up a hotline that will link victims with professional therapists. This will also be a resource for schools that wish to start anti-bullying campaigns and programs.

2   A police department from Baguio, a province located in the northern part of the Philippines, has also been involved in distributing anti-bullying booklets to students. Their agency believes that bullying experiences increase the likelihood of gang involvement, so by preventing bullying incidents they are also hoping to decrease gang-related activities.

3   The Psychological Association of the Philippines (PAP, 2012) has issued a statement addressing bullying, teasing, and harassment of LGBT children and adolescents in families, schools and communities. The PAP is part of the global initiative to remove stigma associated with the LGBT community and the organization has been actively promoting LGBT-affirmative policies and practices in the Philippines by supporting efforts to:

- oppose a public and private discrimination based on perceived sexual orientation, gender identity and expression;
- repeal discriminatory laws and policies and support the passage of legislation that protects the rights and promotes the welfare of people of all sexual orientations and gender identity expressions;
- eliminate all forms of prejudice and discrimination against LGBT in teaching, research, psychological interventions, assessment and other psychological programs;
- encourage psychological research that addresses the needs and concerns of LGBT Filipinos and their families and communities; and
- disseminate and apply accurate and evidence-based information about sexual orientation and gender identity and expression to design interventions that foster mental health and well-being of LGBT.

Role of nurses in bullying prevention

Nurses as advocates and early case finders

Registered nurses play a crucial role in the prevention of bullying incidents. School nurses, for example, are best positioned to screen for and identify bullying experiences among students who visit the clinic. Adolescents who experience bullying and other forms of victimization in school are more likely to use the school health center services (Lewis *et al.*, 2015). Children and adolescents who have been exposed to bullying are at higher risk of developing psychosomatic problems such as tiredness, nervousness, sleeping problems, dizziness, stomach pain, headaches, tension, fatigue, and poor appetite (Feekes *et al.*, 2006; Gini, 2007). Confiding in school nurses about bullying experiences will be more likely because nurses do not have academic or disciplinary roles (Cooper, Clements, & Holt, 2012). As part of their role in promoting the emotional health of an individual, school nurses can develop and implement anti-bullying programs such as bullying support groups. Support groups in school have been shown to decrease the incidence of bullying (Kvarme, Aabø, & Sæteren, 2015). Nurses working in the primary care setting and wellness clinics can include bullying screening questions for children during their health maintenance visit and especially for adolescents who will report smoking, alcohol or drug-use since bullied adolescents are at increased risk to engage in these activities.

Box 23.1 Example of screening questions to identify children involved in bullying:

- How are things going at school?
- Do you enjoy school?
- Do you have friends at school? Outside of school? Tell me the name of one of your friends.
- Has anyone picked on you or been mean to you at school? Outside of school? On the Internet/ your computer or your cell phone?
- Have you picked on anyone or been mean to anyone at school? Outside of school? Using the Internet/your computer or your cell phone?
- Have you ever been in any pushing or shoving fights?

Source: Shetgiri, R. (2013).

Public and community health care nurses should take an active role in disseminating information about the short- and long-term effects of bullying through parent and child workshops. Parents will benefit from learning about their role in protecting their children from harm and the dangers of cyberbullying. Parental support and monitoring, family connectedness, and caring relationships with non-parental adults, have been shown to mitigate incidents of bullying (Jantzer, Haffner, Parzer, Resch, & Kaess, 2015). Nurses can develop and offer classes for parents focusing on how to help their child who is being bullied or involved in bullying activities, how to report incidents of bullying and how to access community resources.

Occupational health nurses can facilitate stress-management classes and implement bullying prevention plans in the workplace. Efforts should be made to foster activities that promote positive self-concept among Filipino children: a healthy self-image not based on skin color or facial features. A dialogue with advertising companies can be initiated by nursing professional organizations to discuss ways to promote healthy self-image through their ads. Nurses can partner with government and non-government agencies in establishing community empowerment programs, which can provide opportunities for youths to participate in mentorship programs, skill building, social networking, sports activities, and other structured extracurricular activities; all of which have been shown to foster improved self-esteem and self-concept (Kort-Butler & Hagewen, 2011).

Nurses in academia

The nursing education curriculum in the Philippines often changes and clinical subjects are heavily focused on the current practice abroad, instead of the present health needs of the community. The Philippines is the leading market in exporting nurses abroad (Brush, 2010). The migration of nurses helped fill the global nursing shortage and at the same time helped boost the economic growth of the Philippines. In 2010, an estimated $21.3 billion were remitted by Filipino service workers abroad, nursing being the largest service sector working group of Filipino immigrants (Brush, 2010; Marcus, Quimson, & Short, 2014). However, migration of nurses abroad declined following the global economic crisis in 2007–2009. Thus, at present, there is a surplus of nurses in the Philippines who are either working as "volunteers" in government or private hospitals, or employed in non-nursing jobs. Nevertheless, most of the new graduates prefer to work in hospital settings in order to gain clinical experience required to work abroad.

The Philippine nursing academic institutions and professional nursing organizations can help support new graduates by creating opportunities for nurses to volunteer and provide leadership in developing community mental health promotion projects such as bullying prevention programs. Nurses in undergraduate and advanced nursing programs can benefit from learning about the prevalence, significance, prevention, and evidence-based interventions for bullying. This topic can be offered and incorporated in health care teaching and community immersion programs. Participation and involvement of nurses in bullying prevention activities can be valuable to nurses who are interested in pursuing a career in psychiatric mental health nursing. Nurses can enhance their clinical interviewing skills, learn how to do mental health assessment and screening, gain knowledge and skills in facilitating therapeutic groups, and develop their communication skills through one-to-one check-ins with children or adolescent participants.

In addition, graduate nursing students majoring in psychiatric mental health nursing can be trained to appropriately screen for symptoms of anxiety and depression associated with bullying experiences, and implement an appropriate plan of care. A validated tool such as the Child Behavior Checklist can be used to screen for emotional, developmental and behavioral problems

(Shetgiri, 2013). Additional materials and tools are also available from the American Academy of Pediatrics' Bright Future website (https://brightfutures.aap.org/), which nurses can utilize.

Nurse-led research around bullying in the Philippines is scarce thus it is difficult to assess the current role and impact of nursing interventions in bullying prevention programs. However, this is a timely and critical area for nurse researchers to pursue.

Nurses as policy advocates

Professional nursing organizations can propose evidence-based bullying interventions to school administrators, local government units, and other stakeholders. A focus on developing and advocating for programs to help remove stigma for members of the LGBT community should also be considered. It is to be noted that the role of registered nurses is not stipulated in the Philippine anti-bullying law. Furthermore, they were not included as members of the Child Protection Committee, a group that is tasked to handle bullying cases for both private and public schools. Psychiatric mental health nurses should offer their expertise and make themselves available in government-led initiatives related to bullying prevention.

Summary

Bullying is a public health concern in the Philippines and 50–65 percent of grade school and high school students have reported bullying experiences. Those who have experienced bullying are at a higher risk for developing symptoms of both anxiety and depression such as fearfulness, hypervigilance, loneliness and sadness, hopelessness, insomnia, and suicidal ideation. Furthermore, bullied adolescents are more likely to engage in unhealthy behaviors such as smoking, drinking, and drug-use. Teasing has been reported as the most common form of victimization. Gay and bisexual males who have been bullied are at a higher risk for having suicidal ideation. Nurses should assume leadership roles in conducting evidence-based bullying prevention interventions for individuals and communities. Outcome-driven projects should be developed and findings should be part of the national dialogue. The development of, and results from, nursing research studies can help direct and guide development of policies around bullying prevention and intervention.

References

Anti-Bullying Act of 2013, Republic Act 10672, House Number 5496, Philippines (2013). Retrieved April 14, 2015 from www.gov.ph/2013/09/12/republic-act-no-10627/.

Brush, B.L. (2010). The potent lever of toil: nursing development and exportation in the postcolonial Philippines. *American Journal of Public Health*, 100(9), 1572–1581.

Calaguas, G. (2011). Forms and frequency of peer aggression and peer victimization among sixth-graders. *Journal of Arts, Science and Commerce*, 2(2), 108–213.

Cooper, G.D., Clements, P.T., & Holt, K.E. (2012). Examining childhood bullying and adolescent suicide: implications for school nurses. *Journal of School Nursing*, 28(4), 275–83.

David, E.J.R. (2013). *Brown skin, white minds: Filipino/American postcolonial psychology*. Charlotte, NC: Information Age.

Feekes, M., Pijpers, F.I., Fredriks, A.M., Vogels, T., & Verloove-Vanhorick, S.P. (2006) Do bullied children get ill, or do ill children get bullied? A prospective cohort study on the relationship between bullying and health-related symptoms. *Pediatrics*, 117(5), 1568–1574.

Fleming, L. & Jacobsen, K. (2009). Bullying among middle-school students in low- and middle-income countries. *Health Promotion International*, 25(1), 1–12.

Gini, G. (2007), Association between bullying behaviors, psychosomatic complaints, emotional and behavioral problems. *Journal of Pediatrics and Child Health*, 44(9), 492–497.

Gladden R.M., Vivolo-Kantor, A.M., Hamburger, M.E., & Lumpkin, C.D. (2013). *Bullying surveillance among youths: Uniform definitions for public health and recommended data elements, version 1.0.* Atlanta, GA: National Center for Injury Prevention and Control, Centers for Disease Control and Prevention and US Department of Education.

Jantzer, V., Haffner, J., Parzer, P., Resch, F., & Kaess, M. (2015). Does parental monitoring moderate the relationship between bullying and adolescent nonsuicidal self-injury and suicidal behavior? A community-based self-report study of adolescents in Germany. *BMC Public Health, 583*, 1471–2458.

Juvenile Justice and Welfare Act, Republic Act 9344, Philippines, (2005). Retrieved July 31, 2015 from www.gov.ph/2006/04/28/republic-act-no-9344-s-2006/

Kort-Butler, L.A., & Hagewen, K.J. (2011). School-based extracurricular activity involvement and adolescent self-esteem: a growth-curve analysis. *Journal of Youth and Adolescence, 40*(5), 568–581.

Kvarme, L.G., Aabø, L.S., & Sæteren, B. (2015). From victim to taking control: support group for bullied school children. *The Journal of the School of Nursing, 32*(2), 112–119.

Lewis, C., Deardorff, J., Lahiff, M. Soleimanpour, S., Sakashite, K., & Brinids, C. (2015). High-school students' experiences of bullying and victimization and the association with school health center use. *Journal of School Health, 85*(5), 318–326.

Manalastas, E. (2013). Sexual orientation and suicide risk in the Philippines: evidence from a nationally representative sample of young Filipino men, *Philippine Journal of Psychology, 46*(1), 1–13.

Manalastas, E., & Del Pilar, G. (2005). Filipino attitudes towards lesbians and gay men: secondary analysis of 1996 and 2001 national survey data, *Philippine Journal of Psychology, 38*(2), 53–75.

Marcus, K., Quimson, G., & Short, S.D. (2014). Source country perceptions, experiences, and recommendations regarding health workforce migration: a case study from the Philippines. *Human Resources for Health, 12*(1), 62.

Mendoza, R.L. (2014). The skin whitening industry in the Philippines. *Journal of Public Health Policy, 35*(2), 219–238.

Ouano, J., Buot, N., & Dela Rosa, E. (2013). A measure of the experience of being bullied: an initial validation in Philippine schools. *Philippine Journal of Counseling Psychology, 15*(1), 14–27.

Plan Philippines (2008). Toward a child-friendly educational environment: a baseline study on violence against children in public schools. Retrieved June 1, 2014 from https://plan-international.org/learn withoutfear/files/philippines-toward-a-child-friendly-education-environment-english.

Psychological Association of the Philippines (PAP) (2012). Statement of the Psychological Association of the Philippines on non-discrimination based on sexual orientation, gender identity and expression. Retrieved June 1, 2014 from www.pap.org.ph/?ctr=page&action=resources.

Roces, A., & Roces, G. (2009). *Culture shock! Philippines: A survival guide to customs and etiquette* (7th ed.). Tarrytown, NY: Marshall Cavendish.

Scott, J., Moore, S., Sly, P., & Norman, R. (2013). Bullying in children and adolescents: a modifiable risk factor for mental illness. *Australian and New Zealand Journal of Psychiatry, 48*(3), 2009–2012.

Shetgiri, R. (2013). Bullying and victimization among children. *Advances in Pediatrics, 60*(1), 33–51.

Synovate Philippines. (2004) *Skin whitening in Southeast Asia.* Pasig City, Philippines: Synovate.

Tan, L., Ujano-Batangan, M., & Cbado-Esanola, H. (2001). *Love and desire: Young Filipinos and sexual risks.* Quezon City, Philippines: UP Center for Women's Studies.

Tan, M. (2013, December). SOGI included in "Anti-Bullying Act of 2013" IRR. Outrage, Retrieved June 1, 2014 from http://outragemag.com/sogi-included-anti-bullying-act-2013-irr/.

Wang, J., Iannotti, R.J., Nansel, T.R. (2009). School Bullying Among Adolescents in the United States: Physical, Verbal, Relational, and Cyber. *J Adolesc Health, 45*(4) 368–375.

24

FAMILY STRESS AND CARE IN SOUTH AFRICA

Authors: Idalia Venter and Lily van Rhyn
Analysis: Ukamaka M. Oruche

Introduction

The identification of mental illness among African people is a low priority, and often only serious mental illnesses and substance abuse disorders are readily identified. This does not mean that the more common illnesses are not present; in fact, the numbers for depression and anxiety disorders are similar to developed countries (Mathers & Loncan, 2006). A case example is presented of a woman who experiences depression with anxiety, a common illness in Africa due to emotional abuse by her husband, along with a lack of family support, circumstances supported by cultural attitudes (Feduka *et al.*, 2014).

Although arranged marriages are no longer common among African people in South Africa, the cultural practice of, for example, *lobola*, paying for the right to marry the woman, is ongoing. It has become a symbolic gesture, but underneath is still the concept that the wife is now the property of the husband and the wife's family has no influence in her life anymore. Men often still think they can treat a woman as property and the women feel powerless when they are dissatisfied with the actions of men (Mawere & Mawere, 2010).

An unfortunate legacy of colonization is the practice of migrant labor. Men often work in the mines far from home and may only visit their families once every few months. During their stay at the mine, many men engage in extramarital relationships. These relationships are usually considered temporary in nature until the man can return home to his wife and family (Zuma, Lurie, Williams, Garnett, & Sturm, 2005). Many women know of these practices, but because of their sense of powerlessness, they remain silent and accepting. The practice of men having a relationship outside the marriage is common, but the HIV/AIDS pandemic has made this practice deadly.

Although these cultural habits are against the constitution of the country, the practice is still rife and the powerlessness felt by women and the impact on their physical and mental health are profound. The following case study will describe a relationship that illustrates a cultural power imbalance between a man and his wife and the mental health consequences that she experienced as a result.

Description of the issue

Biographical details

Name:	Agnes Pitso*
Race:	African (Sesotho)
Gender:	Female
Age:	38 years
Diagnosis:	Depression with anxiety
Occupation:	Clerk at Department of Transport
Education:	High school diploma and 2 years' secretarial and office management training
Marital status:	Married
Children:	Son 16 years, daughter 11 years, son 6 years
Husband's occupation:	Construction site manager
Housing:	Lives in a 4-bedroom house, 2 bathrooms, in an urban area, 3 blocks away from her mother-in-law's home
Habits:	Does not smoke and will have a glass of wine occasionally at a social event. Takes about 4 to 6 Paracetamol tablets per day for headaches, drinks at least three cans of an energy drink with high levels of caffeine per day
Sleep:	Initial insomnia—feels sleepy at work
	Agnes has been admitted to a private psychiatric hospital

* Note: All names used in this case study are pseudonyms.

Main complaint

Agnes was referred for treatment by her employer. According to the employer, Agnes's work and work relationships were suffering. She could not concentrate and had anger outbursts and crying spells. Agnes explained that she had difficulty coping with the added stress in her job resulting from covering for a colleague who was on maternity leave. Upon further investigation it was found that the additional work was shared with two other people who were also coping with the additional load.

Initially the focus of her treatment was on personal stress management, relaxation exercises, diet, and stress-reducing techniques. After one week in the hospital Agnes confided in her designated nurse that she had marital problems. Over the next few days Agnes revealed that her husband Thabo often worked away from home for extended periods. During the past 4 months he had been involved in a construction site in a city 150 miles away. Thabo came home for a weekend every fortnight. When Thabo reduced his visits home, Agnes became suspicious that Thabo was having an affair. Agnes came across incriminating messages when she looked at Thabo's mobile phone. Thabo admitted the affair when confronted by Agnes and said it was to "tide him over" till he was back home again. He reminded Agnes of the long tradition of migrant laborers who have another wife in the city where they are working, but it did not mean that he did not love her and he had no intention of leaving the marriage. Agnes was very upset and after some reflection she started asking Thabo for more information. She was especially concerned about HIV/AIDS and how serious the relationship was. Thabo told her it was not her business and he does not "bathe with his socks on" indicating his refusal to use condoms.

Thabo refused to discuss taking a HIV test and said he was tested 4 years ago when applying for an insurance policy, at which time the test was negative. Agnes was adamant that she wanted to take precautions and asked Thabo to use a condom when having sex with her till he could be tested again. Again Thabo refused and when Agnes suggested she use a female condom or she would refuse to have sex with him Thabo threatened to bring another woman into their bed (while Agnes was there) to satisfy him. As this is not an uncommon practice Agnes believed him (Ekandjo & Motsana, 2014).

She tried to speak to her mother-in-law, who explained that Thabo was a grown man and he had no intention of leaving the marriage. She told Agnes to support him, as it was difficult for him to be away from home for long periods of time to support his family. Not getting any support from her mother-in-law, Agnes tried to speak to Thabo's older brother, Mothibi, who was considered the head of the family, but Mothibi did not want to discuss the issue and said she must solve her own "bedroom" problems. Agnes knew Thabo supported his mother and brother financially and was not surprised at the lack of support from them. Her own family lived in another province and she saw them only twice a year. She tried to talk to her own mother without any success. Her mother also told her to solve her own "bedroom" problems.

Agnes then tried to ignore the problem and just hoped Thabo would not contract HIV. Two months ago she noticed Thabo was not paying the utilities as per their arrangements and stopped providing money for family groceries. When she asked him about it he said he had other expenses. Six weeks ago Agnes received a phone call from Thabo's phone, but a woman spoke to her saying that she would not let Thabo go. Agnes was very upset, she called the woman names and put the phone down. Since then she often got phone calls from this woman (Thabo's lover, Vivienne), often late at night. The calls were abusive and threatening. Vivienne bragged about the nice clothes and jewelry that Thabo bought her.

When Thabo came home for a weekend he was moody and barely spoke to her. Vivienne called at all hours of the day and night. Their eldest son was very upset about this and was in constant conflict with his father. This conflict was threatening to become violent. Their youngest son had started to wet the bed at night and their daughter's schoolwork was suffering. Agnes couldn't take the strain anymore.

Because she couldn't sleep at night Agnes was not functioning well at work, and with the additional load she felt overwhelmed and very embarrassed about her outbursts. At the same time she felt cornered and afraid for her marriage and her life since HIV/AIDS was widespread in their community.

Treatment

Agnes was prescribed a selective serotonin reuptake inhibitor (SSRI) medication for her depression and Molipaxin 100 mg per day for anxiety and insomnia. The health care team wanted to bring Thabo in as part of the treatment regimen. This was a difficult situation because Thabo would likely feel insulted to be considered the cause. The team decided that the psychiatrist should talk to Thabo, since he was also a black man and of a similar age to Thabo. However, Agnes refused to let the psychiatrist talk to Thabo about any of their marital problems or anything about her situation. The psychiatrist then tried to talk to Thabo about supporting Agnes as she was coping with the double burden of the home and the extra load at work. This resulted in a very superficial discussion, which bore no fruit.

Agnes was counselled on her options. During these sessions, Agnes identified the following options: divorce, accepting the situation for the sake of the children, or regular HIV testing.

The counselling also focused on improving her assertiveness and self-esteem as well as developing a support system outside her family.

Brief analysis/aftermath and update

After 3 weeks Agnes was discharged from outpatient services and at her 6-week follow-up visit she seemed visibly more relaxed. Thabo was now working closer to home and lived there full-time. Thabo acted as if the problem was solved and Agnes was just thankful for the peace. She had spoken to Thabo and he had promised to continue to work closer to home so that he could live at home. Agnes felt this was the best for now and trusted the situation would not recur.

Due to the delicacy of the marital affair and consequence for Agnes and the children, the team could only help with medication to treat Agnes's symptoms and by strengthening her coping strategies and improving her self-esteem. In making her stronger, the team believed that Agnes would be in a better position to make decisions for herself. The team remained concerned that the situation would repeat itself since Thabo did not have much control over where he would be working. It was a compromised situation.

Take-home message

Nurses and other health care providers must work in an open, gender-sensitive and culture-sensitive manner with clients, foster their independence, and recognize and respect their involvement and concerns in the planning and delivery of care. Often culture and practices impede the treatment of people, and nurses must learn to work within the limits placed upon them by their clients. Strengthening the individual by enhancing her or his skill set and self-esteem enables the individual to better make decisions in the future. This is a leap of faith that we as nurses must learn to live with.

This case study provides an opportunity for others to view the social and economic context in which individuals live and nurses provide mental health care. Gender issues and cultural norms are evident and their impact on mental health clearly identified. The nurse in this situation provided care that was appropriate to the culture in which it occurred, and placed the patient's wishes at the forefront while offering strategies that would support adaptive coping. However, what follows is a critical analysis of the case study for the reader's broader understanding of the social determinants of mental health and includes nursing considerations.

Critical analysis

Risks for mental disorders are multifactorial and involve many biopsychosocial factors (World Health Organization (WHO), 2013). The influence of Agnes's gender and class are particularly apparent in the case study. Being a woman and having a lower social status or position in her marriage than Thabo fuelled her depression and anxiety as well as a sense of powerlessness to change the life events that led to the psychological distress (Jack, Stein, Newton, & Hofman, 2014; Phillips, 2005; Ostlin, Eckerman, Mishra, Nkowane & Wallstam 2007). Differences in health patterns are also closely linked with social, cultural, and environmental disadvantage (Healthy People 2020; WHO, 2013). We provide a critical analysis of the case study looking at issues of gender, class, and other social determinants of health, including economic factors and stigma, and then we offer some mental health promotion recommendations from a nursing perspective.

Gender

Gender refers to the socially constructed characteristics of men and women, including norms, roles, and their relationships with one another (Afif, 2007; Patel, Abas, Broadhead, Todd, & Reeler, 2001). For example, in most societies across the globe, women are assigned to unremitting caregiving while men are expected to be the primary breadwinners (Afif, 2007). Although these assignments provide some structure, they also create power imbalances between men and women that lead to differential exposure to mental health risks and to gender disparities in the use of mental health services (Phillips, 2005; WHO, 2013). For example, compared to men, women bear a 50 percent greater burden of disease and disability (Marcus, Ysamy, Ommeren, Chisholm, & Saxena, n.d; WHO, 2013). The greater burden of disease is attributed to gender inequalities related to lower social status and class as well as relatively lower social autonomy for women (Jack *et al.*, 2014; Marcus *et al.*, n.d; Ostlin *et al.*, 2007; WHO, 2013).

Class

Women's status and life opportunities worldwide remain low (Jack *et al.*, 2014). Most cultures, especially in low- and middle-income countries in Africa (LMIC) such as South Africa, socialize females into subservient roles and charge them with the responsibility of maintaining the home, bearing and raising children, and taking care of extended family members. Compared to men, women have less time to receive an education, marry at a much younger age, are required to leave their families of origin to join their husbands' families, and are discouraged from working outside of the home. Consequently, women often have limited educational opportunities, little or no economic resources, and little freedom to make life choices, including leaving abusive marital situations. Therefore, many women, such as Agnes in our case study, stay in their marriages and bear the psychological toll of abusive marital relationships. Women who muster the courage to report an ordeal related to their husbands' extramarital affairs are typically admonished, which reflects a lack of the powerfully protective benefits of social support networks.

Economic factors

Mental disorders often lead people to poverty, whereas access to economic resources buffers people from the stresses of daily living and unexpected life events such as extramarital affairs (WHO, 2013). In general, persons with low incomes are relatively more vulnerable to the chronic stress that diminishes mental health (Jack *et al.*, 2014). Women are overrepresented among the poor and depressed across the globe, including in South Africa (Jack *et al.*, 2014; Patel *et al.*, 2001), with a greater burden of disease and disability and limited access to safety and security, education, and a strong social support network (Afif, 2007). People suffering with mental disorders are often unable to work or perform well in the workplace (Jack *et al.*, 2014). Further, poor persons are more likely to live in rural areas with limited access to health or mental health care facilities. And even those who can access facilities may not be able to afford the cost of services. The cost of mental health treatment and loss of productivity due to mental disorders is projected to soar from US \$870 billion to US \$2.1 trillion per year by 2030 in LMIC (Atakilt, n.d.; WHO, 2013). Agnes was fortunate to be employed outside the home and to have people in her social network who recognized the strain she was under and facilitated her access to and use of mental health services.

The lack of mental health resources and trained providers is a major obstacle to mental health care in LMIC such as South Africa (Marcus *et al.*, n.d.; WHO, 2013). It is estimated that between

76 percent and 85 percent of people with mental disorders in these countries do not receive care for their disorders (WHO, 2013). Outpatient mental health care clinics and public mental health hospitals often lack trained psychiatrists and nurses. Private hospitals are reserved for the wealthy, who can afford the care. Furthermore, most mental health facilities or hospitals cannot purchase essential psychiatric medications (Atakilt, n.d; Oruche, 2014).

Mental health research is rarely conducted in LMIC countries such as South Africa (Ostlin *et al.*, 2007; Feduka *et al.*, 2014). Only in recent years have a number of global efforts emerged with the goal of strengthening evidence-based research as part of a broader initiative to expand mental health services in these countries. For example, the WHO Comprehensive Mental Health Action Plan for 2013–2020 outlines targets for strengthening evidence-based care (WHO, 2013). The Programme for Improving Mental Health Center or PRIME runs pilot projects to measure the impact of mental health programs in primary health care settings. PRIME is a consortium of research institutions and ministries of health in Uganda, Ethiopia, India, Nepal, and South Africa, in partnerships with Britain and WHO (Lund, 2012). African Focus on Intervention Research for Mental Health (AFFIRM) is working in Ghana, Malawi, South Africa, Uganda, and Zimbabwe. AFFIRM conducts randomized controlled trials of low-cost, task-sharing interventions such as integration of depression treatment into HIV care (AFFIRM, n.d.). Women like Agnes could benefit from mental health services conveniently located in primary care or women's health clinics for long-term follow-up and monitoring as well as social support.

Stigma

The failure to recognize mental health as a major public health concern that is worthy of economic investment is both a reflection and consequence of the stigma associated with mental illness (Atakilt, n.d.; Jack *et al.*, 2014). Stigma increases discrimination and social exclusion and deters affected persons from disclosing their mental illness or seeking health care services (Egbe *et al.*, 2015; Fitzpatrick, 2015). In fact, most African languages do not have specific words for mental disorders such as depression or anxiety. In the Ibo language of Nigeria, for example, persons with severe and persistent mental illness are described as having *isi-Ngbaka* or *scrambling of the head*. These words connote individual flaws that are not amenable to modern mental health interventions. Persons with overt symptoms of mental disorders are considered aggressive, are maltreated, and excluded from mainstream society by their families, communities, and health care workers (WHO, 2013). Therefore, families keep the mental illness a secret because they fear being ostracized from their communities, which has sustained the stigma and led to grave consequences for future generations. Like most African mothers, Agnes may have feared that public knowledge of her depression could have rendered her children unacceptable as marriage partners.

Implications for mental health nursing practice and mental health promotion within global communities

The multilayered and multifactorial nature of challenges to mental health care in LMIC such as South Africa requires innovation and multipronged, as well as gender-sensitive, approaches (Ostlin *et al.*, 2007; WHO, 2013). Long-established cultural beliefs about mental illness in these countries are not easily amenable to change. Therefore, educational interventions may be most feasible and acceptable in order to create an atmosphere for more comprehensive formalized treatments using pharmacotherapy and psychotherapy that can be scaled up in the long term (WHO, 2009). First, nurses must utilize focused and sustained public health approaches with emphases on building community partnerships and using integrative strategies (Ostlin *et al.*, 2007). To begin, nurses can gain an understanding of the cultural aspects that impact mental health care and client decision-making by partnering with the grassroots community leaders and community lay workers who have trusted relationships with, and intimate knowledge of the cultural values and beliefs of its members. Involving key community stakeholders is necessary to fundamentally "chip off" unfavorable cultural practices including views of women as subservient and as "property."

Mental health researchers and advocates and key world health organizations espouse integration of mental health services into primary care, women's health care, and chronic disease programs, including HIV-AIDs clinics (Feduka *et al.*, 2014; Jack *et al.*, 2014; Marcus *et al.*, n.d.; WHO, 2013). For example, the WHO Comprehensive Mental Health Action Plan for 2013–2020 and the Programme for Improving Mental Health Care or PRIME for 2013–2020 outline targets for member countries including integrating mental health care into community-based settings (Egbe *et al.*, 2015; PRIME, n.d.; WHO, 2013). Integration of mental health services promises a better approach to managing mental health problems, promoting mental health, and preventing mental disorders. Discreet screening and assessment processes in these population-focused settings can alleviate the stigma and discrimination of mental illness and address the lack of outpatient mental health facilities across LMIC such as South Africa (PRIME, n.d.). Likewise, the integration of mental health services into women's health clinics means that nurses can provide individual or group psychoeducation that enables women to share their stories and learn from and support one another on varied topics including sexual health, child rearing, and marital stress (Ostlin *et al.*, 2007). Both access to material resources and social networks are powerfully protective for common mental disorders. Some integration efforts in South Africa and Nigeria have already proved to be successful (Abdulmalik *et al.*, 2013; Egbe *et al.*, 2015; PRIME, n.d.).

In general, the use of medications to treat mental disorders is not widely accepted in LMIC countries such as South Africa. For those groups of patients who need treatment for mental disorders such as depression (Egbe *et al.*, 2015; Patel *et al.*, 2001; WHO, 2013), there are cost-effective treatments that can be easily implemented in primary care settings (Marcus *et al.*, n.d.; WHO, 2013). For example, the WHO Mental Health Gap Action Programme (mhGAP) inter-vention guide provides a treatment algorithm for depression, including psychosocial strategies and medication where indicated (WHO, 2009). There are examples of adaptation of the mhGAP intervention guide for particular communities (Abdulmalik *et al.*, 2013). Nurses can use these examples to adapt the content and delivery of psychosocial interventions so that they fit the culture of the communities they serve (Feduka *et al.*, 2014).

Globally, we have underutilized prevention strategies to mitigate mental health risks (Afif, 2007; Marcus *et al.*, n.d.; WHO, 2013). Preventive strategies include community or population-based approaches aimed at strengthening protective factors and reducing risk factors (Ostlin *et al.*, 2007). For example, nurses could partner with colleagues to design school-based programs targeting cognitive, problem-solving, and social skills for children and adolescents (Jack *et al.*, 2014; Marcus *et al.*, n.d.). Schools would also be a great place to broach the issue of power and gender imbalances, focusing on education about good sexual habits and healthy relationships between genders (Ostlin *et al.*, 2007). Nurses must also leverage the power of media to promote mental health awareness and reduce the stigma and discrimination related to mental illness (Jack *et al.*, 2014).

To increase access to mental health services, nurses must join efforts to train mental health providers in order to expand the workforce capacity needed to meet global mental health needs in sub-Saharan Africa (AFFIRM, n. d.; Marcus *et al.*, n.d.). According to the Comprehensive

Mental Health Action Plan 2013–2020, integration of mental health into general health care requires the acquisition of new knowledge and a redefinition of roles, as well as changes in existing service cultures (WHO, 2013). To start, the educational preparation of all nurses needs to emphasize integration of mental health into primary care throughout undergraduate curricula (WHO, 2013). Additionally, nurses need to obtain continuing education throughout their professional careers. Nursing efforts to build capacity need to include training of community health workers to reach the most rural areas, capitalizing on their trust and familiarity with the cultural norms, beliefs, values, and attitudes of the community dwellers (AFFIRM., n.d; Marcus et al., n.d.). Lay workers will work collaboratively with nurse supervisors, and nurses could partner with global organizations such as African Focus on Intervention Research for Mental Health or AFFIRM and with inter-professional practice teams (AFFIRM, n.d.; Afif, 2007; Jack et al., 2014).

Summary/conclusion

In sum, mental disorders such as depression and anxiety are prevalent in LMIC such as South Africa. Women endure a greater burden of disease because of the power imbalances related to their lower position in society. However, there are global initiatives to combat psychological distress and mental disorders for all, and there is growing attention to gender-sensitive strategies embedded in integrative and multisectoral approaches. These strategies are aimed at mental health promotion as well as prevention and management at individual, communal, and population levels. Nurses have a significant role to play in expanding and scaling up mental health care in LMIC such as South Africa. Nurses in the case study used culturally appropriate strategies to address the needs, concerns and perceptions of Agnes within their current social context, as nurses, we must also assist each other in taking our seats at the table in collaboration with communities, professional colleagues from other disciplines, and international organizations. Through the use of cross-national support, collaboration, and consultation, nurses can stay abreast of, and active in, the design and execution of global mental health efforts with entities such as WHO, PRIME, and AFFIRM. Finally, through mutual support, each nurse can lead in supporting the mental health of those who are most vulnerable.

References

Abdulmalik, J., Kola, L., Fadahunsi. W., Adebayo, K., Yasamy, M.T., Musa, E., & Gureje, O. (2013). Country contextualization of the mental health gap action programme intervention guide: A case study from Nigeria. *PLoS Med*, 10(8), e1001501.

AFFIRM (n.d.). African focus on intervention research for mental health. Retrieved May 12, 2016 from www.centreforglobalmentalhealth.org/about-us

Afif, M. (2007). Gender differences in mental health. *Singapore Medical Journal*, 48(5), 385–391.

Atakilt, M.W. (n.d.). Mental health care in sub-Saharan Africa: Challenges and opportunities: RAND objectives and effective solutions. Retrieved May 12, 2016 from www.rand.org/blog/2015/03/mental-healthcare-in-sub-saharan-africa-challenges.html.

Egbe, C.O., Brooke-Sumner, C., Kathree, T., Selohilwe, O., Thornicroft, G., & Petersen, I. (2015). Psychiatric stigma and discrimination in South Africa: Perspectives from key stakeholders. *BMC Psychiatry*, 14, 191. Retrieved May 12, 2016 from www.biomedcentral.com/1471–244X/14/191

Ekandjo, R., & Motsana, M. (June 11, 2014). Cultural practices among the Sotho. (I. Venter, & L. van Rhyn, Interviewers) Bloemfontein, South Africa.

Fekadu, A., Medhin, S., Selamu, M., Hailemariam, M., Alem, A., Giorgis, T.W., Breuer, E., Lund, C., Prince, M., & Hanlon, C. (2014). Population level mental distress in rural Ethiopia. *BMC Psychiatry*, 14(194), 1–13.

Fitzpatrick, J.J. (2015). The continuing stigma of mental illness. *Archives of Psychiatric Nursing*, 29(3), 133.

Healthy People 2020. (n.d.). *Social determinants*. Retrieved on May 12, 2016 from www.healthy people.gov/2020/leading-health-indicators/2020-lhi-topics/Social-Determinants.

Jack, H., Stein, A., Newton, C.R., & Hofman, K.J. (2014). Expanding access to mental health care: A missing ingredient. *The Lancet, 2*, e183–e184.

Lund, C., Tomlinson, M., De Silva, M., Fedaku, A., Shidhaye, R., & Patel, V. (2012). PRIME: A programme to reduce the treatment gap for mental disorders in five low- and middle-income countries. *PLOS Medicine, 9*(12), e1001359, 1–6.

Marcus, M., Yasamy, M.T., Ommeren, M., Chisholm, D., & Saxena, S. (n.d.). Depression: A global public health concern. Retrieved May 12, 2016 from www.who.int/mental_health/management/depression/who_paper_depression_wfmh_2012.pdf.

Mathers, C., & Loncan, D. (2006). Projections of global mortality and burden of disease from 2002 to 2030. *PLoS Medcine, 3*(11), e422.

Mawere, M., & Mawere, A. (2010). The changing philosophy of African marriage: The relevance of the Shona customary marriage practice of Kukumbria. *Journal of African Studies and Development, 2*(9), 224–233.

Oruche, U.M. (2014). Next generation: The key to sustainable health care? Retrieved May 12, 2016 from www.youtube.com/watch?v=Ek5JEcuP7I4.

Ostlin, P., Eckerman, E., Mishra, U.S., Nkowane, M., & Wallstam, E. (2007). Health promoting challenges. Gender and health promotion: A multisectorial policy approach. *Health Promotion International, 21*(s1), 25–35.

Patel, V., Abas, M., Broadhead, J., Todd, C., & Reeler, A. (2001). Depression in developing countries: Lessons learned from Zimbabwe. *British Medical Journal, 322*, 482–484.

Phillips, S. (2005). Defining and measuring gender: A social determinant of health whose time has come. *International Journal of Equity in Health, 4*(11). Doi: 10.1186/1475–9276-4-11. Retrieved May 12, 2016 from www.ncbi.nlm.nih.gov/pmc/articles/PMC1180842/pdf/1475-9276-4-11.pdf.

World Health Organization (2013). *Comprehensive mental health action plan 2013–2020 (WHA 66.8)*. Retrieved May 12, 2016 from www.who.int/mental_health/action_plan_2013/en/.

World Health Organization Department of Mental Health and Substance Abuse. (2009). *Mental health gap action programme (mhGAP) forum*. Geneva: Switzerland. Retrieved May 12, 2016 from www.who.int/mental_health/publications/mhgap.

Zuma, K., Lurie, M., Williams, B.K.M., Garnett, G., & Sturm, A. (2005, June). Risk factors of sexually transmitted infections among migrant and non-migrant sexual partnerships from rural South Africa. *Epidemiology and Infection, 133*(3), 421–428.

25

AUSTRALIA

Social and emotional well-being of an Aboriginal and Torres Strait Islander population

Rose McMaster, Kerry Mawson and Peter Shine

Introduction: historical background

First Nations, First peoples, Aboriginal and Torres Strait Islander or First Australians are collective names for the original people of Australia and their descendants. Aboriginal and Torres Strait Islander people have lived on this continent for approximately 60,000 years (as the oldest continuing surviving culture on earth) prior to European invasion (NSW Department of Community Services, 2007; NSLHD, 2013). In this chapter the term 'Indigenous' has been avoided wherever possible as some Aboriginal people feel that the term can diminish their Aboriginality. The term Aboriginal is used when referring to Aboriginal people in NSW as the Aboriginal culture was the first and predominant culture.

Aboriginal and Torres Strait islanders view their health holistically:

> Aboriginal health means not just the physical well-being of an individual but refers to the social, emotional and cultural well-being of the whole community in which each individual is able to achieve their full potential as a human being, thereby bringing about the total well-being of their community. It is a whole-of-life view and includes the cyclical concept of life-death-life. Health care services should strive to achieve the state where every individual is able to achieve their full potential as a human being and this brings about the total well-being of their community.
>
> *(National Aboriginal Health Strategy, 1989)*

It has been acknowledged for a very long time that there is an unacceptable level of disparity and health inequity between Aboriginal communities and non-Aboriginal communities. Aboriginal people are one of the most disadvantaged socio-economic groups in Australia and continue to be over-represented in health care systems, child protection systems, welfare systems and criminal justice systems. Levels of homelessness and unemployment are also over-represented in Aboriginal communities (Australian Health Ministers' Advisory Council, 2011; Australian Institute of Family Studies (AIFS), Child Family Community Australia, 2013).

Understanding why Aboriginal people are over-represented within these structures require those who work with Aboriginal people to acknowledge the many historical and cultural factors that have contributed to past and current conditions they experience. Understanding this puts non-Aboriginal workers in a better position to appreciate the complexity of their lives and how we can work with the Aboriginal population in healthier more culturally appropriate ways (NSW Department of Community Services, 2009).

Prior to European contact, their collective sense of spirituality, community, kinship, culture and country, which encompasses mental health or social and emotional well-being, was intact but diminished, particularly in the twentieth century. In addition, disempowerment and marginalisation occurred following colonisation by the British in the 1770s and more prominently after the First Fleet landed in Sydney Cove in 1788.

The removal of children (the Stolen Generation) from Aboriginal families was part of an official government policy on Aboriginal people until the 1970s. The practice by the British government of taking children from their families has had a devastating effect on Aboriginal people and the repercussions have caused further psychological and physical trauma (Parker, 2010; *Working with Aboriginal People & Communities*, 2009).

Aboriginal culture and communities are diverse and there are many different nations, tribes and groups. To meet the needs of the individuals within these groups, professionals need to tailor the way in which they interact and communicate with these diverse cultures and recognise that a 'one size fits all' approach will not work (NSW Department of Community Services, 2009).

Trans-generational transfer of trauma

Trauma and loss can mean different things to different people. Victims of trauma can discount previous history, living conditions and individual circumstances that can be distressing for some but not others (Purdie, Dudgeon & Walker, 2010). Atkinson, Nelson and Atkinson (2010) have argued that a diagnosis such as post-traumatic stress disorder (PTSD) is unable to conceptually capture the level of chronic ongoing stress that Aboriginal people experience in their everyday lives. The stressors are frequently numerous, ongoing and severe. The stressors are associated with multiple factors including the inability to identify and build resilience to single sources of stress, which can then add to other stressors for the individual. Moreover, the victims can experience an added level of stress due to knowing the people who are inflicting them harm (Atkinson *et al.*, 2010).

Trans-generational transmission of trauma from historical events related to colonisation of Aboriginal land has been experienced by elders in the community and then passed from generation to generation through the sharing of those experiences and perceptions (Atkinson *et al.*, 2010; Atkinson, 2013). These negative experiences can also be transmitted across different Aboriginal communities resulting in varied understandings of the trauma and loss with different attributions and meaning (Atkinson, 2013).

Social and emotional well-being and mental health

In Australia, many Aboriginal people and communities have moved towards the term social and emotional well-being (SEWB) as an alternative to mental health as it can reflect a more positive approach to health (Garvey, 2008). An Aboriginal concept of health embraces the social, emotional, spiritual and cultural well-being of the whole community and is extremely important to the health and well-being of each individual in that community. Embedded within this concept is the cultural connection to land (Garvey, 2008). When one of these components becomes disrupted Aboriginal ill health is believed to occur (Swan & Raphael, 1995).

The concept of social and emotional well-being (SEWB) is more consistent with Aboriginal community perceptions of need than are disease-based concepts of mental illness and mental disorder. Aboriginal people have strongly endorsed the concept of social and emotional well-being as being relevant to the conditions of Aboriginal life. The term "social and emotional well-being" is therefore used in preference to the term mental health (NSW Department of Community Services, 2007; NSW Aboriginal Mental Health and Well-being Policy 2006–2010, p. 3).

Substance use

Current levels of alcohol consumption (both chronic and binge) are a concern for Aboriginal and non-Aboriginal Australians alike, and are major risk factors for morbidity and mortality in both populations (Australian Institute of Health and Welfare (AIHW), 2006). Alcohol abuse causes about 7 per cent of Aboriginal deaths and Aboriginal people die at a much younger age from these conditions than do non-Aboriginal Australians. Alcohol also contributes significantly to hospitalization of Aboriginal people and to other significant social problems (Wilkes, Gray, Saggers, Casey & Stearne, 2010). A national approach to co-morbidity issues to help raise awareness, support service providers and improve access to care particularly within primary health care has been established (Aboriginal Medical Services Alliance Northern Territory (AMSANT), 2013).

Polydrug use is common among Aboriginal Australians although there are no comprehensive studies of co-morbidity in the Aboriginal population but evidence of relationships comes from multiple sources (Wilkes *et al.*, 2010). Furthermore, Wilkes *et al.* (2010) emphasised that comorbidity of substance misuse and mental health issues among Aboriginal Australians will continue to be a major problem if the social and structural determinants of good mental health are not addressed.

Child protection

Children from an Aboriginal and Torres Strait Islander background are over-represented in the Australian child protection system. There are a multitude of complex reasons for this including the socioeconomic disadvantage of Indigenous Australians, the intergenerational effects of separation from family and culture, and the varying perceptions arising from child-rearing cultural practices (HREOC, 1997; Stanley, Tomison & Pocock, 2003).

Life expectancy

The Australian population enjoys one of the highest life expectancies in the world if you are from a non-Aboriginal background. For the average non-Aboriginal and Torres Strait Islander population born in 2010–2012, life expectancy was estimated to be 80 years for males and 83 years for females. In the Aboriginal and Torres Strait Islander population, the life expectancy for males is 69 years and for females 74 years (ABS, 2013). Furthermore, the death rates for Aboriginal and Torres Strait people exceeded those for all Australians in every age group, with the risk of death for those aged 35–54 being 6–8 times greater than the national average (HREOC, 2008). In Wilcannia Western NSW the life expectancy of an Aboriginal male is 37 years of age. Alcohol consumption and violence are contributing factors (McCausland & Vivian, 2009).

Importantly, comparisons between the original and revised Aboriginal life expectancy estimates should not be interpreted as a change in Indigenous life expectancy, but should be seen as the result of a revision in statistical methods used to calculate life expectancy (Thomson *et al.*, 2012).

The case of an Aboriginal female

The following case study (we have given her the pseudonym of Ann) illustrates a complex set of issues that impacted the well-being of Ann, a woman of Aboriginal descent. These issues included trauma and trans-generational transfer of trauma, social and emotional well-being, mental health, drug and alcohol use, child protection and life expectancy. Given the complexity of the case, a comprehensive psychosocial assessment and strong treatment alliance was crucial. An assessment tool with culturally appropriate questions is needed and should be used with Aboriginal people.

Ann, a woman in her early twenties, came to the attention of health services when she presented at 22 weeks into her pregnancy at a local public hospital antenatal clinic. She was unemployed and homeless; most of her day was spent looking for somewhere to sleep for the night. Ann would frequently sleep on friends' sofas. She had a long history of drug and alcohol use and her depression and anxiety were exacerbated by substance dependence. The staff at the community mental health and the drug and alcohol centres knew Ann. However, she first came to the attention of the community counselling services after the birth of her baby, but did not initially engage with any of the these services.

It was only after numerous incidents including sexual assaults, domestic violence, substance-related medical admissions, and child protection services becoming involved that she decided to access counselling. Although her motivations to start counselling were the serious issues that had consumed her life in the past, she was able to articulate wanting to make changes in her life in the following ways: (a) manage her depression and anxiety; (b) stop using substances to improve how she felt about herself; and (c) improve her life so that she could have access to her daughter, who was living with her father.

Ann identified that because of substance use, she was unable to finish her studies, which impacted her ability to gain employment and manage activities of daily living, which then contributed to her homeless status. Her situation also resulted in her being a victim of domestic violence and sexual assault. The most severe consequence of her lifestyle was the removal of her daughter due to alleged child neglect and safety concerns. Although Ann was very distressed about the removal of her daughter, at no time did she ever voice suicidal ideation, suicidal plans or threaten violence towards others.

Family and psychological history

Ann lived in the country with a large extended family and moved to the city as a young child to attend primary school. Her parents separated prior to the move to the city. She grew up in a family who displayed a lot of anger towards non-Aboriginal people. This partly explained her anger and blame towards the non-Aboriginal people who were involved in her care. This perceived anger also contributed to her lack of insight regarding her current situation. Although she was estranged from her close family network, she still maintained some connection by attending family get-togethers in country Australia.

Substance use started at a very young age with alcohol being a significant part of the family culture. By the time she was in her early twenties she was alcohol dependent, experienced blackouts when intoxicated and significant withdrawal. Poly-drug use was a continuing feature of her history. She started smoking tobacco in primary school and has continued, with no attempts at quitting.

The complexities of Ann's history included multiple co-morbidities and multiple psychological issues as mentioned previously. She described the trauma associated with being a young person who grew up in a large city yet had a cultural Aboriginal background in Australia. The disconnect from her own cultural background with a subsequent loss of identity, and cultural issues that were not addressed or resolved as a result of living in a predominantly white culture were significant. This contributed to high levels of distress about her current situation. Distress levels were driven by: grief and loss, abandonment, stigma of being Aboriginal along with strong feelings of guilt and hopelessness. She used substances to manage her anxiety rather than work on the underlying factors that contributed to her anxiety. As a result, Ann exhibited limited ability to tolerate her own feelings, which then resulted in blaming others for her experiences.

Past history

Ann had a long history of attending health services including detoxification since the birth of her child, and then after having her child, she was in and out of rehabilitation units. She was seen by a number of different psychiatrists over a number of years and given the diagnosis of anxiety and depression exacerbated by substance use. Pharmacotherapy had been the main treatment with a selective serotonin reuptake inhibitor (SSRI) used for depression and Antabuse (Disulfiram) for her drinking. Taking medication was an ongoing difficulty as she often forgot to take it due to the intoxicating effects of her substance use, but would often also have no money to fill a prescription that resulted in discontinuation syndrome. This had major ramifications for her mental health, which then impacted her ability to present to counselling and keep other appointments. Although counselling was for her, an important adjunct to pharmacotherapy, engaging her in counselling services remained difficult. There were significant medical co-morbidities, resulting in multiple presentations for emergency treatment due to intoxication and medical harm associated with intoxication particularly liver abnormalities and memory loss.

Insight and judgement

It was difficult for her to understand how her behaviour was influencing her current situation and therefore her insight was limited during initial engagement with health services. Recently she started to see that she had control over her behaviour. Being able to see her symptoms as part of the depression, anxiety and substance use was a contributing factor in the change in her insight. Her judgement varied, depending on her relationships at the time with her male partner. For example, she acknowledged that she needed to make changes around her substance use, but her ability to make changes was difficult due to her dependence and the relationship with her current partner. She was very aware of the consequences from continued substance use, which included denial of access to her child by the authorities, health risks associated with substance use and the additional risk to health via domestic violence and sexual assault.

Although she did not have a forensic history herself she was well known to the court system because of multiple assaults from past partners and Apprehended Violence Orders (AVOs) against partners. She was also involved with the family court system for a number of years as she tried to gain access to her child.

Brief analysis/aftermath and update

During the first contact with health services, the individual's family and cultural background must be assessed and understood. This is so the family and individual can have access to culturally appropriate support and the staff can receive guidance on how to work with the client including appreciating and respecting their cultural views and experiences.

When building rapport with the Aboriginal community it is important to remember that time spent with local community organisations, groups, Elders, children and families contributes to the engagement process. Therefore, it is imperative to be aware of and respectful of relevant extended family and kinship structures. Health care providers should ensure that extended family is included (if asked to be present) in important meetings and in making important decisions, in consultation with the client who is receiving direct services.

In Aboriginal cultures, certain customs and practices are performed by men and women separately, often referred to as 'men's and women's business'. It is important that staff working with the Aboriginal population understand this. The Aboriginal woman identified in this case study self-referred to the Community Mental Health and Drug and Alcohol Service and requested a female clinician. Where possible it is preferable for women to speak with women. If the client requested an Aboriginal clinician this would be culturally appropriate Aboriginal women's business. However, Aboriginal health workers are not always available and a non-Aboriginal provider may need to work with the client. When working with Aboriginal people and communities, a practice resource may prove helpful along with consultation with community informants from the specific culture. One example of such a resource is available from the New South Wales (NSW) Department of Community Services (2009).

When Ann's daughter was removed from her care, it was a very distressing time for her and required collaboration with a number of different health services. This included an Aboriginal health worker, mental health services to review the level of depression Ann was experiencing, and drug and alcohol services for detoxification from substances that she had been consuming. In addition, officers from the Department of Community Services worked with her and helped to coordinate the other services to support her remaining in her child's life. Multidisciplinary care was required to address the complexity of her needs.

Implications for mental health nursing practice and mental health promotion within global communities

Mental health nurses must be cognisant of the cultural needs of consumers and maintain professional standards that present as a model of the code of ethics for nurses. Culture and identity are core determinants of health and well-being for all people, including Aboriginal people and are critical to the development of the relationship between the client and the nurse (Stewart & Allan, 2013). It is important for those providing services to Aboriginal people and communities to maintain professional standards including actions that are respectful, courteous and that comply with cultural norms. The service provider needs to comply with local Aboriginal values, and intervention methods and measures used need to be in line with local Aboriginal observances. If research is being conducted, the principles used need to be in line with ethical standards and norms consistent with that of the culture. Expectations need to be realistic and not over exaggerated; outcomes need to demonstrate integrity and professionalism; fairness and equity need to be observed, and intellectual and professional integrity demonstrated. Past reports and dealings have neglected some of these issues and this needs to be rectified through respectful cultural interventions (NSLHD, 2013). Working alongside an Aboriginal client means being aware of their history, developing trust and cultural respect and working towards being pro-fessionally culturally competent. Approaching Aboriginal health holistically means understanding values and traditions of communities that can contribute towards social and emotional well-being for the individual and the community.

The following points summarise important features of engaging with Aboriginal people.

- Be clear and unambiguous with questions and general conversation. Do not use jargon.
- When working with Aboriginal people, be aware of your own communication style. It is important to be mindful of your own body language as you may be giving a message that may not match what you are saying. The goal is to present with a relaxed body position, which may include leaning forward slightly to show you are interested in the person.
- Be aware of your own world-views, prejudices and beliefs, particularly those beliefs that you may have garnered from your peers about Aboriginal people. They will be negative stereotypes that can be dismissed (in most cases) as myth.
- In Western culture the most important indicator that someone is listening is eye contact. However, for some Aboriginal people eye contact can have different meanings. Avoiding eye contact is polite in some communities. It is important not to interpret this as not listening. This is important in cross-gender interactions where it is considered appropriate for women to maintain eye contact with each other and for men to maintain eye contact with each other.
- Facial expressions are important as they communicate who we are. This means that, as a health worker your expressions can help you to engage with an Aborigi-nal person in a more empathic way.
- Gestures are physical movements and are an element of attending that we use both to convey emotion and to emphasise important points. Your gestures should be casual, natural and not distracting. Occasional head nodding for encouragement may be included.
- Just as we can tell much about our emotional state from a person's tone of voice, so too does the consumer make assumptions based on hearing our voice. Being mindful of how we use our voice with Aboriginal people is imperative.
- Physical distance and touching are more vulnerable to cultural differences and ambiguous interpretation. It is important to be aware of the boundaries required in the cultural context.

(Egan, 1998; Indigenous Health Reference Material, 2012; Stein-Parbury, 2005)

Environment

Letting Aboriginal people know they are welcome and providing an environment that is non-threatening gives them adequate time to engage in conversation and answer questions. Creating an environment that is supportive and receptive to what the client is experiencing is very important.

Engagement

When first meeting an Aboriginal client, spend time listening to and building rapport with them so that trust can be developed in the relationship. Avoid writing information down when conducting the initial assessment as this is the most important time to develop and engage with the client. When asking questions, avoid direct questioning, as this can be a barrier to establishing a working relationship. A yarning approach (informal, conversational talking) could facilitate responses that direct questioning would not. Often there can be a lot of paperwork to do when first meeting a client, don't try to do everything during the first visit. Be aware that some Aboriginal people may have difficulties with numeracy and literacy. Providing support with filling out forms and writing information and/or reading information for clients who have difficulties in these areas will be important.

The approach taken by the nurse when assisting with literacy and numeracy is with sensitivity so as not to cause embarrassment or further shame. In Aboriginal cultures shame is a very real component of Aboriginal life. Discussion around substance use, sex, and other issues may seem un-alarming to a non-Aboriginal person, therefore an Aboriginal person may minimize the severity of a problem so as not to lose standing in their community and give them cause to feel ashamed. Prioritise what you will do during the first visit and check how the client is with the process (Indigenous Health Reference Material, 2012).

Therapeutic relationship building

Building rapport with clients also means liaising with Aboriginal health services in relation-ship building, together with and including family or significant others. For example, in this case study, working with Ann and her current partner in numerous sessions promoted the build-ing of insight in a culturally respectful way. In addition, by using motivational interviewing skills, enhanced motivation and insight were achieved.

Confidentiality is an important component of the therapeutic relationship. Aboriginal people can be fearful of information being spoken about in their community, which can be a barrier to not accessing services for help. Make it clear when first engaging in the relationship that you will not be sharing their information with family members without permission. Discussion about confidentiality and family are important parts of this work. The balance is being able to build and maintain a relationship with the client but also with any family member who may be involved without breaking confidentiality (Lee *et al.*, 2012).

Being flexible with follow up

When working with Aboriginal clients who experience challenges to social and emotional well-being or substance dependence issues, be mindful that clients may take 'time out' from being engaged in services. This is important to acknowledge, as the health care worker needs to be patient and flexible. Excessive outreach to the client or leaving multiple messages at these times may compromise the therapeutic relationship. Examples of flexibility may include phone appointments and making appointments scheduled at the end of the day.

Communication styles

Another area of communication that may be interpreted incorrectly is silence on behalf of the client. This may be misinterpreted by the nurse as a sign of other issues such as cognitive impairment, memory loss and/or inattentiveness. The professional nature of the nurse/client relationships typical of Western cultures is not the same as the relationships Aboriginal people prefer to have. There is no professional/personal dichotomy, which means they are quite happy to come and have a yarn (informal, conversational talk) with you in a venue other than the counselling room. Try not to be too prescriptive about what is best for the client. Instead, ask them what they would like help with to improve their social and emotional well-being.

Barriers

Working within a system that is deadline- and time-oriented can often work against Aboriginal people and creates barriers. It is our duty of care to be aware of cultural differences that are present in our health systems and work in ways that assist Aboriginal people in accessing the health care required (Indigenous Health Reference Material, 2012).

Being aware of the past

Clinicians need to be aware of the Stolen Generations being a real experience of the people they are working with. In 2009 the National Aboriginal and Torres Strait Islander Social Survey reported that 8 per cent of Indigenous people aged 15 and over reported being removed from their natural family, with 38 per cent having relatives being removed from their natural family (ABS, 2009). In 2005 The Western Australia Child Health Survey noted that:

> One quarter (24 per cent) of Aboriginal children were rated by their parents as being at high risk for clinically significant emotional or behavioural difficulties. This compares with 15 per cent of children in the non-Aboriginal population. Many families functioned poorly, one-third of children were in the care of a sole parent. About 12 per cent of children were being looked after by a parent who had been forcibly removed from their own natural family.
>
> *(De Maio et al., 2005)*

The Stolen Generations represent a significant cause of trauma and can be trans-generational, meaning the stories and emotions of experiences of trauma that grandparents and parents or other relatives experienced have been passed down to the children. Historical trauma can be embedded in the subjective experiencing and remembering of events in the mind of an individual or in the life of a community (Atkinson, 2013). Complex trauma results from multiple traumas experienced by the individual. These traumas can be over a period of time starting in childhood and spanning the individual's lifespan. Children can experience neglect, maltreatment, psychological and sexual abuse, which then continues into adulthood in exposure to domestic violence, rape, substance use and poor mental health. As trauma and loss can mean different things to different Aboriginal communities, familiarity with community-specific understanding helps with engagement and development of solid relationships.

Sense of self

Aboriginal sense of self is critical as this is connected to spirituality, community, (community means family, if I'm sick my community is sick, if my community is sick I'm sick), culture and country. Kinship is important in defining social roles (together with rules and relationships) for Aboriginal people; therefore these need to be taken into consideration. In addition, recognition and awareness of spiritual beliefs are part of the Aboriginal identity along with a sense of belonging and connecting with kinship, community and country (Parker, 2010).

Summary

This chapter has discussed the case study of an Aboriginal woman with complex health care needs. Background to the case study included discussion surrounding trans-generational transfer of trauma, social and emotional well-being; substance use; child protection and life expectancy. The case study highlighted information concerning this Aboriginal woman's past history, psychological history, family history, forensic history and information regarding her insight and judgement.

Following the case study a brief analysis was given. This was followed by implications for mental health nursing practice. In addition, mental health promotion within global communities discussed issues concerning the environment, engagement within therapeutic relationship building, being flexible with follow-up, communication styles, barriers, being aware of the past and sense of self.

In conclusion, as seen in this chapter mental health (social and emotional well-being) of an Aboriginal and Torres Strait Islander involves the understanding and commitment of health care professionals to deliver services that are of high standards. Concerns surrounding this case study include access and equity issues, human rights issues and health system failures. The aim of health care professionals' involvement in the Aboriginal and Torres Strait Islander population is to have morbidity and mortality outcomes on a par with the rest of the Australian population.

References

Aboriginal Medical Services Alliance Northern Territory (AMSANT). (2013). *Alcohol and Other Drugs and Mental Health Program Support*. Accessed 14 February 2014 at www.amsant.org.au/index.php/aod-and-mental-health-program-support.

ABS (Australian Bureau of Statistics). (2009). *National Aboriginal and Torres Strait Islanders Health Survey 2008*. ABS cat. No. 4714.0. Canberra: ABS. Accessed 14 February 2014 at www.abs.gov.au/ausstats/abs@.nsf/mf/4714.0/.

ABS (Australian Bureau of Statistics). (2013). *Life Tables for Aboriginal and Torres Strait Islander Australians, 2010–2012*. ABS cat. no. 3302.0.55.003. Canberra: ABS. Accessed 14 February 2014 at www.aihw.gov.au/deaths/life-expectancy/.

Atkinson, J. (2013). *Trauma-Informed Services and Trauma-Specific Care for Indigenous Australian Children. Resource Sheet No. 21*. Produced for the Closing the Gap Clearinghouse. Canberra: Australian Institute of Health and Welfare & Melbourne: Australian Institute of Family Studies. Accessed 16 January 2014 at www.aihw.gov.au/uploadedFiles/ClosingTheGap/Content/Publications/2 013/ctg-rs21.pdf.

Atkinson, J., Nelson, J. & Atkinson, C. (2010). Trauma, transgenerational transfer and effects on community well-being, in Purdie N., Dudgeon, P. & Walker, R. (eds), *Working Together: Aboriginal and Torres Strait Islander Mental Health and Wellbeing Principles and Practice*. Canberra: Office of Aboriginal and Torres Strait Islander Health, Department of Ageing, pp. 135–144. Accessed 17 February 2014 at http://aboriginal.childhealthresearch.org.au/media/54847/working_together_full_book.pdf.

Australian Institute of Family Studies (AIFS), Child family community Australia. (2013). *Child Protection and Aboriginal and Torres Strait Islander Children*. Accessed 16 January 2014 at www.aifs.gov.au/cfca/pubs/factsheets/a142117/.

Australian Health Ministers' Advisory Council. (2011). *Aboriginal and Torres Strait Islander Health Performance Framework Report 2010*. Canberra: AHMAC, Canberra. Accessed 16 January 2014 at www.health.gov.au/internet/publications/publishing.nsf/Content/health-oatsih-pubs-framereport-toc/$FILE/HPF%20Report%202010august2011.pdf.

Australian Institute of Health and Welfare (AIHW). (2006). *Australia's Health 2006*. Cat. no. AUS 73. Canberra: AIHW.

De Maio, J.A., Zubrick, S.R., Silburn, S.R., Lawrence, D.M., Mitrou, F.G., Dalby, R.B., Blair, E.M., Griffin, J., Milroy, H. and Cox, A. (2005). *The Western Australian Aboriginal Child Health Survey: Measuring the Social and Emotional Wellbeing of Aboriginal Children and Intergenerational Effects of Forced Separation*. Perth: Curtin University of Technology and Telethon Institute for Child Health Research.

Egan, G. (1998). *The Skilled Helper* (6th edn). Pacific Grove, CA: Brooks/Cole.

Garvey, D. (2008). *A Review of the Social and Emotional Wellbeing of Indigenous Australian Peoples*. Australian Indigenous Health *InfoNet*. Accessed 17 February 2014 at www.healthinfonet.ecu.edu.au/other-health-conditions/mental-health/reviews/our-review.

Human Rights and Equal Opportunities Commission (HREOC). (1997). *Bringing Them Home. Report on the National Inquiry into the Separation of Aboriginal and Torres Strait Islander Children from their Families*. Sydney: HREOC.

Human Rights and Equal Opportunity Commission (HREOC). (2008). *Face the Facts*. Accessed 21 January 2014 at www.humanrights.gov.au/sites/default/files/content/racial_discriminatio n/face_facts_08/FTF_2008_Web.pdf.

Indigenous Health Reference Material. (2012). *Practical Considerations for Health Professionals Working with Aboriginal Clients*. University of Rural Health Website. Accessed 17 February 2014 at www. greaterhealth.org/education training/indigenoushealth/practicaladvice/.

Lee, K., Freeburn, B., Ella, S., Miller, W., Perry, J. & Conigrave, K. (2012). *Handbook for Aboriginal Alcohol and Drug Work*. Sydney: University of Sydney.

McCausland, R. & Vivian, A. (2009). A tale of two towns: A comparative study of Wilcannia and Menindee. *Indigenous Law Bulletin*, 27(13), 7.

National Aboriginal Health Strategy. (1989). Accessed 20 February 2014 at www.health.gov.au/internet/publications/publishing.nsf/Content/mental-pubs-w-wayforw-toc~mental-pubs-w-wayforw-con~mental-pubs-w-wayforw-con-con.

Northern Sydney Local Health District (NSLHD). (2013). *Aboriginal Health Services Plan 2013–2016*. Accessed 13 December 2013 at www.nslhd.health.nsw.gov.au/AboutUs/publications/Documents/Aboriginal%20Health%20Service%20Plan%202013–2016%20Final.pdf.

NSW Aboriginal Mental Health and Well-being Policy 2006–2010. NSW Department of Health policy document. Accessed 20 February 2014 at www0.health.nsw.gov.au/policies/pd/2007/pdf/PD2007_059.pdf.

NSW Department of Community Services. (2007). *Use of Appropriate Language When Working with Aboriginal Communities in NSW*. Research to Practice Notes, Centre for Parenting and Research, DoCS. Accessed 20 February 2014 at www.community.nsw.gov.au/__data/assets/pdf_file/0020/321743/researchnotes_aboriginal_language.pdf.

NSW Department of Community Services. (2009). *Working with Aboriginal People and Communities: A Practice Resource*. Accessed 13 December 2013 at: www.community.nsw.gov.au/docswr/_assets/main/lib 100044/working_with_aboriginal_people.pdf.

Parker, R. (2010). Australian Aboriginal and Torres Strait Islander mental health: An overview. In Purdie, N., Dudgeon, P. & Walker, R. (eds) *Working Together: Aboriginal and Torres Strait Islander Mental Health and Wellbeing Principles and Practice*. Canberra: Office of Aboriginal and Torres Strait Islander Health, Department of Ageing, pp. 3–11. Accessed 13 December 2013 at http://aboriginal.childhealthresearch.org.au/media/54847/working_together_full_book.pdf.

Purdie N., Dudgeon P. & Walker R. (eds) (2010). *Working Together: Aboriginal and Torres Strait Islander Mental Health and Wellbeing Principles and Practice*. Canberra: Office of Aboriginal and Torres Strait Islander Health, Department of Ageing. Accessed 17 February 2014 at http://aboriginal.childhealth research.org.au/media/54847/working_together_full_book.pdf.

Stanley, J., Tomison, A.M. & Pocock, J. 2003. *Child Abuse and Neglect in Indigenous Australian Communities: Child Abuse Prevention Issues No. 19*. Melbourne: AIFS.

Stein-Parbury, J. (2005). *Patient and Person: Interpersonal Skills in Nursing*. Chatswood, NSW: Elsevier.

Stewart, J. & Allan, J. (2013). Building relationships with Aboriginal people: A cultural mapping toolbox. *Australian Social Work*, 66(1), 118–129.

Swan, P. & Raphael, B. (1995). *Ways Forward: National Aboriginal and Torres Strait Islander Mental Health Policy. National Consultancy Report*. Canberra: AGPS.

Thomson, N., MacRae, A., Brankovich, J., Burns, J., Catto, M., Gray, C., Levitan, L., Maling, C., Potter, C., Ride, K., Stumpers, S. & Urquhart, B. (2012). *Overview of Australian Indigenous Health Status, 2011*. Accessed 28 August 2014 at www.healthinfonet.ecu.edu.au/overview.pdf.

Wilkes, E., Gray, D., Saggers, S., Casey, W., & Stearne, A. (2010). Substance misuse and mental health among Aboriginal Australians. In Purdie, N., Dudgeon, P. & Walker, R. (eds) *Working Together: Aboriginal and Torres Strait Islander Mental Health and Wellbeing Principles and Practice*. Canberra: Office of Aboriginal and Torres Strait Islander Health, Department of Ageing: Canberra. Accessed 24 February 2014 at http://aboriginal.childhealthresearch.org.au/media/54847/working_together_full_book.pdf.

Working with Aboriginal People and Communities: A Practice Resource. (2009). NSW: Aboriginal Services Branch in consultation with the Aboriginal Reference Group. NSW Department of Community Services. Accessed 26 February 2014 at www.community.nsw.gov.au/docswr/_assets/main/documents/ working_with_aboriginal.pdf.

26

CHALLENGES TO MENTAL HEALTH CARE IN MALAWI

Location – Central Region, Lilongwe District, Malawi

Author: Katelyn Klein
Analysis: Edilma L. Yearwood

Originally from the United States with a background in intensive care and emergency nursing, I (Katelyn) moved to Malawi to work as a nurse at a rural hospital. I cared for patients on both the adult and pediatric wards with illnesses ranging from malaria to opportunistic infections to mental illness. What I observed was that rural hospitals in Malawi are resource poor, with few oxygen machines, no CT scans, a small number of available laboratory tests, and limited medication access. I spent the first few months of my time in Malawi relearning how to be a nurse with significantly different resources and in a vastly different culture. In addition to my inpatient work, after several months I also began working for an outpatient malnutrition development program. For the malnutrition program, I regularly visited rural health centers that were part of our district and followed up with severe malnutrition cases out in the villages at the patients' homes. I am very thankful to my Malawian colleagues who taught me how to be a nurse in rural Malawi and helped me to better understand the factors—cultural, poverty-related, and otherwise—that impact health care in this beautiful but struggling nation.

Background

Malawi is a small nation in southeastern Africa that shares borders with Mozambique, Zambia, and Tanzania. Malawi is a vibrant country with a predominately agrarian economy. Only 16.3 percent of the population lives in urban areas while the vast majority of citizens live in rural villages (CIA, n.d.). While Malawi used to be densely wooded, deforestation to increase farm land needed to feed a rapidly growing population has left the landscape largely barren in the dry season (May–November) and covered in endless fields of bright green maize in the rainy season (November–May). Malawi has been largely spared from the armed conflicts that have ravaged much of the continent and remains a relatively peaceful land. Malawians proudly refer to their country as "the warm heart of Africa." Though a peaceful nation, Malawi is faced with severe health epidemics, widespread poverty and destitution, corruption, and significant underdevelopment.

Most of the population supports itself with subsistence farming, though in most of the country, rainfall and weather only allow for one major harvest per year as irrigation is not an option for most, and is rarely seen outside of large plantations. There are relatively few paved roads in the country though many dirt paths wind through the fields and hills. Electricity is unreliable; large cities and rural areas alike have frequent outages and only 9.8 percent of households have access to electricity (World Bank, n.d.). Communication can be difficult as less than one-third of the population has a cell phone and only 2.2 percent have internet access (CIA, n.d.). Malnutrition and starvation are significant problems in rural Malawi; 47 percent of children under 5 years have stunted growth from undernutrition and 60 percent of households have poor to borderline food consumption (Wilson, 2014). Poverty and food shortages are exacerbated by the fact that in many households, only the mother is present. While HIV/AIDS and other illnesses account for a portion of single-parent households, polygamy and marital unfaithfulness is commonly seen among men, leaving many women with the responsibility of being both provider and caretaker. Men often provide no support to their first family once they leave the household and engage in a relationship with another woman, often starting a new family. As an average of 5.6 children are born to each woman in Malawi (CIA, n.d.), it is a daunting and often impossible task to perform the manual labor needed for a successful harvest while simultaneously caring for five or six children. Older children often drop out of primary school to stay at home to help care for younger children or assist their mother with housework.

Access to health care in rural areas is extremely limited. The country has a three-tier health system, with rural health centers and outreach clinics being the source of most primary care. However, the primary care facilities are often poorly staffed and frequently run out of medications and supplies. Many of the posts where clinics are held have no electricity or running water. Only 46 percent of the population lives within a 5 km walk of any type of health facility (WHO, 2013), resulting in long and difficult treks for many. While treatment is free at government health centers and clinics, ambulance rides or even public transportation to a higher level of care is often prohibitively expensive for patients in rural villages, preventing them from getting to a hospital, even in an emergency. Malaria, tuberculosis, and HIV are serious health concerns, with over 10 percent of the country (more than 1,000,000 people) being HIV positive. Infant mortality rates are high and the average life expectancy is only 55 years (World Bank, n.d.). Mental health care is extremely limited, with facilities, medications, and trained personnel inadequate in some areas and non-existent in others. Many health care workers in rural areas have received no training on mental illness; in practice psychiatric concerns are often written off as caused by malaria, bacterial infections, or spirits. It is not uncommon for health care workers, particularly at primary care centers in rural areas, to incorporate traditional beliefs into their understanding of mental illnesses.

Introduction

Malawian culture is rich and diverse, with numerous tribes, languages, groups, and religions. The Chewa are the largest ethnic group in Malawi, followed by the Lomwe and the Yao. The Chewa people associate with Christianity while the Yao people are generally Muslim. All ethnic groups incorporate traditional beliefs in spirits, magic, and traditional medicine into their belief system. Traditional healers have been an established part of culture and society since long before official hospitals and health centers were built. Traditional healers have no formal medical training but instead are taught their craft from previous generations or they believe that a spirit medium has come down and imparted the necessary skills and wisdom upon them. Visiting a traditional healer for physical and mental concerns is often more culturally acceptable and geographically convenient than going to an established hospital or health center. Many patients who do come to health care facilities may have first consulted a traditional healer about their malady, and only go on to a hospital if the condition does not improve. Among the Chewa people, there is a strong belief in the power of traditional healers to provide cures or healing for ailments ranging from common illnesses, such as an ongoing cough or severe headaches, to HIV/AIDS, to mental problems. It is believed that many symptoms and diseases, both physical and mental, have spiritual underpinnings, and traditional healers often attribute symptoms to bewitchment or spirits. Treatment techniques vary among healers but common remedies include herbal drinks, powdered roots put on the tongue, or smears of mud and ash applied strategically to the skin. Physical interventions include creating thin cuts in a patient's skin with razor-type tools, sometimes rubbing different mixtures into the cuts, or making small burns on different locations on the body. There is very little collaboration between the traditional healers and the formal health care system, and sometimes, significant animosity. In general, patients are aware that nurses and clinicians look unfavorably upon seeking help from a traditional healer and therefore patients will often lie to staff about their involvement with a healer and the interventions the healer performed on them.

Case presentation

A young man named Mphatso★, approximately 20 years old, was brought to the hospital by his wife Liness★ with a chief complaint of "strange behavior" and talking to people who were not there for several weeks, maybe a month. They were of the Chewa ethnic group and lived in a nearby village, about 4 km from the hospital. They had walked, as they could not afford a bicycle taxi. Their village was not accessible by road, but only by narrow dirt paths. Apparently Mphatso's brother had helped to escort him to the hospital but was not currently present. Liness was thin and appeared tired, repeatedly shooting concerned glances at her husband. The chitenge (traditional fabric) skirts she wore were ragged and her shirt was torn. Mphatso was short and wiry but looked strong and physically fit. His clothing was dirty and his oversized shoes had large holes in the soles. They were quite poor. Upon initial evaluation, the patient was talking quietly and nonsensically to himself, gaze directed downward. With persistent questioning, he was able to give his name. Liness said that he had been having "bursts of anger" where he would suddenly get very mad and run away. The patient usually worked in his fields during the day but his wife reported he had been disappearing on and off for a month, neglecting his crops.

Physical examination showed vital signs within normal limits; weight 50 kgs, height 160 centimeters. Rapid tests for HIV and malaria were both negative. Further physical examination showed mild periorbital and facial edema but was otherwise unremarkable except for several small dark burn marks on his arms and chest. Additionally, in the center of his forehead, slightly above the eyebrows were several small shallow razor-like cuts, which were scabbed over. The patient's wife denied any recent trauma or illness. When asked about the facial swelling, the wife reported that it started about a week ago and was much better now. Upon being asked if any treatment had been attempted prior to coming to the hospital, his wife denied any prior treatment or interventions. When asked about the burn marks and small cuts she said that maybe the patient had fallen down. The patient's wife denied that the patient had seen a traditional healer for his "strange behavior."

At a secondary assessment later in the day, the patient was sitting in bed staring out the window quietly. When asked again about seeing a traditional healer, the patient's wife admitted that the patient had seen one about a month prior because he was hearing voices that were not there. The patient admitted that he still was hearing voices "sometimes" but could/would not give any further specifics. The traditional healer had told them that the patient was bewitched but could be cured. At the initial visit the healer gave the patient some herbs to drink. About a week later, the healer made the burn marks on the patient's arms and chest and created the cuts on the forehead. A week after that, the patient was given "stronger herbs," which caused his facial edema. The wife reported that there was no change in the patient's condition after any of the interventions, except the appearance of facial swelling.

(*Note: All names used in this case study are psyeudonyms.)

Patients and family members in the hospital

It is important to note that interactions between patients, their family members, and hospital staff are very different in Malawi than in Western cultures. In Malawi, when a patient comes to the hospital they are required to have a "guardian" who stays with them. For children, guardians are usually their mother but could also be a father, aunt, or sibling. For adults, the guardian is usually an adult female—a mother, sister, wife, or aunt, though males can be guardians as well. Guardians are responsible for cooking for the patient and often bring firewood, pans, and flour to the hospital and cook outside the patient rooms. The guardian bathes and feeds the patient, turns them to avoid pressure sores, empties bed pans and urinary catheter bags, ensures that the patient takes their medicine when the nurse distributes it, and is present whenever a clinician assesses the patient. When health care staff interview a patient about their illness and how they are feeling, often the guardian will answer for the patient. This is seen as a courtesy that spares the sick patient further stress of having to answer questions. Generally, even when a question is directed at a patient, the guardian will answer, unless the clinician specifically requests that the patient respond. When discussing procedures and treatment, it is often the guardian that will ask the questions and say whether or not they agree. Sometimes patients will be consulted and their opinion will be considered but generally the guardian, in conjunction with the health care staff, has more power in decision-making than the patient does.

Management and outcome

The hospital's mental health nurse spoke extensively with Mphatso and Liness about mental illness, specifically schizophrenia. The patient's wife was unsure about the information and was neither receptive nor dismissive about the idea of her husband having a mental illness that could possibly be helped by medication and treatment at a hospital. She said that the traditional healer had told her that the patient had bad spirits in his head, was that the same thing as schizophrenia? Significant time was taken to answer her questions and explain the medical condition of schizophrenia in plain language. She was given a referral for her husband to the closest psychiatric care facility, which was about 50 km away in the city of Lilongwe. The rural hospital where they were currently did not have antipsychotic medications available. The wife was hesitant to go to the psychiatric facility and said she would first take her husband home to consult her mother and the patient's brother and decide what to do. They were advised to return to the rural hospital in two weeks for follow up if they were not at the psychiatric facility. Mphatso and his wife did not go to the psychiatric facility, nor did they return for follow up.

Discussion

Traditional beliefs and traditional healers have a significant impact on the interpretation of mental illness in Malawi. Widespread beliefs in spirits or bewitchment as the underlying cause of all mental problems permeate much of the culture. Many Malawians, including those who have completed secondary or post-secondary education, have little or no knowledge of the biological roots of mental illness and this can be difficult information for patients and their families to accept. The limited number of psychiatric care facilities, trained personnel, and lack of available psychotropic medications make identification of mental illness, along with education and treatment, particularly challenging. For many patients, accessing hospitals that are far from their home, even if the services are free, is an enormous financial burden and a significant deterrent. The cost of transport alone is often unattainable, and the guardian and patient must also pay for food at large city hospitals, whereas at rural hospitals and health centers they are able to make cooking fires outside the patient's room and walk home to get more supplies if they need to. Socioeconomic factors combined with skepticism about the biological roots of mental illness and lack of infrastructure to support these patients pose significant barriers to diagnosis and treatment and make psychiatric care in Malawi a complicated and challenging undertaking.

Commentary

As an educator, this case exemplar offers opportunities to examine and discuss several critical concepts when nurses and other health care providers work in new, challenging and resource poor environments. Specific issues raised include the intersection of culture and mental health, preparation for cultural immersion, the role of in-country nurse experts, gender roles, competing demands on family members, prioritization of clinical presentations in high volume resource poor clinics, outreach to traditional healers and the culture specific role of families and friends.

Clinicians entering new environments are encouraged to gather as much information as possible about the culture they will be entering and practicing in. These data can be obtained from the literature about the country, state, community, or new health care service. In addition, local clinicians, supportive agencies (such as the local Red Cross, local UN or World Bank services, and local religious groups, clergy and NGOs) and health care organizations may also be sources of information about the culture and health care beliefs and practices. While information obtained in this way can serve as a useful framework to provide familiarity and context, it is also prudent to conduct one's own cultural assessment specific to the individuals for whom you are providing services.

Clinicians in new environments, especially poorly resourced environments are particularly challenged when confronted with large numbers of consumers with complex health and mental health care needs. Establishing priority care needs and realizing practice realities, while important and necessary, may leave the novice nurse feeling less than satisfied or effective in the care delivered. With respect to meeting mental health needs, nurses are encouraged to return to the practice recommendations from the mother of psychiatric nurses, Hildegard Peplau, and work first on developing a relationship with consumers and their families and using yourself as the tool to meeting psychiatric needs (listening, empathy, data gathering, collaboration/patient-centered, educator). Aggressively prescribing interventions that are viewed as culturally discordant may serve as a barrier to trust and impede engagement in treatment by individuals in low-income countries/environments. Slowly working on developing the relationship over a period of time may be a more successful strategy in engaging culturally diverse individuals and families in their care and treatment.

Specific to this exemplar, health care providers in a low-income environment must also seek cultural brokers to assist in gaining a better understanding of the views and practices specific to mental health and mental ill health. If possible, attempts should be made to meet with traditional healers to better understand their practices and to forge potential collaborations/partnerships for joint treatment of individuals presenting with symptoms associated with mental ill health. Nurses and other health care providers providing care are encouraged to take advantage of teachable moments to provide some information that would advance mental health literacy or combat stigma associated with mental ill health. This should by no means focus on lecturing or being dogmatic but should be approached in a respectful, open and participatory way.

Specific to this exemplar, useful sources of mentoring for new clinicians in diverse environments are the nurses from the country. Questions should be asked of these experts and guidance sought as to best approaches to maximize positive mental health outcomes especially given the associated stigma. New clinicians in diverse environments are also encouraged to maintain a journal and reflect on their experiences, what they learned, what were their greatest challenges, how they felt they made a difference and what cultural questions they have. Having a more senior colleague to provide mentorship, guidance and support would assist with the nurse's development from novice toward expert within the specific environment.

Another factor from the case exemplar that bears mentioning is the role of gender within many global families. In this case, discussions and decisions needed to occur within the family with older male siblings and the family matriarch. These processes must be understood and respected but it also provides a clear indication of who should be included when engaging in teaching about mental health and symptom management. In addition, what cannot be underestimated are the competing demands on family members for caring for the individual presenting with symptoms and balancing the agricultural and other needs of the family. Unfortunately, the fact that needed services were only available at a significant distance from the home meant that the wife and other family members could not be spared to travel and stay with Mphatso to provide his day-to-day care. The underlying stigma that had not been alleviated and the competing agricultural needs served as barriers to his receiving necessary care. Nurses must also understand that the use of medications and more specifically psychotropic medications may not be endorsed by some cultures. This needs to be part of the nursing assessment that is conducted followed by clear education in understandable terminology about the type of medication, its intended purpose, risks and benefits. It may take multiple conversations about the benefits of medications before a trial is agreed to. Unfortunately, in low-resource communities, older more side-effect-laden medications are available as they are cheaper than the newer psychotropic medications.

Little research exists with in-country experts in low-resource environments as to their non-pharmacological management of individuals who present to local clinics with psychiatric symptoms. Nurses are also well positioned to establish and conduct inquiry on new models of mental health care in partnership with traditional healers and to evaluate long-term outcomes within poorly resourced communities. These efforts are long overdue and would position nurses at the forefront in increasing mental health care and eliminating mental health inequalities in various global communities (Elliott & Masters, 2009).

References

Central Intelligence Agency (CIA). (n.d.). *The world factbook: Malawi.* Retrieved September 2, 2015 from www.cia.gov/library/publications/the-world-factbook/geos/mi.html.

Elliott, L. & Masters, H. (2009). Mental health inequalities and mental health nursing. *Journal of Psychiatric and Mental Health Nursing, 16,* 762–771.

Wilson, R. (2014). *New anti-stunting drive to begin in Malawi: World Food Programme (WFP).* Retrieved September 25, 2015 from www.wfp.org/stories/promising-approach-end-stunting-malawi.

World Bank. (n.d). *Malawi.* Retrieved September 25, 2015 from http://data.worldbank.org/country/malawi.

World Health Organization (WHO). (2013). *WHO country cooperation strategy 2008–2013 Malawi.* Retrieved September 2, 2015 from www.who.int/countryfocus/cooperation_strategy/ccs_mwi_en.pdf.

27

ARGENTINA

Silvina Malvárez, Patricia Fabiana Gómez
and María Cristina Cometto

Introduction

In this changing twenty-first century, mental health is considered one of the primary health problems and poses a significant impact on the global burden of disease. The reason mental health is so important is its influence on the quality of social life, its strategic position in socioeconomic development, the severity of the damages it may cause to individuals, families and communities, and the barriers it poses to health and development globally.

The world and indeed human life has vigorously changed over the last 30 years. As Prime Minister Shimon Peres said, "The twenty-first century seems not to be the continuation of history, but the future that will allow us to get ahead of danger, and direct our destiny as humanity" (Peres, 1997). Armless revolutions have occurred, frontiers have become blurred and social inequalities and natural disasters have increased around the world. The era of digital information and communication urges a change of mind, a change in lifestyles and a change in human relations. New hopes and new dangers appear and both affect mental health. Mental health problems are increasing around the world including in the Americas. In spite of new and evidence-based strategies and transformed health services globally, the gap between identified problems and effective and accessible treatments remains a significant global challenge (OMS, 2008).

At the same time, because of their mission (human care), the nature of their work (satisfaction of human needs), the proximity to patients and communities, and the size of the nursing profession (the largest within the health workforce in the world), nurses have a privileged place to occupy in societies, a special responsibility, and a great opportunity to help in the complex field of mental health (Malvárez, 1999).

In Argentina, several transformations have occurred in psychiatric services, concepts and practices, since the restoration of democracy in 1983. The traditional custodial psychiatric model is going through a comprehensive change led by a community mental health model, which proposes the substitution of traditional psychiatric hospitals for a community mental health services network. Nurses in Argentina have been involved in such processes from the very beginning, delivering a different kind of nursing care. They have been providing education and management for change, doing new research while exploring new concepts, participating in policy development and implementation, promoting human rights, improving quality of care and facilitating patient reintegration into society (Malvárez, 2007).

This chapter presents community mental health nursing experiences from 14 communities within Argentina, a country located on the southern cone of the American continent. Historically involved with mental health nursing, psychiatric services, and education, the authors have gathered significant experiences from several provinces undergoing transformation within their traditional psychiatric model.

Information was collected through a specific instrument used to describe nursing practices. The method used is the "systematization of practices," developed in Latin America in the 1970s, based on a participatory research process. Research activities include three dialectic moments: practice reconstruction and analysis, theorization, and synthesis. Selected experiences show a variety of interventions related to how mental health nurses are working within communities in activities of mental health promotion, prevention, treatment support, care, and rehabilitation.

The context of the country of Argentina is briefly presented, followed by a description of the selected experiences and their analysis, a conceptual framework and synthesis, and recommendations to promote mental health and well-being of consumers and citizens within the country.

Country context

Argentina is a country located in the southern cone of the American continent. It is made up of 24 provinces and one autonomous city. The autonomous city of Buenos Aires is the country's capital. Its geographic area covers 3,761,274 square kilometers (approximately 1,421 square miles), including a portion of the Antarctic continent (OMS, 2009). Argentina has a population of 41 million people; most of them are of Spanish and Italian descent (as well as from other European countries). Immigration comes mainly from Bolivia and Peru, and almost half a million are part of the original population. The official language spoken is Spanish and the religion is predominantly Roman Catholic. Argentina is considered as a middle-income country (Banco Mundial, 2014) with several areas of poverty located throughout the country. It is an industrialized country with a literacy rate of 97.7 percent.

Argentina experienced a military government regime (1976–1983) that resulted in severe social consequences for the country. It has since had a democratic government since 1983, with strong social policies (OPS, 2013). Current health indicators show that most of the United Nations Millennium Development Goals have been achieved. Life expectancy is 76.3 years-of-age (average), 72.6 for men and 79.9 for women (OPS, 2013). Although considered non-communicable diseases, violence associated with poverty and drug trafficking and substance abuse, are considered to be some of the country's main problems with associated health consequences. Maternal mortality and other health problems associated with social determinants of health remain with moderate positive changes such occurring.

The country is divided into five health regions: the northwest region (including the provinces of Jujuy, Salta, Tucumán, Santiago del Estero, La Rioja, and Catamarca); the northeast region (including the provinces of Formosa, Chaco, Entre Ríos, Corrientes, and Misiones); the central region (including the provinces of Córdoba, Santa Fe, Buenos Aires, and La Pampa); the region of Cuyo (including the provinces of Mendoza, San Juan, and San Luis); and the region of Patagonia (including the provinces of Neuquén, Río Negro, Chubut, Santa Cruz, and Tierra del Fuego).

Development of a health/mental health focus

The overall health system in Argentina has three subsectors: private, public, and mixed. Health insurance is mandatory for workers and retired people. Health insurance is accessible, but may be met with some difficulties for most of Argentinean and immigrant citizens. There are new policies in place for the development of services such as Primary Health Care and Universal Health Coverage, with special attention being paid to social determinants of health. Nursing services are paying increased attention to quality of care, patient safety, and family and community care. Health care management has also been a focus for improving care. The nursing workforce itself comes from a strong education system and there is modern legislation focused on practice and education. However, nursing research and postgraduate education needs to be strengthened. Nursing faces problems such as shortage, resource misdistribution and challenges associated with inequalities.

As relates to mental health trends, there are no known national epidemiological studies conducted. However, preliminary investigations suggest that Argentina experiences the same trends as other Latin American countries. The prevalent mental health problems and concerns include depression, alcohol abuse, anxiety, bipolar and obsessive-compulsive problems, and drug-abuse, among others. In severe situations patients are hospitalized in large traditional psychiatric hospitals and are oftentimes hospitalized for long periods of time (Rodríguez, Kohn & Aquilar-Gaxiola, 2009b).

The answer to serious mental health cases predominantly continues to be the use of traditional models. Treatment in these cases center on use of traditional psychiatric hospitals with custodial and pharmacological treatment, patient isolation and exclusion. In 1983, the new democratic federal and provincial governments defined new policies for mental health services and the national movement towards changing the mental health system began.

These changes in Argentina, as well as in other countries in Latin America, were sparked as mental health gained international status with the Caracas Conference in 1991. It was here that different governments denounced the neglect of people with severe psychiatric problems, the use of psychiatric hospitals as places of confinement, the loss of rights, and lack of treatment that patients faced. They proposed the restructuring of psychiatric assistance (Levav, 1992a).

Subsequently, four Pan American conferences that focused on mental health occurred, Washington 2001, Brasilia 2005, Panama 2010, and Brasilia 2013. Through these efforts, it became evident that progress was being made towards the responsible care of individuals and families dealing with mental health problems and the need to substitute community mental health service networks in place of traditional psychiatric hospitals.

The deinstitutionalization of patients from psychiatric hospitals into the community, the creation of policies and changes in treatment strategies for people with severe mental suffering along with the concern for promotion and protection of mental health, and qualified care provided to people with a variety of problems, led to the creation of a community mental health services network that signaled a new era in the field of mental health in the Americas (Rodríguez, Malvárez, González, & Levav, 2009a).

After 1983 and during a decade of weakness in the 1990s, Argentina began to implement new policies and move towards a community mental health model. Most provinces in Argentina are involved in these new policies and programs, resource mobilization, research, professional and post-graduate education, and in-service training of human resources. The most significant change was the promulgation and implementation of national and provincial legislation on mental health, which restricted the functioning of psychiatric hospitals, assigned budgets, defended the human rights of patients and families alike, and created new services and other supportive initiatives (Malvárez, 1999).

In 2013, the National Department of Mental Health and Addictions of Argentina approved the National Mental Health Plan. It included goals and actions oriented towards guaranteeing the right to mental health care and the protection of human rights for all in the population suffering from mental health challenges. It also guaranteed entitlements based on the rules of the National Mental Health Law Nr. 26.657 and its Regulatory Addendum No. 603/2013 (Ministerio de Salud de la Nacion Argentina, 2013).

Although nursing practices were traditionally concentrated in psychiatric hospitals, new developments have encouraged nurses to generate and practice in new community services and engage in activities as part of multidisciplinary community-focused teams. Nursing care in the remaining psychiatric hospitals is being oriented to facilitating patient discharge and integrating patients back into their communities and family life (Malvárez, 1999; 2002). The following table (Table 27.1) outlines the practices and services that are being developed.

Mental health nursing education in Argentina is also changing its model. Basic education includes mental health nursing in the curriculum of all nursing schools. Postgraduate education is offered through three interdisciplinary master's programs in the country, all of them oriented towards the community mental health model. There are interdisciplinary education work residency programs on mental health that can be accessed by nurses too (Malvárez, 2007). In several provinces, in-service education programs for nurses are also oriented towards mental health policy and legislation. The movement of mental health nursing is growing in that nurses are committed to transformation, quality of care, education, training, and engaging in mental health research.

In the context of a comprehensive and complex process of change, different experiences of mental health nursing and interventions have been selected to illustrate and conceptualize the contributions of mental health nursing in Argentina. Table 27.2 illustrates 15 community mental health nursing observations (activities) taking place within the country. Data and information from each observation was collected using a specific instrument developed in Latin America in the 1970s to describe nursing practices. Our observations and research used the "systematization of practices" of participatory research and included three dialectic moments: (1) practice reconstruction and analysis; (2) theorization; and (3) synthesis. The 15 selected observations demonstrate the variety of interventions and involvement of nurses in Argentina, as well as the country's efforts to transform the traditional custodial psychiatric model to a community mental health model. Each observation in Table 27.2 is an exemplar that evidences how nurses are working with communities in wellness promotion, prevention, treatment, support, care, and rehabilitation. The beneficiaries of each observed intervention were children, adolescents, adults, senior citizens, women, and people with chronic psychological suffering. The observed interventions were oriented to improving people's work and sustenance abilities, mental health needs and psychosocial support. In addition, actions focused on minimization of risk factors,

Table 27.1 Community nursing practices and services

Practices and services	
Mental health service in community health centers	Mental health services in general hospitals
Community mental health centers	Mental health services in specialized hospitals (pediatrics, maternal, infectious)
Family mental health services	
Mobile community mental health teams	Education and work training
Daytime discharged patient services	Recreation and socialization services
Acute mental health services	Mental health residencies, protected homes, and others

supporting orientation and engagement in recreation, cultural activities, bonding, and the reconstruction of social networks. The improvement of interpersonal relationships (nurse–subject, nurse–community, health care team–community) was a focal part of therapeutic care.

Reconstruction and analysis

The information provided by the community mental health nursing intervention experiences in different regions in Argentina, demonstrates advances in the transformation process from that of a traditional psychiatric assistance approach towards the development of community mental health services networks and nurses as integral parts of this process. The names given to most of the experiences highlight the focus of the intervention in the community, with emphasis on the care given to mental health challenges and active consumer participation. The locations where the interventions were conducted were health institutions and universities, representing the different sanitary zones in the country. The professionals were nurses that formed interdisciplinary or nursing teams to carry out the experiences. Many of their activities preceded the new National Mental Health Act No. 26.657 (Legislatura de la Nación Argentina, 2010), others were subsequent to the act and more importantly, most of them are still ongoing.

When analyzing the reasons and background that gave way to the experiences, it can be observed that all of them originated from the identification of needs or situations or problems within the community. Activities are oriented towards health and mental health promotion, and using the community model that respects the needs of populations and people as individuals with legal rights. The psychosocial approach widens the perspective of care, from hospitalized dependent patients with long years of hospital stays, to independent and empowered individuals at risk, with the prospect of a healthy and caring life.

Interventions are oriented to improving people's abilities and emphasizes their healthy aspects; work and sustenance abilities are promoted, assistance is provided with mental health needs and psychosocial support is provided. Risk factors are identified and minimized; orientation is given to providing answers, encouraging engagement in recreation, cultural activities, and reconstruction of social networks. Improvements in interpersonal relationships (nurse–subject, nurse–community, health care team–community) are promoted and are the main therapeutic instrument of care.

This moment of transition highlights a significant distance between the psychiatric custodial nursing profile and the community mental health nursing profile, socially acknowledged, that responds technically and politically to the needs of individuals and the larger community. Some of the concepts used include: health as a social process, resilience, interdisciplinary care, nursing care according to Hildegard Peplau (1992), psychoanalytic theory, mental health promotion and psychic suffering prevention, respect for human rights, understanding of health and mental health according to WHO, concepts on psychosocial rehabilitation, and systemic family theory, among others.

The strategies used include workshop participation (vegetable gardens, sports, recreation); group meetings (of the team and with users, with feedback, along with support and discussion groups led by professionals); role-playing life experiences (dramatizations, re-enactments, simulations, celebrations); interviews (support, follow-up, planning); and home visits, phone support, and other therapeutic techniques. They hold a vision of community mental health nursing that believes in the possibilities of care as a revitalizing and socializing process for the individual and collective perspective and of its ability to promote and protect mental health even in the case of people who suffer from severe and chronic mental conditions.

Table 27.2 In-country exemplars

Place	Beneficiaries	Need	Interventions/strategies	Goals/results
Central Hospital, Río Cuarto, Córdoba (Day Hospital)	Discharged patients	Provide a response to the lack of community support for patients with chronic mental suffering	Workshops and group meetings: organic vegetable garden, audiovisual arts, drama, daily life activities, self-care activities, sports, and recreation	To strengthen the human rights of patients and their right to live and participate within the community. The workshops and meetings promote human relations and occupational reintegration
Municipal Hospital of Cruz Alta, Córdoba	Adults, children, and adolescents Schools	Patient referrals	Nursing office with registration, home visits, school visits	Nurses highlight healthy aspects of patients, provide community support, give feedback, and coaching 3000 visits were conducted during the first year Patient dosages decreased and greater attendance at school was reported
Provincial Hospital Nuestra Senora de la Misericordia, Córdoba (Provincial Hospital of Our Lady of Mercy)	Parents and family members of neonatal hospitalized children	Mental health support and techniques, liaison and advocate between hospital and families	Initial welcome, support in the situation of worsening children's health, provision of education and information, group reflective activities, assessment of mother-and-child relationship	Communication channels were opened between hospital staff and families Mental health services were provided to families during the neonatal experience Visitation hours were modified
The Social and Occupational Rehabilitation Center, Ministry of Health, Córdoba	Patients with chronic mental health suffering	Support and the promotion of skill development (planning, execution, and evaluation)	Group meetings (planning, organization, and execution of events with pre and post reflective activities), commemorative celebrations, and graduations	Occupational and social skills development An increase in interpersonal communication, initiative and involvement, and willingness of patients was observed Patients' and workers' opinions, input, and abilities were appreciated and valued

The Provincial Neuropsychiatric Hospital, Ministry of Health, Córdoba	Hospitalized patients, discharged patients, and community members	Promote social exchange and communal integration and participation	Vegetable garden workshop Bi-weekly meetings welcomed new patients to the garden and group The vegetable garden provided a point of access for integrative activities	Patients worked in teams plowing the earth and growing products that they sold to buy new materials for use in the garden Patients recovered team building and social skills
Mental Health Teaching Hospital, Institutional Group for Alcoholism, Paraná, Entre Ríos	Adults suffering from alcohol addiction	Recovery from alcohol addiction	Group activities, therapeutic care, individual interviews, participative workshops, projects	Group participation was a supportive part of recovery Participants developed new life projects
Health Center of Oñativia, Entre Ríos Ministry of Health	Senior citizens	Support, wellness and improve the quality of life of senior citizens	Two weekly meetings promoted physical activity and motor skills stimulation, health care, and leisure activities (reading, writing, recreation, problem solving, and a memory stimulation workshop) Home visits and support visits were offered to seniors with illnesses	Senior citizens made friendships, learned mental health and wellness skills, and bonded with the community Seniors expressed that the activities improved their independence
Mental Health Teaching Hospital, Geronto Psychiatric Unit, Paraná, Entre Ríos	Long-stay hospitalized patients	Prevent the deterioration of long-stay hospitalized patients	Cognitive stimulation, expressive dance, outdoor recreation and trips, individual interviews, and participation in Victoria's Senior Citizen congress	Affective bonding between patients, senior citizens, nursing staff, and community members was experienced Patients that participated in activities increased their possibility for discharge
National University of Entre Ríos, Concepción	People under ambulatory	In response to the neglect experienced by individuals with	Group meetings, home visits, follow-up care, alternative	Individuals and their primary caregivers gained independence, as well as, knowledge about health promotion and prevention

Table 27.2 continued

Place	Beneficiaries	Need	Interventions/strategies	Goals/results
del Uruguay, Entre Ríos	treatment with difficulty accessing mental health services	severe mental health conditions	strategies (art and music therapy/resources)	Individuals improved adherence to treatment and achieved better group and social insertion
Santa Rosa de Lima Chapel, University of Santiago del Estero, Santiago del Estero	Adult women	Community domestic violence detection and victim protection	The project involves a visit to the Child Nutrition Cooperative, volunteer training, detection, and protection Access to health care professionals	The goals of the project include making home visits, implementing educational workshops, conducting referrals for domestic violence victim assistance, and working with a team to create follow-up protocols
Diego de Rojas School, Santiago del Estero, Santiago del Estero	Teachers, students (ages 10–12), and school personnel	Identifying violence in schools and creating solutions and strategies for beneficiaries	Weekly meetings are held separately for teachers, students, and school administrators Situations of violence are identified and solutions proposed to meet each group's needs Each group writes a proposal for health promotion in schools	Groups identified risk factors that triggered violence in school. Groups found solutions Teachers' predisposed attitudes and responses towards hyperactive children improved
Mental Health Municipal Center, Grupos Abiertos Post-Alta (GAPA), Tandil, Buenos Aires (Municipal Center, Open Groups post-discharge)	Recently admitted patients and their families	In response to frequent patient readmissions, patients with difficulties adhering to psychopharmacological treatment, overcrowding at health service centers, and to remedy the shortage of social insertion spaces for discharged patients	Weekly meetings are a vehicle for sharing and providing support to patients and families Collective solutions and alternatives are discussed	This recent activity uses evaluations to adjust and plan follow-up models for mental health promotion and prevention

Luis Agotte Hospital, Loving You Healthy (Quererte Sano) workshop, Ministry of Health, Chamical, La Rioja	Adolescent school aged children (age 12–15)	Assist rural school aged children around health topics	Two-day participative and creative workshops were organized on hygiene habits, sex education, nutrition, family planning rights and responsibilities	Students actively participated in the workshops and presented a play based on each workshop to the school community
Choel-Choel, Río Negro, Patagonia	Mental health service patients and the community	A part of the Provincial Mental Health Act, No. 2440 (Río Negro Legislature, 1991), the observation was to improve skills and facilitate employment prospects	Activities such as embroidery, fabric painting, and knitting used creative art to communicate and build manual service skills	Patients evaluated their experiences and exhibited their crafts for sale
Mental Health Residence, Ministry of Health, Río Negro, Patagonia	Mental health patients	Provide a resident training program for social and occupational reintegration	Health care professionals conduct in-depth interviews, life story exploration, identify health promotion processes, conduct home visits and strengthen personal bonds	The evaluation acknowledges the therapeutic support and aid in community reintegration Participants described having enriching experiences

Theorizing

New community mental health services network

WHO maintains that mental health care must be delivered through general health services and in community environments. Large and centralized psychiatric institutions must be replaced. The community model favors the integration of mental health services within general health services along with other community services, setting up a coordinated network with the following characteristics: accessibility, acceptability, integrity, coordination and continuity of care, territoriality, effectiveness, fairness and respect for human rights, inter-disciplinarily. and inter-sectoriality (Rodríguez *et al.*, 2009b: WHO, 2013). The model calls for the creation of services and specialized teams for highly complex situations, for counseling and training, the creation of community mental health centers, the installation of mental health services in general hospitals, the integration of comprehensive mental health services in primary health care, support for informal community teams, the promotion of self-care and the strengthening and support of social networks.

It also acknowledges the importance of education and training of human resources to maintain the community model and that participation of patients, families, community members, health personnel, and institutions as necessary for strengthening quality of care and overall effectiveness (Malvárez, 2011). Three groups are identified as requiring prioritization of nursing care: (a) persons hospitalized for a long time in custodial psychiatric hospitals; (b) groups of people who suffer frequent mental health challenges such as those with depression, epilepsy, obsessive-compulsive symptoms, anxiety and panic episodes, alcohol/drugs dependency and violence; and (c) vulnerable groups such as children, senior citizens, the poor, displaced groups, victims of natural disasters and social conflicts, people with special needs, and persons suffering from chronic diseases (Malvárez, 2011).

Synthesis and recommendations

Synthesis of the data allowed the authors to highlight the following conclusions found in Table 27.3.

Recommendations

Based on the experiences of the authors, the following recommendations are identified as they add value to and strengthen development of global community mental health nursing models.

In the area of communication

- Create a virtual sharing and learning environment to connect mental health nurses globally and promote knowledge and experiences exchange.
- Link mental health nursing networks regionally and around the world.

In the area of education

- Establish a community mental health nursing virtual education program.
- Compile psychiatric-mental health nursing programs of basic and post-graduate education.
- Define lines of nursing education for basic curriculum in the area of mental health nursing.
- Define lines of nursing education for post-basic programs in the area of mental health nursing.

Table 27.3 Conclusions

Conclusions
• A change in traditional psychiatric services is occurring in Argentina. It is oriented to building a community mental health services network
• Change is happening at several levels: public policies, legislation, government health programs and services, education, community participation, and daily experiences
• Nursing practices that, for a long time have constituted and supported custodial psychiatric hospitals, are now part of the transition and of the deinstitutionalization programs
• Most of the experiences are interdisciplinary and some are also inter-sectorial, with a strong presence and initiatives taken by nurses
• The variety of community mental health nursing practices illustrated from different provinces in Argentina, supports the idea that building a community mental health-nursing model is possible and ongoing
• The community mental health nursing model moves the focus from centralized hospitals, mental diseases, psychiatric patients, and cure, towards interventions and teams in communities, general health services/social services, that work for individuals, families, groups, and communities
• Social, political, technical and administrative reforms are necessary to allow and facilitate transformation of mental health care systems
• The new approach and paradigm shift emphasizes, recognizes, and supports healthy dimensions of individuals rather than the previous focus on pathology. It also promotes and protects individual, family, and community mental health while identifying risk factors and preventing problems as part of a strong consideration and respect for human rights
• New practices are grounded in ethics, political and legal frames, nursing theories, global concepts of health and mental health, social determinants of mental health, human rights, relational, humanistic, and community nursing theories
• These new practices must continue to be evaluated

In the area of information and research

- Identify main indicators of nursing practices and promote information gathering.
- Promote regular systematization of mental health nursing practices.
- Define mental health nursing research priorities.
- Promote and support multi-centric and inter-disciplinary research.
- Promote research programs of practices in the area of mental health nursing.

In the area of services

- Promote deinstitutionalization processes of traditional psychiatric hospitals.
- Support the creation of mental health services networks.
- Establish in-service education programs on mental health nursing in psychiatric hospitals, general and specialized hospitals, community health centers, and social institution health centers.
- Systematically register, analyze, and conceptualize mental health nursing practices, monitor their epistemological coherence, share and disseminate them.

In the area of policy, legislation, and health programs management

- Stimulate the participation of nurses in the development, promotion, and implementation of mental health legislation and policy.
- Work with Ministers of Health and mental health authorities in the development of community mental health services networks.
- Advise and support health services authorities and personnel to develop renovation strategies towards integrating the community mental health network.
- Help to promote mental health concepts, values and singularity of mental life, social integration of people suffering from mental health problems, and information about mental health services.

Conclusion

As seen in this country profile, nurses are engaged in a variety of actions and contribute to the development of community mental health in Argentina. They provide direct care for consumers, families and communities, assist in formulating and implementing policies, generate mental health promotion and prevention programs, help to create service networks that replace custodial hospitals, manage projects, strengthen and educate health personnel, and produce new information and basic research to support mental health (Malvárez, 2011).

The authors recognize and express their profound gratitude to the nurses and other professionals that contributed with their experiences: Sandra Cerino, Emilce Olivares, Eugenia Mazzoni, Stella Felizzia, and Jorge Possi from mental health services and the National University of Córdoba; Analía Mesquida, Lía Zottola, Malvina Lobos, and Josefa Delgado from mental health services and the National University of Santiago del Estero. María Elena Pérez, Cristina Olivera, Griselda Pabón, Stella Maris Drueto, María Lorena Soria, Cecilia Hoet, and Norma Salvi from mental health services of the province and the National University of Entre Ríos; Luciano Grasso, Constanza Funes, Valeria Giatti, and Walter Ríos from mental health services of Buenos Aires; Agustín Sordo, Fernando Cortés, Claudia Cirera, and María Stella Billazuzu from mental health services of the province of Río Negro.

We wish to thank Dr. Arayna Yearwood, an independent scholar and multilingual editor for her assistance with this chapter.

References

Banco Mundial. (2014). Indicadores económicos de desarrollo. Consultado el 3 de septiembre de 2014 en: http://datos.bancomundial.org/catalogo-de-datos.

Legislatura de la Nación Argentina. (2010). Ley Nacional de Salud Mental No. 26.657. Buenos Aires 2010. Consultado el 3 de septiembre de 2014 en:www.msal.gov.ar/saludmental/index.php/informacion-para-la-comunidad/ley-nacional-de-salud-mental-no-26657.

Legislatura de la Provincia de Río Negro. (1991). Ley Provincial No. 2440, de promoción sanitaria y social de las personas que padecen sufrimiento mental. Río Negro. Argentina. Consultado el 10 de agosto de 2014 en: www.fundacionrecuperar.org/alippi/docsalud/7.pdf.

Levav, I. (1992). *Reestructuración de la atención psiquiátrica en América Latina.* Washington, DC: OPS/OMS.

Malvárez, S. (1999). Construyendo un nuevo paradigma en salud mental. La experiencia Argentina. En: *Enfermería en las Américas.* Publicación Científica 571. Washington, DC: OPS/OMS.

Malvárez, S. (2000). Notas para una concepción crítica de la enfermería en salud mental. En: *Enfermería en salud mental.* Serie Desarrollo de Sistemas y Servicios de Salud No. 19. Washginton, DC: OPS/OMS.

Malvárez, S. (2007). Análisis de la enseñanza de la enfermería en salud mental en las escuelas de enfermería de América Latina. Biblioteca. Facultad de Ciencias Médicas. Universidad Nacional de Córdoba.

Malvárez, S. (2011.) Salud mental comunitaria: trayectoria y contribuciones de enfermería. *Revista Ibero-americana de Enfermería Comunitaria*. Vol. 4, no. 2, octubre 2011. Consultado el 31 de augusto de 2014 en: http://ascane.org/grupo_trabajo_enfermeria/RIdEC.v4n2.22.Especialidades-2_mod.pdf.

Ministerio de Salud de la Nacion Argentina. (2013). Plan nacional de salud mental. Buenos Aires. Consultado el 1 de septiembre de 2014 en: www.msal.gov.ar/saludmental/index.php?option=com_content&view=article&id=2 28:plan-nacional-de-salud-mental&catid=4:destacados-slide228.

Organización Mundial de la Salud (OMS). (2001). *Informe sobre la salud en el mundo 2001. Salud mental: nuevos conocimientos, nuevas esperanzas*. Ginebra. OMS.

Organización Mundial de la Salud (OMS). (2009). *Instrumento de evaluación de sistemas de salud mental: Argentina*. Ginebra: IEMS-OMS.

Organización Panamericana de la Salud (OPS). (2013). *Indicadores Básicos de Salud*. Washington DC: OPS.

Peplau, H. (1992). *Relaciones interpersonales en enfermería*. México: Mason.

Peres, Shimón. (1997). Conferencia dictada en el Salón de Actos de la Universidad Nacional de Córdoba el 8 de abril de 1997. Córdoba, Argentina.

Rodríguez, J., Malvárez, S., González, & R., Levav, I. (2009a) *Salud mental en la comunidad*. Washington, DC: OPS/OMS.

Rodríguez, J. Kohn, R.Y., & Aguilar-Gaxiola, S. (2009b) *Epidemiología de los trastornos mentales en América Latina y el Caribe*. Washington, DC: OPS/OMS.

World Health Organization. (2013). *Mental health action plan 2013–2020*. Geneva: WHO.

28

JAPAN

Disaster mental health care

Pamela A. Minarik and Yoko Nakayama

Because of the volcanic nature of the Japanese archipelago, the Japanese people have experienced many and frequent natural disasters, such as typhoons, volcanoes, earthquakes, and tsunamis. The Japanese have handled disasters in a unique way based on their culture. In this chapter, the case of the Great East Japan Earthquake and tsunami of 2011 will be discussed, focusing on disaster preparedness, disaster response and disaster mental health in Japan in the context of the Japanese culture. Recommendations that are applicable for the future will be addressed.

Introduction: cultural context

Japan is an island country consisting of five major islands and thousands of smaller islands (www.japan-guide.com/list/e1000.html). Based on 2012 data, the area of the country is comparable to California (www.japan-guide.com/list/e1000.html). As of August 1, 2013, the total population of the country was 127,336,000 (Statistics Bureau of Japan www.stat.go.jp/english/data/jinsui/tsuki/index.htm). Figure 28.1 shows the regions and prefectures of Japan's major islands.

Japan is home to a population that is the tenth largest in world. Over 50 percent of Japan is mountainous and forested; most of the land cannot be cultivated because of the presence of mountains. Most of the people of Japan reside in the areas near the coast, which puts them at risk in typhoons, floods and tsunami. It is the thirtieth most densely populated country in the world (www.mapsofworld.com/japan/geography-japan.html). Average life expectancy for Japanese women is 86 years, the highest life expectancy in the world. For Japanese men, the average life expectancy is 79 years. The proportion of older people in the population is the highest in the world.

In 1995, the Great Hanshin-Awaji Earthquake hit the city of Kobe and its surroundings; 6,308 people were killed and 415,000 people were injured. More than 200,000 buildings were destroyed or damaged (www.usgs.gov/newsroom/article.asp?ID=744#.U2VGG4FdVyw; www.japan-guide.com/e/e2116.html). The Great Hanshin-Awaji Earthquake prompted the launch of the Disaster Nursing Society, which promotes disaster nursing scholarship, practice and education (Yamamoto, 2013). Dr. Hiroko Minami, a psychiatric nurse, led the creation of the Disaster Nursing Society. She was concerned about support systems for nurses providing disaster-related care.

Regions and Prefectures of Japan

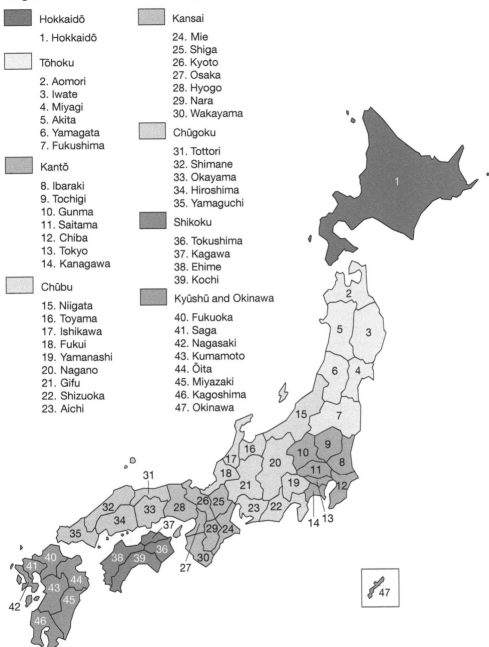

Hokkaidō

1. Hokkaidō

Tōhoku

2. Aomori
3. Iwate
4. Miyagi
5. Akita
6. Yamagata
7. Fukushima

Kantō

8. Ibaraki
9. Tochigi
10. Gunma
11. Saitama
12. Chiba
13. Tokyo
14. Kanagawa

Chūbu

15. Niigata
16. Toyama
17. Ishikawa
18. Fukui
19. Yamanashi
20. Nagano
21. Gifu
22. Shizuoka
23. Aichi

Kansai

24. Mie
25. Shiga
26. Kyoto
27. Osaka
28. Hyogo
29. Nara
30. Wakayama

Chūgoku

31. Tottori
32. Shimane
33. Okayama
34. Hiroshima
35. Yamaguchi

Shikoku

36. Tokushima
37. Kagawa
38. Ehime
39. Kochi

Kyūshū and Okinawa

40. Fukuoka
41. Saga
42. Nagasaki
43. Kumamoto
44. Ōita
45. Miyazaki
46. Kagoshima
47. Okinawa

Figure 28.1 Regions and prefectures of Japan
Source: Image by Yukio Hayakawa.

At the time of the Great Hanshin-Awaji Earthquake, Dr. Patricia Underwood, a psychiatric nursing professor formerly of the University of California, San Francisco School of Nursing, and then at the College of Nursing Art and Science, University of Hyogo near Kobe, Japan, with Dr. Minami, raised her concern about nurses' mental health and the lack of recognition of their needs. She went to hospitals and spoke with nurses, allowing them to talk about their own feelings of guilt (survivor), helplessness and powerlessness. She attended to their acute stress reactions and taught about post-traumatic stress disorder. She received an award from the Japanese government for her mental health work after the earthquake and she was instrumental in the development of psychiatric mental health nursing as part of the twenty-first Century Center of Excellence (COE) disaster nursing program at the University of Hyogo, Graduate School of Nursing (Yamamoto, 2008; 2013). Dr. Minami now leads the recently developed distance learning program of a multidisciplinary consortium of five universities, called Disaster Nursing Global Leader (DNGL) Degree Program, headquartered at University of Kochi (www.dngl.jp/).

Japanese values and beliefs (Dolan & Worden, 1994) contribute to Japanese problem-solving and the management of disasters. In contrast to Western countries that value autonomy, Japanese people value harmony with nature and among people. But a value of harmony does not guarantee harmony and there is tension and competition that must be suppressed. The rights of the individual are secondary, or overridden, to keep society harmonious. Most Japanese people are Shinto or Buddhist religion, which is consistent with the value of harmony. Stigmatizing attitudes toward mental disorders are common in Japan, resulting in greater social distance from people with mental illness and schizophrenia stigmatized more than depression (Ando, Yamaguchi, Aoki, & Thornicroft, 2013; Griffiths, *et al.*, 2006). Recently, the length of stay in psychiatric hospitals has shortened and mental health care systems could change from hospital care to community care, which might have an impact on stigma and social distance. Japanese society is eclectic with a pragmatic and utilitarian approach to problem-solving. The government of Japan is a pluralist democracy with a Parliament (National Diet) and a constitutional monarchy with a hereditary emperor as a symbol of the unity of the people. Policy making is highly centralized. Society emphasizes social interdependence and collective responsibility. These values inform the Japanese approach to disaster management.

In Japanese culture, relationships are governed by amae, a Japanese concept that is not translatable into English (Doi, 1981). Amae conveys an indulgent relationship, a form of love that is telepathic, pre-linguistic and communicated directly from the heart; it is most easily seen in parent–child relationships. Amae does not require talking but results in understanding without talk. Amae also describes how an individual expresses his or her desire (conscious or not) to depend on the goodwill of others. Japanese people intuitively understand how to behave with others in a form of body language. Japanese value silence over talking, and restraint in relationships that are not intimate.

A related concept in Japanese culture is the idea of inner and outer in individual relationships. Inner refers to the group (e.g., family, friends, and colleagues) to which a person belongs. Outer refers to others with whom there are social obligations and complete strangers with whom there are no obligations. The importance of this concept is demonstrated in the Japanese behavior of sharing business cards at the beginning of relationships. Japanese vary their attitude, speech, and behavior depending on whether they are interacting with the inner circle or outer circle, or strangers and the social rank of the people involved. The role of the people (as individuals and group members) and the role of the government are both integral to national disaster planning (personal communication, Mr. Kakuta, former Red Cross administrator, 2011). Plans rely on the power of volunteers and recognition of key Japanese values: jijyo (self-help), kyojyo (help each other), kojyo (help from the government). The three concepts of jijyo, kyojyo, kojyo have been used since Edo-era Japan (1603–1867); these concepts explain the relationship among family (individual), community (place of living), and government (administration). Jijyo is the private level, kyojyo is half private/half public level, kojyo is public level. Developing strategies to actualize jijyo and kyojyo are current foci of nursing research. As a result of these concepts, people have a basic knowledge of disaster planning with a focus on securing one's own safety and helping one's own neighbors. Future planning for disasters will address how to prepare for disaster in large cities such as Tokyo that lack a strong community structure similar to that found in smaller communities where people know each other (personal communication, Mr. Kakuta, former Red Cross administrator, 2011).

Values and beliefs based on the teachings of Confucius include the basic principles in human interaction of obeisance to the superior and benevolence to the inferior creating an obligated trust relationship. Within Japanese society, vertical ranking, based on age and gender, dominates relationships and supports proper social behavior (Nakane, 1970). Older, and usually more experienced, people are at the top of the ranking; men are ranked above women in most situations. People learn from early childhood how to behave based on observation and experiences so that the behavior becomes intuitive. After the Great East Japan Earthquake and tsunami, the hierarchical social relationships were evident in the ways local community leaders (almost always men who were already involved in community leadership roles) took charge and directed activities (Women's Network for East Japan Disaster, Rise Together, 2013). The men had little understanding of the needs, e.g., hygiene, of women, and were not providing for needed supplies or privacy. In some situations, women did make effective leadership efforts to influence women's (and other vulnerable people's) experiences in the disaster aftermath. In such disaster situations, leadership behavior by women was unusual and unexpected. These effective strategies by women can be found on the website of RiseTogether (http://risetogetherjp.org) and are included in Table 28.1 in the sections on the restoration/recovery phase and preparedness.

All of these cultural factors influence how Japanese people have dealt with disasters. In this chapter, the Great East Japan Earthquake and its aftermath illustrate the Japanese approach to disaster management and disaster mental health.

Description of issue: The Great East Japan Earthquake, tsunami, nuclear plant accidents and aftermath

The Great East Japan Earthquake, which occurred on March 11, 2011, at 9.0 magnitude in the Pacific Ocean near Northeastern Japan, was the strongest ever recorded in Japan since the development of modern instruments 130 years ago (www.usgs.gov/newsroom/article.asp?ID=2727&from=rss_home#.U2VCFIFdVyw). It triggered an enormous and devastating tsunami along the Pacific coast of northeast Japan (the Tohoku region and the coasts of Iwate, Miyagi, and Fukushima prefectures). The power of the natural disaster was beyond people's imagination. The massive tides, as high as 7–15 meters, wiped out houses, bridges, buildings, and everything else (Takeda, 2011). As a result, the earthquake and tsunami killed nearly 20,000 people. Of the people who died, 92.5 percent died from drowning and of the 11,108 bodies found, over 65 percent were aged 60 or older (Yamamoto, 2011). Within five hours, 19 medical teams had been dispatched by the Japanese Red Cross, operations centers were set up, and trained staff provided psychosocial support within evacuation centers (Japanese Red Cross Society, 2011).

Before the Great East Japan Earthquake, relief activities for earthquakes initially focused on external injuries, and gradually dealt with chronic conditions and mental care. These activities had been effective in past earthquakes and were assumed to be appropriate responses, but the situation after the tsunami disaster was different. Many of those with external injuries were swept up by the tsunami and passed away, and the people who were actually rescued from the stream of mud were people in a severe condition due to hypothermia, pneumonia, and aggravation of chronic illness (Watanabe, 2012).

Psychiatric mental health services and psychiatric hospitals were challenged by the disaster situation. Some psychiatric hospitals were seriously damaged by the earthquake and tsunami and as a result, some inpatients died. The surviving inpatients were transported to non-damaged psychiatric hospitals within the prefecture or another prefecture. Particularly, the patients hospitalized in psychiatric hospitals within 20 km of the nuclear power plant in Fukushima were transported long distances by bus. Kako, Ranse, Yamamoto, and Arbon (2014) conducted an integrative review of the Japanese literature about the role of nurses in the 2011 Great East Japan Earthquake. Their review included information about psychiatric mental health nursing. Due to the numbers of people who presented for mental health services, local mental health triage services were overwhelmed and continuity of care was difficult due to scarce resources (Kako *et al.*, 2014). Psychosocial support was recognized as an essential aspect of nursing care and psychosocial needs assessed as arguably more important than physical needs, especially after acute issues were managed. The review noted that a nursing role for psychosocial support of all health workers, who may have lost family members, should be considered.

Relief workers worked with ongoing pressure and the stress of relief work. They faced limitations in performing tasks. A psychological conflict between the sense of mission and the limitations of reality caused feelings of guilt or powerlessness (Ishida & Kim, 2011). Some relief workers, firefighters, and local government employees were also disaster victims of the earthquake and tsunami.

Because of the disaster, people of the Tohoku region, where the main industry is fishery and agriculture, lost their vocations and had to change their lifestyle characteristically based on strong family relationships that were weakened by the disaster. The disaster affected all aspects of daily life and brought the residents psychological distress, including anxiety and disturbed sleep, caused by fearful experiences, deaths of family members, evacuation and loss of property, vocations, and relationships. Some of them showed temporary stress responses, and some of them developed sleep disorder, depression, or post-traumatic stress disorder and alcohol dependence (Yabe *et al.*, 2011).

Conflict and distress continues to be experienced by nurses who worked at hospitals, community health and welfare centers, and nursing homes during the disaster. Nurses, who were working when the earthquake occurred, evacuated with and took care of their patients but they felt guilty for not being with their families who were disaster survivors with damaged houses and evacuated to shelters in the community. Other nurses experienced the earthquake at home, evacuated with their families and took care of family, relatives, and neighbors. They knew that the hospital was damaged by the earthquake and tsunami; they felt guilty about not being with their colleagues and patients at the workplace. When nurses experienced the earthquake, they had to make decisions about what to do and experienced a dilemma.

Nuclear power plant accident in Fukushima and resulting stigma

In Fukushima prefecture, the earthquake and the following tsunami hit the Fukushima nuclear power plant and caused nuclear accidents (www.japan-guide.com/e/e2116.html; Yasumara *et al.*, 2012) and radiation hazards, which produced many tragedies and resulted in fear and uncertainty across the country. People living in a 20–30 km radius of the nuclear power plant responded to a government order to move away in order to avoid exposure to radioactive material. More than 210,000 people were evacuated. Triple disasters caused by the earthquake, the following tsunami and nuclear power plant accidents engulfed a broad area, uprooted people and changed victims' lives directly and indirectly. First, the residents in Fukushima Prefecture, including both those who lost their homes and families and those whose homes were barely damaged, had to evacuate due to the dangerous radiation contamination. Public facilities, such as schools, gymnasiums, community centers, or civic halls, were established as evacuation areas but the numbers were insufficient. Due to the government's imprecise public reports of radiation damage, evacuation shelters were established in high-radiation areas. The public did not get enough accurate data in the immediate period and everyone was confused. People thought that if they moved to an area 20–30 km from the electrical plant, they would be safe. Later, it became known that the radiation danger area was not in concentric circles of distance but shaped by wind into a northwest flow that exceed 30 km in specific areas (Hayakawa, 2013) (see Figure 28.2). Many towns near the nuclear power plant, including their administrative functions, were forced to relocate (Niwa, 2012).

Second, according to the report of the Citizens' Commission on Nuclear Energy (2014), social conflicts and divisions occurred as a result of the radioactive contamination. For example, in families and communities, serious internal conflicts arose regarding whether or not to evacuate, or how to prioritize family life and work. Among families and neighborhoods and between generations, opinions diverged regarding how to understand the effects of radiation and how to respond to them, causing interpersonal relationships to worsen. People were divided and isolated by these differences leading to stress due to separation, and decline in physical strength due to being unable to play outside or exercise. The shock of losing their vocations and homes and being unable to envision their future life was particularly great.

Third, the homeland where the family tomb is located is very important for residents. In Japan, belonging to a family, community and/or group is essential to social life. In rural communities, there is a temple and cemetery as well as homes. The tombs represent continuity with ancestors and the future generations, and are key to the identity of the people. Even though their homeland was damaged by disaster, they would never abandon the land that they inherited from their ancestors. However, since their residence of many years had been contaminated by radiation, people lost irreplaceable supports for their lives. They lost their homeland vocations such as agriculture and fishing, and they could not sell agricultural or marine products in Fukushima prefecture due to harmful rumors, causing the economy to decline. People lost meaning in their lives, and they were robbed of the source of their strength (Citizens' Commission on Nuclear Energy, 2014).

Fourth, in addition to the internal and interpersonal conflicts, the nuclear power plant accidents and radioactive contamination caused prejudice and damage by harmful rumors that affected evacuation of people from contaminated areas close to the nuclear power plant. Most people wanted to return to their homeland where they had cultural customs and events, such as traditional festivals, rituals and ceremonies, which were central to their social lives. According to an evacuee opinion survey by the Fukushima Prefecture Evacuee Support Division (administered from January 22 to February 6, 2014; survey subjects included 58,627 households, of which 20,680 households responded, response rate of 35.3 percent), regarding the dispersion of families, 44.7 percent of households all live in the same place together (including people living alone), and 48.9 percent of households that cohabited at the time of the earthquake are living in multiple locations. Because of the damage by harmful rumors, crops that were produced in Fukushima were unsellable and the income was not enough for living. Furthermore, some evacuees from Fukushima Prefecture to other prefectures were warmly welcomed in their destination, but

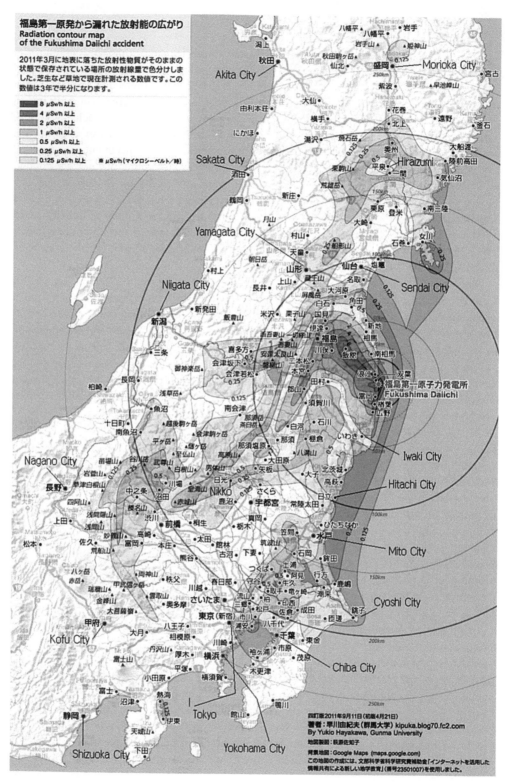

Figure 28.2 Map showing spread of radioactivity from Fukishima Daiichi nuclear power plant
Source: http://kipuka.blog70.fc2.com/blog-entry-613.html. Reprinted with permission from Yukio Hayakawa.

others were treated inhospitably and discriminated against in their destination, causing new anxiety and distress. Particularly, younger people of childbearing age encountered prejudice due to the effects of radiation on the human body, and there were cases where they had to hide the fact that they were from Fukushima Prefecture.

In addition to prejudice, other issues arose. In some cases of victimized families in the childrearing generation, mothers decided to relocate to low-radiation regions within Fukushima Prefecture or outside the prefecture due to anxiety regarding their children's educational environments restricting outside play because of radiation following the nuclear power plant accident. They were uncomfortable in new communities because they did not belong in that group. Other children harassed children from Fukushima; the problem has now diminished. Among the residents whose jobs were lost due to the nuclear power plant accident, and who were paid compensation as a temporary measure, many turned to gambling and drinking to diffuse their stress, anger, and feeling of being overwhelmed, which brought criticism from the residents of their destination.

Fifth, the number of disaster-related deaths is remarkably high in Fukushima Prefecture. The majority are deaths related to the nuclear power plant accident. The fact that the number of disaster-related suicides is increasing annually in Fukushima Prefecture, while they are decreasing in nearby affected coastal prefectures, demonstrates the ongoing impact of the nuclear power plant accident.

Brief analysis/aftermath and update

The 2011 Great East Japan Earthquake and tsunami was an unprecedented compound disaster of the 9.0 magnitude earthquake, resulting tsunami, and consequent nuclear crisis with release of radioactive material into the environment, followed by a strong 7.4 magnitude aftershock less than one month later (Yamamoto, 2011). Assumptions about effective disaster responses developed by nurses (www.coe-cnas.jp/english/index.html) and others since the Great Hanshin-Awaji Earthquake in 1995 were no longer valid and many of the activities were not possible. Because of the simultaneous disasters, wide area and extensive damage, including human casualties, it was difficult to get help from outside with the resultant shortage of food, drink, daily necessities, and medical services. The devastating compound disaster created a health crisis and destroyed a substantial part of the health care infrastructure, especially in the Tohoku area (see Figure 28.1).

"Restoring necessary health services to the affected area has been a national priority and rebuilding is a primary focus of the current government" (The Commonwealth Fund, 2012, p. 71). Yamamoto (2011) identified key issues regarding health care services, which included "what kind of health care services should be provided in evacuation centers or homes, and in what way?" (p. 333). She pointed out that maintaining and improving health required increased discretion (meaning autonomous decision-making) by nurses and systematic dispatch of health professionals to affected areas. This was a bold statement because autonomous decision-making by nurses was not an expected part of nursing practice, working as part of a team was a more normal way of practice.

After the emergency phase, the media were less interested and news reports diminished although many long-term recovery problems remained. Volunteers, such as faculty and students of nursing and health professional schools, from outside the immediate disaster area, have continued to participate in activities, such as teaching English and occupational skills, related to the recovery/restoration phase. This continued activity to aid long-term recovery is an example of kyojyo.

Niwa (2012) suggested the following tasks of mental care in Fukushima prefecture and most of these would be appropriate in other disaster areas: 1) continuation of therapy for mental health patients; 2) early-stage intervention for depression, PTSD, and alcohol dependence that occurred due to the earthquake and nuclear power plant accident; 3) coping with mental problems occurring from the anxiety of radiological contamination; 4) preventing the decline of cognitive and physical functions due to refugee life among the elderly; and 5) suicide prevention. After disasters in Japan, mental health centers are created with local government funding in communities to provide counseling, consultation, home visiting, children's day care, and support groups. The centers are staffed by mental health professionals (nurses, psychologists, social workers, and psychiatrists). These mental health centers are an example of kojyo because they are supported by the Ministry of Health, Labor, and Welfare funding to local governments. Mental health centers created after the Great Hanshin-Awaji Earthquake (1995) continue to operate. It is likely that mental health centers created after the Great East Japan Earthquake will continue for at least 5 years, as long as needed.

Awareness of the importance of post-disaster mental health support and treatment has increased in the past two decades, since the 1995 Great Hanshin-Awaji Earthquake and especially after the 2001 Great East Japan Earthquake and tsunami. Nurses have developed disaster nursing knowledge on the COE website (www.coe-cnas.jp/english/index.html). To promote and organize effective mental health support, The National Information Center for Disaster Mental Health was created in 2011 by the National Center for Psychiatry and Neurology, to benefit the activity of mental health care centers established in the affected prefectures,

Addressing the Great East Japan Earthquake and tsunami as a whole, the Women's Network for East Japan Disaster (Rise Together, 2013) published a booklet about effective and recommended practices to increase the understanding of gender and diversity issues in disaster response. The introduction begins by asserting that people affected by a disaster have different needs and the assistance needed for each person differs "depending on gender, sexual identity, age, disability, nationality, mother tongue, family structure and employment status, and so on. Yet, considering gender and diversity issues have been long been overlooked in disaster response in Japan" (2013, p. 1). The aim of the publication was to "trigger more action towards inclusive disaster response and recovery" (2013, p. 1). The booklet identified the importance of involving women and members of other vulnerable or at-risk groups in decision-making concerning what is needed in the disaster response and recovery process. Although the suggestions related to involvement of vulnerable groups, such as those with mental disabilities, in decision-making are not specifically about psychiatric care, the implementation of the suggestions would enhance the self-efficacy, sense of personal worth and mental health of survivors (see Table 28.1 sections on restoration/recovery phase and preparedness). Much more detail can be found at the website (http://risetogetherjp.org).

Implications for mental health nursing practice and mental health promotion within global communities

Since the Great Hanshin-Awaji Earthquake in 1995, Japanese nurses have studied disaster nursing interventions and developed recommendations for pre-disaster preparedness, emergency phase and recovery/restoration phase. At the University of Hyogo, Graduate School of Nursing, twenty-first century Center of Excellence (COE) program, the education, practice and research focus is disaster nursing and the expansion of the disaster nursing discipline (Yamamoto, 2008, 2013). The COE has systematically integrated disaster nursing knowledge and developed a coherent picture of disaster nursing. The objectives of the COE are to develop mid- to long-term nursing care strategies to develop resilience and regenerate people's health and lives following

Table 28.1 Mental health nursing interventions appropriate to each disaster phase

Disaster phase	Nursing interventions
Emergency phase	• Go to the site as soon as possible because people are more open to help in acute phase • Establish self as member of community by activities such as cleaning and supplying water to establish trust • Respect cherished customs and local lifestyle

In shelters, acute phase	• Provide daily life support and physical care. If physical safety cannot be guaranteed, people cannot feel safe and secure
	• Create a safe and secure environment for disaster response volunteers and staff, with consideration of individual thoughts and feelings
	• Ensure an environment where people can feel safe and secure
	  – Check for lighting, sound-shield, temperature, ventilation
	  – Check for sufficient food, blankets, and clothing
	  – Sufficient space for privacy and for families to stay together
	  – Provide for those with chronic disorders, disabilities, or poor condition
	  – Appropriate medical care without interruption for those with continuing treatment needs—make necessary arrangements
	  – Establish system of response for sleep disturbance
	  – Sufficient number of toilets and cleanliness
	  – Protect from intrusive media
	  – Ensure that women are available in women only meetings to listen to women's concerns and needs such as undergarments and sanitary supplies
	  – Women leaders (usually men are the leaders) may enable children and the elderly to speak about their concerns and needs more easily
	  – Women may need a private women-only place to feel safe
	• Provide opportunities to talk about trauma experience and feelings in a comfortable environment
	  – Use active listening and do not push people who do not want to talk
	  – Respect each person's pace
	  – Communicate while providing physical care, such as taking blood pressure
	  – Develop a relationship through repeated contacts
	  – Listening to disaster victims requires energy, take care of your own mental health
	  – Screen survivors for PTSD
	• Care for the bereaved
	  – Be there and listen attentively if the grieving person wants to talk
	  – If possible, create a quiet setting
	  – Each person needs to grieve in their own way and own time
	  – Attending to a grieving person requires energy, take care of your own mental health
	  – When people reject or avoid support, try to develop a relationship through frequent brief contacts
	  – People are less uncomfortable when asked about physical condition
	• Provide mental health care to elderly, who might feel that they have lost their daily lives in a shelter
	  – Provide attentive support that meets individual needs, based on a full understanding of each person's mental/physical conditions as well as life patterns and values maintained over the years
	  – Encourage them to keep regular hours
	  – Provide support for their family and care-takers

Table 28.1 continued

Disaster phase	Nursing interventions

	• Mental health care for children
	  – Listen attentively to children without denying their feelings and answer their questions in an easy-to-understand manner
	  – Cooperate with adults caring for children to create play space and school activities
	• Mental health care for those with mental disorders
	  – Disaster causing situations are stressful and may exacerbate symptoms
	  – Lack of usual medications may exacerbate symptoms or difficulty with communal living
	  – Talk individually with the person with mental disorder and their family about needs and self-care conditions with a focus on preventing isolation
	  – Talk with community leaders, if necessary, and make arrangements for the person's needs to enable living in a group
	  – Communication should be private with extreme care to not disclose to others the person's mental disorder and cause more isolation
	  – If possible, ensure prescribed medication without interruption
	  – If symptoms exacerbate, refer to a mental health provider as soon as possible

Nurses' mental health care	• Nurses' stress in disasters
	  – Disasters happen unexpectedly. Nurses are no exception.
	  – Nurses may suffer dual traumas of the direct disaster experience and victim support activities
	  – Even if nurses are not primary victims of the disaster, they suffer from the disaster secondarily, by sharing victims' experiences under abnormal conditions and their anguish
	  – In disasters, blocked transportation systems and shortages of resources may occur, possibly leading to frustration, feelings of powerlessness and conflicts with others
	  – Nurses have a strong sense of responsibility and may try to handle everything without asking for help. At shelters, nurses may fail to notice their own physical and mental fatigue. They may be not be able to take a break, or feel guilty for taking time off or being helped by others
	  – Nurses will benefit from checking their own stress reactions
	  – Stress reactions vary among individuals and in different situations. It is important to know one's own stress condition and bodily reactions but it may be difficult to assess oneself. Using a stress measure may help. But if stress goes unrecognized and unexpressed to others, the nurse is at risk of physical and psychological stress reactions, such as listlessness, helplessness, anxiety and sadness. If these stress reactions are intense or continue, PTSD could develop
	• To lessen nurses' stress (to enable supporting others without sacrificing your health)
	  – Ask yourself if you are doing too much and trying to handle everything yourself then recognize your limitations and that stress is natural in a disaster situation
	  – Consider working in pairs or asking others for help
	  – Talk about your thoughts and feelings with your peers or someone close
	  – Begin with what you are comfortable talking about.
	  – Recognize and appreciate your efforts to counter the powerlessness you may feel
	  – Take breaks and relax in favorite ways. Sometimes nurses feel guilty about taking any rest
	  – Attend to own sleeping, eating and families. Talk with family members

	– Receive mental health care as anyone exposed to a disaster might benefit from, especially if suffering from insomnia, anxiety, or recurrent recollection of traumatic experiences
	– Take time to share stories with fellow workers to clarify feelings, thoughts, and problems experienced during the day. Consider inviting a mental health nurse to participate
Restoration/ recovery phase	• Ensure that elderly are not isolated from information and procedures about restoration
	• Deliver women-focused support in the long-term reconstruction process and consider developing "a women's support center"
	• When distributing relief supplies, increase choices to restore dignity for both children and adults
	• At the end of the emergency phase, vulnerable people such as the elderly, single people, disabled people, may need continued assistance into the reconstruction period and afterward. Plan a system that will encourage continued relationships with disaster relief workers and volunteers
	• High-risk areas are often damaged in disaster with many minority people affected. Ensure that minorities are included in development of plans for land use and the complex process of reconstruction
	• In addition to formal meetings to identify needs in the reconstruction phase, hold informal meetings to gain the perspective of people (women, elderly, people with disabilities, and children) who may not be comfortable speaking up in a formal meeting
	• Outside volunteers must understand the local context and develop relationships because mutual trust will allow for effective planning together
	• For safety, arrange two-person teams of man and woman, to go together to homes to check on conditions of those in homes
Preparedness	• Make plans for how to incorporate volunteers from other locales in country and from other countries
	• Develop strategies for supporting vulnerable people such as the elderly, children, pregnant women and child-rearing families, cancer patients, people with chronic diseases, including mental disorders
	• Attend to the safety of volunteers, such as providing changing rooms and separate toilets for men and women
	• Be aware of possible problematic behavior between volunteers, such as sharing personal information or photos
	• Provide workers with training about sexual harassment. Prepare a consulting system for responding to harassment or stalking behavior
	• Establish a conduct code and standards for understanding for both staff and volunteers, especially in mixed-gender situations
	• Provide care for volunteers following tough or shocking experiences
	• Make efficient use of outside volunteers by dispatching people for longer periods in one place; shorter times can lead to inadequate takeover of responsibilities
	• Create a system to match various needs, disclosed by local governments, with available assistance from multiple sources
	• Create a system for information sharing and coordination of various volunteer and local organizations. In disaster preparedness plans, develop a way of providing necessary supplies, such as water, food, diapers, etc. to people who require assistance but may end up at home rather than shelters or temporary housing
	• Hold community disaster drills
	• Encourage foreign residents to participate in community disaster drills and to register with the local government, not only on a foreign resident list

Source: College of Nursing Art and Science (CNAS), University of Hyogo (2006); Women's Network for East Japan Disaster (Rise Together, April 2013).

disasters and to establish information and communication networks. The Center provides an online information base for disaster nursing knowledge and skills to protect lives (www.coe-cnas.jp/english/index.html). After the 1995 earthquake, for the first time, it was recognized that many nurses were working beyond their limits and neglecting their own mental health. On the website can be found mental health care manuals (www.coe-cnas.jp/english/group_psyc/index.html) detailing what can be done at shelters, what to do when you face difficulties at shelters and maintaining nurses' mental health (www.coe-cnas.jp/english/group_psyc/manual/manual01/index.html). Table 28.1 includes many of these recommendations and more details are available on the website. In other global communities, these manuals may be adapted to the local situation.

After a disaster, the most important immediate mental health response is to meet with survivors as soon as possible after the event by visiting them at the disaster scene and evacuation centers. If contact is delayed, people will be left in anxiety, despair, and confusion (Ishida & Kim, 2011). In 2011, many mental health nurses volunteered for this work through the nursing associations. The Japanese Psychiatric Nurses Association sent volunteers of psychiatric nurses to the disaster areas in the Great East Japan earthquake and took care of persons with mental disorders in a 24-hour system in shelters. In some cases, the volunteer nurses found that directly supporting evacuees was difficult because they, the volunteers, were seen as strangers (from outside Tohoku); as a result, the nurse volunteers adapted and provided support to local nurses who were caring for evacuees (personal communication, Dr. M. Tanaka, 2011). In other cultures without such strong insider–outsider relationships, nurse volunteers may not experience this problem. In countries with stigmatized attitudes about mental illness, it may be necessary to approach survivors first in terms of safety and security needs, then physical needs, before addressing psychosocial or mental coping issues.

The National Center for Neurology and Psychiatry (NCNP) provided information about the mental health care response to the 2011 Great East Japan earthquake, tsunami and nuclear disaster (Kim, n.d.). On the third day after the earthquake, NCNP launched a website to provide information. In the guidelines for community mental health, they list cooperating organizations; all hospital and physician organizations. For continued psychiatric care, the NCNP listed these issues: 1) transportation of psychiatric inpatients; 2) provision of medication to psychiatric patients; and 3) onsite treatment by mental health care teams of people with pre-existing mental disorders. Over 1,000 inpatient hospital beds were lost through damage or risk of radio-activity. Through collaborative work of mental health providers with local governments, patients were transported to other areas within 10 days. The supply of psychiatric drugs was affected by the extensive damage to public transportation systems. In addition to providing care in hospitals, nurses were active participants in the mental health teams, which provided care to both people with pre-existing mental disorders and through secondary prevention of mental disorders. The NCNP (Kim, n.d.) described necessary multidimensional care including (in order of lower to higher specialization): 1) rescue and safety; 2) evacuation from catastrophe; 3) societal support; 4) reconstructing living arrangement; 5) medication, as necessary; 6) psychoeducation, counseling; and 7) specialized treatment. After rescue and safety, all must occur in a context of safety, security and sleep (Kim, n.d., p. 19). The suggestions of the NCNP and the University of Hyogo COE may provide guidance for the global community.

Summary/conclusion

In summary, the 2011 Great East Japan Earthquake was a massive and devastating compound disaster in a country frequented by natural disasters. Based on the centuries-old culture of hierarchical social relationships, values of harmony and group belonging, and centralized policy-making, Japan already had a disaster response plan that included roles for local people, volunteers, national and local government, such as development of mental health centers in communities affected by disasters. Because the 2011 disasters were simultaneous and widespread, prior appropriate disaster-related strategies, from the work of the COE and other groups, were either not possible, less effective, or needed further development for the situation.

Nurses were able to use disaster nursing knowledge, including mental health strategies developed since the 1995 Great Hanshin Earthquake, as well as study disaster responses from this compound disaster, such as the multidisciplinary research on the effects of coping with the radiation contamination and evacuation in Fukushima in which the second author of this chapter (Yoko Nakayama) is participating.

Recommendations to promote well-being and recovery

Recommendations to promote well-being and recovery are gathered from published and unpublished literature (Davis, 2014; Yamamoto, 2013; Yamamoto & Watanabe, unpublished), websites, personal communications about experiences of the Great East Japan Earthquake, and from the experience of the second author. Japanese nurses specializing in disaster nursing are sharing their knowledge with the global community at international conferences (personal communication, Dr. Aiko Yamamoto, 2014), on the website from the University of Hyogo, Graduate School of Nursing, twenty-first Century Center of Excellence (www.coe-cnas.jp/english/index.html) and through the work of the Disaster Nursing Global Leader (DNGL) Program (www.dngl.jp/). Doctoral students of the DNGL program are developing mental health-related research protocols such as a qualitative study of needs of Fukushima residents; defining the role of a disaster nursing global leader in and planning holistic end-of-life and grief care; planning for disaster risk reduction in preparation for a predicted Kochi earthquake with emphasis on self-support and community support (jijyo and kyojyo) for elderly Kochi residents with diabetes; and the development of community-level social support programs for disaster risk reduction in natural disasters in Indonesia. More research about continuing care of people with mental illness during a disaster is needed, as well as research about interventions for acute stress reactions and preventing post-traumatic stress disorder. Nurses have discovered new knowledge about disaster nursing and will continue to do so into the future.

Disaster nursing has developed inside and outside of Japan with the creation of nursing support networks, academic societies, and sharing nursing care provision systems for improving organized post-disaster responses (Yamamoto, 2013). More disaster nursing education and training programs are needed to equip nurses with the necessary knowledge, skills, and attitudes to provide immediate, mid-, and long-term follow-up care, including mental health care, to survivors, and these programs need to be evaluated for outcomes (Yamamoto, 2013, p. 165). Future planning would benefit from educating all nurses in disaster nursing, including interventions for acute stress responses and psychosocial support.

Natural disasters happen when you forget about them. Therefore, it is important for community and city residents to promote disaster education including mental health and to establish support networks in cities and smaller communities for disaster preparation and disaster risk reduction in daily living. Disaster produces a crisis situation; both community and city residents are apt to become severely anxious and fearful about loss due to serious damage caused by the disaster. Therefore, support systems and networks in family and smaller communities known as "jijyo (self-help)" and "kyojo (help each other)" will be very effective for increasing social connectedness and mental health.

Disaster planning and disaster recovery by local government leaders and organizations tend to lack vulnerable persons' viewpoint. To prevent this problem and the resultant inattention to needs and accompanying distress, it is very important to include women and other vulnerable groups in discussions of disaster planning and recovery in cities and communities. People with psychiatric disorders and those with mental health problems resulting from disaster experiences can be considered vulnerable persons and their viewpoint is important for future planning. In preparation for the care of those with psychiatric disorders during and after disaster, public education aimed at reducing stigmatizing attitudes among the general population is recommended.

Throughout all disaster phases, an important recommendation is to maintain the care provider's own health, safety and living conditions, while working with knowledge of personal limits and managing stress. See Table 28.1 for recommendations in each disaster phase (pre-disaster preparedness, emergency phase, and recovery/restoration phase). More detailed information can be found in the sources listed below Table 28.1.

References

Ando, S., Yamaguchi, S., Aoki, Y., & Thornicroft, G. (2013). Review of mental-health-related stigma in Japan (abstract). *Psychiatry and Clinical Neuroscience, 67*(7), 471–482.

Citizens' Commission on Nuclear Energy. (2014). *Way to 0 nuclear power generation society.* Tokyo: Citizens' Commission on Nuclear Energy. Retrieved May 26, 2016 from www.ccnejapan.com/.

College of Nursing Art and Science (CNAS), University of Hyogo. (2006). Information base for disaster nursing knowledge and skills to protect lives. Retrieved July 9, 2015 from www.coe-nas.jp/english/group_psyc/manual/index.html.

The Commonwealth Fund. (2012). International profiles of health care systems, 2012: Australia, Canada, Denmark, England, France, Germany, Iceland, Italy, Japan, the Netherlands, New Zealand, Norway, Sweden, Switzerland, and the United States. Commonwealth fund pub. #1645. Retrieved October 11, 2014 from www.commonwealthfund.org/~/media/Files/Publications/Fund%20Report/2012/Nov/1645_Squires_intl_profiles_hlt_care_systems_2012.pdf.

Davis, A.J. (2014). Ethics needed for disasters: Before, during, and after. *Health Emergency and Disaster Nursing 1*(1), 11–18.

Doi, T. (1981). *The anatomy of dependence.* Tokyo: Kodansha International.

Dolan, R.E., & Worden, R.L. (Eds.) (1994) *Japan: a country study.* Washington, DC: GPO for the Library of Congress, 1994. Retrieved July 9, 2015 from http://countrystudies.us/japan/58.htm.

Griffiths, K.M., Nakane, Y., Christensen, H., Yoshioka, K., Jorm, A.F., & Nakane, H. (2006). Stigma in response to mental disorders: a comparison of Australia and Japan. *BMC Psychiatry, 6,* 21.

Hayakawa, Y. (2013). Radiation contour map of Fukushima Daiichi accident. Retrieved 29 May, 2016 from http://kipuka.blog70.fc2.com/blog-entry-613.html.

Ishida, M., & Kim, Y. (2011). Acute mental care policy to the Great East Japan Earthquake and tsunami, Japan, 2011. Retrieved September 3, 2014, from www.ilo.org/safework/whatsnew/WCMS_157149/lang—en/index.htm).

Japanese Red Cross Society. (June 29, 2011). Japan: earthquake and tsunami. Operations Update #4. Glide no. EQ-2011–000028-JPN. Retrieved May 26, 2016 from www.jrc.or.jp/english/relief/110729_001736.htm.

Kako, M., Ranse, J., Yamamoto, A., & Arbon, P. (2014). What was the role of nurses during the 2011 Great East Earthquake of Japan? An integrative review of the Japanese literature. *Prehospital Disaster Medicine 29*(3), 275–279.

Kim, Y. (n.d.). Mental health care response to the Great East Japan Earthquake, Tsunami and Nuclear Disaster (PowerPoint Presentation). Retrieved January 20, 2014 from www.ncnp.go.jp/english/images/Dr.kim.pdf.

Nakane, C. (1970). *Japanese Society.* Berkeley, CA and Los Angeles, CA: University of California Press.

Niwa, S. (2012). Mental health problems after the 2011 Fukushima Daiichi Nuclear Power Plant Accident. *Japanese Society for Social Psychiatry 21,* 195–200.

Takeda, M. (2011). Editorial: mental health care and East Japan Great Earthquake. *Psychiatry and Clinical Neurosciences, 65*, 207–212.

Watanabe, M. (2012). The activity of the Great East Japan Earthquake. *The Bulletin of Japanese Red Cross Toyota College of Nursing 7*(1), 11–20.

Women's Network for East Japan Disaster (Rise Together, 2013). Integrating gender and diversity perspectives into disaster response: the support we wanted! A collection of good practice in disaster response based on the East Japan disaster. Retrieved January 19, 2015 from http://risetogetherjp.org.

Yabe, H., Minura, I., Itagaki, S., Wada, A., Shiga, T., Kaibuchi, T. . . . Niwa, S. (2011). Report on mental care for Tohoku-Pacific Ocean Earthquake and Fukushima Daiichi nuclear disaster: acute situation and future problem of psychiatric service in the Pacific coast of Fukushima prefecture. *Surgery Frontier 18*(4), 19–22.

Yamamoto, A. (2008). Education and research on disaster nursing in Japan. *Prehospital Disaster Medicine 23*(3), S6–S7.

Yamamoto, A. (2011). Experiences of the Great East Japan Earthquake. *International Nursing Review, 58*, 332–334.

Yamamoto, A. (2013). Development of disaster nursing in Japan, and trends of disaster nursing in the world. *Japan Journal of Nursing Science, 10*(2), 162–169.

Yamamoto, A., & Watanabe, T. (unpublished). Disaster nursing competencies. Graduate School of Nursing, University of Hyogo, Japan.

Yasumura, S., Hosoya, M., Yamashita, S., Abe, M., Akashi, M., Kosama, K., & Fukushima Health Management Survey Group (2012). Study protocol for the Fukushima Health Management Survey. *Journal Epidemiology 2012*. Doi: 10.2188/jea.JE20120105.

29

A CANADIAN PERSPECTIVE ON PSYCHIATRIC NURSING CARE

Jason Anuik

Introduction

It's 2000h in the emergency department of a large urban hospital in Alberta, Canada. You are a registered nurse working the evening shift (1515–2315h) in the psychiatric assessment department. The phone rings; it is the local police department informing you they are bringing in a 14-year-old male on a Form 10. You groan—another adolescent assessment. You have never been formally trained to deal with adolescents in mental health, and just the thought of having to do an assessment makes you cringe. You ask yourself, "Will it be another case of a teenager just being a teenager? Or will it be a difficult psychiatric case requiring inpatient admission?" You hope for the best and prepare for the worst. A few minutes later, the police escort the patient into the emergency department.

This scenario occurs more often than not in emergency departments across Canada. An adolescent is brought into the emergency department and it is up to the registered nurse or registered psychiatric nurse to assess whether the behavioural signs and symptoms are normal, or abnormal, possibly indicating a mental illness. If that is not confusing enough, the statutes for involuntary admission differ between the 12 provinces and 3 territories, making it difficult to transfer patients between provinces and territories. Finally, to cap it all off, nursing education in Canada has faced challenges preparing the new registered nurse to work with mental health patients, and those challenges are more significant when it comes to training for work in child and adolescent psychiatry. Nurses, including registered psychiatric nurses are not fully prepared to deal with the complex situations that occur in child and adolescent psychiatry on a daily basis.

The case

Brandon (Brandon is a pseudonym and represents a composite of several adolescent presentations to psychiatry) is a 14-year-old male brought to the emergency department on a Form 10 by the police after threatening to kill himself. The police report states that Brandon made this threat to his parents after they took away his cell phone in response to receiving a $500 phone bill. Brandon is upset at being brought to hospital by police, stating he was just mad at his parents and has no intention of actually carrying out the threat. Brandon is placed in an examination room and the registered nurse, a member of the psychiatric assessment team, completes a psychiatric assessment.

Historically, Brandon has had no previous mental health encounters. He vehemently denies any suicidal ideation, stating "I just lost it when they took my phone away!" Brandon describes his mood as "OK" though he reports feeling "sad sometimes." Brandon denies any homicidal ideation, non-suicidal self-injury, auditory or visual hallucinations, or psychotic symptoms. He reports problems with sleep, specifically not wanting to go to sleep early and problems getting up for school in the morning. On the weekend, Brandon sleeps in until approximately 1pm and does not go to bed until 3am. Brandon reports experiencing irritable mood for the past 6 months and decreased attendance at hockey practices, a previously enjoyed activity in which he excelled. Brandon reports occasional use of alcohol and cannabis at parties but denies any current use. He denies any medical issues or allergies and appears healthy.

Brandon's parents Julie and Mark describe a definite change in his behaviour over the past 6 months. They are very supportive of their only child and are distressed at this change in behaviour. They deny any family mental health history. However, on further questioning, Julie states her mother was "sad most of the time" and Mark reports his father would have periods where he "spent lots of money and then would go away to a hospital for a long period of time." Julie and Mark separated when Brandon was 12 years old. Despite an amicable separation, they struggle with cooperative and consistent parenting of Brandon.

The dilemma: do you recommend Brandon be admitted to the adolescent unit for further assessment or discharge him home with resources and outpatient follow-up? As well, what provisional diagnosis or diagnoses should be given: major depressive disorder, oppositional-defiant disorder, substance use disorder, parent–child relationship problems, or just normal adolescent development? The psychiatric assessment team decides to admit Brandon to the adolescent psychiatric unit. The emergency room physician and the psychiatrist on-call each complete a Form 1. Brandon is transferred to the adolescent psychiatric unit as a formal certified involuntary patient.

Brandon is assessed for 1 week before a provisional diagnosis of major depressive disorder is given. Brandon is started on 10 mg of fluoxetine (Prozac). The dose is increased to 20 mg one week later, which Brandon tolerates well with no side effects reported or observed. Brandon is provided patient education on depression and the use of cognitive behavioural therapy (CBT) for treatment. Brandon is also provided addictions counselling for his alcohol and cannabis use. Family counselling is provided for Brandon and his parents around relationships, normal and abnormal adolescent development, and the medication. Julie and Mark are given information and practice on how to cooperatively and collaboratively parent Brandon.

One month later (typical stay length is 4–6 weeks), Brandon's Form 1 certificates are allowed to lapse, and he becomes a voluntary patient. Brandon continues to make excellent progress and is discharged 6 weeks after being admitted to the adolescent psychiatric inpatient unit. Brandon reports feeling better and attributes this to the combination of CBT and fluoxetine. He is transferred to the adolescent day treatment program for 1 month, and then discharged to outpatient treatment with a community adolescent psychiatrist. At 1-year follow-up, Brandon is still taking 20 mg of fluoxetine, with no side effects experienced. He reports his mood as good, has started playing hockey again, and has not used alcohol or cannabis since admission. Julie and Mark report a positive change in Brandon's interactions with them, with less conflict and more consistency following rules.

This case highlights dilemmas encountered within the Canadian mental health care system, especially for those professionals dealing with adolescent patients such as difficulties with deciphering the involuntary admission mental health statutes between different provinces and territories and whether or not to admit the patient or refer to outpatient services. It also highlights challenges of mental health knowledge encountered in the nursing education system, such as normal versus abnormal development and diagnosing psychiatric disorders in children and adolescents.

Involuntary hospitalization in Canada

Involuntary hospitalization in Canada differs between provinces and territories. Each province and territory has its own statutes with regards to involuntary hospitalization. These statutes can differ in many ways. With regards to transport to hospital for assessment, in some instances a form is required (Province of Alberta, 2013) while in others the patient may be transferred to a facility without any formal documentation (Anuik, 2013; Province of Saskatchewan, 2013). When involuntarily admitting a patient to a psychiatric unit, the differences become even more diverse. First, certificates of involuntary admission can range from a 24-hour hold (Province of Alberta, 2013) to one calendar month admission (Province of Nova Scotia, 2013). As well, each province or territory has different form names and numbers. In Brandon's case, the police to transport him to the emergency department for a psychiatric evaluation completed a Form 10. Two Form 1s were completed to keep Brandon in hospital as an involuntary certified patient. Problems are encountered when attempting to transfer patients between facilities in different provinces or territories. Though this particular situation was not encountered in Brandon's case, it occurs frequently and presents a difficult and confusing process to those professionals who navigate it.

Considering the federal government throughout all provinces and territories in Canada provides that health care, it would be beneficial to standardize this process. This would reduce difficulties and confusion for both nursing staff and the patients they serve.

Psychiatric nursing education in Canada

There are two entries to practice degrees a registered nurse (RN) can possess, a Bachelor of Science in Nursing (BScN) or a Bachelor of Nursing (BN). Both degrees offer similar education and prepare the nursing student to write the Canadian Registered Nurse Examination (CRNE), the registration requirement for Canada (Canadian Nurses Association, 2013). There is no practice difference between a BScN or a BN degree. In the past, a diploma program was offered as the entry to practice requirement. Despite being phased out of the education system, some RNs still possess the diploma level. Certain educational institutions have created a bridging program in which a diploma RN can become a degree RN by completing a variety of university courses.

A major issue encountered by those RNs who choose to work in psychiatry is lack of mental health experiences. Several universities only offer rudimentary exposure to mental health, with many institutions streamlining this course throughout the education process rather than a specific course or practicum experience. Both the amount of psychiatric education offered and the type of degree earned differs from province to province and institution to institution. Within each institution, the volume of time spent on psychiatric education is small, usually comprising one course in a semester (University of Calgary, 2013). Within the mental health course, focus on child and adolescent psychiatry is even smaller at one lecture or less. At other institutions psychiatry is not taught as a separate course, rather the topic is spread across several courses (University of Alberta, 2013). We know that mental health interactions occur in every aspect of nursing care, not just on psychiatric inpatient or outpatient units. For example, RNs provide counselling and support in the intensive care unit, emergency department, and post-anaesthesia recovery room.

Most RNs who aspire to practice mental health nursing need to seek out experience either as their final focus or post-graduation. For those wishing to enter a specialty field, such as adolescent psychiatry, gaining experience becomes even more difficult. There are no specific courses offered on child and adolescent psychiatry during the education process, therefore any additional knowledge must be completed through independent study. Many RNs who practice psychiatry encounter difficulty treating the child or adolescent psychiatric patient due to lack of experience and exposure. Difficulty is encountered when trying to differentiate between normal development and a psychiatric process, as illustrated in Brandon's case. For those RNs with little or no experience, this process can be anxiety provoking.

Western Canada offers a second option for psychiatric nursing education. Registered Psychiatric Nurses (RPNs) specialize specifically in psychiatry and are found only in Western Canada, specifically the provinces of British Columbia, Alberta, Saskatchewan, and Manitoba. Program length is usually shorter than a RN and focuses exclusively on the practice of mental health nursing. RPNs do receive education in medical issues; however it is limited to those situations encountered in psychiatric situations and facilities. Despite psychiatric specialization, institutions offer only limited (Douglas College, 2013) or no exposure to child and adolescent mental health (Grant MacEwan University, 2013). An RPN is better prepared for general psychiatric assessment and care, but would still struggle in the specialty field of child and adolescent mental health.

For both RNs and RPNs, education differs depending on the province in which the institution is located. Standardizing education requirements across the country would allow all students exposure to the same curriculum. Since all RNs in Canada and RPNs in western Canada must write an entry-to-practice examination for licensure, standardized education would better prepare the future RN and RPN.

All RN educational institutions should strive to focus more on mental health education and make it a priority. Child and adolescent mental health education needs to be included for both RNs and RPNs, since diagnosing and treating mental illnesses at a younger age tends to result in better treatment outcomes. Providing better education in child and adolescent development will instill more confidence in the nurse in being able to decipher between normal development and abnormal psychiatric processes. As the nurse is an active member of the assessment team, this knowledge can be used to effectively advocate for the patient during decision-making around hospitalization and treatment.

Summary and recommendations

Not every case that presents to the psychiatric emergency department will be as clear-cut as Brandon's. In most instances, the RN or RPN will be challenged in many ways; from deciphering what is normal and abnormal development and elucidating if mental health issues are present, to dealing with complex family dynamics. A more standardized process for involuntary hospitalization and nursing education will help ease the burden encountered by those nurses involved in psychiatric practice. Better exposure of future RNs to mental health and RPNs to child and adolescent mental health can aid the specializing nurse in providing better care for children and adolescents who present with mental health issues.

Future recommendations include:

1 standardizing involuntary hospitalization statutes across all provinces and territories in Canada;
2 standardizing RN education across all institutions in Canada, with a more comprehensive focus on mental health including child and adolescent mental health;

3 standardizing RPN education across all institutions in western Canada, with a more comprehensive focus on child and adolescent mental health; and

4 providing comprehensive education on normal child and adolescent development, with a focus on what constitutes abnormal development.

By addressing these issues and concerns, RNs and RPNs can be more confident in their nursing care of patients in all settings. For those nurses who choose to specialize in psychiatry, specifically child and adolescent psychiatry, these changes will result in more proficient assessment processes and patient care. The more confidence and proficiency the nurse experiences, the better the outcome for the patient in this challenging and rewarding field.

References

Anuik, J. (2013, August 20). Personal communication.

Canadian Nurses Association. (2013, October 29). RN Exam (Online Document). Retrieved on October 29, 2013 from www.cna-aiic.ca/en/becoming-an-rn/rn-exam/.

Douglas College. (2013). Bachelor of Science in Psychiatric Nursing Program and Diploma in Psychiatric Nursing Program (Online Document). Retrieved on August 24, 2013 from www.douglas.bc.ca/_shared/assets/PNUR_Infobook5/329.pdf?method=1.

Grant MacEwan University. (2013). Course List (Online Document). Retrieved August 24, 2013 from www.macewan.ca/wcm/SchoolsFaculties/HCS/Programs/PsychiatricNursing/CourseList/index.htm#3.

Province of Alberta. (2013). Mental Health Act (Online Document). Retrieved on August 20, 2013 from www.qp.alberta.ca/documents/Regs/2004_136.pdf.

Province of Nova Scotia. (2013). Mental Health Act (Online Document). Retrieved on August 22, 2013 from http://nslegislature.ca/legc/bills/59th_1st/1st_read/b109.htm.

Province of Saskatchewan. (2013). The Mental Health Services Regulations (Online Document). Retrieved on August 20, 2013 from http://rpnascom.jumpstartdev.com/sites/default/files/M13–1R1.pdf.

University of Alberta. (2013). BScN-Collaborative Program (Online Document). Retrieved on August 24, 2013 from www.nursing.ualberta.ca/Undergraduate/ProgramDescriptions/BScNCollaborative.aspx.

University of Calgary. (2013). Summer 2013 Courses (Online Document). Retrieved on August 24, 2013 from http://nursing.ucalgary.ca/courses.

30

TRANSITION

Compassionate nursing care and grief in the United Kingdom

Sue Read

Introduction

The losses associated with living in restricted environments for people with an intellectual disability (PwaID) in the United Kingdom (UK) are likely to be diverse and vast. Such potential losses include loss of independence, freedom, familiarity and autonomy. However, such losses are rarely acknowledged or explored and the evidence surrounding this remains weak. This chapter will introduce and define the client population; integrate a case study to depict the transitional journey of a man with an ID; and critically describe the strategies employed to support him from within a medium secure environment. Finally, the chapter will suggest best professional practice for future, proactive support that promotes well-being and recovery in individuals who have experienced a loss.

Cultural context of learning and intellectual disabilities

According to the DSM-5 (APA, 2013), intellectual disability is defined as 'a disorder with onset during the developmental period that includes both intellectual and adaptive functioning deficits in conceptual, social and practical domains' (p. 33) and is the equivalent to the term Intellectual Developmental Disorder in the ICD-10. The Department of Health in England (DoH, 2001) define people with a learning disability [sic] (intellectual disability) as having a reduced ability to understand new or complex information, or to learn new skills (impaired intelligence) with a reduced ability to cope independently (impaired social functioning), which started before adulthood and with a lasting effect on development (DoH, 2001). While MENCAP (a leading UK charity, described as the 'voice' of learning disability) simplistically define people with an ID as having

> a reduced intellectual ability and difficulty with everyday activities – for example household tasks, socializing or managing money – which affects someone for their whole life. People with a learning disability tend to take longer to learn and may need support to develop new skills, understand complex information and interact with other people.
>
> *(Mencap, 2014)*

Such definitions clearly incorporate a whole range of individuals with differing competencies and personalities; varied communication abilities and styles; and a range of associated (physical and mental) health and social care needs. The prevalence of people with an intellectual disability (PwaID) is estimated to be 10.4/1,000 worldwide (Tomlinson *et al*,. 2014), and the Centre for Disability Research calculates that there will be substantial increased growth in the number of adults with profound and multiple learning disabilities (PMLD), estimated at 1.8 per cent per year until 2026 (i.e. in 2008, there were 16,036 adults with PMLD, *c.*8.8 per cent of adult LD population) in the UK.

PwaID are arguably one of the most marginalized groups in society who often have worse health than the general population, yet have more difficulty accessing appropriate health care (Jackson & Read, 2008). Research and campaign reports have highlighted that when PwaID need to access the UK health care system, they are likely to receive different care and treatment from the rest of the population (Department of Health, 2013; Lin, Wu & Lee, 2003; Local Government Ombudsman, 2009; Mencap 2004; 2007; 2012), but empirical research around this area remains sparse (Jansen, Krol, Groothoff & Post, 2004).

Emerson and Baines (2010) identified five key determinants of health inequalities:

1 greater risk of exposure to social determinants of poorer health such as poverty, poor housing, unemployment and social disconnectedness;
2 increased risk of health problems associated with specific genetic and biological causes of learning disabilities;
3 communication difficulties and reduced health literacy;
4 personal health risks and behaviours such as poor diet and lack of exercise; and
5 deficiencies relating to access to health care provision.

Clearly PwaID are likely to have issues that traverse many of these identified key determinants, which indicate such inequality, including mental health issues. The evidence base regarding psychological interventions is constantly developing and if such therapeutic approaches are modified and adapted to meet the distinct needs of PwaID these may be life enhancing. The lack of access to psychotherapies for PwaIDs has led to their exclusion from much mainstream research (Brown, Karatzias & Horsburgh, 2011). Although the psychological needs of PwaID have been largely overlooked, they experience most of the life crises that potentially impact mental health. These include life transitions such as death and loss. How successfully PwaID cope with these crises is significantly influenced by the professional support they receive.

Clinical context of loss

In the UK secure environments provide treatment to patients with various intellectual disabilities while protecting the public, or the patient themselves, from their own potentially damaging behavior (DoH, 2010). Such patients are detained under the Mental Health Act (1983) at secure hospitals provided according to varied levels of security and the assessed needs of the individual. Because PwaID have increased need for daily assistance and are at higher risk for placement within these secure facilities, they are also at higher risk for multiple losses that result from the transition from familiar surroundings to institutional living.

Loss can be described as a sense of being deprived or being without, and as such can be expected or unexpected (Read, 2014a). While life is characterized by movement and change, therefore by its very nature, it is permeated by transitions, losses and grief (Thompson, 2002).

For most people, loss is dealt with within the individual's immediate social context, with help and support sought from family, friends and work colleagues (Worden, 2008), but for some (particularly marginalized groups such as PwaID), loss can go unnoticed, unrecognized and subsequently unsupported.

People with ID experience the same losses as other members of the population (including loss associated with broken relationships, loss of family and friends, transitional losses due to movement), but many struggle to have their losses acknowledged and actively supported. When losses go unacknowledged and support for grief ignored, self-harm and challenging behaviour can sometimes result (Blackman, 2003; Brown and Beail, 2009), leading to detention in secure settings, or creating a vicious cycle of dependency and disenfranchisement.

Loss is widely acknowledged as a potential explanation for behavioural and mental health problems for PwaID (Dodd, Dowling & Hollins, 2005; Hollins & Esterhuyzen, 1997; O'Hara & Sperlinger, 1997), and having an ID is itself recognized as a significant predictor of mental health problems following bereavement (Bonell-Pascual *et al.*, 1999). People with ID who live in secure environments are more likely to have mental health problems than those who do not (Gore and Dawson, 2009; Hobson & Rose, 2008), perhaps because of their history and catalogue of developing needs over time, and compounded by the fact that they often experience diverse losses throughout their lifespan (Gore & Dawson, 2009; Isherwood, Burns, Naylor & Read, 2007).

Supporting those experiencing loss

PwaID are likely to 'function on a developmental level that is inconsistent with their chronological age' (Lavin, 2002, p. 314) and carry an associated history of marginalization, devaluation and stigma. It is worth remembering that PwaIDs have more similarities to us than differences, particularly within the loss, death and bereavement context (Cartlidge & Read, 2010; Read, 2014a). For one gentleman, loss was very significant in his life, particularly since he lived in a medium secure environment, as illustrated in the following case example.

John: a case example

John (a pseudonym) had lived in the medium secure environment for 6 years. He had an intellectual disability and autism, and recently his mother had died suddenly of a heart attack. John was able to attend the funeral, but several weeks later became very withdrawn, spending long periods of time in his bedroom. The staff referred John to a loss support person, who met with John initially to explore if he wanted help with his loss, and afterwards they began a lengthy support programme to help him to explore the loss of his mother and the impact this had on him and his remaining family.

Autism is a lifelong developmental condition that affects how a person makes sense of the world around them and how they socially interact with other people (Forrester-Jones, 2014), and for John this meant he had many compulsive and obsessive behaviours. Progress was slow and deliberate, but over time John did become able to talk about his mother with an affection tinged with sadness. He knew that she had died and also accepted the finality of death: that she was never coming back. He had many family photographs in albums, but was helped to construct a memory book that focused specifically on his mother, and his family also gave him photos to help him to do this.

Six months into this programme, it was agreed that John was ready to move on, to be in a supported living environment with no additional security, and was much closer to his family.

Although John was delighted at the prospect of moving on, he was also a little anxious about leaving what had become his home for many years, all behind him.

Although everyone saw this move as a positive opportunity for John, many professionals may not fully appreciate the potential impact that transitional loss has on PwaID of any age. Many medium secure environments have a plethora of professional support available (nurses, doctors, psychiatrists, psychologists, etc.) to meet the needs of the individual, but few of these professionals are adequately prepared to proactively facilitate loss in its many guises. Loss is often not perceived as a forensic issue but may be a constant underlying feature of the person's needs. Support for loss is often needed spontaneously and therefore the nurse is often best placed to offer this support when required as the person may not feel able to wait days for his next appointment with a therapist. Also, the nurse can take every opportunity to explore loss and grief in a proactive and reactive way (for example when watching sad programmes on the TV) and usually knows the person well because of the close and regular contact they have together. Therefore the nurse's role is often pivotal for loss support.

John's support person was external to the organization, and over a period of weeks helped him to develop a memory book in anticipation of his leaving. John took pictures of his home environment, places that were important to him, and compiled a loose-leaf ring file of these together with written memories of his time there. This memory book became the focus of his sessions, choosing the right photo to put in the right place; nurturing reflection is cathartic and ultimately can promote heritage and history for a person. Such creative ways of working can produce tangible outcomes that have flexible usage and can move with the person wherever their transition takes them (Read, 2014b). Developing the memory book alongside John provided a regular safe space (with minimal distractions) and time for processing his thoughts and ideas about the past and the future; allowing John to communicate at a pace and rhythm appropriate to his needs. Responding to his questions with honesty, in a straightforward manner in a language that he understood was crucial (Forrester-Jones, 2014). John often talked about his mother while constructing this book, not forgetting the strong bonds he still held with her even though she wasn't physically around anymore.

Comorbidities associated with 'mental health, neurodevelopmental, medical and physical conditions are frequent in intellectual disability' (APA, 2013, p. 41), with the prevalence of some conditions (e.g. mental disorders, epilepsy) being 3 to 4 times higher than the general population' (APA, 2013, p. 41). Mental health professionals need to be able to recognize when the person has an underlying intellectual disability, and be aware of indicators that may lead them to this hypothesis (i.e. an ability to read, write, tell the time, communicate well with others; good memory and recall of life events; social connections, who accompanies them, where they live, where they work, and how they manage social situations) (Royal College of Nursing (RCN), 2010). Collaboration is the key to the effective support of the person with a mental health condition and an underlying intellectual disability and such collaborations include education and training, policy and protocols, and mental health and learning disability specialist services (RCN, 2010).

Conclusion and recommendations

Although the numbers of individuals with intellectual disabilities is significant and organizations such as the Professional Association of Nurses in Developmental Disability of Australia, Developmental Disabilities Nurses Association in the US, the Centre for Intellectual and developmental Disabilities in the UK and the World Health Organization among others identify the importance of nursing as it relates to this underserved population, there continues to be a disconnect between these standards of care and the degree of emphasis on this population's mental health needs in nursing education and nursing practice.

A critical task of supporting the individual during loss is never easy, but remains an important aspect of the nurse's and other health care professional's work when supporting a PwaID, particularly in a medium secure environment where freedom of access and independency is inevitably restricted. Loss for PwaID can go unnoticed, unrecognized and subsequently unsupported, and when someone has restricted movements then accessing additional means of support (such as counselling) may be difficult or impossible. Therefore, a clear understanding of each individual's cognitive abilities and the identification of appropriate supports during this crisis go hand in hand.

To promote holistic well-being and recovery it is crucial that professionals in such environments are able to anticipate the impact that loss might have on the people they care for so that they can be better prepared to deal with these and support people proactively as opposed to solely reactively. Nurses are often best placed to spontaneously support people experiencing loss at the time the person needs that support the most and may be crucial to the consistency of support required at such sensitive times.

Therefore, it is recommended that all professionals need to have some understanding of the meaning of loss and how to make opportunities for creating dialogue for meaningful conversations around this sensitive topic. Nurses and other health care providers need to be able to work creatively, developing memory books and life story books/boxes are important activities for anyone with an ID and are also fun to do. Loss and its impact will not simply dissipate; potentially confusing, emotional responses will stay hidden with the person, bubbling under the surface waiting to explode when an appropriate opportunity arises. Subsequently nurses and other health professionals may hold that important key that unlocks the door to enable these feelings to emerge and provide important help so that the person can understand and deal with these feelings appropriately. Read (2014c) describes this as 'making sense of nonsense' and for some people, trying to understand or make sense of loss is incredibly hard to do, particularly if you have an intellectual disability.

References

American Psychiatric Association (APA) (2013). *Diagnostic and Statistical Manual of Mental Disorders* (5th edn). Washington, DC: APA.

Blackman, N. (2003). *Loss and Learning Disability*. London: Worth.

Bonell-Pascual, E., Huline-Dickens, S., Hollins, S., Esterhuyzen, A., Sedgwick, P., Abdelnoor, A. & Hubert, J. (1999). Bereavement and grief in adults with learning disabilities: a follow-up study. *British Journal of Psychiatry* 175(3/4), 348–350.

Brown, J. & Beail, N. (2009). Self-harm among people with intellectual disabilities living in secure service provision: a qualitative exploration. *Journal of Applied Research in Intellectual Disabilities* 22, 503–513.

Brown, M.H., Karatzias, T. & Horsburgh, D. (2011). A review of the literature relating to psychological interventions and people with intellectual disabilities: issues for research, policy, education and clinical practice. *Journal of Intellectual Disabilities*, 15(1), 31–45.

Cartlidge, D. & Read, S. (2010). Exploring the needs of hospice staff when supporting people with an intellectual disability: a UK perspective. *International Journal of Palliative Nursing* 16(2), 93–98.

Department of Health (DoH) (2001). *Valuing People: A New Strategy for Learning Disability for the Twenty-First Century*. London: Department of Health.

Department of Health (DoH) (2010). *High Secure Design Guide Overarching Principles*. London: DoH.

Dodd, P., Dowling, S. & Hollins, S. (2005). A review of the emotional, psychiatric and behavioural responses to bereavement in people with intellectual disabilities. *Journal of Intellectual Disability Research* 49, 537–543.

Emerson, E. & Baines, S. (2010). *Health Inequalities and People with Learning Disabilities in the UK*. London: Improving Health and Lives (IHAL).

Forrester-Jones, R. (2014). Loss and people with autism. In S.C. Read (ed.). *Supporting People with Intellectual Disabilities Experiencing Loss and Bereavement: Theory and Compassionate Practice*. London: Jessica Kingsley, pp. 165–173.

Gore, N. & Dawson, D. (2009). Mental disorder and adverse life events in a forensic intellectual disability service. *British Journal of Forensic Practice, 11*(1), 8–13.

Hobson, B. & Rose, J. (2008). The mental health of people with intellectual disabilities who offend. *The Open Criminology Journal, 1*, 12–18.

Hollins, S. & Esterhuyzen, A. (1997). Bereavement and grief in adults with learning disabilities. *British Journal of Psychiatry, 170*, 497–502.

Isherwood, T., Burns, M., Naylor, M. & Read, S. (2007) 'Getting into trouble': a qualitative analysis of the onset of offending in the accounts of men with learning disabilities. *Journal of Forensic Psychiatry and Psychology 18*(2), 221–234.

Jackson, S. & Read, S. (2008). Providing appropriate health care for people with intellectual disabilities. *British Journal of Nursing, 17*(4), S6–S10.

Jansen, D.E.M.C., Krol, B., Groothoff, J.W. & Post, D. (2004). People with intellectual disability and their health problems: a review of comparative studies. *Journal of Intellectual Disability Research, 48*(2), 93–102,

Lavin, C. (2002). Individuals with developmental disabilities. In K.J. Doka (ed.) *Disenfranchised Grief: New Directions, Challenges and Strategies for Practice*. Illinois, IL: Research Press, pp. 307–332.

Lin, J.-D., Wu, J.-L. & Lee, P.-N. (2003). Health care needs of people with intellectual disability in institutions in Taiwan: outpatient care utilization and implications. *Journal of Intellectual Disability Research, 47*, 169–180.

Local Government Ombudsman (2009). *Six Lives: The Provision of Public Services to People with Learning Disabilities*. London: The Stationery Office.

Mencap (2004). *Treat Me Right!* London: Mencap.

Mencap (2007). *Death by Indifference*. London: Mencap.

Mencap (2014).What is learning disability? www.mencap.org.uk/definition accessed 24 June, 2014.

O'Hara, J. & Sperlinger, D. (1997) *Adults with Learning Disabilities: A Practical Approach for Health Professionals*. Chichester, UK: Wiley.

Read, S. (2014a). Loss in the caring context. In S. Read (ed.). *Supporting People with Intellectual Disabilities Experiencing Loss and Bereavement: Theory and Compassionate Practice*. London: Jessica Kingsley, pp. 26–35.

Read, S. (2014b). Working creatively to facilitate loss. In S. Read (ed.). *Supporting People with Intellectual Disabilities Experiencing Loss and Bereavement: Theory and Compassionate Practice*. London: Jessica Kingsley, pp. 107–118.

Read, S. (2014c). Living with loss. In S. Read (ed.). *Supporting People with Intellectual Disabilities Experiencing Loss and Bereavement: Theory and Compassionate Practice*. London: Jessica Kingsley, pp. 36–45.

Royal College of Nursing (2010). *Mental Health Nursing of Adults With Learning Disabilities: RCN Guidance*. London: RCN.

Thompson, N. (2002) *Loss and Grief: A Guide for Human Services Practitioners*. London: Palgrave Macmillan.

Tomlinson, M., Yasamy, M.T., Emerson, E., Officer, A., Richler, D. & Saxena, S. (2014). Setting global research priorities for developmental disabilities, including intellectual disabilities and autism. *Journal of Intellectual Disability Research, 58*(12), 1121–1130.

Worden, W. (2008) *Grief Counselling and Grief Therapy: A Handbook for the Mental Health Practitioner* (4th edn). New York: Springer.

PART IV

Empowerment strategies

31

MENTAL HEALTH LITERACY

Vicki P. Hines-Martin and Edilma L. Yearwood

Introduction

The US Institute of Medicine (IOM) identifies *Health Literacy* as

> the degree to which individuals can obtain, process, and understand the basic health information and services they need to make appropriate health decisions. But health literacy goes beyond the individual. It also depends upon the skills, preferences, and expectations of health information and care providers: our doctors; nurses; administrators; home health workers; the media, and many others.
>
> *(IOM, 2004 p. 1)*

However, the IOM in that report also identified that over 90 million Americans had trouble "understanding and acting upon the health information" that was available to them. The World Health Organization (WHO, 2013) identifies that nearly half of the European population have inadequate and problematic health literacy skills. WHO also notes that literacy is a stronger predictor of a person's health status than income, employment status, education level, and racial or ethnic group. The goal of health literacy is person-centered care in which the patient/consumer is an active partner in the attainment of their optimal level of health. This goal can focus on the individual, a population, or a community. Figure 31.1 depicts the WHO conceptual model of health literacy. On the other hand, mental health literacy has been defined as

> knowledge and beliefs about mental disorders which aid their recognition, management or prevention. Mental health literacy includes the ability to recognize specific disorders; knowing how to seek mental health information; knowledge of risk factors and causes, of self-treatments, and of professional help available; and attitudes that promote recognition and appropriate help-seeking.
>
> *(Jorm et al., 1997, p. 183)*

Although there are comparable elements in both the definitions of health literacy and mental health literacy, the expectation that mental health professionals have an essential role in the attainment of the needed information is not explicit in the definition of mental health literacy.

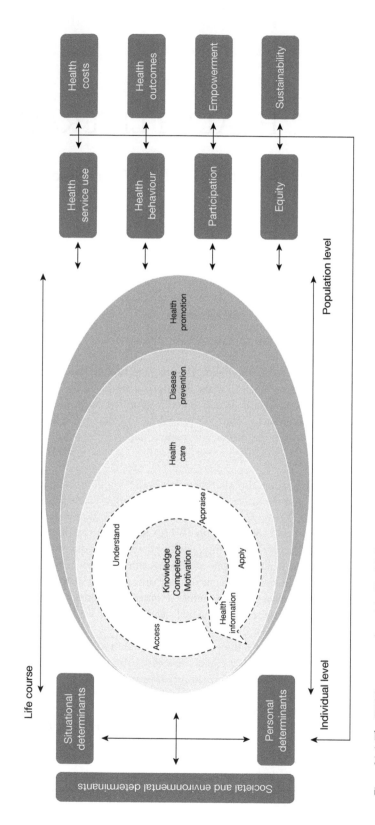

Figure 31.1 The WHO conceptual model of health literacy

Source: © Kristen Sorensen.

A growing body of literature identifies the role of mental health professionals as one of the key influences on the consumer's ability to attain health literacy and improved mental health.

Influences on mental health literacy

The literature about mental health literacy has described influences resulting from individual perceptions and beliefs related to six elements: 1) understanding psychiatric terms and their relationship to symptoms and behaviors; and 2) attribution as to whether behaviors are biological, environmental, psychological, spiritual or under the individual's control. Stigma and uncertainty regarding the help strategies that can be undertaken by nonprofessionals such as the individuals themselves, family and community impact strategies toward mental health literacy. When mental health symptoms are significant, there is a focus on 3) knowledge and 4) perception about the professional help-seeking process (e.g. communicating, identifying and obtaining treatment). Finally, individual influences center on evaluating treatment effectiveness related to 5) outcomes and 6) congruence with values (Byrne, Swords, & Nixon, 2015; Ediriweera, Fernando, & Nagesha, 2012; Ganasen *et al.*, 2008; Jorm, 2000; Jorm *et al.*, 2005; Loureiro *et al.*, 2013; Gaiha, Sunil, Kumar, & Menon, 2014; Marcus & Westra, 2012; Wang *et al.*, 2013). For each of these areas, the literature identifies that the interface between mental health providers, credible and culturally congruent information, and the consumer is critical irrespective of the setting.

Current evidence on mental health literacy

A good deal of research on mental health literacy has incorporated seminal work conducted by Anthony Jorm and colleagues in Australia from the late 1990s to the present. As the originator of the term mental health literacy, Jorm *et al.* concluded that high mental health literacy is positively related to actions and activities designed to manage symptoms of mental ill health (1997). Jorm *et al.* (1997) developed the Survey of Mental Health Literacy in Young People—Interview Version, which has been adapted, expanded upon and used in multiple countries to obtain data from youth and adults about their mental health literacy. The tool, which originally focused on depression and schizophrenia has been updated to include additional disorders such as anxiety disorders (social anxiety, post traumatic stress, obsessive compulsive and generalized anxiety), mania, illicit substance use and suicidal behavior scenarios, and measures all six elements of mental health literacy. Research on mental health literacy has started to yield data that can be used to compare across countries, cultures and groups, ultimately serving as a basis for development of culture-specific interventions (Loureiro, 2015). However, variability of findings exists and points to surprisingly low mental health literacy especially around treatment options and availability, use of psychotropic medications, and fear of individuals with mental ill health disorders. Education level of participants does not correlate to high mental health literacy across all six elements of MHL (Coles & Coleman, 2010; Daniszewski, 2013).

Lam (2014) conducted a population-based cross-sectional health survey study in 2013 in China on 1,678 adolescents ages 13–17. The aim of the study was to assess recognition of mental health problems and intended action to seek help/manage the problem. Data were obtained using the National Mental Health Literacy and Stigma Youth Survey (Reavley & Jorm, 2011). Findings indicated that 15 percent of the sample had moderate to severe symptoms of depression, 25 percent were able to recognize symptoms of depression in the vignette that was presented and 68 percent indicated intent to seek help if they had a problem. The researcher concluded that the young age of the sample might have contributed to low level of symptom recognition.

In another study on youth by Loureiro (2015), the researcher used the Questionario de Avaliacao da Literacia en Saude Mental (QuALiSMental) adapted from the Jorm *et al.* (1997) Survey of Mental Health Literacy in Young People—Interview Version with a Portuguese adolescent population. The research conducted between 2011 and 2012 was conducted in Central Portugal on 4,938 youth with a mean age of 16.75 years of age. The survey was completed in schools and took between 40 and 50 minutes to complete. Findings indicated that the adapted survey is a reliable and valid screening tool that adequately measures theoretical components of mental health literacy in adolescents and young adults.

In a study looking at both community members and village health workers in a rural community in India, Kermode and colleagues (2009) trained data collectors to administer the MHL survey due to concerns about low literacy levels of the participant population. They found that participants had difficulty seeing the vignette depictions as real illnesses and were limited as to what treatment and interventions would be beneficial. They did however identify family and friends as potential sources of help, as did Reavley and Jorm (2011). Study results were used to inform development of a mental health-training program for local community health workers in primary health care environments.

Angermeyer and colleagues (2009) in Germany compared findings from two independent surveys conducted in Germany in 1993 and again in 2001 ($N = 7,119$) with adults that looked at psychiatric labeling, causal beliefs, help-seeking recommendations and beliefs about treatment for major depression and schizophrenia. Respondents in the 2001 sample endorsed brain disease and biological causes of mental illness and recommended use of psychotropic medications and help from mental health providers. In contrast, in a study conducted by Wang *et al.* (2007) in Alberta, Canada, 43 percent of respondents identified weakness of character as the etiology of depression. In the Angermeyer study, however participants also endorsed rejection and social distance from those with a mental illness. Researchers concluded that anti-stigma campaigns are not as robust as exposure to people with a mental illness as a method to promote mental health literacy (Angermeyer, Holzinger, & Matschinger, 2009).

In a review of the literature on MHL in general populations and primary health care workers in developing countries, the researchers concluded that etiology of mental illness is attributed to superstition, poor literacy (low reading, math, and understanding skills), drug use and/or "the will of God" (Ganasen *et al.*, 2008). Strategies identified to promote MHL included increase in government budgets targeting mental health literacy, identifying barriers to mental health policy development and enforcement, an intentional increase in information dissemination, education of traditional healers, use of the internet, and increase in training about mental health for primary health care workers.

Role of health care providers in promoting mental health literacy

There are several recommendations for increasing mental health literacy in individuals, families, and communities by professional and non-specialist health care workers across all income countries. First, training has to start with the workers themselves to develop their knowledge and skills in recognizing and managing individuals who present with mental and behavioral symptoms. Strategies such as the use of the WHO Mental Health Fist Aid curriculum provides workers with basic information on recognizing disorders that include depression, psychosis, anxiety, trauma, eating disorders, drug use, and suicidal behaviors (Kingston *et al.*, 2011).

Riedel-Heller, Matschinger, and Angermeyer (2005) also endorsed the use of the Mental Health First Aid curriculum for use in schools and urged professionals to also work with the media to increase information released to the public about mental health, mental ill health, and promotion of well-being (Jorm, 2000; Reidel-Heller *et al.*, 2005).

A second strategy should target elementary, middle-, and high-school students and teachers to increase their knowledge, influence their attitudes, and provide them with appropriate skills to engage with others presenting with symptoms or behavioral challenges (Daniszewski, 2013; Jorm, 2012; Lam, 2014). In a study using secondary data analysis on 3,913 Grades K–12 teachers, Daniszewski (2013) found four factors that need to be addressed to improve mental health literacy. These included changing the school culture by fighting stigma and increasing communication about social inclusion; providing teachers with guidelines, information and training about common mental health disorders, including management strategies; increasing teacher access to trained professionals who can manage students with mental and behavioral difficulties, and having resources available such as mental health resource materials, targeted curriculum changes to promote discussion of mental health in the classroom, and manageable class sizes to enhance attention to students in need. Of note, Daniszewski also found that teachers have more comfort consulting peers and school administrators, listening to and talking directly with the child/adolescent presenting with symptoms than talking with parents about the child/adolescent.

Health care workers are also strongly encouraged to discuss mental health, mental illness, self-care and crisis management with consumers who come for primary and other health care needs and when working with consumers in the community (Ganasen *et al.*, 2008; Jorm, 2000; Kingston *et al.*, 2011; Lauber, Nordt, Falcato, & Rossler, 2003). Nurses as the largest health care professional workforce globally, and the most trusted health care provider, can and should intentionally provide teaching to all consumers about some aspect of mental health at each encounter. In this way, positive strides can be made to increase mental health literacy and to chip away at the stigma that those with mental ill health currently experience. Given the popularity and reach of the internet, nurses are encouraged to develop teaching modules about specific disorders and use a range of strategies targeting different literacy levels to meet the diversity of learning needs that exist.

The most critical upstream action that nurses and other health care providers can and must engage in is advocacy directed at social and public policy development by local and national government agencies. Nurses can lobby, testify and serve as consultants in the development of policies supporting initiatives that shore up mental health, mental health literacy, workforce training and availability of treatment resources that are accessible to all in rural and urban environments. As financial resources are scarce in low- and middle-income countries in particular, health care providers are also encouraged to approach NGOs and other potential funding entities for support to enhance community mental health literacy and to conduct research on effectiveness.

Resources

As this chapter has indicated, mental health literacy is a critical element in addressing the needs of populations worldwide. Recommendations for improving mental health literacy include development and identification of resources for professional and public use. When providing resources to the public, those resources must be congruent with cultural, social, and literacy contexts experienced by those consumers and therefore must be tailored to those situations. Table 31.1 provides examples of evidence-based resources that can be tailored and used in a variety of settings.

Table 31.1 Examples of evidence-based resources

National/ community initiative focus	Mental Health Commission of Canada Strategy has six values underpinning specific strategic directions in the areas of promotion, prevention, intervention/ongoing care and research/evaluation. The document can be accessed online at http://MHStrategy_strategysummary_ENG_0.pdf. The website also identifies other initiatives developed for the diverse populations in Canada
	The Toolkit for Community Conversations About Mental Health (US) is designed to help individuals and organizations that want to organize community conversations to identify needs and address misperceptions, tailor strategies to community context and utilize existing resources. The toolkit can be located at www.mentalhealth.gov/talk/community-conversation/planning_guide_07–22–13.pdf. The guide also lists multiple resources to facilitate the discussions
School focus	The Centre for Addiction and Mental Health (Ontario) offers an integrated set of web-based resources for teachers, schools, and allied partners to utilize in their prevention/health promotion work with youth. The website at www.camh.ca/en/education/teachers_school_programs/resources_for_teachers_and_schools/Pages/resources_for_teachers_and_schools.aspx also has links for families and public resources
	National Institute of Mental Health (US) is a comprehensive collection of multimedia resources and inquiry-based activities tied to the National Science Education Standards to help teachers and students learn about the structure, function, and cognitive aspects of the human brain. Resources include teacher manual, student manual, DVD of videos, and a CDROM of accompanying materials. The materials can be found at www.nimh.nih.gov/health/educational-resources/index.shtml
Individual/ family focus	Children of Parents with Mental Illness (Australia) offers information for children, parents, families, and professionals who interact or live with adults with mental illness who are also parents. Materials (video and written) are available for each of these groups. This site located at www.copmi.net.au/also has materials translated into several languages
	The National Center on Domestic Violence, Trauma and Mental Health (US) Real Tools kit provide a support group manual and training tools for advocates and other professionals working with women who have experienced domestic violence, sexual assault, substance abuse, and other trauma. This site located at www.national centerdvtraumamh.org/publications-products/real-tools-responding-to-multi-abuse-trauma-a-toolkit/also offers a health care guide for this population
Cultural focus	EthnoMed (US) includes articles and other information for health care providers about topics related to mental health and culture. It provides information about refugee mental health, select populations' cultural perspectives regarding mental illness, and teaching videos about providing culturally competent care and managing stigma. The website located at https://ethnomed.org/clinical/mental-health also includes patient education materials in multiple languages
Workplace	The Mental Health First Aid England: Line Manager's Resource offers a step-by-step framework on creating a healthier environment in the workplace, focusing on key areas such as; managing an employee experiencing mental ill health, reasonable adjustments, returning to work and discussion of key employment legislation. The booklet is located at http://mhfaengland.org/files/5613/9101/5215/MHFA_Line_Managers_Resource.pdf
Other	ScatterGood Foundation (US) is a private foundation that provides grant funding to improve research and resources focused on behavioral health. The site located at www.scattergoodfoundation.org/LiteracyDatabase#.Ves7–33UduZ also lists several resources that support mental health literacy

Conclusion

Mental health literacy is a complex and influential factor that has implications for mental health promotion, early intervention, treatment, and recovery. Nurses and other mental health professionals have an essential role in facilitating improved literacy to support improved mental health outcomes. The ability to perform this essential role requires raising awareness, supporting professional development, training specialist and non-specialist community health care providers, identifying literacy resources, engaging in policy development and advocating for policy implementation. Nurses can provide leadership in this fundamentally important arena regardless of their practice setting.

References

Angermeyer, M.C., Holzinger, A., & Matschinger, H. (2009). Mental health literacy and attitude towards people with mental illness: A trend analysis based on population surveys in the eastern part of Germany. *European Psychiatry*, *24*(4), 225–232.

Byne, S., Swords, L., & Nixon, E. (2015). Mental health literacy and help giving responses in Irish adolescents. *Journal of Adolescent Research*, *30*(4), 477–500.

Coles, M.E., & Coleman, S.L. (2010). Barriers to treatment seeking for anxiety disorders: Initial data on the role of mental health literacy. *Depression and Anxiety*, *27*(1), 63–71.

Daniszewski, T. (2013). *Teachers' mental health literacy and capacity towards student mental health*. University of Western Ontario Electronic Thesis and Dissertation Repository Paper 1165.

Ediriweera, H.W., Fernando, S.M., & Nagesha, B.P. (2012). Mental health literacy survey among Sri Lankan carers of patients with schizophrenia and depression. *Asian Journal of Psychiatry*, *5*(3), 246–250.

Gaiha M.S., Sunil, A., Kumar, R., & Menon, S. (2014). Enhancing mental health literacy in India to reduce stigma: The fountainhead to improve help-seeking behaviour. *Journal of Public Mental Health*, *13*(3), 146–158.

Ganasen, K.A., Parker, S., Hugo, C.J., Stein, D.J., Emsley, R.A., & Seedat, S. (2008). Mental health literacy: Focus on developing countries. *African Journal of Psychiatry*, *11*, 23–28.

Institute of Medicine. (2004). Health literacy: A prescription to end confusion—report brief. Retrieved on August 23, 2015 from http://iom.nationalacademies.org.

Jorm, A.F. (2000). Mental health literacy. *British Journal of Psychiatry*, *177*(5), 396–401.

Jorm, A.F. (2012). Mental health literacy: Empowering the community to take action for better mental health. *American Psychologist*, *67*(3), 231–243.

Jorm, A.F., Korten, A.E., Jacomb, P.A., Christensen, H., Rodgers, B., & Pollitt, P. (1997). Mental health literacy: A survey of the public's ability to recognize mental disorders and their beliefs about the effectiveness of treatment. *Medical Journal of Australia*, *166*, 182–186.

Jorm, A.F., Yoshibumi, N., Christensen, H., Yoshioka, K., Griffiths, K.M., & Wata, Y. (2005). Public beliefs about treatment and outcome of mental disorders: A comparison of Australia and Japan. *BMC Medicine*, *3*, 12.

Kermode, M., Bowen, K., Arole, D., Joag, J., & Jorm, A.F. (2009). Community beliefs about treatments and outcomes of mental disorders: A mental health literacy survey in a rural area of Maharashtra, India. *Public Health*, *123*, 476–483.

Kingston, A.H., Morgan, A.J., Jorm, A.F., Hall, K., Hart, L.M., Kelly, C.M., & Lubman, D.I. (2011). Helping someone with problem drug use: A Delphi consensus study of consumers, carers, and clinicians. *BMC Psychiatry*, *11*, 3.

Lam, L. (2014). Mental health literacy and mental health status in adolescents: A population-based survey. *Child and Adolescent Psychiatry and Mental Health*, *8*, 26.

Lauber, C., Nordt, C., Falcato, L., & Rossler, W. (2003). Do people recognize mental illness? Factors influencing mental health literacy. *European Archives of Psychiatry and Clinical Neuroscience*, *253*(5), 248–251.

Loureiro, L. (2015). Questionnaire for assessment of mental health literacy QuALi Mental: A study of psychometric properties. *Revista en Enfermagem Referencia*, *4*(4), 79–88.

Loureiro, L., Jorm, A.F., Mendes, A.C., Santos, J.C., Ferreira, R.O., & Pedreiro, A.T (2013). Mental health literacy about depression: A survey of Portuguese youth. *BMC Psychiatry*, *13*, 129.

Marcus, M.A., Westra, H.A., Eastwood, J.D., Barnes, K.L., & Mobilizing Minds Research Group (2012). What are young adults saying about mental health? An analysis of internet blogs. *Journal of Medical Internet Research, 14*(1), e17. Doi: 10.2196/jmir.1868. Online publication only.

Reavley, N.J., & Jorm, A.F. (2011). *National survey of mental health literacy and stigma.* Canberra, Australia: Department of Health and Ageing.

Riedel-Heller, S.G., Matschinger, H., & Angermeyer, M.C. (2005). Mental disorders: Who and what might help? Help-seeking and treatment preferences of the lay public. *Social Psychiatry and Psychiatric Epidemiology, 40,* 167–174.

Sørensen K., Van den Vroucke, S., Fullam, J., Doyle, G., Pelikan, J., Slonska, Z., & Brand, H. (2012). Health literacy and public health: A systematic review and integration of definitions and models. *BMC Public Health, 12,* 80.

Wang, J., Adair, C., Fick, G., Lai, D., Evans, B., Perry, BW., Jorm, A., & Addington, D. (2007). Depression literacy in Alberta: Findings from a general population sample. *Canadian Journal of Psychiatry/La revue canadienne de psychiatrie, 52,* 442–449.

Wang, J., He, Y., Jiang, Q., Cai, J., Wang, W., Zeng, Q., Maiao, J., Zhang, M. (2013). Mental health literacy among residents in Shanghai. *Shanghai Archives of Psychiatry, 25*(4), 224–235.

World Health Organization. (2013). *The solid facts: Health literacy.* Copenhagen, Denmark: The Regional Office for Europe of the World Health Organization.

32

MODELS AND FRAMEWORKS OF MENTAL HEALTH CARE WITHIN COMMUNITY ENVIRONMENTS

Sara Horton-Deutsch, Roberta Waite and Maureen Bentley

Introduction

Community mental health services vary depending on the country where the services are provided but in general refer to the systems of care where persons receive treatment outside of a hospital or inpatient setting and close to where they live. According to the World Health Organization (WHO, 2013) community mental health services are more accessible and effective, lessen social exclusion, and are more likely to ensure care and support for human rights. However, many countries have either closed their mental health hospitals, lack adequate mental health services, or have not developed much needed services within their community to meet the expanding mental health needs of the population. As a result, many persons seek treatment from general practitioners, primary care, hospital emergency rooms, traditional healers, or receive no treatment at all.

General practitioners within communities widely accept and often address the importance of prevention, early intervention, and treatment of physical illnesses with their patients. Yet this same conversation related to mental disorders or psychological and behavioral challenges often goes unspoken. Identifying issues that prevent these conversations and empowering both care providers and communities through knowledge of mental disorders and mental health promotion is the initial step to changing actions to improve mental health (Jorm, 2012). Beyond this, integrating mental health services within community services provides the necessary assurance that these services are equally important, worthy of attention, and contribute to overall well-being when adequately addressed.

The demand for and movement toward community mental health services require evidence-based models that demonstrate the effectiveness of services. With the unremitting increase in the number of people experiencing mental illnesses there is an increasing need for service models that provide quality care at a low cost. This chapter will identify pressing issues related to community mental health, identify evidence-based models and frameworks of mental health care developed in several global communities to address these issues, and consider implications and recommendations for the future.

The issues: mental health care in community environments

The importance of mental wellness and mental health care within the global community has gained interest and energy given its impact on overall human health, particularly its effect on risk indicators for cardiovascular disease, stroke, and diabetes (Fricchione *et al.*, 2012). Becker and Kleinman (2013) similarly reinforced the relevance of mental health in reporting that in 2005 the World Health Organization stated there is "no health without mental health," which is critical to recognizing the inherent and central "role of mental health care in health care writ large" (p. 66). To more effectively support the endeavor of mental wellness through early and effective interventions, we need to better understand how mental health disorders are recognized within differing global communities. In addition, we must address knowledge about mental health by professionals and their capacity to address unhealthy states of mental health when working with diverse societies, groups, cultures, and institutions. Strategies that can be used across the lifespan and adapted to diverse cultural groups will help to empower movement towards global mental health.

Recognizing mental health challenges

In order to identify mental health disorders and challenges, we must value the interconnection between mind and body. Traditionally practice and policy implications have supported more of a division than unity (Becker & Kleinman, 2013). This has promulgated lack of economic, social, and scientific investment targeting mental health. Amuyunzu-Nyamongo (2013) asserts that an estimated 14 percent of the global burden of disease is ascribed to mental illness; low-income countries encompass 75 percent of those affected including a broad range of diagnoses from affective disorders to severe forms of psychosis. A mere 2 percent of government health budgets are allocated to mental health care for most developing countries. As one of the top diseases that exceed the economic burden of cancer, diabetes, cardiac disease, and respiratory illness, recognition of mental disorders is paramount to support optimal personal functioning and overall wellness of the community (Becker & Kleinman, 2013).

Since mental health is perceived through a socially constructed and defined lens, diverse societies, groups, cultures, institutions, and professions have varied methods of positing its nature and origins (Amuyunzu-Nyamongo, 2013). Defining ideology of what is mentally healthy and unhealthy, including one's perception of, explanation for, and determination of what interventions are used to support mental health and illness is informed by social and cultural contexts (Arnault, 2009). Therefore, it is essential to understand the meaning cultural groups assign to mental suffering. Importantly, environmental conditions informed by social and economic conditions also play a critical role in recognition of mental health concerns. It is vital to comprehend both anguish and distress associated with mental illness (abnormalities), as well as understand activities that promote mental wellness (ideal states) (Arnault, 2009).

Contextual dynamics stemming from social and economic means must be considered when reflecting on recognition of unhealthy mental states. Social conditions that impede recognition of mental health concerns include natural disasters such as floods and droughts, conflicts causing widespread war, environmental instability, long-term hunger, dislocation, and chronic disease and illness. These experiences do not cultivate good mental health (Amuyunzu-Nyamongo, 2013). However, social conditions that stimulate pride, harmony, and desirability, such as family unity and peace, can be seen as signs of mental wellness. Similarly, poverty is also a significant risk factor for experiencing adverse mental health effects. For individuals who have a propensity for mental health challenges because of genetic factors, poverty can kindle the internal mechanisms and this is often intensified by isolation and lack of appropriate supportive structures (Amuyunzu-Nyamongo, 2013).

Another perspective aligned with recognition of mental health from a social and environmental standpoint requires us to consider cultural variants. For instance, individuals socialized within some Asian nations support the concept that health is a core ingredient of a holistic system of experience whereby the spiritual domain (e.g. ancestors and gods), society, the body, intellectual activities, and emotions are interwoven (Arnault, 2009). Experiences of health therefore implicitly result from an individual's proper relationships with the spirits as well as others. This extends to having appropriate relationships with family, a suitable diet for the season, and thoughts as well as emotions that are pleasant, balanced, and harmonious (Arnault, 2009). Experiences of general wellness are believed to stem from harmonious integration of natural, social, and spiritual forces, and this dynamic directly shapes mental well-being.

King, Fulford, Williamson, Dhillon, and Vasiliou-Theodore (2009) also articulate models of mental disorders including values and beliefs that influence how individuals in communities recognize these disorders. Key factors informing these models that apprise how one views origins of mental illness include: cognitive-behavioral, medical, social, conspiratorial, family interactions, psychotherapeutic, religion/spirituality, and race and ethnicity. King and colleagues (2009) examined some preliminary findings regarding the latter two concepts—religion/spirituality, and race and ethnicity—therefore, information about these are not fully described below. Values are incredibly influential when looking at how mental distress and disorders are understood and recognized. Fundamental features of each model explored by King and colleagues (2009), which inform recognition of states of mental distress, specifically what the nature of the mental disorder is, include:

- *Cognitive-behavioral*: Individuals would recognize mental anguish by levels of poor coping skills and inappropriate behaviors. Psychological factors predominate in this model and treatment focuses on developing self-management skills through an approach like cognitive behavioral therapy.
- *Medical*: Recognition of mental concerns stems from bodily malfunction such as physio-chemical changes in the brain and genetics. Within a Western or European context, pharmacologic interventions would prevail in correcting the problem.
- *Social*: Identifying problems related to mental health through this domain surfaces when persons present with cultural stressors including economic hardship. Social interventions would target this area to for address mental adversity.
- *Conspiratorial*: Concerns regarding mental health in this domain often arise from labeling, specifically use of stigmatizing terms applied to people whose behavior is unconventional, as dictated by the dominate group. Those in political control detect mental problems by creating a myth regarding deviant behavior. The dominant group would see treatment in this domain as abusive rather than as empowering for individuals belonging to vulnerable groups.
- *Family interactions*: Detection of mental distress in accordance with this model would be evident through dysfunctional family dynamics versus dysfunction solely from the individual. Treatment interventions would center on family therapy.
- *Psychotherapeutic*: Recognition of mental distress under this purview is seen in the form of emotional distress most likely arising when the individual is challenged by their own individual personal meaning. Treatment centers on long-term individual therapy and development of self-management skills.

- *Religion/spirituality*: Preliminary pilot research scored religion and spirituality as having a 10 percent influential factor in the recognition of mental illness and both can operate independently of each other. Spirituality allows individuals to understand their mental health concerns, problems, and treatment in a way that transcends any talking or medical treatments. For example, spiritual strategies, including yoga and meditation, are linked with improvements in mental health and reductions in anxiety. Furthermore, spirituality is reported to contribute a sense of comfort in having the individual not feel isolated or alone during their period of illness.

  Religion, a common set of behaviors, beliefs, practices, and values held and identifiable to a group of individuals "provide a way for people to communicate sufferings from a communal, personal, societal or universal perspective" (Mental Health Foundation, 2007, p. 13). Importantly "culture is where religion happens; religion is located within human culture and religion emerges within the cultural phase of evolution" (Mental Health Foundation, 2007, p. 15). Consequently, when a person is managing a mental health issue they may recognize and understand their problem from their own cultural and ethnic perspective. Therefore, beliefs and practices among white practicing Christians can differ from other ethnic groups with similar religious values, such as black Christians. They can all be equally diverse in their perspectives given the multiple overlapping cultural subgroups that overlap for any one individual. It is imperative then that licensed mental health providers understand the role of culture and ethnicity in a patient's life and consider cultural sensitivities and relevant explanations to mental health problems as they relate to spiritual and religious influences (Mental Health Foundation, 2007).
- *Race and ethnicity*: Preliminary pilot research acknowledges that race, racism, and discrimination affect recognition of mental illness; over 80 percent agreed/strongly agreed that these factors contribute to mental illness and its recognition (King et al., 2009).

The thoughtfulness of the mental models shared reflects a significant characteristic of how people understand and recognize mental distress within communities. It illustrates that individuals can shift among diverse models contingent upon the context and the presenting problem. Importantly, we should not attempt to fit individuals in a pre-defined paradigm of how they recognize mental distress. Rather, it is essential to explore what individuals and groups understand and believe causes mental distress and what are the necessary ingredients to promote mental wellness in specific community environments (King et al., 2009).

Capacity of mental health providers

Jack, Canavan, Ofori-Atta, Taylor, and Bradley (2013) report that "strengthening the mental health workforce is a global priority" (p. 1). Low- and middle-income countries need significant help to close the gap of 1.18 million needed mental health workforce employees (Jack et al., 2013). Uniquely juxtaposed to many other areas of medicine, mental health treatment predominantly relies on competent and skilled professionals, rather than technology or tools to manage mental health disorders that account for at least 13 percent of the global burden of disease. Key organizations have acknowledged that mental health workforce expansion is a crucial factor for improving mental health worldwide. These include the World Health Organization's *Mental Health Gap Action Program* (WHO, 2008), *The Lancet* global mental health group, and the Grand Challenges in Global Mental Health Initiative from Canada. Regardless of these appeals for increased attention to this matter, targeted initiatives that focus on how to build this mental health workforce have been unsuccessful.

Fricchione and colleagues (2012) report that in low-income countries the median rate of psychiatrists is 0.05 per 100,000 population, contrasted with 8.59 psychiatrists per 100,000 population in high-income countries. Nurses, the largest workforce in the mental health system, have a rate of 0.42 psychiatric nurses for every 100,000 of the population in low-income countries compared to 29.15 nurses for each 100,000 population in high-income countries. For example, Africa has a median rate of nurses of 0.61 per 100,000 and Europe's median rate of nurses is 21.93 per 100,000. Given the social situation in some contexts such as Liberia with nearly two decades of violence, they have one psychiatrist for a population of roughly 3.5 million people. Similarly, only two psychiatrists for each of the following countries are able to serve their population: Afghanistan's 25 million individuals, Rwanda's 8.5 million individuals, and Togo's 5 million individuals (Fricchione *et al.*, 2012).

Intentional actions are needed to address disparities regarding need for professional mental health providers to build capacity and improve outcomes for country-wide populations. A leader in addressing this was Ghana, a country at the vanguard of mental health policy development among African nations. Ghana's Parliament, in March 2012, passed legislation (Mental Health Act 846 of 2012) to repair the mental health system using broad reforms comprising efforts to strengthen and expand the mental health workforce. This new mental health reform can be used as a model for many other low-income countries given the gravity of human rights provisions in the bill (Doku, Wusu-Takyi, & Awakame, 2012). Examples of some of the innovations Ghana has integrated into their new policy include:

- expanding care from being hospital centric to community focused along with expanding access to mental health services in the communities in which people live;
- contesting discrimination and stigmatization against Ghanaians who are affected by mental illness as well as promoting their human rights;
- regulating the practice of mental health providers both in hospitals as well as in the communities; therefore, both public and private sectors will be monitored including traditional healers;
- clearly describing situations where treatment can be provided, without informed consent, to individuals affected by mental health disorders; and
- encouraging the use of voluntary admission and reserving hospitalization as a last resort.

The international focus needs to be fully supported by stakeholders globally to strengthen the policy reforms that can support effective engagement of more mental health professionals. Taking steps to increase capacity of mental health providers can also improve mental health service delivery for our diverse societies, groups, cultures, and institutions (Jack *et al.*, 2013).

Strategies for prevention and early intervention

Strategies that can be used across the lifespan for prevention and early intervention will help to empower movement towards global mental health. Importantly, Tol, Rees, and Silove (2013) report that pursuing a prevention and early intervention agenda is easier said than actually accomplishing this objective. A fundamental challenge in pursuing this agenda is that many of the systemic determinants of mental health are deeply rooted (e.g., systematic bias and marginalization of racial, ethnic, and/or religious groups, and violence towards women and children) and extend beyond the immediate influence of mental health practitioners. In order to move preventive efforts forward, mental health professionals and anyone else with a vested interest to effect change need to step outside the confines of health centers and disciplines and get involved with advocacy groups, community leaders, policy makers, and other important sponsors that affect social change (Tol *et al.*, 2013). Additionally, prevention and early interventions that focus on global mental health must include the development of an additional skill-set among mental health professionals. They must be taught to integrate broader level elements in prevention efforts, for example, human rights protection efforts, social welfare, and improvement of the education system (Tol *et al.*, 2013). This also demands collaboration across disciplines to align efforts as well as intentionally attending to the needs and opportunities for social action with the aim of eluding the "unidirectional imposition of cultural values from the outside" (Tol *et al.*, 2013, p. 4).

Empowering the community to take action for improved mental health is crucial to promoting overall mental wellness. Knowledge of effective self-help strategies, including increasing levels of mental health literacy and skills in taking interventions to scale including mental health first aid are pivotal steps to prevention and early community intervention. Jorm and colleagues (1997) coined the term mental health literacy to define knowledge and beliefs an individual holds about mental disorders, which help in the recognition, management, and/or prevention of these conditions. Moreover, mental health literacy considers how an individual seeks mental health information including risk factors and causes, self-treatments, accessibility to health providers, and attitudes that stimulate detection and proper help-seeking behavior (Jorm *et al.*, 1997).

When considering life-course development, mental health literacy is especially vital during adolescence and early adulthood since this is a developmental period where there is the greatest risk for the onset of mental disorders. An estimated 50 percent of individuals who will be affected by a mental disorder have their initial episode prior to the age of 18 (Loureiro *et al.*, 2013). It is also during this developmental period when individuals experience substantial changes and transitions; thus, mental disorders influence the individual's personal, social, work-related, physical, and emotional life, and have long-term ramifications for their personal and professional future (Loureiro *et al.*, 2013). Increasing mental health literacy supports early recognition and intervention when faced with mental health challenges (Jorm, 2012).

Early and targeted mental health interventions benefit society as they help to reduce distress in individuals, families, and communities, and promote successful treatment. A key strategy developed to support community members through teaching skills that facilitate individuals to support others with confidence in a systematic and empathetic way is mental health first aid training. According to Hart, Jorm, Kanowski, Kelly, and, Langlands (2009) the mental health first aid program, an action-plan model to mental illness, was developed in 2001 because there was a need for public education about mental disorders, its management and treatment. Thus, it increases the public's mental health literacy through knowledge development about the different types of psychological disorders (e.g., depression, anxiety, psychosis, and substance abuse disorders), the causes of mental illness, as well as diminishing mental health stigma (Morawska *et al.*, 2013). The distinct goal of this approach is to provide help to a person developing a mental health concern or in a mental health crisis until suitable professional treatment can be accessed (Borrill, Jarman, & Agudelo, 2012; Hart *et al.*, 2009). These programs have been used and adapted for diverse cultural contexts including organizations in England, Finland, Hong Kong, Aotearoa/New Zealand, Canada, Northern Ireland, Scotland, Japan, Singapore, Thailand, United States of America, and Wales (Hart *et al.*, 2009).

Evaluation of mental health first aid programs has established that this approach is effective with cultivating mental health literacy, shifting beliefs about treatment, diminishing social distance among persons affected by mental illness with those who are not, enhancing confidence for being able to help another person affected by mental illness, and positively affecting the mental health of those receiving help (Borrill *et al.*, 2012). As responsible citizens of our global community, we all have a responsibility to guard our own mental well-being as well as the well-being of those around us (e.g., colleagues at work, family, and friends).

Community-based mental health movements, programs, and models

Beyond mental health first aid training there are other in-depth community models of mental health care developed to address the increased demand for systemic changes in mental health care services globally. For example, from a historical perspective, in the United States a large-scale system change was initiated with a well-known and landmark national policy, the Community Mental Health Act of 1963. This national policy change was revolutionary for its time, and resulted in a system change by establishing federally funded community mental health centers (CMHC) to provide community-based mental health care. President John Kennedy signed the bill into law with the goal of treating individuals in their communities where they lived and worked. This important movement for change in national policy, which is now 50 plus years old, started a shift to change and improve mental health care services globally (Drake & Latimer, 2012). This movement for improved mental health services remains a catalyst for models and frameworks of care to improve availability, access, and quality of mental health service that are delivered in less restrictive and community-based environments.

Currently, the global concern is how to organize and deliver high-quality, cost-effective, community-based mental health care in resource-poor countries and communities. Given the impact of mental illness on the health and functioning of the individual, there is a growing demand for effective models of mental health care within community mental health and delivered by adequately trained providers. Individuals with mental illness are at an increased risk for comorbidities and chronic illness and have poorer physical health in comparison to the general population (Wiley-Exley *et al.*, 2013). As emphasized earlier, good mental health is important to maintain family and social relationships, successfully attain a high level of education, afford decent housing, and to be able to compete successfully for jobs.

The following section provides resources for the development of community-based models of mental health care and a sample of evidence-based models from around the world.

A resource for the development of community-based models

The World Health Organization's *Mental Health Gap Action Program (mhGAP)* promotes networking, sharing of research, collaboration among international partners, and support and guidance in changing national policies (WHO, 2008). The program promotes the development of community models and frameworks in order to improve accessibility and quality of services for treating mental health disorders, and thereby reducing geographic, financial, and system factors that impede access to care. The goal is to increase access to care for individuals diagnosed with mental, neurological, and substance use disorders around the world, with particular attention to countries with economic constraints that impede treatment and care (WHO, 2008). The focus of this program is to provide resources for the development of innovative models of care and reshape health care delivery in communities worldwide. This in turn improves people's lives by decreasing hospitalizations, providing for continuity of care, keeping individuals in their communities, reducing barriers to care, improving quality of care, and decreasing the cost of care. The advantages for individuals are that they stay in their community with support services, and have the additional support of friends and family, which leads to improved outcomes for consumers and their families.

Sample of community-based models

Tables 32.1 and 32.2 present examples of community mental health care models, which promote recovery within the community, providing the opportunity to live, work, and take part in community support services. Search strategies used to identify community mental health models were conducted in PubMed, OVID, and GOOGLE Scholar databases. This is not an exhaustive list and there are undoubtedly others that have value for providers. Additional sources included in the community models came from the reference lists of Substance Abuse and Mental Health Services Administration (SAMHSA) and the National Association of State Mental Health Program Directors (NASMHPD).

Strengths and challenges facing community-based mental health models

The models in Tables 32.1 and 32.2 were grouped by where services are provided including community-based, home-based, or integrated into primary care. The first models focus exclusively on services in the community to reduce hospitalizations, improve quality of care, link consumers to community resources, and reduce health care costs. Community outreach teams provide services solely in the community through interdisciplinary mobile teams. Outreach teams improve crisis stabilization within the community; decrease the likelihood of consumer emergency department visits or inpatient psychiatric admissions. The team provides services on-site and links consumers to community support partners for health care, housing, and other support services (Farrell *et al.*, 2005). For example, the assertive community treatment (ACT) model helps to ensure consumers remain in the community and avoid hospitalizations. ACT teams also help to reduce the number of emergency room visits and decrease health care costs. However, ACT teams are challenged to meet physical health needs and there is further research needed to look at the integration of primary care physicians and nurses within the teams (Wiley-Exley *et al.*, 2013).

In another example, the community mental health center (CMHC) model provides comprehensive mental health services within the community and aims to meet the gap in service in underserved areas and for underinsured consumers. The services provided include 24-hour crisis response, outpatient services for all age groups, home-based programs, school-based programs, skills development services, job training and employment services, and peer-led recovery services. Peer recovery specialists provide consumer support by sharing their life experiences. The peer-led services reduce barriers by assisting consumers to navigate health care systems, promoting use of preventative care services, providing resources for community partner services and providing individual support and crisis stabilization (Lander & Zhou, 2011).

Finally, skill development represented by the money management model aims to improve money management skills to assist consumers improve their independence, self-efficacy, quality of life, and increase access to health care. A direct correlation has been found between financial resources and outcomes of mental illness (Elbogen, Tiegreen, Vaughan, & Bradford, 2011).

In response to the global trend to move care to the community, researchers and community members of Goa, India developed an innovative approach to address anxiety and depression by incorporating health counsellors recruited from the local community into a collaborative health care team (Patel *et al.*, 2010). The program, called *mana shanti sudhar shodh* (MANAS), means, "search for mental peace" in Konhani, the local language of Goa. Integrated into primary care, MANAS takes a stepped-care approach with a collaborative team of three care providers including: lay health counsellor, primary physician, and a mental health clinical (a consulting psychiatrist) (Patel *et al.*, 2010). The health counsellors are recruited from the local community, receive two

Table 32.1 US models of mental health care within communities

Model	Conceptual base/framework	Evidence-base	Approach to care	Program goals
Home-based model Primary care and behavioral care	Collaborative care model that offers improved coordination and integration of primary health care and behavioral health care systems Links consumers to other community resources and supports	SAMSHA-HRSA Center for Integrated Health Solutions (n.d. a)	Team-based clinical approach to care Comprehensive coordinated care for persons with multiple health conditions (mental health and substance abuse disorders included) Across the lifespan	Improve health care quality Reduce health care costs
Chronic care model Primary care	Patient-centered medical home structure and collaborative care approach delivering on-going treatment and support Delivery service via self-management support, decision support, care management, delivery system redesign, community linkage	SAMHSA-HRSA Behavioral health homes for people with mental health and substance use conditions (2012)	Integrated/comprehensive approach Coordinated care for persons with multiple disorders to include mental health and substance abuse disorders Across the lifespan	Improve health care quality Reduce health care costs
Health homes (including primary and behavioral care)	Collaborative care model that improves coordination of behavioral health care and primary care Coordination and management of full range of health care services	Miller, J.E. (2012)	Integrated care Targets people with serious mental illness Coordinates and manages integrated care of medical, mental health, and substance abuse disorders Across the lifespan	Improve health care quality Improve access to health care and services Reduce health care costs
Accountable care organizations (ACOs)	Designed to manage and coordinate care for Medicare fee for service beneficiaries Comprehensive home and community-based services	Miller, J.E. (2012)	Comprehensive and integrated care Coordinated care for persons with multiple mental health and substance abuse disorders Recipients of Medicare benefits	Improve quality of care Reduce health care costs

Table 32.1 continued

Model	Conceptual base/framework	Evidence-base	Approach to care	Program goals
Primary and Behavioral Health Care Integration Program (PBHCI)	Coordinates supports and integrates primary care services into publicly funded community-based behavioral health settings for adults with serious mental illness	SAMSHA–HRSA center for integrated health solutions (n.d.b); Scharf et al. (2013)	Integrated comprehensive care Serious mental illness and substance abuse Adults	Improve quality of care Improve access to primary care services
Money management model	Significant link between finances and outcomes of mental illness The more financial resources/income one has the better health care access one receives	Elbogen, E., Tiegreen, J. Vaughan, C., & Bradford, D.W. (2011)	Targeted population individuals with mental health disorders Across the lifespan	Improve money management skills Maximize self-determination and independent functioning Improve quality of life Improve access to health care
Implementation partnership	Model is based on Wells' evidence-based community partnership model The implementation partnership is structured according to the 12 guiding principles outlined by Jones and Wells: 1) shared decision-making and power between academics and community stakeholders; 2) use of written agreements and standard operating procedures; 3) frequent communication and direct forms of conflict resolution; 4) transparency; 5) understandability; 6) resource sharing; 7) respect for community values and timeframes; 8) scientific integrity; 9) academic productivity; 10) mutual reliance; 11) awareness of history and culture; and 12) development of capacity and leadership among community stakeholders	Hunt, J.B et al. (2012)	Community initiatives with active partnerships across a variety of agencies, to ensure complementary actions	Community partnerships for adoption and adoption of mental health EBPs

Model	Description	Author	Approach	Goals
Integration Models—3 Managed care organizations (MCOs) Primary care case management programs (PCCMs) Behavioral health organizations (BHOs) Primary care and community	Coordinated delivery of physical and behavioral health care Alignment of financial incentives across physical/behavioral health systems Real time information sharing across systems Accountability for coordinating the full range of medical, behavioral and long-term supports and services PCCMs Aligned with the development of accountable care organizations Less flexibility for providers to tailor benefits BHOs Specialized capacity around managing behavioral health services Both physical and mental health	Hamblin, A., Verdier, J., & Au, M. (2011)	All –3 Integrated and comprehensive Coordinated care for persons with multiple health conditions Across the lifespan	Improve quality of care Continuity of care
Assertive community treatment model (ACT) Community based	ACT is a model in which services are provided exclusively in the community through mobile teams comprised of psychiatrist, nurses, social workers, case managers, addictions specialist, peer support workers, and other staff	Wiley-Exley et al. (2013)	Integrated team approach Coordinated care for persons with multiple disorders to include mental health and substance abuse disorders Across the life span	Improve quality of care Reduce hospitalizations
Integrated community health services model Community based	Collaborative care model (CCM) can improve mental and physical outcomes for individuals with mental disorders Provides a strong framework for care integration	Bauer et al. (2011)	Integrated approach Coordinated care for persons with multiple disorders to include mental health and substance abuse disorders Across the lifespan	

Table 32.1 continued

Model	Conceptual base/framework	Evidence-base	Approach to care	Program goals
Community mental health center model (CMHC) Community based	CMHC provide comprehensive mental health services in the community; 24-hour crisis response; outpatient services including services for children and the elderly; home-based, school, job training and employment services; and community programs	Rochefort, D.A. (1984)	Integrated and comprehensive Mental health disorders and co-morbidities Across the lifespan	Improve quality of health care Reduce hospitalizations
Peer-delivered wellness recovery-oriented service Community based	Peer specialists are individuals in recovery employed in community mental health centers, to provide consumer support by sharing their life experiences with consumers	Lander, G.M., & Zhou, M. (2011)	Peer-led services Mental health disorder and substance abuse Across the lifespan	Improve quality of care Crisis stabilizations Reduce psychiatric hospitalization

Table 32.2 International models of mental health care within communities

Model	Origin	Conceptual base/framework	Evidence-base	Approach to care	Program goals
Strength-based therapy	China	Mental health recovery oriented intervention Tailored to persons suffering from addiction Adopted the 12 guiding principles from SAMHSA Key traits needed for success in recovery: resilience, respect, empowerment, and impact of the stigma	Tse, S., Siu, B. W. M., & Kan, A. (2013)	Recovery process within the context of Chinese communities uses stages of recovery Target area: persons with addictions Adults	Recovery Gaining understanding of recovery in a cultural realm
Chronic care model Wide variety of care settings	United Kingdom and United States	Uses the chronic care model Based on a process model for access to care via three levels: community engagement, address the quality of interactions in primary care, the development and delivery of tailored psychosocial interventions	Gask et al. (2012)	CCMs provide a strong framework for integrated care CCMs can improve mental and physical outcomes for individuals with mental health disorders Across the lifespan	Improve health care quality Reduced health care costs
Balanced care model Hospital/ community care	Global	Balance between hospital and community care as well as all active service teams	Thornicroft, G., & Tansella, M. (2013)	Integrated/comprehensive Mental health recovery Adults	Service development in low-, medium-, and high-resource settings globally

Table 32.2 continued

Model	Origin	Conceptual base/framework	Evidence-base	Approach to care	Program goals
Psychiatric outreach team model Community based	Canada	Outreach team provides on-site mental health screening, assessments, and intervention as well as links to services for housing and other community services Meets clients in their current environments to assess present level of functioning and abilities	Farrell, S.J., Huff, J., MacDonald, S., Middlebro, A., & Walsh, S. (2005)	Integrated care Homeless and marginally housed individuals with mental illness and substance abuse disorders Across the lifespan	Prevention Reduced hospitalizations Reduced cost of care Improved quality care
Home clinic program Community based	Australia	Discharges clients from hospital into community within specified time frame (maximum 14 days' hospitalization) and clients visited by mental health registered nurses (RNs) RNs provide continuity of care between the clinic and the client	Blacklock, E. (2006)	Study targeted adults with a diagnosis of depression	Improved health care quality Improved continuity of care Reduced health care costs
Model for rural mental health Community based	Australia	Model for the delivery of mental health care to rural areas based on the concept of integrating mental health professionals into rural general practices, to assess and treat clients referred from GPs in that practice setting	Campbell, A. (2005)	Integrated and comprehensive Mental health disorders and co-morbidities Across the lifespan	Improved quality of care Coordination of service

months of training, and take the role of case manager at primary health care centers for patients screened for and diagnosed with anxiety or depression. The health counsellors provide psychoeducation, address psychosocial concerns, and connect patients with local community resources and referrals. The MANAS model achieved the goals of a collaborative by improving recovery rates and reducing barriers to primary health care (Patel, *et al.*, 2010).

Community models of treatment are embracing comprehensive and coordinated care to improve the quality of care, promote recovery, and reduce health care costs. Integrating mental health care into primary care settings increases access to care and optimizes the use of resources. Building bridges between the public and private health sectors utilize resources to the best possible advantage. When consumers go without preventative services, their acuity is often higher when they do enter a health care system, which increases the use of resources and the cost of care. Collaborating with community resources and establishing partnerships humanizes consumers and families and builds a sense of belonging and connection with the community.

The focus of recovery within the consumer's community creates an increased need to provide services at sites outside of psychiatric institutions. The important elements are coordinated continuing care, integration of care and partnerships with community entities to reduce gaps in service to deliver high-quality, cost-effective, and community-based mental health care. Models of care that promote partnerships with community services expand the landscape of mental health care providers and services for consumers and families. The utilization of services in the public sector expands the venue of health care outside of traditional care settings, reducing barriers of transportation, hours of operation, and location. Through the sharing of knowledge, accessing the expertise of community resources, and maximizing the utilization of available resources, health care costs can be reduced and outcomes for consumers and their families improved.

The delivery of quality and appropriate community mental health care remains an ongoing challenge, due to obstacles to implementation of new models and maintenance of existing community models. Obstacles to overcome in the community to meet the complex health care needs include commitments for change from governments, health care systems, communities, and other stakeholders to engage in to change, provide financial funding for programs and education and training of mental health care providers. There is a need globally for a skilled workforce of adequately trained care providers and a need for financial resources to develop the infrastructure to support the models, especially in countries with low economic resources (Chee, Fraser, Goding, Paroissien, & Ryan, 2013, WHO, 2008).

Implications for mental health within global communities

Before employing a model to guide care, considering the value of community engagement and its implications for establishing mentally healthy and unhealthy states for individuals living within the global community is essential. In addition to calling for greater resources and for professional involvement to address prevention and early intervention, community participation is also needed to achieve the goals of enhancing overall mental wellness (Jenkins, Baingana, Ahmad, McDaid, & Atun, 2011). This has significant implications for diverse communities when addressing prevention and early intervention measures since understanding community norms and integrating effective services are more likely to be approved if community members acknowledge and are responsive to explanatory models of mental illness/mental health and social realities of their environment (Petersen, Baillie, & Bhana, 2012). Implications for community participation extend to the practical value of involvement of community members in self-help actions plus the fact that community contribution offers opportunities for greater individual and collective control of mental health (Petersen *et al.*, 2012).

When individuals and communities are involved collectively in thinking, deliberating about, and assisting one another with mental health and social difficulties, there is also greater probability of increasing collective agency to act on their problems. This influences the level of adeptness to address any issues related to mental health within their communities. Using informal social controls helps to establish public health actions that generate more health-enabling environments. Formal conduits, however, afford opportunities to initiate discussion that speaks to structural drivers of mental ill health. Regardless of which stance is taken, community engagement stimulates increased influence over mental health, individually and collectively. Moreover, implications for community engagement embraces potential for improving social inclusion and limiting stigma and biased judgment through allowing those with mental disorders and their families to manage and alter their social settings towards being more socially inclusive.

Summary and recommendations

The landscape of mental health care within the world's communities is changing with the knowledge that mental disorders contribute significantly to the global burden of disease; the increased demand for improved access and quality of care and positive treatment outcomes; the need for optimal use of limited resources; and the need to reduce the cost of health care (Chee et al., 2013). Within the United States community mental health centers have undergone numerous changes within the past 50 years with advances in evidence-based practice and recovery models and they continue to provide comprehensive mental health services within communities; caring for people where they live and work (Drake & Latimer, 2012), however the need for services repeatedly outweighs the availability and affordability of this care. The gaps in services have garnered international attention; leading to the development of new opportunities to develop community models to deliver care within fragmented and resource-poor health care systems. Partnering to develop the next generation of service providers can help to increase knowledge among general practitioners, share limited resources, facilitate early treatment and/or referral, reduce barriers to care, and assist families and persons suffering from mental illnesses to navigate complex health care systems.

The models identified in this chapter promote the use of preventative services, help consumers meet service care needs where they live, aim to improve quality of care, and reduce the cost of health care. The types of services offered through these models were also developed to empower persons with mental illness and their families as well as promote a culture of community engagement and person-centered care. Services are extended to individuals living in urban, rural, and economically underserved communities. The services include preventive care, outreach, connection to other community support services; transportation services, nutrition programs, and housing services. However, for these models to be effective, providers must value the interconnection between mind and body, appreciate the meaning cultural groups assign to suffering and mental illness, and be responsive to the influence of social and economic factors on mental illness.

Psychiatric mental health nurses are well positioned to model the way for the future of mental health care within communities. With expertise in collaboration, person-centered care, and compassion as well as knowledge of mental health, mental illness and prevention, these practitioners are poised to facilitate the team building and partnership required to successfully implement and pilot new models of care. Advanced practice psychiatric nurses in academic settings are also needed to support the development of future psychiatric-mental health nurses and other health care providers through interprofessional education that will model and facilitate the development of partnered health care services within communities around the world. Through interprofessional education, faculty must actively engage learners in teamwork and collaboration in classroom and practicum settings while threading the essential areas of cultural inclusion and sensitivity, integrated and person-centered care, wellness, and recovery into the student experience. Helping students to embody this knowledge, and these skills and values while in their training supports the development of practitioners prepared to address global mental health needs holistically. Psychiatric-mental health nurse researchers are also needed to lead in knowledge development through theory generation, creative problem solving, and the systematic use of cognitive, rational logic, and other ways of knowing. Together psychiatric mental health practitioners, academicians, and researchers are poised to develop, engage in, and evaluate innovative treatment models to meet the continuously expanding and complex community mental health needs.

However, for any of these recommendations to be successful all health care practitioners must move beyond their professional confines to more visibly advocate for and address unjust societies, which promulgate mental despair through lack of action. Globally the socio-political construction of mental dejection is undeniable, yet the human right for the pursuit of mental health and wellness is unequivocal. Psychiatric-mental health nurses are well prepared and positioned to lead this call to action by role modeling advocacy, protecting the most vulnerable, speaking out against injustice, and endorsing models of care that empower individuals, families and communities worldwide.

References

Amuyunzu-Nyamongo, M. (2013). The social and cultural aspects of mental health in African societies. Commonwealth Health Partnerships. Retrieved May 10, 2016 from www.commonwealthhealth. org/wp-content/uploads/2013/07/The-social-and-cultural-aspects-of-mental-health-in-African-societies_CHP13.pdf.

Arnault, D. (2009). Cultural determinants of help-seeking: A model for research and practice. *Research Theory and Nursing Practice*, 23(4), 259–278.

Bauer, A.M., Azzone, V., Goldman, H.H., Alexander, L., Unutzer, J., Coleman-Beattie, B., & Frank, R.G. (2011). Implementation of collaborative depression management at community-based primary care clinics and evaluation. *Psychiatry Services*, 62, 1047–1033.

Becker, A., & Kleinman, A. (2013). Mental health and the global agenda. *The New England Journal of Medicine*, 369, 66–73.

Blacklock, E. (2006). Home clinic programme: An alternative model for private mental health facilities and sufferers of major depression. *International Journal of Mental Health Nursing* 15, 3–9.

Borrill, J., Jarman, P., & Agudelo, J. (2012). Course helps keep first aid in mind. *Occupational Health*, 64(4), 27–29.

Campbell, A. (2005). The evaluation of a model of primary mental health care in rural Tasmania. *Australian Journal of Rural Health*, 13, 142–148.

Chee, N., Fraser, J., Goding, M., Paroissien, D., & Ryan, B. on behalf of the Editorial Group of the Asia-Pacific Community Mental Health Development Project Stage 2. (2013). Partnerships for community mental health in the Asia-Pacific: Principles and best-practice models across different sectors. *Australian Psychiatry*, 21(1), 38–45.

Doku, V., Wusu-Takyi, A., & Awakame, J. (2012). Implementing the mental health act in Ghana: Any challenges ahead? *Ghana Medical Journal*, 46(4), 241–250.

Drake, R.E., & Latimer, E. (2012). Lessons learned in developing community mental health care in North America. *World Psychiatry*, 11, 47–51.

Elbogen, E., Tiegreen, J. Vaughan, C., & Bradford, D.W. (2011). Money management, mental health, and psychiatric disability: A recovery-oriented model for improving financial skills. *Psychiatric Rehabilitation Journal*, 34, 223–231.

Farrell, S.J., Huff, J., MacDonald, S., Middlebro, A., & Walsh, S. (2005). Taking it to the street: A psychiatric outreach service in Canada. *Community Mental Health Journal*, 41, 737–746.

Fricchione, G.L., Borba, C.P., Alem, A., Shibre, T., Carney, J.R., & Henderson, D. C. (2012). Capacity building in global mental health: Professional training. *Harvard Review of Psychiatry*, 20(1), 47–57.

Gask, L., Rogers, A., Waheed, W., Dowrick, C., Bower, P., Lamb, J., & AMP Research Group. (2012). Improving access to psychosocial interventions for common mental health problems in the United Kingdom: Narrative review and development of a conceptual model for complex interventions. *BMC Health Services Research, 12*(1), 249–249.

Hamblin, A., Verdier, J., & Au, M. (2011). State options for integrating physical and behavioral health care. Retrieved May 10, 2016 from, www.integration.samhsa.gov/integrated-care-models/Integrated_Care_Briefing_Paper_models_of_integration_analysis_10–6-11.pdf.

Hart, L., Jorm, A., Kanowski, L., Kelly, C., & Langlands, R. (2009). Mental health first aid for Indigenous Australians: Using Delphi consensus studies to develop guidelines for culturally appropriate responses to mental health problems. *BMC Psychiatry, 9*, 47–59.

Hunt, J.B., Curran, G., Kramer, T., Mouden, S., Ward-Jones, S., Owen, R., & Fortney, J. (2012). Partnership for implementation of evidence-based mental health practices in rural federally qualified health centers: Theory and models. *Program Community Health Partnership, 6*, 389–398.

Jack, H., Canavan, M., Ofori-Atta, A., Taylor, L., & Bradley, E. (2013). Recruitment and retention of mental health workers in Ghana. *PLoS One, 8*(2), 1–8.

Jenkins, R., Baingana, F., Ahmad, R., McDaid, D., & Atun, R. (2011). Social, economic, human rights, and political challenges to global mental health. *Mental Health in Family Medicine, 8*, 87–96.

Jorm, A. (2012). Mental health literacy: Empowering the community to take action for better mental health. *American Psychologist, 67*(3), 231–243.

Jorm, A., Korten, A., Jacomb, P., Christensen, H., Rodgers, B., & Pollitt, P. (1997). Mental health literacy: A survey of the public's ability to recognise mental disorders and their beliefs about the effectiveness of treatment. *The Medical Journal of Australia, 166*(4), 182.

King, C., Fulford, B., Williamson, T., Dhillon, K., & Vasiliou-Theodore, C. (2009). Model values: Race, values and models in mental health. Mental Health Foundation. Retrieved May 10, 2016 from www.mentalhealth.org.uk/content/assets/PDF/publications/model_values.pdf.

Lander, G.M., & Zhou, M. (2011). An analysis of relationships among peer support, psychiatric hospitalization, and crisis stabilizations. *Community Mental Health Journal, 47*, 106–112.

Loureiro, L., Jorm, A., Mendes, A., Santos, J., Ferreira, R., & Pedreiro, A. (2013). Mental health literacy about depression: A survey of Portuguese youth. *BMC Psychiatry, 13*, 129–137.

Mental Health Foundation. (2007). *Keeping the faith: Spirituality and mental health.* London: Mental Health Foundation. Retrieved May 10, 2016 from www.mentalhealth.org.uk/content/assets/PDF/publications/Keeping_the_faith.pdf?view=Standard.

Miller, J.E. (2012). Taking integration to the next level: The role of new service delivery models in behavioral health. Retrieved 10 May, 2016 from, www.nasmhpd.org/docs/publications/docs/2012/Taking IntegrationtotheNextLevel.pdfs.

Morawska, A., Fletcher, R., Pope, S., Heathwood, E., Anderson, E., & McAuliffe, C. (2013). Evaluation of mental health first aid training in a diverse community setting. *International Journal of Mental Health Nursing, 22*(1), 85–92.

Patel, V., Weiss, H.A., Chowdhary, N., Naik, S., Pednekar, S., Chatterjee, S., & Kirkwood, B.R. (2010). Effectiveness of an intervention led by lay health counsellors for depressive and anxiety disorders in primary care in Goa, India (MANAS): A cluster randomized trial. *The Lancet, 376*, 2086–2095.

Petersen, I., Baillie, K., & Bhana, A. (2012). Mental Health and Poverty Research Programme Consortium. *Transcult Psychiatry, 49*(3–4), 418–437.

Rochefort, D.A. (1984). Origins of the "third psychiatric revolution": The Community Mental Health Centers Act of 1963. *Journal of Health Politics, Policy, and Law, 9*(1), 1–18.

SAMHSA-HRSA. (2012). Behavioral health homes for people with mental health and substance use conditions: The core clinical features. Retrieved from, www.integration.samhsa.gov/clinical-ppractice/CIHS_Health_Homes_Core_Clinical_Features.pdf.

SAMHSA-HRSA. (n.d. a). Center for integrated health solutions. Retrieved May 10, 2016 from, www.integration.samhsa.gov/integrated-care-models/health-homes.

SAMHSA-HRSA. (n.d. b). Center for integrated health solutions. Retrieved May 10, 2016 from, www.integration.samhsa.gov/resource/pbhci-program.

Scharf, D.M., Eberhart, N.K., Schmidt, N., Vaughan, C.A., Dutta, T., Pincus, H.A., & Burman, M.A. (2013). Integrating primary care into community behavioral health settings: Programs and early implementation experiences. *Psychiatric Services, 64*, 660–665.

Thornicroft, G., & Tansella, M. (2013). The balanced care model for global mental health. *Psychological Medicine, 43*(4), 849–815.

Tol, W., Rees, S., & Silove, D. (2013). Broadening the scope of epidemiology in conflict affected settings: Opportunities for mental health prevention and promotion. *Epidemiology and Psychiatric Sciences*, 1–7. Retrieved May 10, 2016 from http://journals.cambridge.org/abstract_S2045796013000188.

Tse, S., Siu, B.W.M., & Kan, A. (2013). Can recovery-oriented mental health services be created in Hong Kong? Struggles and strategies. *Administration and Policy in Mental Health*, 40(3), 155–158.

Wiley-Exley, E., Domino, M.E, Ricketts, T.C., Cuddeback, G., Burns, B.J., & Morrissey, J. (2013). The impact of assertive community treatment on utilization of primary care and other outpatient health services: The North Carolina experience. *Journal of American Psychiatric Nurses Association*, *19*, 195–201.

World Health Organization. (2008). *Mental health gap action programme (mhGAP): Scaling up care for mental, neurological and substance abuse disorders*. Geneva: World Health Organization.

World Health Organization. (2013). *World Health Statisics*. Retrieved July 24, 2016 from www.who.int/gho/publications/world_health_statistics/2013/en/.

33

CONCLUSION AND RECOMMENDATIONS

Edilma L. Yearwood and Vicki P. Hines-Martin

Lessons learned

Mental health challenges and disorders impose significant social and economic burden, not just on individuals with the disorders but also on households, communities, employers, health care systems, and governments. Studies demonstrate that untreated mental health and behavioral problems in childhood and adolescence can have profound longstanding social and economic consequences into adulthood. Specifically, untreated symptoms effect interpersonal relationships, impede educational attainment, increase potential for contact with the criminal justice system, lower employment and earning capacity, and erode self-concept and competence.

The 2007 *Lancet* series on global mental health was a pivotal moment in the movement to raise awareness, provide epidemiological data on mental health, and urge low- and middle-income countries to increase their efforts in providing treatment services for individuals challenged by mental ill health. The subsequent 2011 Lancet journal series offered specific strategies related to treatment but also focused on the educational and training needs of the provider to deliver that treatment, while highlighting the urgency for research and evaluation of strategies used across various environments.

Three main approaches have been shared that have been used to improve mental health in low-, middle-, and high-income countries. These include strategies that focus on a combination of prevention and treatment of common mental health disorders; delivery of mental health services within the context of current health service systems such as primary or medical care settings; and placing mental health within social, cultural and economic contexts, which have broad implications for human rights with a focus on advocacy, equity, and policy development. Authors within this book have demonstrated their involvement and commitment to each of these common areas.

As has been illustrated in each chapter and exemplar, nurses are engaged in support of individuals, populations and communities through direct care, advocacy, education, research, and policy development. Many barriers to mental health care are encountered. Two of the largest and most prevalent barriers are stigma and a lack of resources. Resources include people, services, treatment structures, print materials, affordable medications, and modes of transportation to access services.

Development of mental health literacy across nursing specialties, health care professionals, consumers, families, policy makers, and communities is a priority tactic that would begin to combat stigma. Lack of resources in low- and middle-income countries has prompted development and use of new strategies such as training non-specialist community workers, among others, to deliver basic mental health care and social support within their own communities, where they are viewed as trusted cultural brokers.

While there have been strides made in uncovering neurobiological causes of mental, neurological, and substance use disorders, scientists in the field of mental health are equally aware that social determinants of health/mental health serve as incubators for mental ill health and barriers to achieving well-being. Unfortunately these structural impediments are harder to combat and have long been out of the usual purview of nurses and their health care provider colleagues. Therefore, in addition to providing direct treatment, health care providers must also engage in actions directed at tackling the social determinants of health and may need additional training and guidance for advocacy roles, policy development, community engagement, and to increase effectiveness when working in low-resourced environments.

Global roles for nurses

The ability to function as nurses in partnership with individuals and groups is affected by the context in which one works. Barriers and facilitators that are related to social, economic, human rights, and political challenges affect current and future roles of nurses (see Table 33.1). Even as these barriers exist in varying degrees across the globe, contributors to this text identify some essential components that can support mental health nursing roles. These components include a mechanism for sharing best practices that can be utilized in low- to high-resource countries, the value and necessity of forming partnerships with consumers along with colleagues within and outside of the health care profession, and the need to assertively inject the voice and presence of nurses in legislative efforts and when creating and revising policies.

In 2011, Horatio, the European Psychiatric Nurses Association pointed out that throughout Europe, there is limited regulation of mental health nursing. They recommended that training of psychiatric mental health nurses become responsive to cultural context and prepare this specialty nurse to address complex changes impacting overall health when delivering quality mental health care (Ward, 2011). Table 33.1 illustrates some challenges and opportunities for nurses in the area of mental health promotion.

The Mental Health Action Plan

The Mental Health Action Plan (2013–2020) provides the necessary framework and guidance for initiatives to improve global mental health. The four goals of the plan and approaches to achieve the goals are included in Table 33.2 below.

Table 33.1 Current challenges and opportunities for nurses

Challenges	Opportunities
1) Tremendous need exists globally for adequately trained mental health nurses	1) Nurses are prepared to fill the existing void as service providers
2) Competing priorities in resource-poor environments with a usual default to meeting physical health needs over mental health needs	2) Given global number of nurses, an intentional and organized effort to improve mental health treatment, literacy, and human rights protection by nurses will have an impact
3) In some environments, there is a lack of buy-in from consumers with antiquated views about mental ill health	3) Nurses are trained to provide care

Table 33.2 The Mental Health Action Plan—goals and strategies for achievement

Goals	Strategies for goal achievement
1) Strengthen effective leadership and governance for mental health	a) Support equity by providing universal health coverage
2) Provide comprehensive, integrated, and responsive mental health and social care services in community-based settings	a) Endorse and champion human rights through compliance with the Convention on the Rights of Persons with Disabilities and other human rights promotion policies
3) Implement strategies for promotion and prevention in mental health	a) Disseminate evidence-based practice guidelines derived from well-conducted research
4) Strengthen information systems, evidence, and research for mental health	a) Provide guidelines and strategies specific to lifespan stage (children, adolescents, adults, and older adults)
	a) Operate from a multisectoral/multidisciplinary/ partnership perspective
	a) Empower persons with mental disorders and psychosocial disabilities

Source: (2013). Reprinted with permission.

There are several examples of best practices that are in place and can serve as models and templates for other countries. First, The Rio Political Declaration on Social Determinants of Health: A Snapshot of Canadian Actions 2015 is a report card that chronicles the Canadian government's response to the crisis associated with the social determinants of health. The government focused on improving governance, participating in policy development and implementation, reducing health inequities, fostering collaboration, taking responsibility for monitoring pro-gress, and increasing accountability. Interventions include better communication, structural changes, endorsing inclusivity, promoting self-determination, building capacity, and championing health equity (Government of Canada, 2015). A second example is the Emerald Program organized and delivered in six countries, India, Nepal, South Africa, Ethiopia, Nigeria, and Uganda. The program centers on improving mental health outcomes by focusing on capacity building to increase service-user and caregiver support of systems strengthening (Semrau et al., 2015). Barriers to effective mental health service delivery were identified and culture-specific solutions enacted.

The imperative for capacity building

When human and material resources are poor and treatment gaps exist, social scientists and others recommend use of capacity building strategies to develop tools that can be used to provide needed interventions. Capacity building involves identifying specific needs, assessing available resources, and engaging in development of skills in your resource population to then meet identified needs. An example would be efforts placed on workforce development and supervision of non-specialist community workers who would then provide mental health care in low-resource communities (Fricchione et al., 2012).

Strategies to promote capacity building also include task shifting, scaling up and providing education and training. Strategies such as Psychological First Aid and Mental Health First Aid are simple, structured and evidence-based tools that can be used to teach lay community members about common mental and behavioral health presentations and ways to provide basic interventions to manage consumer symptoms (Armstrong, Kermode, Raja, Chandra, & Jorm, 2011; Bond, Jorm, Kitchener, & Reavely, 2015).

Task sharing/shifting is a capacity building strategy in which tasks are given to individuals or groups with less training or narrow/specific training because of their availability and interest (Kakuma, Minas, & Dal Poz, 2014) in meeting existing needs. Teachers, clergy, and primary care providers are examples of individuals and groups that can be trained to assist with providing basic mental health care and other as needed interventions.

Scaling up refers to increasing the impact of innovative services or research findings in order to benefit larger number of individuals. Scaling up prompts development and enforcement of policies and programs that have worked, while looking for stakeholder support to maintain sustainability (Eaton *et al.*, 2011). Scaling up relies on existing evidence that interventions are effective.

Education and training

Lastly, providing education about mental health is a fundamental need across all constituencies, including mental health nurses, non-specialists, consumers, traditional healers, native nurses, caregivers, health professionals, and lay community members. Providing knowledge of the subject area contributes to improved mental health literacy and again serves to erode stigma.

All nursing programs globally must practice inclusion of mental health nursing content including strategies for working in complex environments where challenges to overall health associated with social determinants of health exist. In addition, content on mental health promotion and prevention should be provided to both undergraduate and graduate nursing students to assist them in meeting needs across all settings and environments. Educational opportunities should exist across all income countries to support mental health nurses who want to pursue additional focused training in the specialty or who want to obtain advanced and/or terminal nursing degrees to enrich their clinical practice or to conduct research.

Collaboration and partnerships

Collaboration in mental health care is an imperative and can be accomplished at many levels. Each chapter identifies that the goal for nursing care at the individual and family level is collaboration with individuals to ameliorate mental health risks and address pressing mental health needs. Authors clearly assert that nurses can, and do, work closely with consumers in an effort to assist them in recognizing and acknowledging personal strengths and challenges, identify choices and goals, and to develop and implement strategies to restore, attain, or maintain emotional and social functioning and well-being. However, barriers to this collaboration have also been described, which include stigma and limited understanding of mental health influenced by cultural beliefs and literacy level.

Contributors to this text also emphasize that nurses are increasingly collaborating as part of interprofessional groups and with paraprofessionals and lay groups to provide mental health services. In these collaborations, multiple workers from different professional backgrounds provide comprehensive services by working with targeted groups and communities to deliver an enhanced quality of care regardless of setting. Teams are able to combine their resources and coordinate knowledge, skills, and strategies to provide needed services. Cited literature from low- to high-resource countries all identifies that this approach maximizes resources and focuses on empowerment of targeted populations to make decisions that are informed and culturally and socially appropriate. Even as progress is made in improving collaborative efforts, continued efforts will require increased numbers of nurses across settings and a reconceptualization of how nurses are educated, function, and serve as leaders within interprofessional teams.s.

Co-location of services, minimizes consumer non-adherence to their mental health needs. In co-located services, the primary care clinician can refer to mental health services and complete a hand-off to his/her mental health colleague at the same site following the primary care visit. This seamless transfer can decrease stigma and support help-seeking behaviors. Collaborative practice models support practice partnerships for which there is evidence of effectiveness (Rebello, Marques, Gureje, & Pike, 2014).

Funding mental health initiatives and research

It has been well documented that mental health conditions and poor mental health result in significant global disability-adjusted life-year burden that has implications across the life span. The WHO has published extensively on mental health emphasizing the need for targeted efforts to improve literacy, service access, mental health resources, service delivery research/innovation, and dissemination of best practice models. Many high-resource countries have identified research priorities according to population/condition, treatment modalities (especially related to use of technology, psychopharmacology, and genetics), and influences on mental health decision-making (primarily stigma and mental health literacy).

Low- and middle-income countries are moving forward in their identification of the burden of mental health disease and risk factors, and conditions especially those that have onset in childhood and adolescence. Across low- to high-resource countries, an increasing emphasis has been placed on maximizing the limited mental health resources. Those initiatives that utilize collaborations between services such as integrated care and those that involve use of lay or community members to educate about mental health and promote early identification are increasingly being investigated. Even as research priorities have been identified and a variety of nursing organizations have spoken out to identify that nursing is critical to advancement in these areas, there continues to be disparity in the number of nurses educated to conduct research, who receive funding to conduct research, or who become members of mental health research teams. As the largest group of health care providers and as providers who have first contact and sustained interactions with consumers who experience poor mental health, nurses have unique insights that can enhance any mental health research from the conduct of research through the translation of research into practice. Governmental policy and limited governmental and nongovernmental budgetary resources continue to be barriers to mental health research. The priorities identified for allocated funding may serve as unintended barriers to nursing as a full partner in the development of new knowledge.

Anti-stigma campaigns and visibility

At the heart of barriers to mental health care and violations of human rights is stigma. Nurses and other health care workers can promote mental health and well-being if they confront stigma and participate in anti-stigma campaigns. Disparities exist with respect to anti-stigma campaigns across different income level countries. High-income countries such as the United States, Australia, the United Kingdom, Japan, Germany, and Canada have fairly robust anti-stigma campaigns using various social media tools. A list of global organizations fighting stigma can be found at uhaweb.hartford.edu/owahl/stigmaorg.htm. In addition to public education efforts to decrease stigma, high-income countries conduct research periodically to assess changes in stigma and effectiveness of the public awareness/education efforts. There is a need for developing similar strategies that are culturally congruent for use in low- and middle-income communities. However, efforts in these communities may require targeting multiple information dissemination strategies, as technology may be spotty or inaccessible in some environments. Anti-stigma campaigns should begin in early childhood and continue into adulthood to support effectiveness.

Visibility can be achieved by keeping issues related to mental health in public awareness, using strategic dosing and encouraging conversations that break down barriers and challenge biases and misconceptions. For example, in the United States, October is recognized as depression awareness month, and depression screening, making available information sheets, and eliciting mental health professionals to provide consumer education on the topic, serve to de-stigmatize depression. Opportunities for structured exposure to individuals with mental health challenges accompanied by processing time with a mental health provider remains a good strategy for breaking down the barriers of stigma and changing negative beliefs and behaviors.

Leveraging collective nurse resources

As stated throughout this book, nurses are in a unique position to make a difference in the effort to improve the mental health of individuals and communities. A recommendation would be establishment of an intentional and strategic global alliance among mental health nursing organizations to develop a work plan for collective action around specific mental health initiatives. The mental health nurses alliance could also establish interprofessional work with the WHO, the United Nations, the World Bank, and the International Council of Nurses (ICN) to name a few organizations working in low-, middle-, and high-income countries. Leveraging collective nurse resources promotes increased visibility and recognition that the specialty is working well towards providing the best evidence-informed mental health care across the lifespan.

The issue of gender

Gender has implications for mental health and mental health care. The WHO identified that "gender determines the differential power and control men and women have over the socio-economic determinants of their mental health and lives, their social position, status and treatment in society and their susceptibility and exposure to specific mental health risks" (WHO, n.d). Because gender is enmeshed with cultural, historical, and social meanings linked to generation, culture, and race, women and girls are more likely to experience gender-based violence, and socially constricted roles, which have significant implications for their mental health. The WHO also identifies that "gender differences occur particularly in the rates of common mental disorders—depression, anxiety and somatic complaints. These disorders, in which women predominate, affect approximately 1 in 3 people in the community and constitute a serious public health problem" (WHO, n.d). Authors within this text clearly present the need for nursing advocacy for social change, mental health promotion and treatment in addressing the needs of women and girls to improve global mental health, thereby affecting mental and physical well-being across generations. International collaboration among nurses and interprofessional partnership are greatly needed to address this significant mental health problem.

Nursing remains a predominantly female field, although the number of men in nursing has increased. The predominance of women in nursing and in mental health practice is a double-edged sword. As women, nurses can bring feminist insights to practice, policy, and research. Conversely, nursing can also encounter barriers to equality in power, politics, and leadership. In mental health, service development and delivery is based on the way in which gender is perceived within the context. Gender can affect both the focus of care and research. High-resource countries are leading in the generation of literature focused on nursing advocacy and leadership. Globally, however, nurses consistently provide leadership in consumer environments often without needed resources, supportive infrastructure, and deserved recognition.

Empowering individuals, communities, and governments

Involving consumers in the development and delivery of mental health care is the centerpiece of person-centered care. Person-centered care has been described as more comprehensive, socially and culturally informed, and respectful of the consumers with whom we work. One of the critical elements of person-centered care is empowerment. Empowerment has been discussed in terms of access and comprehensive exposure to information (mental health literacy), having options that are compatible with beliefs and values, and some degree of control over factors that affect mental health and mental health care. The process through which empowerment occurs is engagement, which focuses on the mutual exchange of information, respect, and shared power in decision-making. Person-centered care can be focused on the individual, a population, or a community.

The process of engagement becomes even more powerful when the target is community and used to minimize risk and promote wellness. Initiatives focused on engaging local people in actions to improve health-seeking gives the community influence over which issues are to be prioritized for action, what the action is to be, who delivers it, and how it is to be delivered. The greater the emphasis on giving communities more power and control over decisions that affect their lives, the more likely there can be enhancement of service quality, social cohesion as related to the targeted issue (such as bullying, disaster management, and suicide), community empowerment, and ultimately improved population mental health. Empowerment and engagement (especially for communities) are strongly tied to resources, public policy, and the political/social environment.

Research about mental health and its impact (personal, social, and economic) has generated new perspectives about the importance of this topic. Public policy is evolving and nursing organizations are an integral part of this change. However, change in discourse has not been readily translated into action. Mental health continues to receive disproportionately fewer resources globally and the burden of poor mental health remains significant. Innovative practices such as use of trained lay community members in mental health promotion and screening is one best practice that supports empowerment in environments in which there is a disconnect between resources and policy. Nurses as advocates for populations and through involvement in innovative practices have demonstrated skill and success in care delivery and those efforts need scaling up and broadening in scope to better meet the needs that exist. The current emphasis on mental health provides a unique opportunity for nurses to advocate for and partner with individuals, communities, groups, and governments to effect change.

Although diverse perspectives have been presented, a limitation of this text is the absence of nurse authors from India and China, two of the largest populations in the world. In addition, input from the LGBT, immigrant and refugee communities are also not represented. Future editions of the book will strive to encompass these important voices. This beginning effort to describe realities of the conditions in which persons with mental illness exist and then offer solutions for improving the well-being of individuals in low-, middle-, and high-income countries is informed by practice, advocacy, and research. Nurses are an untapped resource and are well positioned to provide essential mental health care.

References

Armstrong, G., Kermode, M., Raja, S., Chandra, P., & Jorm, A. (2011). A mental health-training program for community health workers in India: Impact on knowledge and attitudes. *International Journal of Mental Health Systems, 5*. Retrieved April 3, 2016 from www.ijmhs.com/content/5/1/17.

Bond, K., Jorm, A., Kitchener, B., & Reavley, N. (2015). Mental health first aid training for Australian medical and nursing students: An evaluation study. *BMC Psychology, 3*. Doi 10.1186/s40359–015–0069–0.

Eaton, J., McCay, L., Semrau, M., Chatterjee, S., Baingana, F., Araya, R., Ntulo, C., & Saxena, S. (2011). Scale up of services for mental health in low-income and middle-income countries. *Lancet, 378,* 1592–1603.

Fricchione, G., Borba, C., Alem, A., Shibre, T., Carney, J., & Henderson, D. (2012). Capacity building in global mental health: Professional training. *Harvard Review of Psychiatry, 20*(1), 47–57.

Government of Canada. (2015). Rio political declaration on social determinants of health: A snapshot of Canadian actions 2015. Retrieved May 23, 2016 from publications/science-research-sciences-recherches/rio/alt/rio2015-eng.pdf.

Kakuma, R., Minas, H., & Dal Poz, M. (2014). Strategies for strengthening human resources for mental health. In V. Patel, H. Minas, A. Cohen, & M. Prince (Eds.). *Global Mental Health Principles and Practice* (pp. 193–223). New York: Oxford University Press.

Rebello, T., Marques, A., Gureje, O., & Pike, K. (2014). Innovative strategies for closing the mental health treatment gap globally. *Current Opinions in Psychiatry, 27*(4), 308–314.

Semrau, M., Lacko, S., Alem, A., Ayuso-Mateos, J., Chisholm, D., Gureje, O., Hanlon, C., & Thornicroft, G. (2015). *BMC Medicine, 13*. Doi 10.1186/s12916–015–0309–4.

Ward, M. (2011). *Educational preparation for nurses working with the mentally ill: The case for Cyprus.* Horatio: European Psychiatric Nurses.

World Health Organization (WHO). (n.d). Gender and women's health. Retrieved October 21, 2015 from www.who.int/mental_health/prevention/genderwomen/en/.

World Health Organization (WHO). (2013). *Mental health action plan.* Geneva, Switzerland: WHO.

Snowflakes

We are all like snowflakes
Delicate, vulnerable and no two alike
Floating thru life on our own path
Mixing in, gathering together, yet separate
Put into the wrong environment, we melt away
Together we are strong, lasting, a thing of beauty
Alone we can go un-noticed, unappreciated
But when joined we can affect our world

By Kenneth Martin ~1992

INDEX

The following italicized abbreviations have been used after relevant page numbers: *b* for boxes, *fig* for figures, *m* for maps, and *t* for tables.